The Long-Term Care

Legal Desk Reference

Understanding and Minimizing Risk for Nursing Home Managers

Barbara Acello, RN, MSN

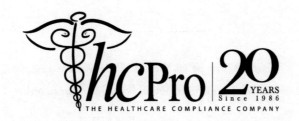

The Long-Term Care Legal Desk Reference: Understanding and Minimizing Risk for Nursing Home Managers is published by HCPro, Inc.

Copyright 2006 HCPro, Inc.

ISBN 1-57839-826-6

HCPro, Inc., provides information resources for the healthcare industry.

HCPro, Inc., is not affiliated in any way with the Joint Commission on Accreditation of Healthcare Organizations, which owns the JCAHO trademark.

Barbara Acello, RN, MSN, Author

Elizabeth Petersen, Senior Managing Editor

Noelle Shough, Executive Editor

Paul Amos, Group Publisher

Mike Mirabello, Senior Graphic Artist

Paul Singer, Layout Artist

Jean St. Pierre, Director of Operations

Shane Katz, Cover Designer

Advice given is general. Readers should consult professional counsel for specific legal, ethical, or clinical questions.

Arrangements can be made for quantity discounts. For more information, contact:

HCPro, Inc.

P.O. Box 1168

Marblehead, MA 01945

Telephone: 800/650-6787 or 781/639-1872

Fax: 781/639-2982

E-mail: *customerservice@hcpro.com*

Visit HCPro at its World Wide Web sites:

www.hcpro.com* and *www.hcmarketplace.com

Contents

Contents

Chapter three: The litigation process 35

Chapter four: Standards of care 51

Chapter five: Most common causes of survey deficiencies 65

The Long-Term Care Legal Desk Reference

Chapter six: Survey outcomes **85**

Chapter seven: Conflict resolution/managing complaints **97**

Contents

Contents

Chapter fourteen: Infection-related complications.....................................269

Chapter fifteen: Progressive injuries related to nutrition and hydration ...299

©2006 HCPro, Inc.
The Long-Term Care Legal Desk Reference

Chapter sixteen: Injuries precipitated by progressive failures and omissions of care 335

Chapter seventeen: Rights of the resident 365

Contents

Chapter eighteen: Medication monitoring 383

Chapter nineteen: Employee lawsuits...419

Chapter twenty: Self determination 445

Chapter twenty one: Quality assurance/benchmarking 459

Chapter twenty two: Financial fraud and abuse 471

Contents

Chapter twenty three: Documentation **483**

Introduction

This book is designed to assist nurses and nurse managers working in long-term care facilities, hospital skilled nursing units, and long-term care subacute centers. Most legal nursing books do not combine nursing practice with legal theory. The reader is expected to learn the law, then apply it to the health care setting. The text is written with an emphasis on "real world" clinical practice, and provides awareness of and solutions to potential legal problems that nurses encounter in the long-term care setting. More is expected of the nurses than ever before in the history of long-term care. To help you meet the ever-increasing expectations and demands of sicker, less stable, and increasingly fragile and complex residents, this text is designed to assist you in learning and identifying the pitfalls and problems that lead directly to the courtroom, and how to avoid them. *The Long-Term Care Legal Desk Reference* is designed to parallel the federal long-term care requirements, upon which many state laws are based. Although the federal requirements are standardized, each state has the flexibility to adjust their own laws to meet regional needs. If there is a discrepancy, follow your state laws.

The Long-Term Care Legal Desk Reference uses a practical, reality-oriented approach to lawsuit prevention based on need to know information in the long-term care facility. Current trends and issues in health care are emphasized, and when appropriate, real world solutions to problems are presented. The text is designed to assist nurses to practice as strong, proactive clinicians. This book was developed to be a nursing reference of up-to-date information that will help you survive and thrive in avoiding the sometimes litigious long-term care facility environment of the twenty-first century. It is not meant to be an exhaustive or comprehensive source of long-term care or legal information. A typical legal nursing book explains the law to you. This book explains the law as it applies to long-term care facility administration, nursing management, and nursing practice. The book was written using current clinical information and standards of practice that are useful to nurses and will complement more exhaustive sources of long-term care nursing and legal information. The purpose in using this format was not to recite the law to readers. Rather, issues and problems were selected that are common components in long-term care-related litigation. The book discusses principles of the law and provides nursing principles and practices that will assist the reader in complying with the law.

As an experienced nurse, consultant, and author, I am considered an expert in some areas, including long-term care. I have been called upon to assist in many long-term care-related lawsuits as an expert witness and legal nurse consultant. An expert witness assists the attorneys, judge and jury by explaining technical nursing information and operational aspects of long-term care. Much of the information in this book is based on my experience with the legal system, both in chart reviews, and as a testifying expert at deposition and trial. With today's litigious society, I believe that nurses must stay informed regarding legal issues affecting nursing practice. Sadly, resident acuity has increased, some areas of the United States have a nursing shortage, and caring for the residents has become much more difficult than it was in the previous decade. The number of lawsuits against long-term care facilities has increased over the past decade as well. Some law firms virtually survive because of lawsuits against long-term care facilities and their employees. I write about some of the issues here in hopes that you will benefit from the information in your personal practice, and stay out of the courtroom, which is usually not a fun place to be.

I have wanted to write this book for several years. There is so much important information to share and there are commonalities in lawsuits involving long-term care facilities. All of the information here is relevant to nurses in long-term care practice. The format consists of information grouped in chapters by subject with various legal opinions, expert reports, standards of practice, diagrams, charts, lists, and tables so that you can readily access and apply or implement the information. Everything in the book is material for which the long-term care nurse is accountable and may have potentially serious legal exposure.

In the author's opinion, the resident is the most important individual in the long-term care facility. All care is directed to providing the highest quality of life possible for facility residents. Nurses are important members of the interdisciplinary team and will receive a great deal of personal satisfaction from working in a long-term care facility. The staff at HCPro, Inc. Publishers are committed to helping you succeed by providing quality educational materials to assist with your important responsibilities in the long-term health care delivery system.

The federal long-term care rules make it clear that each resident must be admitted to the facility with physician approval. Each resident's care must be supervised by a physician. State and federal regulations also stipulate the frequency of physician visits, progress notes, and availability of physicians in an emergency. The initial face to face medical visit must be made by a licensed physician. However, after this every other required (60-day) visit may be made by a nurse practitioner (NP), clinical nurse specialist (CNS), or physician assistant (PA) who works in collaboration with the physician. Today, non physician practitioners are increasingly assuming primary health care duties that were formerly the exclusive province of physicians. The author and publisher acknowledge the many positive contributions that these non physician practitioners make to quality resident care. However, for ease of reading and grammar, this book uses the terms "doctor" and "physician" when referring to the health care provider. This is not meant to devalue the contributions that nurse practitioners, clinical nurse specialists, or physician assistants make to facility operations and resident care. Facilities are encouraged to use the services of these practitioners in keeping with state and federal laws.

To protect the privacy of the individuals involved, names of residents and facilities have been changed in the case histories and all example legal documents included in this book. All names pseudonyms, and any resemblance to any individual, alive or dead, is purely coincidental. Where published legal opinions are quoted, the case style, number, and identifying information is factual.

Information in this book should not be construed as legal advice. This material is for informational purposes only. Always consult an attorney if legal assistance is needed. The forms, suggested procedures, checklists, and actions plans are not designed or intended to include or address all possible legal or risk management exposures or solutions. Advice given is general, and readers should consult professional counsel for specific legal, ethical, or clinical questions. long-term care facility readers should consult attorneys who are familiar with federal and state health laws. Facilities are encouraged to retain your own legal advisors to assist you in developing policies, procedures, guidelines, practices, and a risk management plan specific to your own activities and services delivered.

Acknowledgments

The Long-Term Care Legal Desk Reference was written with professional collaboration from my legal nurse consultant and expert witness colleagues. I am grateful for the cooperation of my colleagues on the Peer2Peer (ACHCA), Texas Legal Nurse, Medical Legal Consultants, Litigated Disability Professional, and LNC Exchange listservs.

I owe a huge debt of gratitude to Ken Reynolds, a licensed nursing facility administrator. Ken dedicated many hours to reviewing this manuscript and providing helpful comments throughout the text development. His input was invaluable, and I sincerely appreciate his resident advocacy, cooperation, and dedication. Appraising the facility from the administrator's perspective is an awesome responsibility, and I greatly admire Ken and others who willingly give of themselves to ensure quality care and nursing support.

Janie Krechting completed an exhaustive peer review of the first draft of the book while it was in manuscript form and provided many helpful comments to assist me with manuscript development.

The following individuals and organizations have directly contributed to the development of this book, and I sincerely appreciate their cooperation:

- Jeni Gipson, MS, RN, National Network of Career Nursing Assistants

- Martha Ryan, RN, Health Occupations Credentialing, State of Kansas

I spend many hours at my computer, and could not do so without the love, support, and capable assistance of my family, Fran, Jon, J.R., and Chris. You are always there for me when I need help, and you always go the extra mile in the patience and cooperation departments.

Elizabeth Petersen, the HCPro editor, has nurtured this project through manuscript development to the completed book you hold in your hand. Her foresight, acumen, and close contact with the industry identified a need for this manual. I sincerely appreciate her vision of excellence in long-term care nursing publishing, as well as her vote of confidence and responsiveness to many questions and concerns. Elizabeth is truly an author's treasure, and I sincerely appreciate her long hours, dedication, and always making herself available.

Many unnamed individuals at HCPro handle the manuscript as it makes its way through the production process. Each individual makes a contribution that ultimately enhances the value of the book, and I am eternally grateful for their efforts.

Barbara Acello

bacello@spamcop.net
April 2006

Introduction to long-term care

> "All the results of good nursing, as detailed in these (notes) may be spoiled or utterly negatived by one defect, viz: in petty management, or in other words, by not knowing how to manage that what you do when you are there, shall be done when you are not there."[1]
>
> —Florence Nightingale, 1859

Introduction

Holding an administrative or nursing management position in long-term care is the toughest job you'll ever love. To be successful, you must have an inherent love for the elderly, or the types of clientele your facility serves. Other useful qualities are respect for your staff and others, good communication skills, adequate management skills, good organizational skills, a basic understanding of employee behavior, and an understanding of state and federal requirements. Think about the old adage, "The mark of a good manager is not how well the facility runs when the manager is present." The well-managed facility will also run well when the manager is not on the premises. Work with and teach your staff to achieve this goal.

Some days, you will be stressed, feeling as if you are spread too thin. On others, you wonder how to be all things to all people. However, the job is so rewarding and gratifying that on many days, you are proud of your facility, staff, and residents, bragging about them as a parent brags about a child.

Strive to be the best at what you do. Work to make your facility the best in the area. Set long- and short-term goals for your department and facility, and strive to meet them. If you blow it, don't quit. Determine to do better next time. Accept responsibility for your own actions. Avoid internalizing each and every problem. However, you must strike a balance to avoid blaming others for every problem that occurs in the facility. You may have to do a great deal of positive self-talk, such as telling yourself that "failure is not an option." Be proactive. See if you can find a better way of doing things. You will find that fire prevention is easier than firefighting. By striving to be the best and taking a proactive approach to facility management, you will do a great deal to reduce your facility's legal exposure, as well as your personal legal exposure.

New trends and concepts in caregiving

Long-term care facilities operate under a set of laws enacted by the Omnibus Budget Reconciliation Act (OBRA) of 1987. The OBRA rules have always stressed the importance of providing a homelike environment.

For many residents, the facility is their home. The focus is on the holistic model of care. The medical model is discouraged. An understanding of nursing care versus medical care (Figure 1-1) helps explain the focus. "Nurses have a different perspective on providing care compared with physicians, and it starts with the definition of our professions. Physicians diagnose and treat illness. Nurses, on the other hand, diagnose and treat the human response to illness. From day one, a physician's education is focused on the disease, illness, or injury, while a nurse's education is focused on how that same disease, illness, or injury affects the person."[2]

Figure 1-1 *Nursing versus medical care*

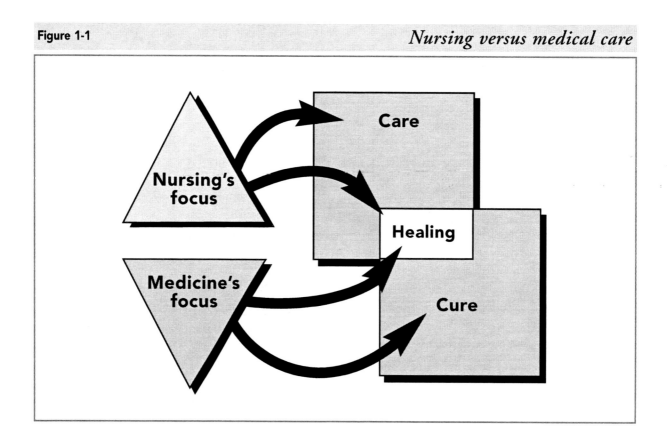

Because the focus of care is holistic, staff must view each resident as a whole person, with many strengths and needs. Residents are entitled to make decisions about their lives, their care, their living conditions, and daily routines. Even residents who are confused have some decision-making ability, and most have a means of expressing satisfaction or displeasure. Many facilities have broken away from the medical model by providing formal systems, such as the Eden Alternative, Wellspring, the Greenhouse Project, and Pioneer Network. Other facilities provide care in small communities, or neighborhoods, that are self-governed by the residents. Permanent staff are assigned to each community. Some facilities have implemented change gradually by switching to buffet meal service and family dining. These alternative models of care have proven successful in improving care, improving resident satisfaction, reducing turnover, and reducing legal exposure while improving quality of life.

Facility advertising and marketing materials

Your advertising and marketing materials are designed to promote your facility and to fill the beds. Maintaining the census is essential to paying the bills and meeting the payroll. However, you must be honest with your advertising and the promises you make. Review your advertising and marketing materials carefully to ensure they are not inviting a lawsuit. For example, a life care community has a residential (independent living) unit, an assisted living unit, and a skilled nursing unit. They are in separate buildings on the same property and operate autonomously. A resident in the assisted living unit became ill late Friday evening, and the unlicensed staff failed to recognize the magnitude of the problem. By Monday, his condition had worsened markedly, and he was transferred to the hospital, where he died several hours after admission. The facility was named in a lawsuit. Their marketing brochure noted that "24-hour nursing care" was available. However, they failed to note that this applied to the skilled unit only. The assisted living unit was routinely staffed with unlicensed personnel, and no provision was made for a nursing assessment if residents became ill. Medication aides administered medications. Although the state law required the medication aides to be "remotely supervised" by a licensed nurse (the nurse does not have to be on the premises), none was available on the unit. The medication aide did not even consider asking a nurse from the SNF to assess the resident because of the autonomous method of facility operations. The assisted living unit did not routinely interact with the nurses on the skilled unit. The jury in this case took this into consideration, and the plaintiff was awarded a high-six-figure judgment.

Making unrealistic promises in marketing materials and contracts may fall under the fraud statutes in your state. Some marketing pitfalls are made innocently. While it is good that an administrator wants to brag about his or her facility, statements such as "We are the best" or "We offer the best care" can come back to haunt you in a courtroom. There is a differ-

ence between a desire to provide excellent care and a declaration that you are providing excellent care. Quality of care and safety/security issues can be especially problematic. In fact, some of these promises may be easily refuted by reviewing the facility's survey history. In lawsuits involving false advertising, monetary damages can be hefty. Negligence is a more common charge. If an injured party can prove fraud, they most likely will qualify for punitive damages. Although the plaintiff is compensated for his or her medical problems, the punitive damages are assessed to punish the facility and the corporation. Damages can meet or exceed the corporation's assets. An example of a verdict of this nature is $200,000 for negligence, plus $100,000 in punitive damages. The facility may be required to pay an additional penalty, such as $75,000 for breach of contract.

Meeting expectations and understanding nursing facility care

Long-term care facilities are commonly misunderstood by the community at large. Because they are misunderstood, they are often unfairly maligned by the public and the press. Most private citizens view them as an extension of the medical model provided by the hospital. They do not understand that the philosophy and type of care provided is vastly different. Some do not realize that "24-hour nursing care" does not mean the residents need or will receive 24-hour care by licensed nurses.

Taking time to thoroughly explain the services offered and what the customer can expect prior to the time of admission goes a long way toward avoiding lawsuits down the road. Explain that residents usually need and receive approximately two to four hours of licensed nursing time each day. Most care is given by paraprofessionals who will inform the nurse if further assessment is needed.

The many problems associated with the aging process provide additional grounds for misunderstanding. Make sure residents and families are aware that skin becomes more fragile, bones become osteoporotic, and reaction time will slow down with aging. None of us likes the aging changes, but they are inevitable, and the residents' abilities must be evaluated realistically in light of the aging process. Dissatisfaction may be expressed over the resident care, when in fact the real problem is loss of control over aging changes that are occurring to the resident. An understanding of the aging changes, and what can be done to help compensate for them will help to reduce dissatisfaction.

Residents and families must also be tactfully informed that there are no guarantees in long-term care facility care. This is difficult, at best. For example, despite the best care possible, falls and injuries can and do occur. From the time of admission, residents and responsible parties should be taught that the facility cannot protect the residents from the normal risks of living, such as falls, choking, and skin tears. However, the facility should provide a reasonable explanation regarding how they will address risk factors and abate the risks as much as possible. In the event of adverse outcomes, or if an untoward event occurs, the resident or responsible party has a right to know how the facility will respond. The response to an adverse occurrence substantially affects the decision to file a lawsuit. Staff must know facility policies and procedures, be well-prepared and tactful, and be taught to apply critical thinking in emergencies.

Customer service and guest relations

You probably chose healthcare as a career because you genuinely like and want to help other people. Being nice, empathetic, and responsive to everyone will go a long way toward preventing litigation. Make sure that all staff are aware of the facility's commitment to customer service and guest relations. Provide inservices and role-playing activities to teach "people skills." Most people find it difficult to sue someone whom they respect and like. They find it difficult to sue people who are perceived to be helping them. Keeping the residents' best interests in mind is your ethical responsibility. Adhering to this ethical code also protects you from potential liability. Residents and families are less likely to file a lawsuit if they believe staff are sincere and conscientious, and if they are confident in your ability. Because of this, being nice to everyone and gaining resident and family support should be high priorities.

Keeping residents and families informed

Strive to develop and maintain positive relationships with families, and encourage frontline staff to speak to all visitors they encounter in the facility. Keeping residents and families informed of changes in residents' conditions is critical. The law requires the facility to notify the responsible party when a significant change has occurred. In this situation, notification must be prompt and timely.

However, it may behoove you to inform the responsible party of changes even when they are not considered significant. Verify the contact information for the responsible party at each care conference. Encourage the resident or responsible party to communicate with you if he or she has problems or concerns. Make sure he or she is aware of support groups, resident and family councils, and other resources. Teach the personnel on the units how to respond to complaints. Half of all complaints are made to direct-care staff, so they must understand how to manage them. Using role-playing is an effective method of presenting this information. Focus on the importance of providing good customer service. Keeping the lines of communication open will do much to enhance resident and family satisfaction.

Importance of staffing

Each long-term care facility must have sufficient staff to provide nursing and related services to attain or maintain the highest practicable physical, mental, and psychosocial well being of each resident, as determined by resident assessments and individual plans of care. What constitutes "sufficient" is very subjective. Keeping the facility properly staffed is often the greatest stressor experienced by nurse administrators. Discussing the problems associated with staffing issues in depth is well beyond the scope of this book. Even when the facility is staffed according to budget, floor workers may undermine the facility by complaining to residents, families, and others about "short" staffing. Unfortunately, there are few good answers and no quick fixes to resolving staffing problems. Many facilities have been successful in forming committees of staff members to address turnover and staffing problems. Turnover is expensive, and it typically takes three to four weeks to replace a worker. Staff members are expected to work overtime, or agency staff are brought in. One study showed that 13% of the staffing budget was spent on overtime, compared with 5% in hospitals.[3] Paying overtime and using agency personnel are expensive options that increase your legal exposure. Resident security is also affected, because of the bonds they form with staff members. Reducing and stabilizing turnover and staff stability is an admirable goal.

A certain amount of staff education may help you. To begin with, staff must understand that your staffing is at or above state minimum requirements. (This is the case in most facilities.) Even if a worker calls off and cannot be replaced, the facility is not breaking the law. Most people work in long-term care by choice. Environment has a profound effect on worker morale. For some, the facility will be the nicest environment they come to each day. The environment must also foster worker respect, security, comfort and safety, and the facility must ensure that staff have adequate resources to do the job. Educational opportunities and inservices should be available. Wages and benefits should be competitive. Some staff grumble about inadequate wages, although this is often an excuse for their unwillingness or inability to discuss the real issues. However, staff should also be educated on the value of their benefits. Most are unaware of the value of the employer's contribution to withholding taxes, paid vacations, holidays, and insurance programs. This is often the equivalent of one-third to one-half of the salary.

Computing budgets

Long-term care facilities use a ratio to determine budgets. Thus, if you ask how much staff the nursing department has, you may be given an answer, such as 2.5. This does not mean that the entire department has 2.5 staff members. When staffing is presented in this manner, it means that the nursing department is budgeted for 2.5 hours of labor per patient (resident) day (HLPPD). In English, this means that the staffing is adjusted so that each resident receives 2.5 hours of nursing care each day, on an average. Obviously, some residents require less, and some require more. Budgets are determined using this method because the number of staff allowed is based on the census. Staffing varies with occupancy. It is easier to calculate staffing that varies from week to week in this manner. If the census decreases or increases significantly during the month, your budgeted hours will change proportionately. Minor variations, such as a resident being in the hospital overnight, do not usually affect staffing.

The formulas for converting staffing are as follows:

A. Formula for number of staff hours per patient (resident) per day:

   1. Total number of staff in the department for a 24-hour day.

   2. Multiply this number by the number of hours worked. Some employees may work 7.5 hours, and others work eight hours. If this is the case, multiply the number of employees working 7.5 hours x 7.5, and the number of employees working eight hours x eight. Add the totals together.

   3. Divide this number by the census for the day to determine the number of hours per resident per 24 hours.

Example: A facility has 100 residents. Thirty-one nursing assistants care for the residents in a 24-hour period. Nursing assistants work 7.5 hours a day. There are 13 assistants on days, 10 on second shift, eight on nights. The licensed nurses work eight hours a day. There are seven nurses, excluding supervisory personnel (three on days, two on second shift, two on nights).

31 (nursing assistants) x 7.5 (hours a day) = 232.5

Seven (nurses) x 8.0 (hours a day) = 56

232.5 + 56 = 288.5, or 289 total hours of labor per 24 hours

289 hours ÷ 100 (census) = 2.89, or 2.9 hours of labor per patient (resident) day

Note: Some facilities count supervisory personnel into the HLPPD figure, and some count them separately. Your number of direct-care hours per day will be determined by your facility's practice.

B. Conversion by hourly figures:

   1. Add the total number of hours for a 24-hour period.

   2. Divide the number of hours by the daily census to compute the 24-hour number.

Example: A facility uses 375 hours a day in the nursing department. The census is 140.

375 (hours per day) ÷ 140 (census) = 2.67, or 2.7 hours of labor per patient (resident) day.

C. To use the budgeted hours to determine the number of personnel for a 24-hour period:

   1. Multiply the budgeted HLPPD figure by the census.

   2. Divide this number by hours of work (per shift) to determine the number of personnel required.

Example: The facility has a census of 100. The nursing department is budgeted for 2.8 HLPPD. This facility includes the Director of Nursing (DON) and Assistant Director of Nursing (ADON) into the total HLPPD figure. The DON and ADON are budgeted at 5.8 hours each for seven days (they work eight hours a day for five days, which is the equivalent of 5.8 times seven days). The nurses in the facility work eight hours a day. The nursing assistants work 7.5 hours a day.

2.8 (HLPPD) x 100 (census) = 280 total hours per day

5.8 (DON) + 5.8 (ADON) = 11.6 hours

Six licensed nurses a day x eight hours = 48 hours

11.6 (DON/ADON) + 48 (licensed nurses) = 59.6 hours

280 (total hours) - 59.6 (total licensed hours) = 220.4 (hours remaining for Nursing Assistants [NA])

220.4 (total NA hours) ÷ 7.5 (hours per shift) = 29.38 (total number of NA for 24 hours)

Due in part to public awareness of staffing challenges, new laws have been developed to require facilities to publicly post daily staffing hours. It is extremely important that you know and can defend the numbers you post.

Supply budgets

Supply budgets are also calculated by using an equation. You are told that you have $1.20 to spend. This means that you can spend $1.20 per patient (resident) per day, for supplies in a month. If the census decreases or increases significantly during the month, your budget will change proportionately.

A. To determine the budgeted amount:

   1. Multiply the budgeted amount per patient day by the average daily census.

   2. Multiply this figure by the total number of days in the month to obtain the total monthly budgeted amount.

Example: The nursing supply budget is $1.20 PPD (per patient day). There are 30 days in the month. The average census for the month is 150.

$1.20 PPD x 150 (census) x 30 (days in the month) = $5400 (total amount for the month)

B. To determine the amount you spend per patient (resident) day (PPD):

   1. Multiply the average daily census by the total number of days in the month.

   2. Divide the figure by the total amount spent in the month.

Example: The average daily census in the facility is 110. The nursing department spent $3500 in April.

110 (census) x 30 (number of days in April) = 3300

3300 (total resident days in April) ÷ $3500 (amount spent) = $0.94 PPD

Using the PPD method is a useful tool when comparing expenses from facility to facility. While dollar amounts may vary greatly between a 100- and 300-bed facility, the PPD amounts will be comparable.

Need for insurance

Insurance has become so expensive that some facilities have voluntarily dropped it. Some insurers have stopped offering long-term care coverage, particularly in the South. Insurance rates vary, depending on facility location. However, the starting rate is commonly $1,000 to $2000 per licensed bed. Premiums increased an average of 130% between 2000 and 2001, and 143% between 2001 and 2002. Providers today are paying substantially more money for less coverage than they did in the past. Coverage excludes existing claims. If the facility wants coverage for fines, penalties, and punitive damages, the cost of the policy increases.

Some insurers use a rating system to determine insurance costs. The insurer determines the degree of risk the facility poses to the insurer by reviewing lawsuit history, surveys, and whether or not the facility has a sound risk-management program. This type of system rewards facilities with a good history and charges higher premiums to facilities with a history of problems. Alternatives such as self-insurance, group self-insurance, and joint underwriting agreements have made insurance more affordable for some facilities, but these types of programs are not available for all providers. The insurance industry contends that increases in premiums are needed to cover losses, but activist and consumer groups assert that inadequate oversight allows insurers to overcharge customers. During the recent explosion of tort reform laws, the Center for Medicare Advocacy did a study to evaluate the impact of frivolous lawsuits on insurance premiums. The study concludes that cases of abuse in the court system are not frivolous, and tort litigation is necessary to hold facilities accountable. Because the civil justice system complements the public regulatory system in its efforts to improve the quality of care, tort litigation can lead to significant improvements in care. This study also revealed that multi-million dollar payouts are unusual, which is why they receive so much publicity. The study also demonstrates that tort litigation is not the cause of rising liability insurance premiums.[4]

Going without liability insurance may be referred to as "going bare." Some facilities and healthcare providers advocate this method, believing that without insurance, no one will be interested in suing them. This may or may not be the case, because assets can be seized to satisfy a judgment. Interestingly, state law may prohibit jurors from being told about presence or lack of insurance. Your state law may require jurors to determine damages, whether or not they are covered by insurance. Another consideration is insurance on the building itself, for fire and other damage. Going completely bare is risky business.

Personal malpractice insurance

The facility and the nurses are separate entities with separate interests. Neither wants to be the scapegoat for interests divergent from their own. Some employ-

ers discourage nurses from purchasing personal malpractice coverage. This recommendation is made based on the belief that having additional coverage increases their legal exposure; that potential plaintiffs will sue anyone with "deep pockets." The plaintiff attorney usually determines whom to name in the lawsuit based on information in the medical record. Early in the game, when the suit is filed, he or she is probably unaware of which individuals (if any) have personal malpractice coverage. The opposing attorney learns of your coverage after the suit has been filed. One large plaintiff firm routinely names the administrator, director of nursing, and a charge nurse from each shift when they file a lawsuit.

They also routinely name the MDS nurse and some supervisory nursing personnel. Their belief is that the facility will defend its employees, even if these individuals are no longer employed by the entity. If they fail to defend the employees (or former employees), they may become witnesses for the plaintiff, and their inside knowledge of facility operations may be very damaging. By naming both corporate entities and individuals, the plaintiff is increasing the potential damage award substantially. Nurses should consider the following when determining whether to purchase a personal malpractice policy:

- A jury will deliberate and recommend a verdict based on information presented in the courtroom only. Information from other sources should not be considered. Most jurors know little to nothing about the nuances of nursing practice or long-term care. Their deliberations are based on the information and expert witness testimony given at trial. The medical record will be admitted into evidence, and will be available for juror review. The record may or may not be helpful to your case.

- If criminal charges are involved, your employer's policy will probably not cover you. Allegations of abuse, neglect, and drug diversion may have both civil and criminal penalties in your state.

- Regardless of the outcome, being sued is extremely stressful. Your insurance carrier will designate your attorney. You will probably not have the freedom to select an attorney. You will be the only client (associated with the facility) that this attorney represents in this lawsuit. You cannot talk about the lawsuit with other nurses, who would normally serve as your support system. The only one you can discuss the case with is your attorney and his or her employees.

- If you do not have a private insurance policy, the facility's attorney usually will represent you. However, you must remember you are the "secondary" client. The facility is the "primary" client. By defending your actions, the attorney helps to mitigate the case against the facility.

- If the facility does not pay for your attorney, you will be forced to pay privately to defend yourself. You will be expected to make a deposit on the front end, and add to the legal fees as they are exhausted. You may pay additional fees for expert witnesses, paralegals, legal nurse consultants, and other researchers working on your case. You will be billed for time you spend on the phone with your attorney and his office.

- Regardless of the outcome, being named in a lawsuit may completely deplete your finances. Some states have laws protecting jointly held assets, or assets such as a house that are also owned by your spouse.

- Some county and public facilities are privileged to "governmental," "sovereign," or "charitable" immunity, and cannot be sued without consent.

The doctrine of governmental immunity originates in old English law, and is based on the premise that "the king can do no wrong." If a resident is grievously injured, he or she is unable to sue the facility for compensation for medical expenses or punitive damages. In this case, the plaintiff will name personnel individually. Usually, multiple healthcare workers are named, including the physician, nurses, pharmacists, and paraprofessionals. Since the facility is not a party to this lawsuit, it may not defend its employees.

- Some states have enacted tort reform, which caps punitive damages in medical malpractice actions. In these states, the plaintiff may name as many individuals as possible in the lawsuit, to derive maximum financial benefit. As the nurse's individual legal exposure increases, so does the need for malpractice insurance benefits.

- Occasionally, other workers or managers sue nurses for libel and other situations. If this type of suit is filed, the facility's insurer may not cover you.

- Some healthcare facilities have been found negligent in malpractice suits because of the actions or omissions of their employees. These facilities have later sued their employees (or former employees) to recover their costs. If your employer's policy does not contain a subrogation clause, you may be personally sued to cover the damages your employer had to pay as a result of your actions or omissions in the lawsuit. A subrogation clause is a provision in the insurance policy or contract. It gives one party the right to act on behalf of another person in legal actions related to the subject of the contract or insurance policy.

- If your name is not individually listed on your employer's insurance policy, the insurer may refuse to defend you. However, your employer cannot drop you from his or her policy if you elect to purchase a private malpractice policy.

- If your employer's policy is "claims based," you are covered by the policy only during your employment. If a resident names you in a lawsuit after you have resigned, you may not be covered. Most personal malpractice policies are "occurrence based." These policies cover you during the specified policy period. If an individual files suit after the policy lapses, you will be covered for injuries that occurred while it was in effect.

- Depending on your insurance policy, you may have no say in how your case is defended or settled. You may prefer to fight things out in an attempt to clear your name. However, the facility or insurer will settle the claim, because doing so is cheaper.

In simplistic terms, an employer's insurance will defend you if you are acting within the company's policy and procedures. Personal malpractice insurance will defend you only if you are acting within reasonable and professional guidelines. Some professionals refer to personal malpractice insurance as "painting a target on your back," while others consider it protection of their own personal finances.

Policies and procedures

Having up-to-date facility policies and procedures is essential. If you add a policy or teach staff to use a new piece of equipment, add the information to your manuals. In addition to maintaining a master set of manuals in the office, copies should be available in designated locations, such as nursing stations and offices for staff review and reference. Review the manuals in their entirety annually. Make sure they are current. Since lawsuits often reflect care given several

years after the fact, maintaining a set of manuals by year is helpful.

In a lawsuit, all applicable policies and procedures will probably end up in the courtroom and be available to jurors for review. These manuals usually show that the facility and its staff were familiar with and had access to resources related to applicable standards of care. Other materials, such as videotapes, handouts, and other visual aides presented to staff for inservice, may also be used, and reviewed by the jury. Staff are expected to be familiar with and to follow facility policies and procedures. If an inservice videotape presents a procedure to be followed by staff, this establishes a standard of care. When staff attend continuing education programs, particularly if the class is mandatory, the court may rule that the class(es) established an additional standard that they are required to meet. Verdicts are usually not favorable when staff are not familiar with facility policies and procedures, or fail to follow them.

Delegation, responsibility for monitoring subordinates' performance

Delegation is a management principle used to obtain desired results through the work of others, and it is a legal concept used to empower one to act for another. The nurse who can effectively work through others can expand access to nursing care, maintain and promote quality healthcare, and facilitate the effective utilization of healthcare resources. The appropriate use of delegation allows better use of licensed nurses' time in the provision of safe nursing care. Professional skill and expertise in delegation have a positive impact on resident care. Individuals to whom responsibility is delegated must have the ability to accept and perform delegated activities.[5]

Each state board of nursing addresses delegation in the nurse practice act, or elsewhere. The American Nurses Association also addresses delegation.

All long-term care managers work through other people. State and federal nursing home laws require managers to ensure that employees are competent in their responsibilities. The National Association of Directors of Nursing Administration/Long-Term Care (NADONA) and American College of Healthcare Administrators (ACHCA) also describe delegated quality-of-care activities in their professional standards of practice. Because the art of delegation is so important, managers must ensure that delegation is appropriate and that delegated activities are properly and regularly monitored. We entrust the residents' lives to the hands of our employees. Managers have both an ethical and a legal responsibility to ensure delegation is appropriate. You will find additional delegation information in Chapter 2.

The importance of the nursing process

The nursing process is used as a model for long-term care assessment. This process consists of four separate and distinct steps. Each is equally important in the care of the residents. These steps are:

- assessment and formulation of nursing diagnoses

- planning

- implementation of the plan, and

- evaluation of the resident's care plan. Development and maintenance of the care plan is an ongoing process.

Long-term care facility care is designed to maintain or improve the residents and prevent deterioration in each resident's condition and ability to function. The long-term care nursing facility must use the nursing process to accurately assess the residents, then develop and implement a plan of care to meet each resident's needs. The plan directs the nursing care of each resident, and is revised as often as necessary to ensure it reflects the resident's current condition, problems, and nursing care needs. Revising the plan infrequently, and failing to use the plan in daily care of the residents, are probably the greatest contributing factors to nursing legal exposure.

The American Nurses Association (ANA) Code for Nurses notes the following: "The nurse assumes responsibility and accountability for individual nursing judgment and actions. The nurse is responsible and accountable for individual nursing practice and determines the appropriate delegation of tasks consistent with the nurse's obligation to provide optimum patient care. The nurse acts to safeguard the client and the public when healthcare and safety are affected by the incompetent, unethical, or illegal practice of any person."[6] The ANA Code for Nurses is not open to negotiation in employment settings. The Code for Nurses encompasses all nursing activities and may supersede specific policies of institutions, of employers, or of practices. Therefore, the Code for Nurses with Interpretive Statements is nonnegotiable.[7]

Most expert witnesses and legal nurse consultants will tell you there is a breakdown in the nursing process in each and every healthcare lawsuit in which negligence is proven. If you think the nursing process is unrealistic, "pie in the sky" information, think again. The nursing process is the foundation for solid, sustainable nursing practice, and using it correctly provides a high degree of protection from legal exposure.

References

1. Nightingale F. (1859). Notes on nursing. London: Harrison and Sons, 1859.

2. Carroll, Patricia. (2004). What nurses know. New York. Perigree Publishing.

3. Lacey LM, and Nooney JG. (2005). Turnover rates and related spending among nurse employers. Online. *www.nursenc.org/research/empsurv2004/turnover%20%20statewide.pdf.* Accessed 11/04/05.

4. Center for Medicare Advocacy. (2003). Tort Reform and Nursing Homes. Online. *www.medicareadvocacy.org/snf_TortReformSummary.htm*

5. Delegation: Understanding the concepts and decisionmaking process. *Insight*, Volume 7 Number 1, 1998. Chicago. National Council of State Boards of Nursing.

6. American Nurses Association. (2002). *Code for Nurses with Interpretive Statements.* Washington. American Nurses Publishing.

7. American Nurses Association. (2002). *Code for Nurses with Interpretive Statements.* Washington. American Nurses Publishing.

Employee issues

> The DON displays knowledge of the Nurse Practice Act and the state and federal regulatory guidelines. The DON is fully aware of the state board of nursing rules and regulations and utilizes these guidelines in managing registered and licensed practical (vocational) nurses and certified nursing assistants. The DON does not, in any fashion, violate or perform in opposition to those rules and regulations specified by the state board of nursing. In effecting positive change in the nursing facility, the DON uses his or her professional guidelines as instruments for achievement.[1]

Nurse practice act

Each state has a nurse practice act which describes the roles, responsibility, and code of conduct for nurses in that state. Your state nursing board is responsible for protecting the health, safety, and welfare of the public as it pertains to nursing practice. Nursing Practice Acts and Nursing Administrative Rules/Regulations apply to all nursing roles in all settings. Because of the importance of your state board of nursing, you will be practicing under state nursing rules and laws, and state and federal nursing home rules, when you work in a long-term care facility. Nurses are responsible for knowing and following their state nurse practice act. This is a situation in which ignorance of the law offers no excuses if your state nursing board takes disciplinary action.[2]

The practice of nursing means

- assisting individuals or groups to maintain or attain optimal health

- implementing a strategy of care to accomplish defined goals

- evaluating responses to care and treatment

The practice of nursing includes, but is not limited to

- initiating and maintaining comfort measures

- promoting and supporting human functions and responses

- establishing an environment conducive to well-being

- providing health counseling and teaching

- collaborating on certain aspects of the health regimen

The practice of nursing is based on understanding the human condition across the life span and the relationship of the individual within his or her environment.[3]

Code of conduct

Each facility must have written standards of conduct and professional services that have been endorsed by the facility's senior management and governing body. This is a separate code from the ANA *Code for Nurses*. Licensed nurses are in the unique position of having to be familiar with both codes. A *code of conduct* is a brief, readable, and general expression of the facility's fundamental values and operating principles. The code should be translated into other prevailing languages in the community and written at an appropriate reading level so that it is accessible and readily understood by all employees. The code functions as a constitution, by detailing the fundamental principles, values, and framework for action. It helps define the organization's culture. All relevant operating policies are derivative of its principles. Because of this, the code is of real benefit only if it is meaningfully communicated and accepted throughout the organization. If the code of conduct reflects the organization's ethical philosophy, then its policies and procedures represent the organization's response to the day-to-day risks that it confronts while operating in the current healthcare system.[4]

These standards of conduct are binding on all employees and professionals, consultants, independent contractors, and volunteers performing services for the facility. The written standards also apply to ancillary providers operating under the facility's control, such as therapy companies, durable medical equipment suppliers, laboratories, and x-ray companies. Having sound standards is crucial to regulatory compliance, and to deterring fraud and abuse. The standards of conduct are in the form of written policies that articulate the specific procedures facility staff (and the other individuals listed above) must follow. The nursing facility administrator or his or her designee acts as the compliance officer for the facility to ensure that standards and policies of the governing body are adhered to.

Policies and procedures

Facilities are required by law to have policies and procedures on a variety of subjects, covering a broad range of employee issues, facility operations, and resident care. Both the plaintiff and defense attorneys will request policies and procedures in the event a lawsuit is filed. A *policy* is a written plan specifying a course of

action. Policies designate a process of formal rules. They are usually written based on laws, standards of care, and best practice or clinical practice guidelines. Policies usually elaborate on programs and actions of various individuals, and describe how the business of the facility will be conducted. They usually include statements describing how the facility will achieve its goals and objectives. They provide useful information for judging individual and facility performance.

Procedures assign, prioritize, and order responsibilities. They are the practices and processes used to implement the policies, manage the various departments, and provide resident care. To develop procedures, evaluate the functions and tasks needed to make processes effective and determine appropriate roles of staff members. It may also be helpful to identify the facility's mission statement. The *mission statement* conveys the facility's philosophy and serves as a reference for decision-making. It is a brief, global statement identifying the organization's purpose, population served, guiding principles, and distinguishing characteristics.

The goals and objectives of the facility, as well as the objectives of various services, are listed in the policies and procedures, as are the roles and responsibilities of staff, components of clinical care, care processes, regulations, and standards and guidelines important to the provision of long-term care facility care. The policies and procedures direct the activities of all staff members. Facility staff are a group of diverse providers, representing an interdisciplinary team. When defining issues and drafting documents, it is a good idea to invite residents and employee representatives from each affected discipline. These individuals are entitled to provide on input issues affecting them. You will also find that involving residents and employees improves satisfaction and promotes quality of life.

For your protection, make sure all employees are familiar with facility policies and procedures, and have signed an acknowledgment. Make sure relevant policies and procedures are accessible to employees for reference. Avoid locking them in an inaccessible area. Stress the importance of following facility policies and procedures to employees. You may be surprised to learn that most never look at them. Most are unfamiliar with state long-term care laws. Many do not understand the liability associated with failure to follow your established procedures rather than those they learned in school or at another facility. This is an area in which continuous education is essential.

Implementing policies and procedures

Orientation, educational, and inservice sessions are used to introduce staff to policies and procedures that are new to them. Specialized content inservices may be required for some personnel, depending on the subject matter. This may be a perpetual process, because as the facility grows and changes, additional policies and procedures will be needed for expanding services, adopting new treatments and therapies, or implementing new regulations. An important management responsibility is establishment and maintenance of an internal control structure that monitors performance to ensure the staff are adhering to facility policies and achieving stated objectives.

Facilities may also have a *Code of Conduct* that employees are expected to follow. Ethical requirements and behavioral rules are listed in the code. The various policies, procedures, and written documents should cover the basic laws, rules relating to the job, clinical practice guidelines, and standards that employees must follow.

Evaluating the effectiveness of policies and procedures

In some facilities, evaluating policies and procedures is a quality assurance activity. The easiest method for evaluating policies and procedures is to develop an audit tool to determine whether they are being followed. Develop an additional tool to evaluate the outcomes. Outcomes will be desirable if the policies and procedures are effective. A template entitled, "QA & A AUDIT" is on the CD that accompanies your book. Complete the templates by adding your audit criteria, and maintain them as permanents records of your reviews. Use your audit findings to make suggestions, provide constructive feedback, and modify the policies and procedures.

Employee turnover/employee retention

Having a stable staff is essential to providing excellent resident care and reducing the facility's legal exposure. Facilities that are successful in reducing turnover have lower costs and more satisfied residents. A goal of zero turnover is unrealistic. Some turnover is expected and is healthy. A high absenteeism rate also contributes to the perception of "working short" and having high turnover, so concurrent with addressing turnover, be attentive to rates of absenteeism and its effect on staff morale, as well. One well-done study recommends tracking both turnover and stability rates.[5] For the purposes of this study, stability was length of employment, and most turnover occurred in positions with fewer than two years' seniority.

Problems with calculating the turnover rate are many and varied, but lack of a standard formula is sometimes an obstacle. Turnover can be calculated by facility, by department, by unit, by quarter, or by year using this simple formula:

$$\frac{\text{number of terminations}}{\text{total full time equivalents (FTE)}}$$

Recordkeeping

Maintain employee records and schedules as required by law. If your facility is involved in a lawsuit, you can expect the plaintiff to subpoena all employee schedules, sign-in sheets, time cards, and daily assignment records. They may also request payroll data to verify your paper records. Analyze your staffing budgets and data to ensure they comply with the law and are adequate to meet resident needs. In a lawsuit, the defense often focuses on the medical issues of the suit, ignoring the impact that short staffing has on resident outcomes. The plaintiff will use staffing data to his or her best advantage. Inadequate staffing is often used by the plaintiff as a tool to exacerbate medical and nursing issues in the lawsuit. Another area to consider is employees who work excessive hours. You may be grateful for the employees who volunteer for overtime, but allowing them to work many extra shifts without adequate rest may place the facility in a position of disadvantage if you face a court challenge because these individuals had lapses in judgment or made serious errors.

Staff empowerment

Beyond the cost savings associated with turnover, employee dedication and satisfaction are increased when turnover is reduced. Likewise, resident satisfaction and quality of care are improved. Reduced turnover is often a byproduct of providing education and tools to empower staff in resident care. However, it is a long-term commitment or goal. There are no quick fixes. Each facility must develop an individual plan for providing 21st-century care. This includes finding a means of empowering your staff. Examples of programs that have been effective are listed below:

Good Samaritan Center (Lyons KS)

Open dining 24 hours a day.

Menu choices available at meals, or residents can request take-out meals.

Residents choose the color of their room and can personalize their room as desired.

The call system has been replaced by a vibrating pager system.

Residents participate in prospective employee interviews.

Residents choose from 25 to 30 activities or list their own preferences.

The facility has a day care center for employee children.

Care is provided in neighborhoods, in which central nurses' stations have been replaced with living rooms.

The main dining room has been changed to a classroom, beauty shop, computer room, and community room. A soda shop was also added.

Each neighborhood is staffed by a team from all departments.

Team leaders learn interviewing, mentoring, conflict resolution, and other skills.

Each neighborhood develops its own work schedule.

Personnel in each neighborhood are cross-trained.

Turnover has dropped to 48 percent annually from 77 percent.

Barry Community Care Center IL

Certified nursing assistants (CNAs) select the community in which to work; they do not float.

Upon admission, each resident is adopted by a CNA advocate. He or she provides general assistance, helps the resident create an individualized care plan, and assists in issues of concern to the resident, such as decorating the room, planning outings, and arranging for special meals.

CNAs assist with the interviewing, hiring, and orientation of new staff and provide feedback for performance evaluations.

CNAs serve as team leaders to coordinate staffing schedules and assignments and act as mentors for new staff.

Creative empowerment

Other suggestions that have been effective in promoting resident and staff satisfaction, reducing turnover, and empowering staff are:

- Creating a nursing assistant advisory council

- Creating career ladders with varying levels of education, responsibility, and pay

- Conducting staff satisfaction surveys

- Improving orientation, assigning mentors to new employees

- Creating float positions so assistants are not pulled from their assigned units to cover for absences

- Instituting sign-on and recruiting bonuses, in which the incentive money is split between the referring staff member and the new hire

"The current and anticipated changes in the healthcare delivery system will have a tremendous effect on the practice environment for nursing. It is critical to the survival of organizations that they recognize the creative and innovative talent at every level. The focus of purpose for all healthcare is successful individual healthcare management. The majority of work related to this purpose is done on patient care units, in clinics, emergency departments, operating rooms, long-term care units, specialty units, etc. The best strategy for the future is to involve those who are most affected by the changes. The long-term care nursing executive and the staff nurse do make a difference in patient care and will make a significant difference in the planning of the future delivery of cost-effective quality patient care."[6]

Coping with change

Change is a constant in healthcare. The culture of long-term care is changing dramatically. As a rule, people are resistant to change, which can be challenging for the most pliant employee. However, change often provides opportunities for growth and positive transformation that would otherwise be missed. Workers have a certain degree of self-confidence and autonomy that they have developed by making decisions and performing routine tasks day after day. Because of this, workers usually project an image of competency and confidence, and feel a certain degree of security in their jobs. Change is always unknown, and venturing into unknown territory can be threatening. Change increases the risk of exposing deficits and may unmask our weaknesses. With each change, we risk failure. It is easier to avoid and resist change than risk exposing oneself to criticism or facing other potentially negative consequences.

Each of us is responsible for effecting change. Managers must understand that we change no one. Each individual must be motivated to change and accept responsibility for changing. The motivation is internal. We can educate and instruct employees about the benefits of change. We can threaten them with consequences for not changing. However, employees must ultimately make the personal decision to make change work. Empowering employees is an effective method for successful change. Invite employees to use the change as a means of using their knowledge and skills. Share information with them.

Sharing information without withholding details implies that your employees can be trusted. However, several studies have shown that employees prefer to receive information about change from their immediate supervisors, not department heads or senior managers.[7] Many changes take place at the individual unit level. In addition to trusting charge nurses and other nursing supervisors to communicate information, you also trust them to implement and oversee the change. Think about it. Communicating information and implementing change go hand in hand. The success of any major change largely depends on how well these low-level managers influence attitudes and behaviors of employees.

Change is often stressful. Before *introducing* an organizational change, think about how the employees and residents will cope, and provide tools to assist them in preserving self-esteem, managing stress while maximizing flexibility, and finding opportunities for growth. Employees will probably need the opportunity to ventilate and describe feelings when change is anticipated or experienced. Provide an outlet for employees to ventilate, such as small group meetings in which information can be shared and employees will feel safe expressing concerns. Teach charge nurses to facilitate these groups so they remain positive and do not become "gripe sessions." Always solicit staff suggestions. Remember, change will be much more acceptable and manageable if employees have some control over the variables that accompany the change.

> "Nursing Staff at all levels within the organization must accept the challenges and opportunities of the future design of the healthcare system and its implications for how and where they will practice professional nursing. Accepting the challenge is a choice that all must make. The risks are high . . . and . . . the potential rewards for continued and enhanced quality patient care and for the professional practice of nursing are without limits. It is the nurses, after all, who are the backbone and the lifeline of patient care delivery. Nurses CAN make a difference!"[8]

Before *initiating change*, you must have a solid plan. Developing a plan based on employee (and resident) input is always best. If staff have ownership in the change, they are much more likely to make it work. Massive changes in the facility should be made slowly. The old question "How do you eat an elephant?" (one bite at a time) applies here. Always consider how proposed changes will affect residents and staff before beginning. Carol Kinsey Goman identifies six qualities common to those who thrive on change and provides tips on how to develop these qualities in your staff in her article, "How to Develop a Change-Adept Workforce."[9] She suggests:

- Self-confidence is an important quality in coping with change. Avoid focusing on employees' weaknesses. Instead, identify and develop competencies and accomplishments based on the person's strengths.

- A positive attitude is essential to success. Cultivate employees' optimism. Although acknowledging the stress, uncertainty, and disruption associated with change, it is also essential to accentuate the opportunities for growth, challenge, and reward.

- Employees with good coping skills are probably skilled at adapting to complex, rapid change. Avoid taking things so seriously that you lose your sense of humor. Combine your sense of humor with a spirit of fun and teamwork.

- Employees with a variety of outside interests (beyond their professions) are more resilient under stress and may be more effective on the job. Encourage staff to offset the stress and work-related demands by balancing them with enjoyable recreational activities.

- Nurture, nourish, and empower employees' cre-

ativity. Creative individuals espouse changing conditions that provide opportunities for gaining new knowledge, meeting new people, and doing new things.

- Promote teamwork and collaboration. You cannot demand teamwork, but you can teach and inspire employees to work as a team by using games and role playing to develop team-building skills. None of us succeeds alone. As you know, many different long-term care employees and departments are needed to care for each resident. You can persuade staff members to collaborate and share their ideas by creating an environment in which it is safe, enjoyable, and beneficial to do so.

Goman lists other important suggestions for making successful change:[10]

- Develop and nourish an atmosphere of trust. If employees don't trust management, share in your vision, understand the reasons for change, and are not included in preliminary planning, they may thwart your plans.

- Appreciate your staff, and let it show. Up to 75 percent of all major restructuring fails because of human problems.

- Remember that there is an emotional side of change. Transformation requires a redefinition of who we are and what we do. It may be unpredictable, and staff are often required to respond to unforeseen circumstances. This can be unnerving and highly emotional. To lead a team through change, you must touch them emotionally. Transformation leadership is about creating meaning. Employees must have a vision, then be inspired to attain that vision. Managers must have a solid grasp of human emotion and the ability to see or perceive the intangibles.

- Be honest. Avoid sugarcoating the truth. Doing this augments the trust gap between management and workers. Honesty involves sharing all details, whether positive or negative.

- Remember that workers will discuss the proposed change among themselves, with residents, and others. "Official communication" from management is not the only source of information.

- Avoid "command and control" tactics. Doing this places an unfair burden on managers and implies that team members don't have anything worthwhile to contribute. Solicit feedback. Listen to your team and implement their suggestions! During transformation, the primary challenge is to link these components as tightly as possible. The most successful change strategies are highly collaborative.

> The DON assesses the educational and training needs of the staff for which he or she is responsible and assures appropriate education and training to satisfy those needs. Further, the DON assures that care personnel do not administer care until such personnel can demonstrate the necessary skills and knowledge for such activity.[11]

Job descriptions

Since the long-term care facility hires the nursing assistants and others, the facility (versus the individual nurse) is responsible for

- developing or obtaining appropriate and acceptable job descriptions

- hiring people who are qualified for and capable of doing the job

- providing appropriate orientation and ongoing education

- determining and evaluating the competency of each worker

- communicating information about the employee's stage of learning and individual competency to the nurse who is directly responsible for supervising the employee

- if necessary, terminating the employee for substandard performance

Each employee should be given (and acknowledge receipt of) a job description that outlines his or her role and responsibilities in the facility. Maintain records showing that employees are competent in the responsibilities listed. Review the job descriptions periodically to ensure they are accurate and in compliance with the standards of practice in your state. Avoid asking employees to function outside their job descriptions or assigned scope of practice. This seems like common sense, but it occasionally happens. Do not put yourself or the employee in a position with potential legal ramifications. (For example, the nursing assistant job description lists responsibilities such as, "Other, as assigned by supervisor." A nursing assistant is a diabetic and injects herself and her young son with insulin each day. Despite her advanced knowledge of diabetes, the supervisor would not ask her to administer insulin to diabetic residents.)

Delegation

Delegation is a means of transferring the responsibility for a procedure or other task from a licensed nurse who is qualified and authorized to perform the activity to another person who does not possess the authority.

After a task is delegated, only the person to whom the authority has been given may perform the procedure. This means that this person cannot delegate or assign someone else to do the task. The nurse is accountable for the task and its outcome. He or she does this by first assessing the resident and believing that the resident is stable and the outcome of the activity is predictable. Second, the nurse must be familiar with the scope of practice, qualifications, and competence of the individual to whom the task is being delegated. In some situations, such as when the resident is unstable, delegation may be inappropriate, even if the task is a simple one.

Some states provide further definitions for the terms "delegation" and "assignment." *Assigning* means advising, instructing, or informing a subordinate to complete a task. The person making the assignment must possess the authority to do so. Delegation is only made to licensed personnel. In states that make a distinction between assignment and delegation, "*delegate*" means to authorize or entrust another to do the task. The person doing the delegation entrusts another and authorizes him or her to take the responsibility for seeing it is done.

The nurse is responsible and accountable for individual nursing practice and determines the appropriate delegation of tasks consistent with the nurse's obligation to provide optimum patient care.[12] Delegation is a management principle used to obtain desired results through the work of others, and it is a legal concept used to empower one to act for another. Professional skill and expertise in delegation have a positive impact on resident care. Individuals to whom responsibility is delegated must have the ability to accept and perform delegated activities. The outcomes of effective delegation include

- allowing protection of resident safety
- achieving desirable resident outcomes
- facilitating access to appropriate levels of healthcare
- delineating the spectrum of accountability for nursing care
- decreasing nurse liability

The effective use of appropriate delegation promotes positive resident outcomes with efficient use of resources. Emphasis must be placed on evaluation, the often-missing link in delegated activities.[13] Your state board of nursing and the National Council of State Boards of Nursing have delegation guidelines available. Check both sources for a comprehensive overview of nursing responsibilities. In most states, the nurse is responsible and accountable for his or her individual nursing practice and determines the appropriate delegation of tasks consistent with the nurse's obligation to provide optimum patient care.[14] The Director of Nursing is responsible for overseeing activities and ensuring that delegation in the nursing department is safe and appropriate.

Five rights of delegation

The National Council of State Boards of Nursing has developed a guide titled *The Five Rights of Delegation*.[15] The nurse must verify the delegation is appropriate. Appropriate delegation assures the following:

- The nurse is certain that delegating the activity is not against the law.

- The person to whom the task is delegated has been taught to perform the procedure. He or she can demonstrate the procedure correctly, if necessary.

- The resident is stable, and frequent, repeated assessments are not necessary.

- The resident's response to the activity is reasonably predictable.

- In the nurse's opinion, the person to whom the task is delegated will obtain the same or similar results as the nurse in performing the procedure.

In some situations, delegation is inappropriate. For example, an unstable resident needs the assessment skills of a licensed nurse during a procedure. In this case, the procedure cannot be delegated. Inappropriate delegation of activities that are routinely done by unlicensed personnel provides potential legal problems. Assessment is an activity that cannot be delegated to an LPN or nursing assistant. Part of the assessment consists of organizing, analyzing, prioritizing, evaluating, and synthesizing data. This must be done by an RN. However, other caregivers can assist with the collection of assessment data by obtaining vital signs, height, weight, and other information. The RN will use this information to develop an overall plan. Other caregivers may contribute to the plan, but the responsibility for its development cannot be delegated.

Orientation and regular inservice education

Orientation of your employees may be your most important risk-management tool. When employees are hired, the natural tendency is to try to get them on the units as soon as possible, theoretically to save money and ensure that staffing is sufficient. Invest in a solid, thorough orientation program. This protects the facility legally and ensures the residents receive optimum care. In fact, having a commitment to solid orientation and meaningful, ongoing staff development is an excellent way of reducing the risk of legal exposure. Getting a new job is stressful for everyone, and the stress increases tenfold if the employee is ill-

prepared for the position. Explain facility policies during orientation. Avoid the trap of showing a video or handing the employee a stack of papers to read. Tell them and show them. Augment and reinforce the verbal lessons with audiovisuals. Make sure to provide reference information, such as where additional information and policies and procedures can be located. Upon completion of the orientation, give a written quiz to verify that employees have retained the information. Keep good records of the content presented and employee attendance. Make sure to tell employees how much you value the facility residents and staff. Be sincere! They are your most important assets!

Depending on the position, on-the-job orientation is essential after classroom information is covered. This is a strength in facilities with staff-mentoring programs. Carefully pair the new employee with a staff member who will teach him or her well and set a good example. Ideally, the length of orientation will be based on employee need. We all learn at different rates. Evaluate the new employee's competency and ability to function independently before turning him or her loose. Even highly competent employees will have questions when they begin to work independently. Make sure they have a resource person to turn to. Having a resource person debrief them at the end of each shift for several weeks may also be helpful.

Learning

Action learning occurs when students immediately read, view, and do activities learned in the lesson. This list of teaching methods is not all-inclusive. Your objective should be to recognize that everyone is different, and vary your teaching methods, stimulating as many senses as possible. Remember to apply the old Chinese Proverb, *"Tell me, I forget. Show me, I remember. Involve me, I understand."*

People learn in many different ways. Some use primarily one learning style, and others use a combination of styles. When teaching, try to satisfy as many styles as possible through a variety of creative teaching methods. The *visual learner* learns by seeing and watching. The *auditory learner* learns by hearing an explanation of the subject. The *cognitive learner* learns by reading, studying, then working with the material until he or she figures it out. The *kinesthetic learner* learns by trial and error.

Importance of follow-up inservice monitoring

The federal long-term care facility rules require facilities to evaluate staff competency and address deficiencies through the inservice program:

F497: The facility must complete a performance review of every nurse aide at least once every 12 months, and must provide regular inservice education based on the outcome of these reviews. The inservice training must be sufficient to ensure the continuing competence of nurse aides, but must be no less than 12 hours per year. It must address areas of weakness as determined in nurse aides' performance reviews and may address the special needs of residents as determined by the facility staff; and for nurse aides providing services to individuals with cognitive impairments, also address the care of the cognitively impaired.

F498: The facility must ensure that nurse aides are able to demonstrate competency in skills and techniques necessary to care for residents' needs, as identified through resident assessments, and described in the plan of care.

Ensuring that learning has occurred

Managers are legally responsible for ensuring staff are competent in their responsibilities. Facilities and states interpret the method for verifying staff competence in many different ways. Most facilities complete a written evaluation tool on each staff member annually. These tools evaluate issues such as appearance, attendance, and dependability. Most do not evaluate technical performance or skills used in resident care. Because of this, some facilities verify nursing assistant competency by checking each assistant off on the skills required by the state nursing assistant program.

CMS is aware that verification of skills is not always done and may not be adequate. They are aware that facilities have no specific documentation that proves that inservice "addresses areas of weakness as determined in nurse aides' performance reviews..." Because of this, they are reviewing their procedures and requirements and plan to close this loophole in the future.

Some facilities also validate competence and learning after each inservice. They prepare a list of skills or theory information presented, then observe staff performance as unobtrusively as possible to ensure that learning took place. If not, remedial individual or group education is done. These are both excellent methods of verifying staff competence and learning. Whatever method is selected, the facility is responsible for the outcome of the learning and for ensuring the residents receive proper care.

Overtime and use of agency staff

Studies have shown that rotating shifts, working permanent nights, and excessive overtime disrupt physiological circadian rhythms, as well as personal social activities. Working under these conditions has been identified as a work-related stressor.[16] A great deal has been written on creative scheduling and reducing these negative effects on employees.[17] It should come as no surprise that many managers identify short staffing and call-offs as the most stressful, ongoing problem that they routinely contend with.

Paying overtime is a quick way to exceed the budget. It also causes staff burnout, and safety is sometimes questionable when staff members are tired from working a great deal of overtime. On the other hand, employing agency staff is costly, and although the registry personnel are competent, they are usually not familiar with your facility and its policies. Agency personnel have been known to recruit facility staff, singing the praises of higher agency wages and self-directed schedules. Suddenly, you find many of your personnel have resigned and return to you working for the agency. Also, remember that agency staff can and do call off. They are not always available to fill the open shifts.

Nursing boards do not become entangled in employer-employee disputes, but they do investigate charges of *resident abandonment*, which is a violation of the nurse practice act. Nurses are required to maintain a safe environment for residents and others. This is a legal and ethical standard. No physician's order or facility policy can relieve the nurse of this responsibility. Generally speaking, walking off the job without notifying anyone and without ensuring that another qualified nurse assumes the responsibility for resident care is abandonment. Even if a supervisor has been notified that the nurse is leaving unexpectedly, the nurse still abandons the residents if he or she leaves the premises before some kind of handover is done, and another qualified nurse assumes responsibility for care of the residents.

Where staffing is concerned, there are no pat answers. Some facilities do well with staff-directed scheduling,

or creative schedules, such as 12-hour shifts. If your personnel routinely work eight-hour shifts, you may be able to get them to cover 12 hours in an emergency. The open shift is covered by having a person from the previous shift work four hours overtime, then a person from the next shift comes on duty four hours early. Another consideration is to develop an in-house pool to cover open shifts. In-house personnel usually receive 10% to 20% higher salaries. However, they have no guaranteed hours or benefits. In most facilities, they are also required to make specific weekend and holiday commitments to ensure adequate staffing.

If you routinely have one call-off per shift, consider creating a float position. This person is scheduled as an extra, and is sent to work on the unit where the call-off occurred. Some facilities have mandatory overtime policies to ensure the units are covered. These policies are not popular, but may be a necessary evil. Avoid mandatory overtime, if possible. The nursing board does not get involved in facility business. However, it does hold the nurse individually accountable for accepting only those assignments that are within his or her physical and emotional ability. If a licensed nurse accepts an assignment, he or she is responsible for the care delivered. The nurse has a duty to recognize when he or she is unfit to practice secondary to physical, mental, and/or emotional fatigue. Nursing judgment and provision of nursing care may be impaired if a nurse is physically, mentally or emotionally exhausted, which could lead to nursing errors.[18] Anticipating occasional scheduling problems and forming an employee staffing advisory committee to address them is usually the most sound solution.

One more key consideration for using an in-house pool or outside agency personnel is to make sure you have a method for communicating essential information about residents and their care plans to temporary personnel. This is in addition to the change-of-shift report. A supervisory person or charge nurse should brief the pool person at the beginning of each shift. Make sure he or she understands where to find resident care plans and other resources. However, he or she will probably not have time to do extensive reading about resident care. Verbal instructions are usually the most effective method of communicating with direct care staff. Determine who instructs the pool staff and the mechanisms for reporting problems. Make sure they know who is in authority, how and to whom to report concerns, and who can answer questions about resident care. Be sure they are adequately supervised.

Orientation

All personnel, including agency staff and students, must receive orientation to the facility, including fire and disaster policies and procedures. Verification of the employee's skills may also be appropriate. Some facilities and agencies also require drug testing.

When agency staff are used to cover for staffing shortages, you must meet the legal requirements for your state in regard to verifying licensure or certification information and criminal background check, or ensure the agency has done so. You must also meet public health requirements, such as ensuring that tuberculin testing has been done to verify the individuals are free from communicable disease. These requirements also apply if students, consultants, and others work in the facility periodically.

Some nurses participate in substance abuse recovery programs. In some states, these nurses are prohibited from working as travel nurses or through a contract agency. The consistent belief is that recovery is best achieved through stable monitoring in a stable employ-

ment setting, by the same manager. Follow-up is not always possible in a travel or agency environment.

The facility must adhere to EEOC, OSHA, ADA, and other guidelines when using contract agency employees. Some states have specific requirements for orientation when agency personnel are used. Make sure orientation is adequate for them to do the required job. Having another resource person on duty with them is best. Make sure the agency workers have a contact number for questions or emergencies. If you use agency personnel regularly, you may wish to consider developing a handbook or list of frequently asked questions for them.

Employee discipline

Employees are accountable for following facility policies and procedures. Your policies should include a progressive discipline policy for infractions of various rules. A progressive discipline policy usually begins with an oral warning, then progresses to a series of written warnings, suspension, and termination for policy violations. Allegations of abuse and theft often bypass the mechanisms of the progressive discipline policy because of the potential severity of the offense and risks associated with allowing the employee to remain on duty. In this instance, the person in charge has the authority to suspend the employee without pay until the allegations have been thoroughly investigated. Other violations, such as "no call, no show" behavior may be considered and written up as a voluntary termination instead of a deviation from the attendance policies. (However, employees should be informed of this procedure in advance.) In any event, facility policies should address discipline, and employees must be aware of policies, procedures, and the penalties for violations.

Oral and written warnings

Your human resources department most probably has a tool to use for documenting employee discipline. One of the most effective is a one-page template on two-copy NCR paper. This enables the supervisor to retain the original and give the employee a copy for his or her records. This format may also be used to maintain a record of oral warnings, or another format may be used. Employees are usually not receptive to receiving a "write up," and may be so defensive that any opportunities for teaching and performance improvement are lost. Some facilities use other terminology for the discipline process, such as "employee memorandum" or "teachable moment." Although these are documented in the same manner as any other progressive discipline, the terminology is more aesthetically acceptable and does not conjure up as many negative emotions.

When issuing a written warning, be as specific as possible. Identify the policy infraction. Objectively state how the employee violated this policy. You may also wish to list corrective action to take, or consequences if the employee violates the policy again. Present the warning to the employee in a private area. Always praise in public, and counsel or discipline in private. Remember to criticize the employee's action, not the person. Tell the employee that you value him or her and will provide an opportunity to correct the behavior. Verbally state the consequences if the problem persists. Sign and date the warning. Ask the employee to sign the warning. If he or she refuses or disagrees with the warning, document the refusal to sign. Invite the employee to state the disagreement at the bottom of the warning. Give him or her a copy.

Employee termination

Employee termination is a sensitive, difficult task for most managers. Rightfully, it should be. Use your written warning form as a precursor to termination. Follow your policies for an aggregate of offenses. For example, as a manager you should be aware of how the progressive policy is implemented. Most facilities require several infractions of the same policy before termination occurs. Thus, the employee could theoretically receive three warnings about tardiness, three about attendance, and three for violating the smoking policy before termination occurs for any of these offenses. One violation for tardiness, one for attendance, and one for improper smoking does not warrant termination in most facilities. However, you must know how your facility policies are interpreted before proceeding. In some facilities, the administrator or human resources director must approve all terminations. Know and follow your facility policies. Remember that your employees are your greatest asset. Salvaging/retraining them is often preferable to termination and the potential backlash that may occur as a result.

Exit interviews

Your facility policies should state your expectations for notice of resignation. Most facilities require notice equivalent to the length of one pay period for direct care staff, and two pay periods for managers and department heads. Make sure employees are familiar with these requirements. Exit interviews are an excellent method of obtaining employee feedback, along with employee satisfaction surveys. Unfortunately, this valuable tool is often overlooked in long-term care. Besides obtaining information about the reasons for termination, the interview is also a valuable tool that provides insight into what it takes to do the job. When done correctly, an exit interview is mutually beneficial for both the facility and the former employee. The facility retains and uses the employee's knowledge. The employee can articulate his or her unique contributions, and leave his or her mark.

Exit interviews can be conducted over the phone, in person, over the Internet, or by using a written questionnaire. However, the return rate is not usually as good when you depend upon the employee to complete and mail or email a written survey. Make it clear to the employee who will use the exit interview information and how it will be used. Explain that the purpose of the interview is to collect information that the facility will use.

Employees may be more likely to participate and may be more honest when someone who is not connected with the employer asks the questions. Another alternative is to have a department head from another department or a member of the employee attendance committee conduct the interview. Whoever conducts the interview should be taught to do it properly, however. A nursing assistant may say he or she is leaving for higher pay. What the employee really means is, "You can't pay me enough to work for that charge nurse." Employees tend to identify tangibles, such as salary because they are easier to discuss than intangibles, such as feelings and emotions. The interviewer should be skilled in drawing the employee out.

Study the data collected at exit interviews. Look for trends in age, length of employment, position, assignment, and other variables. Use the information to examine hiring patterns and trends, and to benefit existing and future employees of the facility.

Employee dissatisfaction and retaliation

Sadly, current and former employees sometimes retaliate against the facility for real or perceived slights. Their actions vary widely from doing things such as causing all the care plans to disappear to calling the state hotline and making complaints. Disgruntled employees or former employees may speak negatively about the facility in the community, making remarks such as, "I wouldn't admit my dog to that facility." A body of evidence also exists suggesting that characteristics such as skill use, skill variety, and autonomy are associated with both motivation and individual mental health.[19]

Poor leadership may exacerbate work-related stress by isolating individuals and denying access to social support. Managers who have a tendency to be abusive, aggressive, or punitive, and those who lack appropriate leadership skills, increase employee stress.[20] The authors of one study describe the lack of leadership skills in this type of manager as "passive leadership." This management style is a combination of the "laissez-faire" and "management-by-exception" styles of transformational leadership. Those applying the management-by-exception (passive) style ignore problems until the problems are either brought to their attention or become serious enough to demand action. Managers using the laissez-faire style avoid decision making and the responsibilities associated with their position. Control, autonomy, and decision-making latitude have been identified as factors that affect positive (or conversely, negative) job performance. For many years, researchers have identified control as being the most critical element in promoting positive performance and worker mental health.[21] Karasek and Theorell assert that a healthy workplace is one in which the worker's level of demand on the job is met with appropriate levels of control, promoting growth and development. Conversely, a job in which demands are high and control is low is theorized to cause stress and burnout.[22]

Obviously, the ideal solution is to manage the facility correctly to prevent conditions from deteriorating in the first place. However, you may be a new manager who inherited a mess from someone else. In this situation, the facility probably has a history of one or more managers using aggressive behavior as a means of controlling subordinates. Your only option is to try to identify and correct the problems, and this is seldom easy. Conditions cannot be changed overnight. One thing is certain: disgruntled, dysfunctional employees are your worst enemy. They are sabotaging the facility internally and in the community. The situation cannot be ignored. Use the progressive discipline process to manage individual problems until a more satisfactory, global solution has been implemented.

The nurse administrator fosters a professional environment. The nurse administrator acquires and maintains current knowledge in administrative practice. The nurse administrator systematically evaluates the quality and effectiveness of nursing practice and nursing services administration. The nurse administrator evaluates his or her own performance based on professional practice standards, relevant statutes and regulations, and organizational criteria. The nurse administrator's decisions and actions are based on ethical principles.[23]

Poor leadership

Staff job satisfaction is often proportionate to the leadership style of the manager. In healthcare, there is a close relationship between quality of care, staff morale and productivity, and the effectiveness of nursing management. Before the 1950s, leadership traits such as personal stability, intelligence, and self-confidence were studied and believed to directly affect worker satisfaction. Since then, we have learned that manager behaviors have a greater impact on employee morale. Managers can freely change their behavior to meet the needs of changing situations. Markham describes a *transformational management style*, in which the manager is collaborative, consensus-seeking, and consultative.[24] This manager attributes power to interpersonal skills and personal contact. Transformational leaders exhibit four characteristics in their interactions with employees: idealized influence, inspirational motivation, intellectual stimulation, and individualized consideration. A literature review is beyond our current scope. It is clear that managers' transformational leadership style is positively associated with employee commitment to the organization.[25]

Transactional leadership is based on the belief that the organization is all-powerful. The transactional manager relies on the power of his or her position and formal authority to punish and reward employees. Rosner suggests there are gender differences in management styles. Females seem to prefer the transformational style of leadership.[26] Since the vast majority of nurse managers are female, we will discuss transformational leadership here. Kouzes and Posner[27] identify five key practices in transformational leadership:

- Challenging the process
- Inspiring shared vision
- Enabling others to act
- Modeling the way
- Encouraging the heart

Whatever your management style, these are excellent steps to follow in effecting organizational change and garnering employee support. Transformational leaders have strong values, ethics, and standards. They set long-term goals. The manager motivates and empowers staff to aspire to higher standards and goals. This management style is characterized by an open, empowering culture. Mutual respect, good communication, and strong ethics and values are fundamental. Transformational leaders articulate the mission and vision, then create and maintain a positive image in the minds of employees. The manager is much like a cheerleader, motivating and encouraging employees, and sharing the long-term vision. Sometimes simple slogans, like "Together we can make a difference" serve as reminders. Your management style is one of the most powerful forces in the nursing facility. A positive style tends to "flavor" the facility, and motivates employees to do well. The manager provides direction and purpose, causing team members to act. Through empowerment, communication, and motivation, the nurse manager optimizes resident care and reverses negative employee attitudes and behavior.

Charge nurses

Remember that the position and job description for the charge nurse describes an individual who is in charge. If you approach the nurses on your units and ask them to increase supervision of the nursing assistant staff, they will most likely say they are too busy and don't have time. For a charge nurse, supervising nursing assistants is not an option. It is a job requirement.

If your quality assurance or survey team identifies problems on a nursing unit, the charge nurses are likely to tell you they cannot correct the problem without more staff. If you are desperately short of staff, this is probably true. However, if the unit runs at or near its budgeted PPD most days, look for other problems. Often, charge nurses will ask for more help because they *don't know how* to solve the problem. Just remember to analyze the issues. Throwing money at a problem is not a good solution, yet it is usually the first thing nurses suggest. In fact, you may find that personnel, practices, and procedures are so disorganized that solving the problem is impossible. To

solve the problem, you must first focus on unit efficiency and organization. This takes a commitment and can be very time consuming. In fairness to the charge nurses, however, most have never been taught how to manage a unit. Their education focuses on doing total patient care in a hospital, using the medical model. Comparing that position with being a charge nurse in a long-term care facility is like comparing oranges and tomatoes. Spend some time reviewing the operations, organization, and efficiency of your nursing units. Then develop a plan for assisting the charge nurses to improve their management skills. Residents and staff will benefit from your efforts!

It doesn't work!

This book is about legal aspects of the long-term care managers' jobs, not management theory. You may wish to check the references and study management styles. Find a style that is comfortable and learn to use it. You may also find useful management books on maintaining employee motivation, such as those written by Zig Ziglar. Ziglar's books are not written specifically for healthcare, but they are easy reading, and his principles are effective. For additional information, go to *www.ziglartraining.com/*.

Over the *short term*, investigating the reasons for employee dissatisfaction and sabotage, and changing the facility management style, will probably not change much. These are very effective *long-term* strategies. Over the short term, it may be necessary to develop policies regarding information that can and cannot be released to the public (including residents and families). This should include opinions about "short" staffing, salaries and benefits, care given, and other facility business. After educating staff about these policies, put some teeth into them by utilizing the progressive discipline system, if necessary. This is an effective short-term approach, but the best long-term plan probably involves modifying the department management style.

Providing references

Giving out post-employment references is considered a risky business. This is an area in which the laws need to be strengthened to protect the employer, who gives out honest performance information in good faith. Fearing defamation suits, most facilities will verify only the former employee's position and dates of employment upon reference checks. However, *defamation* means damaging or harming someone's reputation by libel (in writing) or slander (verbally). If you are truthful in providing reference information and do not use graphic, subjective terms to describe the former employee, defamation should not apply. Providing a reference is not defamatory unless the employer discloses information he or she knows is false or makes the disclosure in violation of the employee's rights.

Attorneys regularly advise facilities to say as little as possible, even if a worker has been terminated. There is no national data bank for reporting problem employees. Charles Cullen is an example of how the system failed to protect patients (the public) for sixteen years. Coworkers complained about him. He had been fired by several hospitals and nursing homes, and left others under a cloud of suspicion. Prosecutors investigated his involvement in suspicious deaths dating from 1993, but no charges were filed. Instead, Cullen easily found new nursing jobs.[28] "Mr. Cullen would soon tell the authorities an astounding story of his 16 years as both caregiver and killer: claiming to have fatally poisoned 12 to 15 patients at Somerset, at least half a dozen at St. Luke's, and 10 to 20 at other stops. When he was arrested, Mr. Cullen went quietly.

His nursing licenses were in order. He was, in theory, ready to be hired somewhere."[29]

On the other hand, some human resource professionals fear that withholding or concealing negative information about a former employee increases their legal exposure under a *negligent reference* theory. Because of this, some employers will respond to specific questions about performance, work habits, and attendance. When considering the negligent reference theory, a facility may be held liable if it conceals information and the former employee repeats injurious behavior. For example, if a nursing assistant is terminated for willfully injuring a resident and this is accurately documented, the information would be disclosed to a potential employer if the employee has applied for a position in which the behavior is likely to be repeated, injuring other residents. If the employee is suspected of abuse but this has not been verified, the reference would be answered by noting the employee is not eligible for rehire.

Establish a policy and procedure on giving references. Reference information must be accurate and objective. In some facilities, department heads are authorized to answer questions the prospective employer asks. They are not permitted to volunteer information. Identify individuals who are authorized to provide reference information. Consider the pros and cons of the various methods of providing reference information, then have your legal counsel approve your policies and procedures. After formulating a policy and procedure, inform all employees of how the facility will handle requests for post-employment references. Teach department heads and supervisors how to manage reference requests and inform them of the consequences of deviating from the policy. Both the individual giving the reference and the facility have liability if a former employee alleges defamation. The laws in some states specify that the employer must inform the parting employee of the truthful reason for the termination. At the time of this writing, these states include Arizona, California, Nebraska, Minnesota, Missouri, Montana, and Texas.

Make sure the former employee has signed a consent to release employment and reference information, and keep this consent in the personnel file. If you are contacted for a reference request, ask for the caller's name and phone number and return the call to verify the information. Make sure you contact a business and not an individual. Verify the phone number, if necessary. Doing this will help ensure that you provide reference information only to an authorized individual. Have the employee personnel file in front of you when providing information. When providing a telephone (verbal) reference, it is a good idea to document the questions and your responses. Retain a copy in the personnel file. Retain a copy of your response to written requests for information as well.

If employees are terminated due to census decrease or reduction in the workforce, clearly state this on the reference. (In fact, you may wish to give each of these employees a letter noting this reason for separation.) Facilities should also consider their position on providing letters of reference for current employees. It is not unusual for employees to ask their coworkers, charge nurse, or supervisor to write them a letter of recommendation. The letter is given to a prospective employer in lieu of a reference from the department head or human resources department. In most cases, the person who has authored the letter does not have the authority to represent the facility or to provide reference information. The letter of recommendation may provide vastly different information compared with the department head's evaluation.

Although you may be tempted to bypass reference checks because you know you may receive nothing other than dates of employment, skipping the reference check entirely presents a new set of problems. If an employee injures a resident accidentally or deliberately, you may be sued for negligent hiring. In a *negligent hiring* claim, the employer may be held responsible for the employee's misconduct (or other criminal act) if the employer did not adequately investigate the employee's background and qualifications at the time of hire. Negligent hiring claims usually involve employees who are in a position to cause injury to others, such as the vulnerable, dependent residents. To successfully establish this type of claim, the plaintiff must prove that the

- employer did not use reasonable care in hiring the employee

- employee posed a risk or danger to others (usually the residents); the risk would have been apparent if the employer had used reasonable care in screening and hiring

- the employer placed the employee in a position in which he or she could injure a resident (or another person)

Eligibility for rehire

Some facilities have rigid employment policies. In these facilities, employees who leave employment through resignation may never return. Other facilities are slightly more relaxed. If the employee's performance was average or above, he or she may be rehired in the future, if a suitable position exists. Employees who have been terminated for cause, as well as those who do not give adequate notice of resignation, are not eligible for rehire. Eligibility for rehire is often used as a carrot to get employees to give adequate resignation notice. If they give notice, the prospective employer is given this recommendation. If no notice is given, only dates of employment are verified. Employees are usually pretty savvy. They correctly view eligibility for rehire as a positive recommendation. If you have a stringent policy and refuse to release information beyond dates of employment, the carrot is lost. How you act on this information is between the managers, the policies of the facility, and your legal counsel.

So, how do I get reference information?

Like most managers, you are probably struggling with turnover and trying to hire the best employees possible. Responses to your ads are sometimes abysmal and are seldom encouraging. Again, the best solution is a long-term one. Network with other nurse managers in your area. If there is no networking organization, start one! As your peers get to know and trust you, you will find they are much more willing to share references and other information with you. You can write your own local rules, such as not hiring each others' employees unless proper notice of resignation is given.

Beyond this suggestion, the best thing to do is to contact former employers by phone and obtain whatever reference information you can. Faxing them an employee consent to release information immediately before calling may be helpful. At the end of the phone conversation, ask if the employee is eligible for rehire. You may be surprised to find that you get the information 50% of the time. The same is not true when requesting a written reference. In any event, this is one of those tips that is worth a try! Remember that persons listed as references by an applicant were selected by the individual, and most probably will provide a positive reference.

Also, remember to verify active nurse licensure. Check with the nursing assistant registry in each state in which a nursing assistant applicant has worked to ensure there are no abuse or neglect charges on file. In some states, both checks may be done online. Verification with the licensure board or registry is essential. Never depend on the paper copy of the certification or license alone.

References

1. National Association of Directors of Nursing Administration/Long Term Care (NADONA) (eds). (2000). *Standards of Practice* (4th edition). Cincinnati, OH. National Association of Directors of Nursing Administration/Long Term Care.

2. Green A, Cady C, Waddell L and Fitzpatrick O. (1995). Are you at risk for disciplinary action? *American Journal of Nursing*, 95, 41-45.

3. National Council of State Boards of Nursing. Nursing regulation: Nursing practice. Online. *www.ncsbn.org/regulation/nursingpractice.asp.* Accessed 01/06/06.

4. Office of Inspector General and American Health Lawyers Association (Eds.). (2003). Corporate responsibility and corporate compliance: a resource for health care boards of directors. Rockville, MD. U.S. Department of Health and Human Services.

5. Remsburg RE, Armacost KA, Bennett RG. Improving nursing assistant turnover and stability rates in a long-term care facility. *Geriatr Nurs* 1999;20:203-8

6. Zagury CS. Making a difference: Strategic planning for the director of nursing in long term care. The Director. Online. *www.nadona.org/media_archive/media/media-238.pdf.* Accessed 08/25/04.

7. Larkin, T.J. and Larkin, S. (1996). Reaching and changing front line employees. *Harvard Business Review*, May-June, 1996, (a) p 97, (b) p101.

8. Zagury CS. Making a difference: Strategic planning for the director of nursing in long term care. The Director. Online. *www.nadona.org/media_archive/media/media-238.pdf.* Accessed 08/25/04.

9. Goman CK (2005). How to develop a change-adept workforce. Online. *http://ezinearticles.com/?How-to-Develop-a-Change-Adept-Workforce&id=90792.* Accessed 11/06/05.

10. Goman CK (2005). How to develop a change-adept workforce. Online. *http://ezinearticles.com/?Have-We-Learned-Nothing-About-Managing-Change?&id=90789.* Accessed 11/06/05.

11. National Association of Directors of Nursing Administration/Long Term Care (NADONA) (eds). (2000). *Standards of Practice* (4th edition). Cincinnati, OH. National Association of Directors of Nursing Administration/Long Term Care.

12. American Nurses Association. (2002). *Code for nurses with interpretive statements.* Washington. American Nurses Publishing.

13. Delegation: understanding the concepts and decision-making process. *Insight,* Volume 7 Number 1 1998. Chicago. National Council of State Boards of Nursing.

14. American Nurses Association. (2002). *Code for nurses with interpretive statements.* Washington, DC. American Nurses Publishing.

15. National Council of State Boards of Nursing. (1995). *Delegation concepts and decision-making process.* Online. *http://www.ncsbn.org/regulation/uap_delegation_documents_delegation.asp.* Accessed 11/04/05.

16. Ettner, S. L., & Grzywacz, J. G. (2001). Workers' perceptions of how jobs affect health: A social ecological perspective. *Journal of Occupational Health Psychology*, 6, 101–113.

17. Tucker, P., MacDonald, I., Folkard, S., & Smith, L. (1998). The impact of early and late shift changeovers on sleep, health, and well-being in 8- and 12-hour shift systems. *Journal of Occupational Health Psychology*, 3, 265–275.

18. Texas Board of Nurse Examiners. (2005). FAQ - practice. Online. *http://204.65.35.7/faq-practice.htm.* Accessed 11/13/05.

19. Parker, S. K., & Wall, T. D. (1998). *Job and work design: Organizing work to promote well-being and effectiveness.* Thousand Oaks, CA: Sage.

20. Kelloway, E.K., Sivanathan, N., (MSc Graduate) Francis, L., & Barling, J. (2005). *Poor leadership.* In J. Barling, E.K. Kelloway, & M. Frone (2005) (Eds.) *Handbook of work stress* (pp. 89-112) CA: Sage Publications.

21. Hackman, J. R., & Oldham, G. R. (1980). *Work redesign.* Reading, MA: Addison-Wesley.

22. Karasek, R., & Theorell, T. (1990). *Healthy work: Stress, productivity and the reconstruction of working life.* New York: Basic Books.

23. American Nurses' Association (eds). (1995). *Scope and Standards for Nurse Administrators.* Washington, D.C. American Nurses' Publishing.

24. Markham G (1998) Gender inleadership. *Nursing Management.* 3,1, 18-19.

25. Barling, J., Weber, T., & Kelloway, E. K. (1996). Effects of transformational leadership training on attitudinal and financial outcomes: A field experiment. *Journal of Applied Psychology,* 81, 827–832.

26. Rosner J. (1990). *Ways women lead. Harvard Business Review.* Harvard MA, Harvard Press.

27. Kouzes J, Posner B. (1997). *The leadership challenge.* San Fransisco CA, Jossey Bass.

28. How dangerous employees continue to get new jobs. (3/22/04). *USA Today.* Online. *www.usatoday.com/news/opinion/editorials/2004-03-22-our-view_x.htm.* Accessed 11/09/05.

29. Perez-Pena R, Kocieniewski D, George J. (2/29/04). Death on the night shift: through gaps in system, nurse left trail of grief. NY Times. Online. *www.nytimes.com/2004/02/29/nyregion/29NURS.html ?ex=1393390800&en=042467b20cd853af&ei=5007& partner=USERLAND.* Accessed 11/09/05.

The litigation process

Governing body

Under federal law, all Medicare- and Medicaid-approved long-term care facilities must have a *governing body* or designated persons functioning as a governing body. The governing body is responsible for determining the mission, goals, and objectives of the facility. These individuals are legally responsible for establishing and implementing policies for facility management and operations. The owner may serve on the long-term care facility's governing body, but this is not required.[1] The governing body must ensure that all written policies and procedures are formally and regularly revised, adopted, and dated. These policies and procedures specify and govern the provision of all services. The formal policies and procedures must be available to all of the governing body's members, the staff, the residents, family or legal representatives of residents, and the public.

The governing body is responsible for securing a licensed nursing home administrator (LNHA) or licensed nursing facility administrator (LNFA). The administrator is accountable to the governing body for overall management of the nursing facility. Final responsibility for the operation of a long-term care

facility lies with its governing body, which is the legal entity licensed by the state to operate the facility. The governing body sets policies, adopts rules, and enforces them for the healthcare and safety of the residents. The nursing facility administrator or designee acts as the *compliance officer* for the facility to ensure that standards and policies of the governing body are adhered to. The compliance officer has the authority to review documents and all other information that are relevant to compliance, survey, and quality assurance activities. Facility management is structured to ensure that there is an open line of reporting from management to the governing body. The structure must ensure timely and candid reports. The Office of the Inspector General (OIG) reinforces their belief that compliance officer must have sufficient personnel and financial resources to implement all aspects of the compliance program.[2]

Quality of care

Many people who file lawsuits state they did not file suit because of money. They list reasons such as preventing the suffering of others and teaching the facility (and governing body) a lesson. One hospital patient was misdiagnosed with pneumonia. The patient's daughter stayed at her side and continually called for help as her mother deteriorated. The hospital was very short of staff and the nurse did not respond until the patient experienced a cardiac arrest. She was successfully resuscitated, but experienced brain damage. The daughter sued successfully. She stated, "I wanted them, as I wheeled my mother into that courtroom, to see what their decision to run the hospital shorthanded cost somebody."[3]

The OIG emphasizes quality of care and protection of resident dignity in its guidance for nursing facilities. They recommend that facilities include a statement affirming a commitment to quality of care and providing the care necessary to attain or maintain the resident's "highest practicable physical, mental and psychosocial well-being" in the policies and procedures. Quality of care is also an issue when the facility is investigated for fraud and abuse under the False Claims Act. The government, fiscal intermediaries, and various insurers pay facilities to deliver a certain quality or standard of care. If care is not delivered, or if the care given falls below this standard, the facility may be prosecuted for fraud. Clearly, the commitment to delivering high-quality care should not be taken lightly.

Negligence is the most common charge filed in civil suits against long-term care facilities. However, punitive damages are often higher if the plaintiff proves fraud. Fraud charges are usually filed when the injured party wishes to seek damages from the governing body and corporation. State and federal governments have also filed fraud and abuse charges against facilities, resulting in the execution of search warrants, individual charges against personnel, and protracted legal battles.

"The long term care facility administrator is assigned the administrative authority, responsibility, and accountability necessary for carrying out his or her assigned duties by the governing board (a.k.a. governing body) of the facility. The primary purpose of this position is to direct the day to day functions of the facility in accordance with current federal, state, and local standards, guidelines, and regulations governing long term care facilities to assure that the highest quality care is provided to the residents at all times. To do this, the administrator must plan, organize, monitor, evaluate, and direct the operations of the facility in a responsible manner. He or she must be responsive to family members' concerns and follow up to ensure they are promptly and properly resolved. He or she must ensure that sufficient, qualified staff are in place to meet the residents' needs. The nursing facility administrator is expected to delegate department management to qualified personnel, supervise department heads, and direct the general nursing facility operations. He or she must monitor and evaluate performance of all departments to ensure regulatory objectives are met. John Doe neglected his responsibilities as administrator in failing to recognize, identify and correct the system-wide breakdown in the delivery of needed care to Mary Smith. John Doe failed in his responsibility as administrator as summarized in this report.

Elizabeth King, RN, was the Director of Nursing (DON) for QRS Convalescent Center during the time in which Mary Smith was a resident in the facility. In absence of the Medical Director, the DON is responsible and accountable for carrying out the resident care policies established by the facility. The primary functions of the DON position involve planning, organizing, monitoring, evaluating, and directing the overall operation of the Nursing Services Department in accordance with current federal, state, and local standards, guidelines, and regulation governing the long term care facility, and as directed by the Administrator and Medical Director, to ensure that quality care is delivered at all times.

The professional standard of practice for a Director of Nursing and state regulations governing participation in the Medicaid Program held Elizabeth King, RN responsible for the care and services provided to Mary Smith. Elizabeth King, RN neglected her duties as DON in failing to recognize, identify, and correct the system wide breakdown in the delivery of needed care to Mary Smith. Elizabeth King, RN failed in her overall responsibility as DON in this facility. Issues that are problematic and of concern regarding the failure to meet the standards of care and professional nursing practice include those listed in this report."

(From a petition of an actual lawsuit alleging progressive failures and omissions of care.)

Elements of a lawsuit

Nurses and other healthcare professionals have certain responsibilities to residents for whom they care. *Negligence* is the failure to act as a reasonably prudent nurse would in the same or similar circumstances. It is failure to exercise the degree of care considered reasonable under the circumstances.[4] Malpractice is a legal situation that exists when resident injury occurs as a result of negligence. For a malpractice claim to be successful, four elements of negligence must be proven. These are

- *Duty*—To have legal exposure, the nurse (or facility) must have a *duty* to care for the resident. The facility accepts the duty when it

admits and agrees to care for the resident. The facility has a duty to ensure its personnel are competent in their responsibilities. The nurse and other personnel accept the legal duty of care when they receive report and assume responsibility for the care of the resident. Duty always supersedes facility policies or physician orders. If a nurse knows, or should have known, that a resident was potentially in danger, the nurse's duty is always to act in the resident's best interest. One of the nurse's major duties is to comply with the applicable standards of care. A nurse also has a duty to exercise independent skill and nursing judgment within his or her scope of practice, and activate the chain of command, when appropriate, by notifying a supervisor, physician, or other party. In a healthcare lawsuit, there is no single duty. Duty to care must be individualized to the resident in light of his or her physical and mental condition. In a lawsuit, failure to fulfill one's duty is perceived to be failure to follow applicable laws/professional standards.

- Another, less common term that may be used in place of duty is beneficence. When written in this manner, *beneficence* (duty) is an ethical principle that requires healthcare providers to do what will further the resident's interest. All nurses are expected to practice in keeping with their board of nursing rules and nurse practice act. Your board of nursing probably has a document explaining the client's vulnerability and the nurse's "power" differential over the client. The board of nursing rules take into consideration the client's status with regard to age, illness, mental infirmity, and other factors and the nature of the nurse/client relationship, in which the client typically defers decisions to the nurse and relies on the nurse to protect him or her from harm. The nurse is accountable to the board of nursing to ensure that nursing care meets standards of safety and effectiveness. Because of this, the board holds the position that nurses must practice within the parameters of the nurse practice act and board rules. Each nurse must be able to support how his or her clinical judgments and nursing actions were aligned with the nurse practice act and board rules.

- *Breach of duty*—The standard of care for the procedure or practice must be consulted to determine whether a breach of duty occurred. Breach of duty implies a deviation from the standard of care. The breach is an act of omission or commission that causes harm or damage to the resident. Nurses cannot hide behind the "I was just following physician orders" excuse. Professionals are taught current practices and have a legal and ethical obligation to question physician orders, especially if resident welfare is at stake. In a courtroom, the jury will most probably believe the expert witness who testifies that no reasonable clinician would have followed an unsafe, unacceptable, illogical, or unreasonable order. There are no guarantees of successful outcomes in medical and nursing care. A negative result in and of itself is not necessarily an indication that someone committed malpractice. Because of this, each situation must be studied individually, and the applicable standards of care identified and applied.

- *Proximate cause or causation*—In malpractice litigation, the plaintiff must show that the damages were *proximately* caused by the malpractice of the defendant. This means that a connection must be present between the act or omission and the harm or damages to the resident. An act of simple negligence is not enough for a plaintiff to prevail. The plaintiff must prove the negligent act was the cause or a contributing cause of the injury. Causation must be proved to a *reasonable degree of medical (or nursing) probability*. This is the likelihood or chance of occurrence of a medical or nursing phenomenon. A mere *possibility* is not sufficient. If the documentation and testimony reveal that a given outcome might or "possibly would" (as opposed to "probably would") have been avoided by a treatment, there is generally a failure of proof.

- *Damages*—Damages are injuries, including pain and suffering or mental anguish, sustained by the resident as a result of the breach of duty (omission or commission). Damages or injuries can take many forms, and can be either physical or mental. They can subject the resident to additional medical treatment, surgery, and the associated risk factors. The damages must be legally compensable. For example, in a wrongful death suit, the damages are usually things such as loss of wages, fringe benefits, and other non-economic losses associated with losing a family member. However, in other cases, the damage may not be present. If a resident develops a Stage II pressure ulcer, which nurses identify, treat, and heal within a week, the damage element is missing.

- *Risk factors* are conditions that indicate or suggest a problem may develop. These conditions have the potential to cause the resident's health to worsen.

Other legal terms that long-term care facility personnel must be familiar with are:

- *Respondeat superior*—"The master is liable for the acts of his agent." "Let the master answer."

This is a Latin expression meaning that the facility is responsible for the actions of its employees who are acting within their scope of duties in the course of employment.

- *Plaintiff*—the injured party, or his or her personal representative or heirs, who are suing for damages.

- *Defendant*—an individual or entity (such as a facility) who is being sued. In a long-term care facility, the facility and its ownership, governing body, administrator, and personnel may all be named as defendants in a lawsuit.

- *Standards of care*—Practices and actions that are considered reasonable under the circumstances. These are actions that a reasonable, prudent caregiver would take in the care of the resident. Standards may vary over short periods of time, depending on research and available technology. Standards are established by professional organizations, nursing board rules and nurse practice acts, textbooks, government statutes and regulations, journal articles, facility policies and procedures, manufacturer's instructions (including information from the PDR and other drug books for medications), JCAHO accreditation standards, opinions of reputable experts, common sense, and other relevant sources. The standard of care that applies is what was current when the incident or injury occurred. Facilities are expected to keep up with current standards and practices. Thus, it is important to provide care that is in keeping with current trends. In a lawsuit, the expert witnesses usually define the standard of care applicable to the current situation.

- *Expert witnesses*—Individuals who are considered experts in their field. They are retained by the plaintiff and defense to advise the attorneys, judge, and jury regarding the standards of care at issue in a legal action. In long-term care-related lawsuits, the expert witnesses are usually considered experts in long-term care and geriatric practice. They may be physicians, nurses, surveyors, and others. However, one expert cannot generally address the standard of care for other professionals. For example, a physician cannot address the nursing standard of care, and vice versa. States have varying requirements for the use of expert witnesses. A physician expert is almost always required to testify to causation, but in many jurisdictions, nurse experts can testify to causation related to nursing issues and problems. Experts can express their professional opinions in a trial, whereas most witnesses are permitted to testify only to facts.

- *Ordinary care*—is the degree of care that a long-term care facility (or nurse) of ordinary prudence would use under the same or similar circumstances.

- *Proximate cause*—is the cause which, in a natural and continuous sequence, produces an event. Without this cause, the event would not have occurred. In order to be a proximate cause, the act or omission complained of must be such that a long-term care facility (or nurse) using ordinary care would have foreseen that the event, or some similar event, might reasonably result from the act or omission. There may be more than one proximate cause of an event.

- *Clear and convincing evidence*—The measure or degree of proof that produces a firm belief or conviction that the allegations are true.

Malice

Malice is an important legal concept. The legal defini-tion of malice is not like the definition that people commonly use. When we use the word "malice" in conversation, it usually refers to a deliberate action to harm another person. It is often done as a means of retaliation. When we speak of an action that was done maliciously, this means it was done deliberately or on purpose. In the legal definition, malice is a specific intent by the defendant to cause substantial injury to the plaintiff. However, it is also an act or omission by the defendant, which, when viewed objectively from the standpoint of the defendant at the time of its occurrence, involved an extreme degree of risk, consid-ering the probabilities and magnitude of the potential harm to others. *The defendant has actual, subjective awareness of the risk involved, but nevertheless proceeds with conscious indifference to the rights, safety, or welfare of others.* A simple example of malice, when used in this context, is leaving a confused, unstable resident in the bathroom alone. The nurse knows there is a risk the resident may fall and get injured, but he or she leaves anyway. The nurse may be busy, preoccupied, or not consider or think of the risk. He or she may believe injury to the resident is not likely. When he or she walks away, the nurse gambles that the resident will not fall. In this situation however, the nurse is wrong. The resident falls and breaks a hip. Another example is failure to reposition a bedfast resident every two hours. Turning the resident is difficult and time consuming. We know that there is a risk of skin break-down unless pressure is relieved regularly. However, we are busy and disregard the risk. The resident develops a pressure ulcer. According to the legal definition of the term, disregarding the risk factors of the residents constitutes malice. The nurse is aware of the risks, but takes a chance, trusting that no complications will occur, and consciously disregards them.

"KRP Hospital Skilled Nursing Unit was aware of measures to prevent falls. However, they did not provide these basic services. They did noth-ing to assess or plan for continuity of care on the resident's behalf. The KRP Hospital Skilled Nursing Unit was aware that this resident was at high risk for falls. Despite this knowledge, however, they failed to assess her for restraint alternatives, restraints, or environmental modifi-cations to prevent falls. There is no evidence that they assisted her with ambulation. No plan of care was developed to direct the staff in how to care for the resident or meet her needs. The resident's response to care was not evaluat-ed. The nurses' notes do not reflect adequate observation, assessment, planning, or continuity of care. Therefore, in my opinion, The KRP Hospital Skilled Nursing Unit acted with malice and disregarded the rights, safety, and welfare of Alice Smith, resulting in serious injury, pain, and mental anguish."

(From an expert report of an actual lawsuit alleging omissions of care.)

Consideration of resident risk factors

Malice becomes an issue when we consider risk fac-tors. Remember the definition of nursing practice from Chapter 1: Nurses diagnose and treat the *human response to illness*. The ANA standards make the responsibility for acting on risk factors very clear: "When making clinical judgments, nurses must base their decisions on consideration of consequences, which prescribe and justify nursing actions."[5] We identify risk factors in many different ways. Some are just common sense, such as knowing the skin will break down if exposed to excretions for a prolonged period of time. Thus, incontinence is a risk factor for skin problems.

Many different tools identify residents' risk factors. The most prominent of these are the Minimum Data Set

(MDS) and the various assessments, such as skin assessments and fall assessments. The Resident Assessment Instrument (RAI) is the formal name for the resident assessment, of which the MDS is the main component. The Resident Assessment Protocols (RAPs) are tools to guide the facility through an assessment of the resident's functional status. "Triggers" are bridges leading from the MDS to various RAPs. Facilities are responsible for assessing areas that are relevant to residents, regardless of whether these areas are included in the MDS. The RAI is the minimum assessment tool, not the only assessment tool. Completion of the MDS does not remove the facility's responsibility to document a more detailed assessment of particular issues of relevance for the resident.[6]

> "The STE Health Care Center failed to adhere to acceptable standards of nursing practice regarding the nursing process and care plan. The plan did not accurately reflect Mr. Smith's individual problems, needs and risk factors. Thus, personnel did not take appropriate steps to address or monitor his high-risk conditions. They were unprepared to deal with the needs of this resident. Their approach was a reactive one, rather than a proactive one. Despite knowing that the resident was at risk for certain complications, they took no effective action to prevent complications from developing. Once complications developed, they attempted to treat them. This type of care defies nursing ethics and the principles upon which nursing practice is based. Absence of assessments and lack of a complete, proper, accurate, and timely care plan deprived Mario Smith of uniform, timely, goal-directed care."[7]
>
> *(From an expert report of an actual lawsuit alleging progressive failures and omissions of care.)*

When risk factors are identified, they are often listed on the care plan. As the process of problem identification is integrated with sound clinical interventions, the care plan becomes each resident's unique path toward achieving or maintaining his or her highest practicable level of well-being.[8] Nurses are responsible for taking action to reduce the residents' risk factors, once they have been identified. (However, you are not relieved of your responsibilities if certain risk factors are not listed on the care plan. You are expected to use common sense and solid nursing judgment to identify actual and potential problems.) If you know residents have certain high-risk conditions, but choose to gamble that no complications will occur, you may be accused of acting with malice, or conscious indifference to the resident's welfare. The penalties are often much more severe in a lawsuit, if the plaintiff proves malice. Malice is a component of abuse and neglect charges, which are often attached to additional criminal penalties.

Adhering to standards of practice

If you read the definitions carefully in this chapter, you will see that you must use the nursing process in order to adhere to professional standards of nursing practice. The ANA notes, "Gerontological nursing practice involves assessing the health and functional status of aging adults, planning and providing appropriate nursing and other healthcare services, and evaluating the effectiveness of such care. Emphasis is placed on maximizing functional ability in activities of daily living (ADLs), promoting, maintaining, and restoring health, preventing and minimizing disabilities of acute and chronic illness; and maintaining life in dignity and comfort until death. Gerontological nursing focuses on the client and the family."[9]

> "The director of nursing was not competent in his responsibilities as manager of the nursing department. He failed to establish standards of nursing service that facilitate the provision of quality nursing care. He failed to establish indicators for monitoring the effectiveness of nursing care. He failed to monitor the quality and effectiveness of care delivered. The failures in the nursing process and departmental direction and oversight, including observation, assessment, planning, intervention, evaluation and delivery of basic nursing care caused injury to Louis Doe."
>
> *(From an expert report of an actual lawsuit alleging progressive failures and omissions of care.)*

Statute of limitations

The *statute of limitations* is the time frame allowed by statute within which a lawsuit must be filed, or legal action taken to enforce the plaintiff's rights. Crimes such as murder often have no applicable statute. However, other actions have varying time limits. In most medical cases, this time frame is two years from the time the incident or injury occurred, although there are exceptions to the rules. For example, if an instrument is left in the patient's body after surgery, and is discovered three years later it would appear that the discovery of the instrument has exceeded the applicable statute. Because of this, the statute allows two years from the time the person first learns that he or she is injured to file the lawsuit.

Filing the lawsuit in court, serving a summons and complaint, or in some cases writing a letter expressing your intent to sue within the time set by the state for the statute of limitations preserves the right to sue. If these procedures are not followed, the case will expire due to the passage of time, regardless of the legal merits of the lawsuit. However, the courts have considerable latitude in the interpretation of the case and may elect to use one limitations period rather than another, depending on the inciting event. Because of this, the plaintiff (and defendant) should consult knowledgeable legal counsel before assuming that the applicable statute of limitations has expired.

Defense strategy

When defending a long-term care facility, the defense attorney commonly uses one or more of these strategies:[10]

- The standard of care was followed.

- The resident's injury/death was caused by a pre-existing medical problem.

- The resident's condition deteriorated even though proper care was provided.

- The resident was frail, old, and sick, and was about to die anyway.

- It did not happen here or it did not happen the way the plaintiff said it did.

- The plaintiff was negligent.

- It was an accident (or) it happened so quickly that we could not stop it.

- We did the best we could.

- The pressure ulcers (or other problems) were unavoidable or caused by pre-existing medical problems.

- Our records are incorrect. He really was given the care in question, but it was not documented.

- The facility uses "Charting by Exception" to document care, which is why you do not see documentation that this care was routinely delivered.

- The family did not visit very often. Now they want money.

- The _____ (experts, family, other witnesses) are simply not credible.

- We admit we did something wrong, but we did not cause the resident's injury (or death).

Pre-existing medical conditions, weakness, frailty, and an anticipated short life expectancy are the basis of the defense in many lawsuits. The focus is that the injury was the inevitable product of a compromised health status. This removes the emphasis on foreseeing, identifying risk factors, and acting on risk factors to prevent negative outcomes. This argument forces the plaintiff to show that the injury was most likely a result of external factors for which the defendant is responsible instead of the resident's pre-existing medical problems. To counteract this defense, the plaintiff will emphasize that the underlying medical problems and risks were known to the facility at the time of admission. They did not have to accept the resident, and in doing so, confirmed they could meet the resident's needs. The plaintiff will also emphasize that the resident's chronic medical problems were stable for many years while he or she was at home or in another facility. The conditions became unstable as a result of poor care after admission to this facility. Because the defense may try to obfuscate the significance of other, irrelevant medical problems, the plaintiff attorney will emphasize the underlying conditions affecting the current injury. He or she will try to show that the facility accelerated the resident's deterioration, and that the magnitude or severity of the injury was caused by the facility's negligence. If the facility accelerated the time of death by even one minute, it caused the outcome. This refers to the "playing God" argument below, which contends that no one has the right to modify God's plan regarding

the length of life. They will strive to get the jury to answer "No" to this question: "Absent the wrongful conduct, would the adverse condition (or death) have occurred *at this time?*"[11] To prevail in the lawsuit, the attorneys and experts must prove the deterioration was probable as a result of the defendant's conduct. *Probability* means the event *was likely* to occur. Compare this with the definition of possibility, which means the adverse event *might have occurred.* The AAOS says this succinctly: "Possibility is a less than 50% chance that something occurred. Contrast with 'probability,' a more than 50% chance."[12]

When all else fails, the defense attacks the integrity of the plaintiff witnesses, such as family members and expert witnesses. They typically investigate every facet of the witnesses' backgrounds. If there is a skeleton in the personal or professional closet, they will find and expose it while the witness is testifying and it is least expected. This an effective tactic to destroy the witnesses' credibility. It causes individuals who routinely do expert witness work to develop a thick skin or leave the testifying expert business.

The plaintiff's response

To counteract the strategies used by the defense, the plaintiff will:

- remind the jury that the resident was someone's mother; a much-loved family member

- contend the long-term care facility's care was profit-driven

- advise the jury that the facility knew what it was getting when it agreed to accept the resident

- advise the jury that the sickest residents have the most nursing needs, and the facility had agreed to meet the resident's needs in the admission agreement

- contend the facility was playing God, and despite the resident's potentially short life span, no one has the right to play God and shorten the life further

- remind the jury that life is already too short and the actions of the facility reduced the length of the resident's expected lifespan, robbing the resident and family of precious time together

- remind the jury that making a decision to place a loved one in a facility is a difficult one, but the family should be able to take comfort in the fact that the facility will provide the best care possible, keeping the loved one safe and secure; the facility violated this trust

- inform the jury that all residents have a right to quality care and should not be discriminated against because of age, race, religion, marital status, sexual preference, etc.

The plaintiff will try to prove that the negligence is a condition for which the resident was known to be at high risk, or one that occurred as a result of prolonged neglect. For example, a burn happens quickly. However, pressure ulcers, malnutrition, and hydration develop over a long period of time.

The plaintiff may also use the pre-existing condition rule, which states: *"If a man be sick of some disease which possibly, by course of nature, would end his life in half a year, and another gives him a wound or hurt which hastens his end by irritating and provoking the disease to operate more violently or speedily, this hastening of his death is homicide or murder, as the case may be. In such case the victim doth not die simply by the visitation of God, but as a result of the hurt that he received which hastened death, and an offender of such a nature shall not apportion his own wrong."*[13]

Contributory negligence and comparative fault

Contributory negligence and *comparative fault* are legal concepts that mean that an act or omission of the plaintiff is a contributing cause of the injury and a bar to recovery. In this case, the jury assigns a percentage of responsibility to both the plaintiff and defendant. The courts are given the power to reduce the award of damages in proportion to the claimant's share of the blame. For example, the jury finds the plaintiff bears 50% of the responsibility for the negative outcome because he inconsistently followed physician orders. The jury finds the physician 50% responsible because he made several errors. The jury awards a judgment of $100,000. The physician must pay the plaintiff $50,000. The plaintiff is responsible for the other $50,000.

Negligence per se

Federal and state rules require conduct and care in keeping with professional standards. *Negligence per se* is negligence that occurs as a result of neglect of duty to the resident(s) by action or omission(s). It is generally thought of as a violation of the rules, or OBRA regulations. If the plaintiff establishes that the defendant was negligent in violating a statute, little other proof is required to prove negligence per se.

Mediation and arbitration agreements

After years of unpredictable, costly lawsuits, some healthcare facilities and managed care companies now require prospective residents and patients to sign mandatory mediation or arbitration agreements at the time of admission. The purpose of the agreement is to reduce the potential cost of protracted litigation. Mediation and arbitration are *not interchangeable* terms. In mediation, a neutral third party facilitates communication and works with the opposing parties to assist them in reaching an agreement. Depending on the original agreement, the results may be binding or not binding. If they are not binding, the parties are not required to reach an agreement. If they are binding, both parties must adhere to them. When using this type of agreement, make sure the person who signs the admission paperwork has the legal authority to do so. This is a complex area of discussion, but you want to avoid getting into the middle of disputes between family members. Also, remember that a designated durable power of attorney (healthcare proxy) can legally make medical decisions on behalf of the resident. He or she is not authorized to make financial decisions, and some of the admission agreements are financial in nature.

Arbitration is a form of alternative dispute resolution in which a neutral third party (the arbiter) settles and disposes of the matter. Binding arbitration is the most common method, but non-binding arbitration may be used. The arbiter can rule in favor of either side, or establish a compromise. The disputing parties agree in advance to accept and be bound by the arbiter's decision. The arbiter (or a panel of arbiters) serves as a private judge in a closed court. He or she reviews evidence and hears testimony.

Persons who serve as mediators and arbiters are usually more knowledgeable than the average juror, and are in a better position to evaluate the legitimacy of the complaint. Attorneys and retired judges may provide this service. A mediator or arbiter will make a decision based on the facts of the case and is unlikely to be sympathetic. Damage awards are usually substantially less than jury verdicts. Juror sympathy often increases the damage award.

Legal issues surrounding arbitration

Arbitration is governed by state law. In some states, healthcare providers can refuse to care for residents and patients who will not agree to binding arbitration. The statutes in some states permit the courts to determine whether an arbitration agreement is acceptable, based on contract law. In other states, a form of non-binding arbitration may be ordered by the courts, but is not mandated. Binding arbitration agreements are usually presented for signature at the time of admission, before an adverse event occurs. If state law allows, the resident may be denied admission if he or she refuses to sign the agreement.

Mediation and arbitration agreements should be carefully written by the facility's legal counsel and approved by the governing body. Some states have voided arbitration agreements because of the way they were worded, depriving residents of their rights. An agreement may be declared unconstitutional if it

- revokes, discredits, or undermines a statutorily created right

- contains fraudulent language

- discriminates against either party

For example, the Tennessee Court of Appeals has ruled that upon admission to the long-term care facility, a spouse cannot voluntarily waive the resident's right to pursue a jury trial. This is based on a ruling in which a facility presented a waiver to a resident's husband as a condition of admission to the facility. The husband signed the form, agreeing to submit potential claims for mediation and, if necessary, binding arbitration. The resident was mentally alert but ill at the time of admission, and the husband signed all admission documents. He stated that he felt pressured to sign the arbitration agreement because he was unable to care for his wife at home. The resident subsequently was injured and died. The daughter alleged the injuries were the result of facility negligence. When the daughter sued for damages, the trial court ruled her stepfather had signed away the right to sue. The appellate court ruled that there was no evidence that the resident's husband had the express authority to sign a mediation or arbitration agreement on her behalf, and voided the agreement. "Contrary to the admissions coordinator's testimony that the resident's husband was aware of what he was doing, the daughter testified that her stepfather 'was very upset, very agitated (and) very confused' after he signed the agreement," the appellate court said in its decision. "The daughter also testified that her stepfather told her that his 'only choice' as to have his wife admitted to the long-term care facility because he was physically unable to take care of her."[14]

In a Florida case, a resident's son filed a lawsuit for negligence and wrongful death, based on care given to his mother. He named 10 companies that owned, operated, or consulted to the long-term care facility in his lawsuit. These companies had various contracts with the long-term care facility for consulting and financial services. The contracts contained an arbitration agreement. The attorney for two of the defendants moved to compel arbitration because they stated that the resident was an intended third-party beneficiary of the consulting and financial agreements. The trial court granted their motion. Because of this, the son was told he was required to submit to binding arbitration. The resident's son immediately appealed, claiming the arbitration requirement was an error, because his mother was neither a signatory to nor a third-party beneficiary of any contract that would subject her to arbitration. The Court of Appeals of Florida ruled that the resident received nothing more than an incidental or consequential benefit from the contracts nor was she the intended

third-party beneficiary. Because of this, her estate was not bound to the arbitration provisions of the agreements, overturning the trial court's ruling.[15]

The litigation process

A *lawsuit* is any proceeding in a court of justice by which an individual pursues a remedy which the law affords.[16] Civil procedure is the body of rules and practices by which justice is meted out by the legal system.[17] It is the written set of rules that sets out the process that courts will follow when hearing cases of a civil nature (a "civil action"). These rules explain how a lawsuit or case may be commenced, what kind of service of process is required, the types of pleadings or statements of case, motions or applications, and orders allowed in civil cases, the timing and manner of depositions and discovery or disclosure, the conduct of trials, the process for judgment, various available remedies, and how the courts and clerks must function.[18] Civil procedure includes the rules and process by which a civil case is tried and appealed, including the preparations for trial, the rules of evidence and trial conduct, and the procedure for pursuing appeals.

Complaint

A lawsuit begins, or *commences*, when a complaint is filed. The *complaint* defines the lawsuit and serves as notice to the defendant that he or she is being sued. This must be within the applicable statute of limitations. An attorney files the complaint, in person or by fax or mail, with the clerk of the court. The complaint lists the facts upon which the lawsuit is based. It begins with a listing of the name of the court, docket number, and all the parties of the lawsuit. Next, it lists numbered facts that the plaintiff alleges. It ends with a prayer for relief and request for a jury trial. After filing the complaint, the plaintiff's attorney must make arrangements to have it *served*, or formally delivered to the defendant. This can be done by means of a process server, or certified mail, depending on the rules of the local jurisdiction. The plaintiff's attorney must arrange for service to take place during a specified period of time.

After the complaint has been served, the defendant has a brief period of time (approximately 20 to 30 days, depending on state law) during which to file a response or a motion to dismiss. Judgment may be entered against the defendant by default if he or she fails to answer. A *motion to dismiss* lists the defendant's bases for dismissal. These are reasons such as improper venue, lack of jurisdiction, and failure to state a claim. A judge will have to rule on this motion. Dismissal is not automatic.

In filing an answer to the complaint, the defendant must respond to every numbered item listed in the complaint. He or she may include additional or alternative defenses, such as the statute of limitations and comparative negligence.

Discovery

Discovery is the process by which the parties to the lawsuit gather information held by the other side by obtaining various documents and other evidence, including requiring oral testimony in deposition. The discovery rules are fairly liberal. The objective is to give all parties an opportunity to review the information and negotiate a settlement, if possible. Old television shows such as *Perry Mason* and *Matlock* are filled with suspense, and almost always end with courtroom surprises, such as admissions of guilt. In today's litigation atmosphere, there are few surprises. In fact, one purpose of the liberal discovery rules is to prevent surprises at trial.

Motions

Requests for action by the court are always made in the form of oral or written *motions*. The subject matter of the motions varies from motions to dismiss, to motions for continuance, and motions for judgment.

Depositions

Depositions are sworn testimony and carry the same weight as testimony in a court of law. A deposition is commonly done in an attorney's office, but can be done anywhere. Anyone can be deposed. After the witness is sworn in, the opposing attorney has the opportunity to question him or her. The attorney may also issue a subpoena duces tecum requiring the witness to turn over certain things, such as his or her notes. A court reporter documents the testimony and makes a transcript. The deposition may be videotaped or audiotaped. No judge is present during the deposition. Depositions are the most powerful form of obtaining evidence under the discovery rules. Your attorney may meet with you prior to the deposition and explain the process to you. He or she may ask you various questions and critique your performance to assist you in learning to testify and following the court rules.

Trial

Many factors affect how lawsuits are settled. If the two parties can come to a mutual agreement, the lawsuit will be settled amicably before ever going to trial. A judge presides over every trial. He or she ensures proper procedures are followed and determines what evidence may be used. In healthcare lawsuits, most trials are *jury trials*. This means that a panel of jurors is selected to be the finders of fact. They review the evidence and render a verdict. In a *bench trial*, the judge is the only finder of fact and will render the verdict based on the evidence.

Damage awards, trial outcomes, and appeals

As you can see, it takes a long time for a lawsuit to move through the legal system. The plaintiff has a prolonged period of time in which to file a lawsuit, depending on the statute of limitations. The court system is often backlogged. Lawsuits are fraught with delays, and move through the system slowly. It may be a lengthy period of time before a lawsuit gets to trial. This can be very expensive to defend, so the defendant or insurer may attempt to settle the case rather than paying ongoing legal fees. If the case proceeds to trial, the jury verdict will list recommended amounts for compensatory and punitive damages. *Compensatory damages* are awarded to reimburse the plaintiff for the actual injury or loss. They may also include fees for expenses, loss of time, bodily suffering and mental suffering. They do not include punitive damages. *Punitive damages* are a separate figure that commonly exceeds the economic losses. They are intended solely to punish the defendant because of reckless or malicious acts. Compensatory damages are usually covered by insurance unless they exceed the limits of the insurance policy. In most jurisdictions, the judge usually has the authority to reduce awards that are unreasonably high given the facts of the case. Punitive damages are not covered by insurance.

A defendant has the right to appeal the jury verdict to a higher court. The higher court can let the verdict stand or reverse the verdict, sending it back through the system for yet another trial. Depending on the circumstances, the case could be appealed to the Supreme Court. These appeals can tie up damage awards for years, although the plaintiff may be able to collect interest on the jury award.

Many factors affect the amount ultimately awarded

to the resident. Since most long-term care facility residents do not earn a paycheck or support a young family, damages may be less than a comparable injury to a younger person. Most people are not aware that there is a provision in health insurance policies, as well as the Medicare and Medicaid rules, that requires you to repay the cost of your medical care if you are awarded damages in a lawsuit. This further reduces the award to the plaintiff. In 2005, the U.S. Supreme Court ruled that when a plaintiff's recovery constitutes income, the income includes the portion of the recovery paid to the plaintiff's attorney as a contingency fee. The Court rejected the taxpayer's argument that because the value of the plaintiff's claim is speculative when he signs the contingency fee agreement, the anticipatory assignment doctrine is not applicable.[19]

> "Evidence at trial showed that the owner of XYZ Healthcare Corporation, while operating Marybrook in a chronically understaffed condition, managed to amass a net worth for XYZ Healthcare of over $648 million, with revenues exceeding $1.7 billion. Following a two week trial, a jury awarded the estate $2.3 million in actual damages and $90 million in punitive damages. As a result of "tort reform," state law limits the amount of punitive damages to four times the amount of actual damages unless the damages are the product of intentional conduct. Because the jury didn't find that the defendant, Marybrook Nursing Home, acted with malice, the trial judge reduced the jury's verdict of $90 million punitive damages award to approximately $9.5 million."
>
> *(Auld v. Horizon Healthcare. (1999). PRNewswire. www.mrltc.com/. Accessed 12/10/99.)*

State laws and damage caps all affect the award amount. Of this, the attorney will probably receive 40%. Additional payments will be deducted from the award to pay the costs associated with expert witnesses, various filing fees, duplication of medical records, and the like. Most medical malpractice actions are brought on a contingency basis. *Contingency* is an action conditioned upon a certain event. When an attorney accepts a lawsuit on contingency, he or she is expected to pay these incidental costs. The attorney is not repaid for these costs, or for his or her own time, until the lawsuit is ultimately settled and damage awards are made. The cost of bringing a lawsuit to trial can easily be between $25,000 and $100,000. There is never a guarantee of the outcome or an award. Because of this, only the most egregious instances of malpractice causing serious injuries result in viable malpractice litigation. Claims of "frivolous lawsuits" overloading the courts are largely a hoax perpetrated by the insurance industry whose stock market investments did not bring adequate returns. It is not economically feasible for any plaintiff's attorney to accept and pursue anything other than the most meritorious claims.

See your CD-ROM for additional information on lawsuit warning signs, actions and precautions you can take, and nursing board investigations.

References

1. *How to contact nursing home owners about problems.* Atlanta Legal Aid Society. Online. *www.law.emory. edu/alas/fact2.htm.* Accessed 9/11/02.

2. Office of Inspector General and American Health Lawyers Association (Eds.). (2003). *Corporate responsibility and corporate compliance: A resource for health care boards of directors.* Rockville, MD. U.S. Department of Health and Human Services.

3. Marquez L. (2006). Nursing shortage: How it may affect you. Family awarded $2.7 million over alleged nursing neglect at Kansas hospital. ABC News. January 21, 2006. Online. *http://abcnews.go.com/ WNT/Health/story?id=1529546.* Accessed 01/30/06.

4. *The American heritage® dictionary of the english language,* Fourth Edition. Copyright © 2000 by Houghton Mifflin Company.

5. American Nurses Association. (2002). *Code for Nurses with Interpretive Statements.* Washington. American Nurses Publishing.

6. Morris, J.N., Murphy, K., Nonemaker, S. (2002). *Long-term care facility resident assessment instrument (RAI) user's manual.* Des Moines. Briggs Corp.

7. Nursing encompasses the prevention of illness, the alleviation of suffering, and the protection, promotion, and restoration of health in the care of individuals, families, groups, and communities. Nurses act to change those aspects of social structures that detract from health and well-being. *The Code for Nurses,* published by the American Nurses Association, is the standard by which ethical conduct is guided and evaluated by the profession. It provides a framework within which nurses can make ethical decisions and discharge their professional responsibilities to the public, to other members of the health team, and to the profession. *The Code for Nurses* is not open to negotiation in employment settings, nor is it permissible for individuals, groups of nurses, or interested parties to adapt or change the language of this code. *The Code for Nurses* encompasses all nursing activities and may supersede specific policies of institutions, of employers, or of practices. Therefore, the content of the *Code for Nurses with Interpretive Statements* is nonnegotiable (American Nurses' Association (Eds.). *Code for Nurses.* (2002). Washington, D.C. American Nurses' Publishing).

8. Morris, J.N., Murphy, K., Nonemaker, S. (1996). *Long-term care facility resident assessment instrument (RAI) user's manual.* Des Moines. Briggs Corp.

9. American Nurses' Association (eds.). *Scope and Standards of Gerontological Nursing Practice.* (1995). Washington, D.C. American Nurses' Publishing.

10. Modified from Laska, L. (Ed.). (2003). *Medical Malpractice Verdicts,* Settlements and Experts. Nashville, TN.

11. Marks DT. (1996). People at risk: Neglect in nursing homes. *Trial Magazine,* February 1996.

12. American Academy of Orthopedic Surgeons. Orthopaedic Knowledge Online. Online. *http://www5.aaos. org/oko/vb/online_pubs/professional_liability/glossary.cfm.* Accessed 12/29/05.

13. State v. Morea, 2 Ala. 275; People v. Moan, 65 Cal. 532, 4 Pac. 545; Commonwealth v. Fox, 7 Gray, 585; State v. Castello, 62 Iowa, 404,17 NW 605; People v. Ah Fat, 48 Cal. 61.

14. No. E2003-00068-COA-R9-CV Lynn Raiteri ex Rel. Mary Helen Cox V. NHC Healthcare/Knoxville, Inc., et al.

15. Case No. 2D04-2623. Fenton H. Germann, as Personal Representative of the Estate of Irene A. Germann, Appellant, v. Age Institute of Florida, Inc., Age Institute Holdings, Inc., Senior Health Management Llc, Extendicare Health Services, Inc., Extendicare, Inc., Partners Health Group-florida, LLC, Partners Health Group, LLC, Bart Wyatt, Daniel Davis, Richard G. Moss, and Frances Rich.

16. *91 U.S. 376, 375.*

17. Gifts S. (1984). *Law dictionary.* Page 368.

18. Wikipedia. (2005). Online. *http://en.wikipedia.org/ wiki/Civil_procedure.* Accessed 11/10/05.

19. *Commissioner v. Banks,* 125S.Ct. 826 (Jan. 24, 2005).

Standards of care

Florence Nightingale, the mother of modern nursing, believed nursing to be a special calling, and more than a century ago, advised nurses to make nursing *"less a matter of business and more of the noble calling that it is."*[1]

Standards of practice

A *profession* is an occupation or career, such as law, medicine, or engineering, that requires advanced educational preparation and specialized study. A *professional* is an individual who is engaged in certain careers, such as *lawyers, doctors,* and *nurses.* Professionals are educated and qualified, and often must pass a licensure exam, pay a fee, and be licensed to perform these duties. Most professions change regularly due to new research, technology, and other information. Continuing education is necessary to maintain the professionals' knowledge and learn new trends and standards of practice. In some states and professions, continuing education is mandatory to maintain licensure. However, it is usually necessary, even if it is optional in your state. *Professional behavior* involves assuming responsibility and conforming to the standards of the profession. A professional may be considered a skilled practitioner or expert.

Professional responsibility

Professional responsibility is assuming responsibility for your own actions, abiding by the law, knowing and applying current standards of practice, and keeping the residents' best interests primary. "Professional responsibility is a paradigm case of the moral responsibility that arises from the special knowledge that one possesses. It is mastery of a special body of advanced knowledge, particularly knowledge which bears directly on the well-being of others, that demarcates a profession. As custodians of special knowledge which bears on human well-being, professionals are constrained by special moral responsibilities; that is, moral requirements to apply their knowledge in ways that benefit the rest of the society."[2]

Adhering to *professional standards of practice or standards of care* protects the residents from injury. This protects both the professional and healthcare facility from liability. Because of ongoing changes and new information, this is an area in which your knowledge must constantly be updated. One important professional responsibility is to do what is necessary to maintain knowledge of professional standards of practice and proficiency in the necessary skills. For example, a resident who is a full code goes into cardiac arrest. None of the nurses on duty has a current CPR card. Should you start CPR or wait for EMS? Neither choice is a good one. Your employer is not responsible for keeping your CPR card current, although they likely will be sanctioned if you fail to fulfill your

Chapter four

professional responsibility in maintaining your certificate. CPR is a skill you need to meet the standards of care for the residents for whom you are responsible. A long-term care facility must provide services in compliance with accepted professional practices and standards. As part of the nurses' professional responsibility

- The nurse assumes responsibility and accountability for individual nursing judgment and actions.[3]

- The nurse promotes, advocates for, and strives to protect the health, safety, and rights of the residents.[4]

- The nurse exercises informed judgment and uses individual competence and qualifications as criteria in seeking consultation, accepting responsibilities, and delegating nursing activities to others. The nurse collaborates with members of the health professions to meet the health needs of the public.[5]

- The nurse is responsible and accountable for individual nursing practice and determines the appropriate delegation of tasks consistent with the nurse's obligation to provide optimum resident care.[6]

Adhering to professional standards

All professions have *standards* and practices for their members. The standard of care is the degree of care or competence that one is expected to exercise in a particular circumstance or role.[7] In the nursing profession, the American Nurses Association (ANA), professional organizations, and state licensure boards identify standards for nurses to follow. Failure to provide care that meets or exceeds these standards may cause resident harm and is cause for disciplinary action against the licensee. The old adage "Ignorance of the law is no

excuse" can be applied to professional standards. Ignorance of professional standards is no excuse, either. Nurses must become familiar with the standards for their area of practice. You do not have to join a professional organization to learn and apply the standards. You will be held accountable to the standards of professional organizations, such as the American Nurses Association (ANA), even if you are not a member.

The standard of care is what a reasonable, prudent professional would do based on his or her education, experience, institutional policies and procedures, standards set by their professional organization(s), textbooks, research, and professional literature. Remember that many individual standards apply to the care of each resident. The standard of care is not what the *best professional* would do, but rather what *any reasonable professional* would do in the same or similar circumstances. Technology and practices change rapidly, and professionals must remain current and keep up with these changes. Facilities must strive to keep their policies and procedures up to date. If the facility policies and procedures are outdated, research and evidence-based practices will supersede them if a lawsuit is filed. For example, in the early 1990s, government research indicated that nurses should not massage red areas to stimulate circulation.[8] Prior to this, massaging was an age-old method of pressure ulcer prevention. A nurse documents that he or she vigorously massaged a red area daily, according to facility policy. If the area subsequently ulcerates, the evidence-based government research and information supersede the outdated practice of massaging. The nurse and facility may be found liable for contributing to pressure ulcer development.

If a professional holds certifications and advanced education, he or she is held to the same standard as other professional individuals with like qualifications.

For example, if a registered nurse holds a certification in gerontologic nursing care, he or she is held to a higher standard than nurses without this certification.

The long-term care facility laws are quite clear regarding the applicable standards of care:

- §483.20(k)(3) The services provided or arranged by the facility must (I) Meet professional standards of quality and; §483.20(k)(3)(ii) Be provided by qualified persons in accordance with each resident's written plan of care.

- Interpretive Guidelines §483.20(k)(3)(i) "Professional standards of quality" means services that are provided according to accepted standards of clinical practice. Standards may apply to care provided by a particular clinical discipline or in a specific clinical situation or setting. Standards regarding quality care practices may be published by a professional organization, licensing board, accreditation body or other regulatory agency. Recommended practices to achieve desired resident outcomes may also be found in clinical literature.[9]

Protocols and routine practices

Some facilities have a set of protocols or standards used in the care of all residents. Because these are routine practices, they are usually not listed on the care plans. The care plans list only additions and exceptions to the usual routines. (How care plans are managed is a facility determination.) If your facility decides to implement protocols and standards for routine resident care, avoid writing the standards yourself. Involve appropriate staff, including residents and nursing assistants (and others) where appropriate, in the development and adoption of standards and protocols that affect overall resident care. Staff are much more likely to make this type of system successful if

they have ownership in protocol development.

An experienced medical/legal reviewer can easily identify the various components of the nursing process during a medical record review. Years ago, nurses neglected documentation when they were busy, focusing instead on resident care. "Put the patient ahead of the paper" was a common expression. Today, management must support nurses in finding a way to do both. *Documentation is part of the resident's care, and nurses no longer have the luxury of choosing between providing care and keeping records.*[10] Documentation validates that care was given. Sometimes, it proves that the facility was providing care it was paid to provide. It proves that standards of care were met. Documentation is an essential element of communication. Accurate and complete documentation is essential so others can determine what has been done. All healthcare practitioners rely on having accurate and thorough data on the medical record when they are completing their individual assessments and planning future clinical approaches to resident care.

Healthcare professionals have a broad knowledge of many subjects. We have additional, specific, specialized knowledge in our selected areas of expertise and practice. Nevertheless, knowing all we need to know about every subject is impossible. For the most part, our generalized knowledge sustains us, but sometimes the nurse must learn more about applicable, current standards in subjects outside the specialty area. At the very least, professionals must familiarize themselves with the actions, uses, side effects, indications, contraindications, and precautions for new drugs. Aside from that, you may be faced with situations in which you will need to research standards, even if you think you know them cold. Some of the simplest standards may be the most difficult to find, and you may need to be resourceful to find what you need. Published standards of practice come from many different sources. The Internet has become another important source. Thousands of standards can be accessed online, quickly and painlessly. Knowing and following the standards of practice for your profession and employment setting will ensure that residents receive quality care. Applying professional practice standards

- protects resident (and employee) safety

- achieves desirable resident (care) outcomes

- facilitates access to appropriate services and levels of healthcare

- identifies the scope of accountability for nursing care

- reduces nurse and facility liability and legal exposure

See your CD-ROM for more information on the ANA Code for Nurses with Interpretive Statements, an overview of gerontological nursing practice, and standards of gerontological nursing care.

Quality of care

The Director of Nursing (DON) in long-term care maintains a constant vigil to assure that the physical, mental, and social needs of the residents are met. The DON develops systems for appropriate staffing, appropriate medical supervision, and appropriate therapeutic attention.[11]

Each resident must receive, and the facility must provide, the necessary care and services to attain or maintain the highest practicable physical, mental, and psychosocial well-being, in accordance with the comprehensive assessment and plan of care. *Highest practicable* is defined as the highest level of functioning and well-being possible, limited only by the individual's presenting functional status and potential for

improvement or reduced rate of functional decline. Highest practicable is determined through the comprehensive interdisciplinary resident assessment, and by competently and thoroughly addressing the physical, mental, or psychosocial needs of the individual. The facility must ensure that the resident obtains optimal improvement or does not deteriorate within the limits of the right to refuse treatment, and within the limits of recognized pathology and the normal aging process.[12] When a resident shows signs of decline, surveyors will review the record to determine whether the decline is unavoidable. A physician statement that the decline is unavoidable will be considered, but is not accepted at face value without a detailed investigation of the situation. An accurate determination of unavoidable decline or failure to reach the highest practicable well-being may be made only if all of the following are present:

- An accurate and complete assessment

- An assessment-based care plan that has been consistently implemented

- The resident's response to care has been evaluated, and the care plan revised as necessary

Nursing process breakdown

The Director of Nursing (DON) in long-term care advocates for the assessment and evaluation of outcomes in the long-term care facility and develops implementation strategies for negative outcomes.[13]

The medical model of operations (care) is designed to promote staff efficiency and provide for the residents' medical needs. Under the medical model, mealtimes usually dictate daily schedules and routines. Care may be driven by the third-party payers. Residents are not always involved in making the decisions affecting their care. Many facilities are finding that for holistic care, wellness, and optimal quality of life, care must reflect an integration of various models of care, including the medical model, the holistic, resident-centered model, the participatory model, and the wellness model of care.

When the nursing process breaks down in long-term care, it is usually due to one or more of the following:

- lack of functional understanding of the nursing process itself

- lack of understanding of the OBRA regulations

- inability to differentiate between the medical model of care and holistic, resident-centered care

- feeling stressed, overwhelmed, and spread too thin

Nurses must deliver competent care as demonstrated by the nursing process, including assessment, diagnosis, outcome identification, planning, implementation, and evaluation. The nursing process encompasses all significant actions taken by nurses in providing care to all clients, and forms the foundation of clinical decision making.[14]

Frequently, the nursing process breaks down in the assessment stage. Occasionally, assessment is not done at all. More commonly, the resident is assessed, but personnel fail to act on the results of the assessment by calling the physician, providing continued reassessment, or taking whatever other actions are necessary. Sometimes assessment is not timely. The resident may have been deteriorating slowly for several days, but he or she is not assessed and physician notifications are not made until the situation is emergent or the resident unstable. Remember, once data have been collected, the nurse and facility are responsible for the information. Use the clinical assessment data and medical record information to take appropriate action

based on your appraisal and evaluation of that data. When you collect data, you are obligated to use it.

Care planning

When making clinical judgments, nurses must base their decisions on consideration of consequences, which prescribe and justify nursing actions. The recipients of professional nursing services are entitled to high-quality nursing care.[15] The gerontological nurse collects data through assessment, analyzes the data, plans nursing care, implements the Plan, and evaluates the effectiveness of the Plan of Care. The process is fluid and ongoing to ensure quality nursing care. The gerontological nurse systematically evaluates the quality of care and effectiveness of nursing practice. The gerontological nurse considers factors related to safety and effectiveness in planning and delivering client care.[16]

Another area in which nursing process breakdown commonly occurs is care planning. This is usually because many nurses have mental blocks against care plans stemming from bad experiences in nursing school. Some nurses subscribe to the myth that the care plan is a means of paper compliance only, and is not an essential document in the care of the residents. Additionally, there are many fallacies about how care plans are to be structured and the format for identifying problems and needs. In truth, the facility is required to develop a comprehensive care plan, but there are no requirements for a prescribed format. Many facilities use the medical model of care to construct their care plans. This seems somewhat incongruent in a homelike environment. It also results in the "problem-need" format. It does not identify or use resident strengths to overcome needs.

The care plan cannot be separated from the nursing process. Facilities that keep the care plan in front of staff, update it as often as necessary, and use the plan as a tool for directing all resident care activities seldom deliver bad or dysfunctional care. Successful managers really do make this happen, and it shows in the quality of care delivered by the entire health care team. The care plan is probably the single most important document on your chart. It is much more than paper compliance. In fact, keeping the care plan on the chart limits its utility and accessibility. Using a Kardex format is often much more useful.

The probes for §483.20(k)(1) (the care planning rules) ask the following questions. As you can see, these are all issues discussed in your book as being important in reducing the risk of legal exposure:

- Does the care plan address the needs, strengths and preferences identified in the comprehensive resident assessment?

- Is the care plan oriented toward preventing avoidable declines in functioning or functional levels? How does the care plan attempt to manage risk factors? Does the care plan build on resident strengths?

- Does the care plan reflect standards of current professional practice?

- Do treatment objectives have measurable outcomes?

- Corroborate information regarding the resident's goals and wishes for treatment in the plan of care by interviewing residents, especially those identified as refusing treatment.

- Determine whether the facility has provided adequate information to the resident so that the resident was able to make an informed choice regarding treatment.

- If the resident has refused treatment, does the care plan reflect the facility's efforts to find alternative means to address the problem?

Converting the system from one in which the care plan is considered paper compliance to one in which the care plan is a dynamic document requires considerable managerial time and effort. It also takes staff commitment. Without this commitment, the results may be abysmal. Staff resistance to change is a normal human phenomenon, but this document often evokes such strong feelings that some staff members may do all they can to actively resist change. Using the care plan is a worthwhile endeavor, and will make a difference in quality of care, quality of life, and reduced legal exposure.

To be viable, the care plan must be initiated on admission. All assessments will not be complete, but your preliminary plan should identify any obvious problems, risk factors, or conditions for which the resident was hospitalized. At this point, no one expects the plan to be perfect. It should be functional and should direct initial care until you know the resident better. Add to the plan as new information becomes available. The residents' conditions are not static. Changes in condition, problems, needs, strengths, and approaches must be added to the plan as often as necessary to ensure the plan is kept current. Like our residents, the plan evolves and changes. Care planning considerations include

- The services provided or arranged by the facility must meet professional standards of quality. There should be evidence of assessment and care planning sufficient to meet the needs of newly admitted residents, prior to completion of the first comprehensive assessment and comprehensive care plan.[17]

- Facilities are responsible for assessing areas that are relevant to residents regardless of whether these areas are included in the *Resident Assessment Instrument* (RAI; MDS). The RAI is the minimum assessment tool, not the only assessment tool.[18]

- The care plan is a dynamic document that needs to be continually evaluated and appropriately modified based on measurable outcomes. This continual evaluation takes into consideration resident change relative to the initial baseline—in other words, if the resident has declined, stayed the same, or improved at a lesser rate than expected, then a modification in the care plan may be necessary.[19]

- As the process of problem identification is integrated with sound clinical interventions, the care plan becomes each resident's unique path toward achieving or maintaining his or her highest practicable level of well-being.[20]

- When the care plan is implemented in accordance with the standards of good clinical practice, then the care plan becomes powerful and practical, and represents the best approach to providing for the quality-of-care and quality-of-life needs of an individual resident.[21]

Developing an initial plan and updating the care plan are particularly problematic for long-term care facilities, which (technically) have up to 21 days to develop a comprehensive plan of care. A lot can happen in the first 21 days. In fact, this period is when the resident's risk factors may be greatest, because they are unfamiliar to staff. The resident is not familiar with the facility. During the first 21 days, safety risks, weight loss, inadequate fluid intake, and risk of skin breakdown can be particularly problematic. Leaving the vulnerable resident without a plan for a pro-

longed period exposes him or her to serious hazards, and exposes the facility and its staff to the potential for liability. Having an interim plan that is imperfect (and not comprehensive) is certainly better than no plan at all. Using this plan is a key to successful care. Having a perfect piece of paper doesn't translate into excellent care, but you can make this happen. Use the plan for developing assignments and giving reports. Keep it in front of the staff. Update the plan promptly if the problems, goals, or approaches change, even if changes seem minor. Avoid discouraging unit staff from making changes to the plan. It is their plan for the resident's care. In some facilities, only the MDS nurse can change the plan. Facilities are encouraged to rethink this strategy. The MDS nurse most probably does not know of changes immediately after they occur, and is probably not on duty during the second and third shifts. Staff nurses and charge nurses are in a much better position to change and develop the plan.

After the MDS (Minimum Data Set) is done and the comprehensive long-term care plan is developed, the natural tendency is to bury the plan in the chart and not look at it until it is time for quarterly review. Although residents in this setting are more stable than those in acute care, the plan must be updated for changes in condition or it will be ineffective and inaccurate for directing care. Even stable residents are likely to require minor care plan changes during the three-month period between quarterly care plan reviews. Used correctly, the plan evolves throughout the individual's stay in the facility. Information should be added or removed as often as necessary. If a change involves a single department, that department may make the change and implement the plan. If a change involves two or more departments, you may wish to bring the plan into care conference for a quick review and update. For example, the nurse nicks the skin slightly when clipping a resident's fingernails. This information should be added to the plan by the nurse on duty, because care for the cut is given only by the nursing department. However, if the resident experiences an unplanned, undesirable weight loss, the nurse who identifies the loss should add the information to the plan of care. He or she should flag the plan for update at the next available care conference, because dietary, activities, and social services may also have responsibilities for managing the resident's weight loss. Whether you invite the resident and family to this update conference is a facility decision. Many facilities handle updates at the end of each regular care conference, with only staff members in attendance. Since updating the plan normally involves only minor changes, outside parties are usually not invited. However, they should be advised of the need for a change in the plan, and their suggestions (if any) included.

Additional care plan considerations

Although the MDS drives the long-term care facility comprehensive plan, consider all other assessments, as well as other contents of the medical record when developing the plan. List any potential risk factor, medication, treatment, or other order that modifies or increases a risk factor or requires special monitoring. For example, a nursing assessment or MDS may not identify problems related to medication interactions or side effects. A review of the physician's orders or medication record will identify potential problems in this area. Drugs such as anticoagulants interact with many other foods and drugs, and almost always increase the resident's risk of adverse outcomes. Because of this risk, the drugs and special monitoring should be listed on the care plan. Use your professional judgment to ensure this information is added to the plan. Avoid assuming that all other caregivers know what you know. They probably don't. Write it down!

Most nursing boards have rules that require nursing

diagnoses to be the basis of the care plan. Nursing assistants and other paraprofessional workers usually do not understand nursing diagnoses terminology. If you list nursing diagnoses on the care plans to comply with the requirements of the state nurse practice act, you may wish to write a simple problem in parentheses next to it. For example, if a resident has a nursing diagnosis such as "deficit fluid volume" or "risk for deficient fluid volume," you may wish to write "dehydration" or "risk for dehydration" or "inadequate fluid intake" next to it so all caregivers understand the problem.

Consider the care plan location. In many states, the long-term care rules require facilities to make the plans available to all direct care staff. Burying the plan in a medical record with hundreds of other documents makes it inaccessible, and staff will be less likely to sift through the charts each shift to review the care plans. In some facilities, nursing assistant staff are not permitted to read the charts. This is somewhat incongruous if the chart contains the only copy of the plans of care! Some facilities have had problems with care plans disappearing. Sadly, this is usually done in retaliation for perceived managerial injustices, because staff know that developing new care plans requires a great investment in management time and effort. Copying the care plans after care conference is a simple task. Store the copies in an office or secure medical records file. Although the copies are not updated when changes occur, they are a good starting point if you must rewrite an entire plan. For day-to-day unit operations, using a notebook or Kardex for care plans may be a more useful approach. Some facilities make copies of the care plan and store them in notebooks with flow sheets, according to team assignments. The original plans are maintained in the medical record. Consider the options that work best for your facility, but do all you can to ensure the plans are accessible to, and used by floor-level staff.

Care plan checklist

The care plan should be

- created upon admission, listing potential safety problems, high-risk conditions, and obvious medical and psychosocial problems

  – Use common sense when developing admission problems. If the resident fell at home, list him or her as being at risk for falls. If he or she has an indwelling catheter, list the potential for catheter infection. Formal written assessments are not needed to identify these potential admission risks. The problem can be removed later if it does not pertain to the resident's current needs.

- further developed and refined after the MDS and other admission assessments have been completed

- interdisciplinary

- individualized to the residents' unique problems, needs, and risk factors

- reflective of the residents' strengths

- reflective of the care being given

- updated as often as necessary to ensure the plan is current

- readily and freely available to direct caregiving staff

- used as the basis for making assignments and giving report to staff

- reviewed each shift with direct care personnel (problems, goals, approaches)

- implemented consistently by all staff (problems, goals, approaches)

- regularly evaluated (effectiveness of problems, goals, approaches)

- revised if approaches are ineffective, inappropriate, or no longer relevant, or if new problems develop

Documentation should reflect observations, care given and resident response, and evaluation of care listed in the plan. Consistent, individualized care is crucial to positive resident outcomes and safety. Documentation in one area of the medical record should be consistent with other areas of the record. Take care to ensure information is not contradictory. Make sure care is in keeping with the full plan. For example, physical therapy is working with a confused resident and determines he can safely ambulate independently for short distances, such as with a walker in his room. Nursing documentation should not state, "restrained in chair at all times for safety." This defeats the purpose of the therapy, and probably contradicts the therapists' professional judgment and physician orders. Additionally, you are being paid to provide therapy and supervise the resident's ambulation in his or her room. A managed care payer source may deny payment for the entire month because the care was not delivered as ordered, and according to the prescribed and approved plan of care.

The care plan keeps everyone apprised of the resident's strengths, problems, and needs. Your commitment to developing and using the plan is a key to success. Changing the system and making it care plan–driven takes time and effort. However, over the long term, it saves time and energy. Most important, it ensures resident safety, improves satisfaction, enhances the quality of care, and improves quality of life in your facility.

Chapter four

Quality of life

The Director of Nursing (DON) in long-term care continuously seeks out those indicators which will define quality of life in the long-term care facility and monitors or develops tools which will monitor those indicators. The DON seeks collaboration with other disciplines in the development and monitoring of such indicators.[22]

Along with the quality of medical care residents receive, the quality of each individual's life is an important way to measure the success of a facility's caregiving. *Quality of life* is the state of being that results from the reconciliation of one's abilities and resources with one's collection of perceptions and beliefs that define meaning and purpose for life. Remember personal indicators as well as medical ones when measuring quality of life. Ask residents and family members how they measure the quality of care, quality of life, and customer satisfaction.[23]

Making a distinction between quality of clinical care and quality of life is appropriate, because these aspects of facility care are monitored and assessed very differently. Quality of care is quantitative, whereas quality of life is qualitative. Measurement of clinical care tends to be a matter of objective observation and examination of the person and comparison of that person's data to an established clinical standard of practice. Quality of life, on the other hand, depends on the subjective view of each individual, a far more difficult thing to measure. Two residents could receive comparable clinical care, yet one resident views his quality of life as good, and the other rates his quality of life as poor. Projects such as participating in pet and music therapy, environmental and art enhancement, and multi-generational activities involving local elementary school children, are things that enhance the quality of many residents' lives. Interpersonal interventions that reduce learned helplessness and restore the residents' sense of autonomy and control also enhance quality of life. Residents who believe they are receiving good quality of care, and those who are satisfied with the quality of their lives, are not likely to complain to the state or file a lawsuit. In fact, they are apt to praise and defend the facility when questioned by surveyors.

Cultural change in long-term care

The Eden Alternative®, Pioneer®, and other culture-changing programs have been very successful because they view aging as a distinct stage of human development. The medical model of care reinforces the defeatist attitude that declines are not optional in aging and that we must learn to live with the deterioration. According to the medical model, the greatest problems facility residents face are disease, disability, and decline. Undoubtedly, many declines accompany the aging process, but the human spirit can and does continue to grow. The culture-change movement approaches care for all residents, including those with dementia, with the attitude that everyone has the capacity for continued personal growth if provided an environment that supports and nurtures that growth. Eden is based on the belief that the major problems of aging are loneliness, helplessness, and boredom, which cause a disintegration of the residents' spirit. Many of the principles are based on an ethical framework and broad thinking about social responsibility, ecology, and anthropology. They promote autonomy and control over the everyday matters in residents' lives, noting that some residents thrive when given small challenges, such as making food choices or tending a plant. Eden and other alternative movements promote the philosophy that the focus of long-term care should be on "care" rather than on the notions of "treatment" or "therapy" inherent in a medical model. Whether you agree or disagree with this philosophy, it is evident that many elderly individuals thrive in this type of environment, and the quality of their lives appears to be excellent. Borrowing successful ideas from the culture-change movement and implementing them in your facility may be very beneficial to the residents.

Determining whether life is worth living is a highly subjective and personal viewpoint, particularly when an individual is faced with physical or mental impairment and protracted dependency and institutionalization. The current long-term care laws are based on an activist vision that includes the reduction or elimination of restraints, therapeutic activities using music, art, pets, plants and intergenerational exchanges, architectural and design alterations that enhance safety and autonomy, an emphasis on rehabilitation and discharge, and other options. Assisted living has become a very popular option for higher functioning individuals. These things all promote the philosophy that life is worth living.

Many facilities do not have the means or desire to change their philosophy or culture of care. Suggestions for enhancing quality of life in the traditional long-term care facility are

- Providing choices, such as

  - When to get up

  - When does the resident want to eat and drink

  - What does he or she want to eat and drink

  - When does the resident want to bathe or shower

- Facility response to resident needs

  - Flexible staffing schedules

  - Cooperation among staff

  - Everyone pitches in; cross-training

  - Assigning a staff person to advocate for each resident's wants and needs

  - Providing support

- Additional suggestions

  - Teach staff about aging and increase their capacity to understand individual residents' perspectives

  - Promote and enable a normalization of social relationships

  - Recognize how aging affects things such as diet, identity, and relationships

  - Treat each resident as an individual; avoid stereotyping

  - Provide continuity of care through use of the care plan

  - Treat residents as your equals; work with them toward a common goal

The relationship between the nurse manager and paraprofessional caregivers is also believed to affect the quality of residents' lives. Residents do well in an environment in which the supervisor and paraprofessional have developed skill in

- Empathy

- Reliability

Resident quality of life is also enhanced when facility staff

- Nurture personal relationships with the residents

- Know residents' needs and assign fair workloads

- Mentor other staff

- Can delegate

- Can turn to the Administrator for advice

- Communicate well and share information

- Eliminate obstacles that prevent supervisors from doing their work

Residents with dementia

In years past, providing reality orientation (RO) was a very popular care plan intervention. Most facilities have "RO Boards" that are changed daily, and list information such as the day and date, season, weather, and holiday facts, when appropriate. Although the daily bulletin boards are helpful, formal reality orientation is often unsuccessful and may upset some residents. Staff must learn to relate to cognitively impaired residents' reality, instead of imposing their reality on the residents. For example, if the resident worries that the children need to be fed, reassure her that someone has taken care of that. Or ask the resident about what she likes to cook and how she prepares it. Doing this restores the state of mind she is seeking, reducing her anxiety. These are not lies. It is true that someone has tended to things the resident is worried about, although the issue is probably no longer relevant. Restoring the resident's state of mind is an excellent way of relieving agitation. Understanding our reality is not a realistic goal for most residents with dementia. Entering into their reality is a therapeutic measure that improves and enhances quality of life!

References

1. Nightingale F. (1859). *Notes on nursing.* London: Harrison and Sons, 1859, p. 74

2. Mann M. (2000). *Research ethics glossary.* University of Nebraska. Online. *www.unmc.edu/ethics/words.html.* Accessed 11/13/05.

3. American Nurses Association (Eds). (2002). *Code for Nurses with Interpretive Statements.* Washington, D.C. American Nurses Publishing.

4. American Nurses Association (Eds.). (2002). *Code for Nurses with Interpretive Statements.* Washington, D.C. American Nurses Publishing.

5. American Nurses Association (Eds.). (2002). *Code for Nurses with Interpretive Statements.* Washington, D.C. American Nurses Publishing.

6. American Nurses Association (Eds). (2002). *Code for Nurses with Interpretive Statements.* Washington, D.C. American Nurses Publishing.

7. *Merriam-Webster's dictionary of law* (1996). Merriam-Webster's, Incorporated.

8. U.S. Department of Health and Human Services (Eds). (1992). *Pressure Ulcers in Adults: Prediction and Prevention.* Rockville, MD. Agency for Health Care Policy and Research.

9. Centers for Medicare & Medicaid Services. (2004). *State Operations Manual.*

10. Richards, M. (2001). Documentation - a vital and essential element of the nursing process. *Survey Savvy.* Des Moines, Briggs Corporation.

11. National Association of Directors of Nursing Administration/Long Term Care (NADONA) (eds). (2000). *Standards of Practice* (4th edition). Cincinnati, OH. National Association of Directors of Nursing Administration/Long Term Care.

12. §483.25 *State Operations Manual* Revision 8 (2005).

13. National Association of Directors of Nursing Administration/Long Term Care (NADONA) (eds). (2000). *Standards of Practice* (4th edition). Cincinnati, OH.

National Association of Directors of Nursing Administration/Long Term Care.

14. American Nurses Association. (1998). *Standards of clinical nursing practice.* Washington, D.C. American Nurses Publishing.

15. American Nurses Association (eds.). *Code for Nurses.* (2002). Washington, D.C. American Nurses Publishing.

16. American Nurses Association (eds). (1995). *Scope and Standards of Gerontological Nursing Practice.* Washington, D.C. American Nurses Publishing.

17. *State Operations Manual.* Probes for §483.20(k)(3)(i).

18. Morris, J.N., Murphy, K., Nonemaker, S. (1996). *Long-term care facility resident assessment instrument (RAI) user's manual.* Des Moines. Briggs Corp.

19. Morris, J.N., Murphy, K., Nonemaker, S. (1996). *Long-term care facility resident assessment instrument (RAI) user's manual.* Des Moines. Briggs Corp.

20. Morris, J.N., Murphy, K., Nonemaker, S. (1996). *Long-term care facility resident assessment instrument (RAI) user's manual.* Des Moines. Briggs Corp.

21. Morris, J.N., Murphy, K., Nonemaker, S. (1996). *Long-term care facility resident assessment instrument (RAI) user's manual.* Des Moines. Briggs Corp.

22. National Association of Directors of Nursing Administration/Long Term Care (NADONA) (eds). (2000). *Standards of Practice* (4th edition). Cincinnati, OH. National Association of Directors of Nursing Administration/Long Term Care.

23. Wisconsin Department of Health and Family Services. (2000). *Care planning 2000 guideline.* Madison. Bureau of Quality Assurance and Wisconsin Board on Aging and Long-term Care. Online. *www.dhfs.wisconsin.gov/rl_DSL/Publications/care2000.pdf.* Accessed 3/15/04.

Common causes of survey deficiencies

> "If a patient is cold, if a patient is feverish, if he is sick after taking food, if he has a bedsore, it is generally the fault not of the disease, but of the nursing."[1]
>
> —Florence Nightingale, 1859

Government regulation

Long-term care facilities are highly regulated. Many agencies have regulatory authority over the long-term care industry. Government agencies with regulatory authority have the freedom to inspect the facility. Most agencies do this annually, but the survey frequency varies with the agency. Each agency has its own focus and set of rules to follow. For example, the Occupational Safety and Health Administration (OSHA) is the government agency charged with overseeing worker safety. The Centers for Medicare & Medicaid Services (CMS) is responsible for long-term care facility regulation and inspection.

Payment for care

Most long-term care facilities (approximately 93.1%) accept state/federal money as payment for providing care. *Medicaid* is the government agency that pays for the care of residents who meet certain low-income guidelines. Residents receiving Medicaid are expected to contribute to the payment by using their pension or social security (SSI) checks. They are permitted to keep a small amount, usually $30 to $50 a month to pay for incidental expenses. The remainder is paid to the facility.

Medicare is a federally funded program for elderly and disabled individuals. Medicare pays for certain services in the hospital, long-term care facility, and home healthcare setting. Residents must meet very specific criteria in order for Medicare to pay for their stay, and payment is time-limited. *Medicare Part A* pays room and board for residents with qualifying conditions who have spent at least three consecutive midnights in the hospital. Upon facility admission, the resident may remain on Medicare for up to 100 days if he or she needs a daily skilled service, intervention, or observation. The first 20 days are paid at 100% of the Medicare fee. From days 21 through 100, the resident must pay a substantial daily copayment. Medicaid covers this fee for eligible residents. The Medicare payment to facilities is substantially higher than payments from other sources. This is because it is an all-inclusive fee. The facility is expected to pay for the resident's medications, treatment supplies, therapy, and all other services with the Medicare fee. Because the Medicare rate is higher, the copayment for days 21 through 100 may also be higher than the facility's private-pay fee. This is because residents who pay privately pay separate bills for their medications and other services. While the resident is on Medicare, the fee remains all-inclusive. Each facility has a separate Medicare rate based on the cost reports and other expenditures. These are submitted to the government, and the fee to the facility is set. There is no universal Medicare payment rate or fee.

The Medicare program pays for 100 days per *spell of illness*. A spell of illness begins with the first day of care in the facility and ends when the resident is either discharged for 60 consecutive days, or does not require daily skilled care (according to the Medicare criteria) for 60 consecutive days. There is no limit to the number of spells of illness for each resident, and the resident does not have to use all 100 inpatient Medicare days before breaking one spell of illness and beginning a new spell of illness. This is a source of great confusion for both residents and facilities. *Medicare Part B* pays for certain supplies, ancillary services, diagnostic tests, and therapy. Part B is a voluntary program. Residents must agree to having a deduction from their social security check each month to pay for part B. There is an annual deductible. In addition, the resident has a 20% copayment for Part B services. Because Part B is voluntary, some residents do not pay for or have Part B coverage.

The Medicare Drug Program is called *Medicare Part D*. Each Medicare beneficiary is eligible for the drug plan. He or she selects a payment plan to use. The various plans pay for a substantial part, but not all, of the medications. There is an annual deductible, and the resident is expected to pay a copayment or a fixed amount for each prescription. The benefits vary, depending on the plan each individual selects. For most plans, the beneficiary will pay 100% of the drug costs after the total spent on prescriptions reaches $2,250 a year. After the beneficiary spends an additional $3,600 out of pocket in medication expenses (for the year), the plan picks up again.

Although the drug program is available to all beneficiaries, there is an additional charge for it, depending on the benefits of the plan the beneficiary selects. There is also an enrollment period. If the resident does not enroll during the specified time frame, he or she will pay a penalty for enrolling late. If the resident does not enroll by a specified date, he or she cannot participate in the plan until the next open enrollment period. In some circumstances, a third party has designated the Medicare drug plan for the resident. This has become problematic because the resident's routine drugs may not be on the plan formulary, or a local pharmacy may not accept the elected plan, so there is no one available to fill the prescriptions. Selecting a plan from the many available is very confusing and can be overwhelming to the resident. The long-term care facility may not select the drug plan on behalf of the resident. However, the pharmacy/long-term care facility may go to the Medicare site online and enter the resident's routine drug regimen. The computer will provide an analysis of how each plan will (or will not) meet the resident's needs. Based on this information, the resident or responsible party can select the plan to use. Entering the data into the computer is considered an "objective assessment" that is "based on the individual's needs." At the time of this writing, CMS is permitting facilities and pharmacies to assist the residents in this manner. Since Medicare Part D is a new program, you can expect it to change periodically during the first few years until the bugs are worked out.

Medicare and Medicaid do not pay for incidental expenses, such as telephone, cable television, beauty shop, clothing, or other special items. These are the residents' responsibility. There are limitations on some Part B benefits for recipients residing in long-term care facilities.

For example, Part B will cover 80% of the cost of a wheelchair for an eligible individual living at home. There is no wheelchair payment benefit available for long-term care facility residents. In most states, Medicaid will not cover these costs, either. The long-term care facility is expected to absorb certain costs, including the cost of wheelchairs for Medicaid and Medicare recipients.

Many states have passed laws enabling them to recover Medicaid money spent for long-term care upon the resident's death. For example, if the resident owns a house that is sold after death, the state will put a lien on the property to recover the cumulative cost of the resident's medical care. State laws vary, but when a resident is a Medicaid recipient, the Medicaid state agency will review and consider the transfer or sale of all real property during the two-to-five-year period immediately before the resident's admission to the facility. If they attach a lien, it is usually to a valuable item. The liens often cover any property that was transferred into the name of another person (such as an adult child) within a designated time frame prior to the resident's admission into the facility. (If the resident dies leaving a surviving spouse, he or she will also be entitled to a portion of the proceeds from the sale of a house and other property.)

If the resident receives a judgment or jury award as a result of a lawsuit related to his or her medical condition, the resident is expected to repay Medicare and Medicaid (and also most private insurers) out of the proceeds of the damage award. Many individuals are not aware of the repayment provisions of the law.

State and federal regulations

State laws vary regarding facility designations, classifications, and licensure. Different types of facilities meet different levels of quality inspection standards.

Each long-term care facility holds a state license, which permits it to conduct business. Facilities possessing a license must follow the state long-term care licensing rules. Some facilities also possess a certification. *Certification* is necessary to collect money from the Medicare and Medicaid programs. Certified facilities must follow both the state licensure rules and federal certification rules.

The OBRA rules

OBRA is an abbreviation for the *Omnibus Budget Reconciliation Act*. There is an OBRA legislation of some sort written annually. The OBRA Legislation of 1987 was written to provide sweeping reforms in the long-term care industry. The OBRA long-term care rules have been modified and updated, but remain in place to this day. OBRA was designed to improve the quality of life, quality of care, health, and safety for residents in long-term care facilities. Residents' rights are emphasized. Facilities must provide a homelike environment, and are expected to maintain or improve the quality of the residents' lives. Physical and mental declines are not permitted unless they are medically unavoidable.

Common problems, such as contractures, pressure ulcers, and incontinence are considered declines under the OBRA laws. Generally speaking, the state and federal long-term care rules represent the minimum required standards of long-term care facility care. (Facility nurses must also follow the state nurse practice act and rules of the state board of nursing.)

OSCAR

The Online Survey Certification and Reporting System (OSCAR) has been online since October 1991. CMS uses OSCAR to monitor state survey agency and provider performance. OSCAR contains data for the current and three previous surveys. Deficiency data is tracked historically. CMS also tracks the scope and severity of deficiencies. Part of the information in the OSCAR database is self-reported by facilities and provides information about the facility and its residents. The remaining information is generated by surveyors based on deficiencies. The federal regulations detailing survey requirements are classified into 17 major categories. The specific survey requirements within these categories were consolidated from 325 individual items to 185 items effective on July 1, 1995.

Understanding the inspection (survey) process

Periodic surveys are done by representatives of your state health department or human service agency to ensure care is acceptable, and the facility is meeting the standard of care in compliance with the long-term care rules. Survey teams are interdisciplinary, and typically have four to seven members, such as nurses, dietitians, social workers, pharmacists, and sanitarians. A typical certification inspection takes three to four days. If the facility is licensed and certified, the state surveyors will inspect using both sets of rules (state and federal).

In addition to the regular survey process there are "special" and "extended" surveys. Special surveys may be conducted within two months of any change in ownership, administration, management, or director of nursing to determine if the change is having an effect on the quality of care in the facility. Extended surveys are performed immediately or within two weeks after the standard survey completion on those facilities found to have provided substandard quality of care. The survey team reviews the policies and procedures that produced the substandard care, expands the size of the sample of resident's assessments, reviews staffing, in-service training, and if necessary, contracts with consultants.

Sometimes CMS conducts the facility survey. However, it is more common for them to entrust the state surveyors to conduct the survey, by following the federal rules. If federal surveyors visit, the survey is based only on federal long-term care rules. They do not survey for compliance with state rules. CMS personnel validate the survey results of 5% of the facilities in each state. This means they will arrive unannounced and do another complete survey using only the federal rules. The reinspections are done within two months of the state survey. CMS is also piloting a project in which they jointly inspect the facility with the state team. When these surveys are done, the survey involves two concurrent, independent surveys. One team is checking for compliance with state regulations, while the other is monitoring federal compliance.

Federal validation surveys can be very stressful, and it is not unusual for the outcomes to vary greatly from the state survey teams' findings. One outcomes study revealed that CMS surveyors identified problems in about 20% of the facilities that state surveyors had deemed deficiency-free. In almost 19% of a sample of nursing facilities considered free of deficiencies after state surveys, federal surveyors wrote serious deficiencies, such as failing to prevent pressure ulcers, failing to adequately monitor pressure ulcers, and failing to notify physicians and obtain treatment orders. The outcomes studies also identified a pattern of understatement of problems that should have been classified as actual harm or higher. Federal inspectors found actual harm or higher-level deficiencies in 22% of homes in which state surveyors hadn't found such deficiencies.[2] State survey agencies are required to refer facilities with a pattern of harming residents to CMS for immediate sanctions. Many states did not fully comply with the requirement. In fact, states failed to refer hundreds of nursing facilities for immediate sanction, according to one study.[3] Because of this, CMS takes the responsibility for conducting validation surveys very seriously. Anecdotal reports say that each year, a formula is used to identify facilities for survey validation. For example, the 5% sample will be selected from a combination of homes that are deficiency free, homes that have many deficiencies, homes that are very large or very small, and those that offer highly specialized services, such as ventilator care or pediatric care.

Other types of surveys

Some long-term care facilities are also accredited. *Accreditation* is a voluntary process that healthcare facilities undergo to ensure they are meeting high quality standards. Gaining accreditation is difficult, but is very prestigious. Representatives of the accreditation agency will also survey the facility. In the past, these reviews have been scheduled and known in advance. The accrediting agencies are now conducting unannounced surveys. At one time, facilities had hoped that, by achieving accreditation, they might receive "deemed" status. This is a process used for acute care hospitals in which accredited facilities do not have to undergo annual state or federal surveys. By meeting the requirements for accreditation, they have satisfied the state that the facility meets or exceeds the conditions for participation. However, CMS refused to grant long-term care facilities deemed status, and, therefore, a survey waiver. Accredited facilities undergo an annual survey just as all other facilities do. Despite the lack of this waiver, however, accreditation continues to be a prestigious, worthwhile endeavor and helps ensure that residents will receive quality care.

Other governmental agencies, such as OSHA, may also survey the facility. Long-term care facilities overall have a high incidence of employee injuries. OSHA has specific requirements for posting the injury rate

and notifying the agency of employee injuries. OSHA selects facilities with a high incidence of injuries, as well as businesses in which risk of employee injury is high, and randomly surveys them. (Long-term care facilities are known to have a high risk for employee back injuries, so usually are included in the targeted survey group each year.)

Surveyors in some states also visit the facility periodically to evaluate the quality of care that Medicaid recipients receive. This type of survey is commonly called *inspection of care* (IOC). The IOC survey verifies that residents are receiving the services for which Medicaid is paying. If the facility has other special agency contracts, those groups will inspect as well. For example, if they have a contract to accept Veterans' Administration (VA) residents, The VA will also conduct periodic inspections.

Type, frequency, and duration of long-term care facility surveys

Long-term care facilities routinely have a licensure (or combined licensure and certification, if applicable) survey every nine to 15 months. This visit can occur at any time of the day or night, or on a weekend. In addition to annual licensure and certification inspections, surveyors respond to and investigate complaints filed by residents, family members, facility employees, and interested others, such as the facility ombudsman. Occasionally, a hospital will phone in a complaint based on a resident's condition upon his or her arrival at the hospital. Because of the many different types of surveys in long-term care, most facilities have two or more surveys a year. State surveyors come to the long-term care facility unannounced and spend several days to a week. The length of time spent in the facility is determined by facility size, whether complaints are also being investigated, and the nature of the problems identified during the first few days of the visit.

If the facility is very large or if the nature of potential deficiencies is severe, the surveyors will remain in the facility for a longer period of time.

An extended survey is done when surveyors remain in the facility longer than originally anticipated to investigate conditions. This is potentially very serious. In an extended survey, surveyors examine facility practices and conditions in great detail to determine whether a danger to residents exists.

By virtue of having an extended survey, the facility is banned from conducting nurse aide classes for two years, even if the eventual outcome of the extended survey is not negative. This creates quite a hardship in some facilities and communities. Fines, or civil monetary penalties, may be imposed up to $10,000 per day until the surveyors revisit and determine that deficiencies have been corrected.

Surveyors will return a month or two after the annual survey to see whether deficiencies have been corrected. They also make unannounced visits in response to complaint calls from residents and families. Long-term care facilities are required to post a state "hotline" or complaint line number in a visible location so residents and family members can call if they are dissatisfied with care.

Survey preparation

Preparing for a long-term care facility survey is virtually impossible. Surveys are irregular and unannounced. Laws provide for severe penalties or jail terms for individuals who alert the facility of an impending licensure, certification, or other type of survey. The element of surprise is crucial to the process. Surveyors want to see resident care and facility routines on a normal day. *Knowing this, facilities must strive to be survey-ready every day.* This means that staff deliver care that meets the minimum acceptable standards.

Documentation must be accurate and reflect the care given and resident response. Correcting ongoing or longstanding documentation problems is impossible during a survey.

Survey team preparation

Surveyors research, review, and thoroughly familiarize team members with the facility history prior to the survey. Thus, they know a great deal about the facility and its residents before they arrive. Much of their information is derived from MDS data, which facilities are required to submit electronically. Surveyors also review deficiencies written during past surveys, and will check closely to ensure they remain corrected. They study the OSCAR database. Repeat deficiencies may be considered more serious than new deficiencies. Fines may be higher for repeat deficiencies. However, each deficiency is also rated for scope and severity, including actual injury or potential injury to the residents. The matrix for determining scope and severity of deficiencies is featured on your CD-ROM.

During the survey, surveyors review cumulative issues that develop over a period of time, such as contractures, pressure ulcers, weight loss, and resident falls and injuries. Being survey-ready and meeting the standard of care every day will help prevent cumulative problems.

The entrance conference

There will be little preparation time from the moment surveyors arrive until they make rounds on the nursing units. One surveyor usually conducts an entrance conference with facility administration. The purpose of this meeting is to advise management of the reason(s) for the survey, and nature of any complaints they will be investigating. The identity of individuals who register complaints will be concealed. While one surveyor conducts the entrance conference, others may go directly to the nursing units to make rounds and observe care. Doing this prevents staff from correcting problems before the survey begins, which is another reason why you must be survey-ready every day. The review of cumulative outcomes is a central issue to the survey, but it is not the only issue reviewed. Facility conditions and atmosphere during the first four hours of the survey often set the tone for the remainder of the survey.

The initial facility tour

During the first round (initial tour) of the facility, surveyors will make observations of residents and facility conditions. Surveyors often split up and make rounds simultaneously on separate nursing units. They will write down information, then return later to examine certain residents and conditions in greater detail. The first round has a major impact on the survey. If conditions are not acceptable, strong odors are present, or surveyors suspect serious problems, they may immediately change to extended survey mode.

Notifications, interviews, and the survey process

Surveyors will post a sign at the entrance to the facility informing all who enter that a survey is in process. Any resident, family member, or worker may speak with the surveyors at any time, and they are usually very good about accommodating requests for private meetings. Surveyors will also interview alert residents. They will conduct a resident council meeting so they can question residents in detail about facility conditions. Staff are not invited to attend this meeting. Surveyors will also question staff, residents, and families whom they encounter on the units. They often select nursing assistants and staff nurses to respond to their questions. The nature of the questions will vary, from questions such as "If there were a fire in the hallway right now, what would

you do?" to questions about individual residents' problems and needs. They are trying to determine whether staff have been prepared to do the job. They often avoid questioning managers and department heads, believing they have been trained to respond to surveyor questions. They will carefully review residents' medical records and plans of care. They may question staff about their familiarity with each resident's care plan goals, and inquire how the staff member provides care to meet the goals. They will monitor one or more medication passes. Expect surveyors to watch licensed nurses and nursing assistants while doing treatments, wound care, range-of-motion exercises, and other aspects of care. The surveyors will evaluate and verify the level (intensity) and quality of care provided to the residents. They will evaluate how well staff communicate with residents by explaining procedures and maintaining an ongoing dialogue while they are in the residents' rooms. They will monitor staff members' approaches to residents, such as knocking before entering the room, to ensure resident rights are respected. Surveyors look for positive outcomes of resident care. They observe residents to see whether the facility is providing services to maintain and improve residents' conditions and prevent declines whenever possible.

Meal service and food preparation will be closely monitored. The survey team will split into groups and observe one or more meals. They will review menus, dietary department storage procedures, cleanliness, and sanitation, and watch food preparation and delivery in different areas of the building. Serving food at the proper temperature is important to reduce the potential for food-borne infection. Food is more palatable and is accepted better when served at the proper temperature. (Temperature requirements vary according to state law. Cold foods must be below 40° F and hot foods above 140° F in most states.) Surveyors will also check for the need and provision of adaptive feeding devices, and watch staff to ensure they are providing adequate mealtime assistance. They will observe staff feeding residents and evaluate their techniques for maintaining resident dignity, and providing safety and infection control measures. They will evaluate how well staff verbalize and interact with residents during the meal. Surveyors will also evaluate pre- and post-meal grooming and hygiene, sanitary food service practices, and how facility staff manage mealtime problems, such as caring for residents who are incontinent during meals and those who request to be toileted during or immediately after the meal.

Surveyors will evaluate use of catheters and restraints. They will evaluate the facility's overall pressure ulcer program. They will closely evaluate prevention, development, treatment, and documentation of pressure ulcers for each resident. They will check care plans to ensure they reflect preventive care for high-risk problems and conditions. They will evaluate resident hygiene and grooming, and management of incontinence. Surveyors will monitor the overall environment for safety, control of odors, infection control practices, and general facility cleanliness. One or more surveyors will examine incident reports, review falls and injuries, and evaluate how well staff protect resident rights. They will evaluate quality of life to ensure that staff are meeting residents' physical and psychological needs and that residents are overall satisfied with the care they receive.

As you can see, a survey is an exhaustive process that is usually very stressful for staff. Viewing the survey as a routine daily event will help relieve your stress. Think about it. Someone is evaluating your performance every day of the year. Residents, families, physicians, supervisors, administrators, and other staff all watch and review your performance. Their evaluations are often more important than those of the state surveyors, because they affect your continuing employment, performance evaluations, and salary. Residents and family members make decisions regarding whether residents will remain in the facility or move elsewhere. Facility management determines who will work at the facility. In any event, keep survey stress in perspective and remember that you are being evaluated every day.

Survey completion

A *deficiency* is a written notice of inadequate care or substandard practices. Resident rights violations and infection control problems are major causes of deficiencies in surveys. However, surveyors review every area of the facility. They will stay as long as necessary to thoroughly observe resident care, staff preparation and education, ongoing inservice training, record keeping, infection control, food preparation, safety, and facility cleanliness. They also review facility policies and procedures, and determine whether staff are complying with them.

Surveys identify specific areas in which care is deficient or outcomes are negative. *Surveyors are instructed not to be consultants to the facility.* They are responsible only for identifying deficiencies. The facility is responsible for hiring its own consultants and finding ways of correcting the problems. Surveyors follow a prescribed format during most surveys. Procedures may vary slightly depending on the circumstances of the survey, but you can expect surveyors to do basically the same things each time they visit the facility.

Exit conference

Upon conclusion of the survey, surveyors conduct an *exit conference.* During this meeting, surveyors will advise the administrator of their findings and the nature of any deficiencies. The administrator will specify who attends the exit conference. Commonly, the director of nursing and other department heads are invited to attend.

The exit conference is sort of like a verbal report of the surveyors' findings. Some surveyors may provide a preliminary written report. The surveyors will return to their office, have a conference, and submit their findings and validation (proof) of the findings to their supervisors. The supervisors ultimately make the decisions regarding whether proposed deficiencies will stand. Surveyors may write two types of deficiencies. *Resident-centered deficiencies* are violations of minimum standards of care for each resident, such as failure to prevent pressure ulcers or contractures, failure to protect dignity, or failure to adequately assess the residents. *Facility-centered deficiencies* are systemic problems, such as lack of an adequate infection control program, odor problems, an unclean environment, or inadequate staffing.

If you receive deficiencies

- Notify your attorney or corporate office of survey findings.

- Begin your plan of correction (Chapter 6) immediately after surveyors exit.

- Document all corrections and activities undertaken and by whom.

- Begin inservices and competency verifications, as needed.

- Collect monitoring data to prove staff are doing things correctly.

- Collect monitoring data to prove staff competence.

- Collect needed information from physicians and others.

- Sort and organize correction data in a clear,

understandable manner to prove your activities and compliance data.

Final survey report

The final survey report is a collaborative effort that results from a meeting of the survey team and their supervisory personnel. They will discuss the prospective deficiency list, give examples, and agree on scope and severity designations. If supervisory personnel do not attend this meeting, they will review this report or the report will be sent to state regional supervisors or a centrally located enforcement committee. Changes can be made at any time during the review process by adding, deleting, or substantially changing the deficiencies. Deficiencies identified by surveyors are seldom removed from the final data, although they may be modified. The most common reason for changing or removing a deficiency is a failure to meet the specified documentation requirements. Surveyors have rigid principles for documentation so that the deficiency can be supported on appeal. Each state has a process for notifying facilities when deficiencies are finalized and cited, and they are sent a copy of the survey report (2567). **A description of each category of deficiencies is on your CD-ROM.**

Penalties

The facility must correct immediate jeopardy deficiencies within two days of receiving notice, or penalties will take effect. Deficiencies with no immediate jeopardy may have a 15-day correction window before penalties begin. If deficiencies are considered severe in nature, if actual harm has occurred to one or more residents, or the potential for serious harm to residents exists, the survey agency will take further action against the facility license, certification, or accreditation. They may issue a probationary license or even revoke approval. Fines as high as $10,000 per day may be imposed. The facility may lose approval to conduct nursing assistant classes. Facility payment for Medicare and Medicaid recipients may be withheld. If conditions are extremely poor, or if the safety or welfare of the residents is jeopardized, they may require and designate an independent overseer to manage the facility. In extreme situations, the monitor will be required to remain in the facility for a prolonged period of time, until surveyors are satisfied that corrections have been made and will be maintained, and overall conditions have improved.

Unfavorable surveys have caused some facilities to close. At the very least, they create a financial hardship, and increase stress on staff. The newspapers are often merciless in criticisms of facilities following surveys, and the negative publicity creates another set of image and public relations problems. *CMS is required to notify the nearest daily newspaper and all local physicians of their findings when they determine an immediate jeopardy situation exists.* Following the appropriate standards of care and documentation every day will help ensure positive survey outcomes. In the long run, doing things correctly is much easier than trying to clean up the after-effects and negative outcomes.

Common causes of survey deficiencies

The most recent statistics about nursing facility deficiencies are from the year 2004.[4] The five categories with the highest number of deficiencies were given for failure to

- ensure sanitary food (31.5 percent)

- ensure quality of care (26.2 percent)

- remove accident hazards in the environment (19.9 percent)

- meet professional standards of quality (22.1 percent)

- prevent accidents (19.2 percent)

Failure to prevent pressure ulcers and failure to prepare comprehensive care plans are intermittently on and off the top five list. Knowing and adhering to the regulations are the best means of reducing legal exposure. Since there is a strong correlation between factors that instigate lawsuits and survey deficiencies, facilities should always have a goal for maintaining regulatory compliance. Aside from reducing legal exposure, if a lawsuit does go to trial, chances are good that facility surveys will be produced into evidence. Depending on the results, they can help or hurt the facility.

Approximately 75% of the repeated violations of federal standards from 1999 to 2003 were at long-term care facilities in 12 states. They are Arkansas, Illinois, Indiana, Kansas, Mississippi, Missouri, New Jersey, North Carolina, Oklahoma, Tennessee, Texas, and Washington. These violations include failure to protect residents from mistreatment, hiring staff without conducting criminal background checks, and allowing residents to be abused, neglected, and physically punished. In some of these facilities, problems were isolated. However, in others poor conditions were widespread.

Common causes of lawsuits

Family members initiate most lawsuits against long-term care facilities. They commonly do this because of festering guilt and anger, not greed.[5] Among the most common reasons for litigation are problems that are largely preventable, such as

- pressure ulcers

- contractures (usually in combination with pressure ulcers)

- falls and fractures or other injuries, such as subdural hematoma

- inappropriate restraints (which cause agitation,

injury, and other complications such as incontinence, pressure ulcers, contractures, loss of will to live, and death)

- failure to follow physicians' orders

- failure to notify the physician of a change in condition in a timely manner

- failure to provide proper monitoring and care for an acute illness or other medical condition

- failure to monitor diabetes accurately

- medication errors

- inadequate medication monitoring, resulting in serious complications

- wandering resident inadequately monitored and elopes from facility and is killed or seriously injured

- improper use of equipment, resulting in resident injury

- failure to sufficiently monitor resident/failure to sufficiently monitor staff

- infections (pressure ulcer and intravenous infections are common)

- sepsis and septic shock

- dehydration

- weight loss

- malnutrition

- the conditions listed here are often seen in combination

Peripheral issues are also commonly identified during the course of a lawsuit, such as

- failure to accurately assess the resident

- failure to order diagnostic tests ordered by physician; and/or failure to report abnormal

results of diagnostic tests to the physician in a timely manner

- incomplete, altered, or missing documentation

- inadequate staffing

- staff unqualified or not properly trained

- staff not adequately supervised

- poor hiring and screening practices, including

  - failure to perform reference checks

  - hiring employees with criminal histories

  - failure to screen employees for drug or alcohol use

- inappropriate delegation

- abuse/neglect, other resident rights violations

- pattern of negligent or intentional acts causing injury or the death

- inadequate or ineffective equipment and supplies

- insufficient budgeting or inadequate resources to provide care for the residents.

- causing pain, mental anguish, and reduced quality of life

Occasionally, criminal charges are filed as a result of the lawsuit.[6]

Public sentiment

In some areas of the country, aggressive attorneys have advertised extensively seeking long-term care facility cases. This is especially true in communities in which there is much public sentiment against nursing homes, or when a purported case of nursing home abuse or neglect has recently received extensive news coverage. In an advertising blitz such as this, both for-profit and nonprofit nursing homes are targeted. Facilities owned by large corporations may be especially vulnerable, because they appear to have "deep pockets" for large punitive awards. In most states, survivors of a resident can file a claim if the statute of limitations has not expired. Even a legal guardian who is unrelated to the resident can initiate litigation on behalf of the resident and receive reimbursement.[7]

Admissibility of survey reports as evidence in a lawsuit

The subject of the admissibility of surveys has been an argument upon which several appeals are based. Facilities have argued fiercely that the results of state surveys should not be admitted. One of these went all the way to the Texas Supreme Court, which ruled that the survey was admissible. The facility challenged a verdict on several grounds, including the admissibility of state nursing facility certification and complaint investigation surveys. (The facility also argued that a cap on civil liability verdicts applies equally to compensatory damages and punitive damages, which would have reduced the judgment against them substantially.)

This lawsuit was filed due to allegations of substandard care resulting in multiple (17) severe pressure ulcers and flexion contractures. The plaintiff also alleged malnutrition and dehydration. The surveys were introduced by the defense to support the testimony by three of their witnesses. These individuals stated that the facility had not given improper care to this resident. They contended that, if they had given poor care, the state would have cited them on the resident's behalf during a survey. The surveys were admitted to validate their testimony. The facility had not been cited in the care of this resident. If the trial court had not allowed the survey reports into evidence after defense witnesses testified in this manner, the jury would be left with the false impression that the facility was deficiency free. In fact, they had been cited for

rendering improper care, but this resident was not listed in the survey sample group. The plaintiff was simply not targeted for review during these surveys.

The defendant presented several arguments to support the appeal. They contended that the survey reports were inadmissible because the surveyors who wrote the deficiencies were not present for cross examination. They also stated the surveys were inadmissible because they were not relevant to the standard of care. Even if they were relevant, any relevance was substantially outweighed by the prejudicial impact of the reports. The Supreme Court of Texas found for the plaintiff on two counts: a) that the defense did not request a limiting instruction at the time the trial court admitted the reports; and b) that the defendant opened the door for admission of the survey reports into evidence, although they were admitted in support of another issue.

At the time the surveys were admitted, the defendant waived any complaint concerning their admission. When evidence is admissible for one party or for one purpose, but *not admissible* to another party or for another purpose, the court (upon request) restricts the evidence to its proper scope and instructs the jury accordingly. If a limiting request is not made, the court's action in admitting the evidence without limitation is not grounds for complaint on appeal. Thus, if the survey reports were admissible by any party or for any purpose, the court of appeals did not err in affirming the trial court's admission of the reports. The court affirmed the surveys *were admissible by any party or for any purpose*. They further noted that when considering the entire record except for the survey reports, both sides presented evidence regarding how the nursing home treated the plaintiff. Therefore, the survey reports by themselves probably did not cause the rendition of an improper judgment.[8]

The defendant in this case had good reason to try to keep the surveys out of the courtroom. Many deficiencies had been written addressing quality-of-care issues. Keeping unfavorable surveys out of the courtroom provides yet another reason that facilities should be survey-ready every day.

Dietary and food deficiencies

Food is more than "just something to eat." We eat for pleasure and enjoyment. Food also represents love, security, and comfort. It has both positive (happy times, holidays, parties and social events, family gatherings, hospitality) and negative (foods we dislike or were forced to eat as children, restrictive diets, emotions about food preparation, such as pureed food being for babies, not adults) associations. Religion, ethnicity, and culture also affect eating habits. Common expressions such as "My eyes were bigger than my stomach" or "We eat with our eyes" tell us that the aroma and appearance of food are also important and affect appetite and food acceptance.

The body's sensory response affects the resident's ability to eat, as well as the ability to derive pleasure from eating. The brain's sensory response to food is complex. In addition to smell and taste, the brain correlates and interprets sensory signals for sight, temperature and texture. Aging often causes changes in the senses of smell and taste. Smell is diminished, and taste buds are lost, beginning with sweet and salt. Bitter and sour taste buds are not affected. Residents may compensate for the loss of taste buds by adding sugar and salt to food. By age 70, about one-third to one-half the taste buds are lost. Taste may also be affected by certain medications, smoking, and wearing dentures. Keep the importance of the residents' sensory response in mind when evaluating meal service.

Residents who complain about food often complain about other conditions as well. Facilities that have switched to buffet meals and family-style dining often have fewer complaints about food. Buffet lines and other non-traditional methods of serving meals have been well-received by facility residents. However, this type of food service is much more expensive than traditional meal service. The increased cost often pays dividends in improved resident satisfaction, improved quality of life, improved community image, and positive public relations. Another consideration is to ensure the menus are properly rotated. A short rotation, such as every three weeks is probably not appropriate in this setting. A three-month rotation may be more acceptable to the residents. The food should also be culturally appropriate. For example, some large chains have dietitians throughout the country. The dietitians in the southern states may plan to have grits for breakfast, and red beans and rice for dinner on a regular basis. These items are staples of the southern diet. Residents in northern states may reject these food items.

Consider soliciting suggestions from residents and staff to make meals as pleasant as possible. Explore what other facilities are doing to enhance resident satisfaction with meals, and determine whether any of their ideas will work in your facility. Some facilities routinely use liberalized diets instead of therapeutic diets. For example, they routinely serve a no-added-salt (NAS) rather than 2-gram-sodium diet, or no concentrated sweets (NCS) instead of calorie controlled sugar-free diets. Liberalized diets are much more palatable and usually closer to what most residents were eating at home. The administrator of a Milwaukee, WI, facility that was featured in a television documentary titled *Almost Home* notes, "If a resident wants to eat greasy bacon five times a day, we let them do it. I mean, who cares? They're 90 years old. What's a reduced-salt, low-fat diet going to do for someone who's lived a full life? Why feed them bland, miserable food if that's not what they want?"[9] Regardless of whether therapeutic diets are served, both the director of nursing (DON) and dietary services manager (DSM) should pay close attention to meal service and make regular meal rounds. Adopt the viewpoint that you are the host or hostess for an important get-together. The residents are your honored guests, and you must do all you can to impress them.

Meal Rounds

- Check menus and stock on hand to ensure that all food items are available.

- Taste the food, including mechanical soft and pureed diets. Evaluate all food for flavor, texture, and seasoning.

- Plan and prepare meal substitutes.

- Check the dining room for cleaning or repair needs.

- Make the dining environment as pleasant as possible. Check to make sure tables are clean and ready, trash picked up, and the floor clear.

- Set the tables in an attractive manner. Consider place mats or tablecloths. Decorate tables with seasonal decorations.

- Check the dishes, silverware, and flatware. Make sure it is attractive, clean, and free from defects.

- Make sure staff have assisted residents in preparing for meals by assisting with toileting, washing hands, and applying dentures, glasses, and hearing aid, if used.

- Transfer residents from wheelchairs into dining room chairs with arms, if possible.

- Seat residents with others with whom they can relate and socialize. Avoid social isolation, such as seating one alert, talkative resident with three

nonverbal, confused residents. Avoid positioning residents so they are looking at the wall.

- Monitor the residents' position at the table. Make sure they can reach the food and that table height is not too high or low. Residents should be positioned upright, in good alignment. Make adjustments, if necessary.

- Apply a clothing protector, if used by the resident.

- Coordinate between the dietary manager and director of nursing to ensure resident arrival in the dining area is timely and meal service efficient.

- Check food temperatures before serving.

- Check the time. Note when food carts leave the kitchen and arrive in the dining room, and when the last resident is served.

- Regularly put a test tray on carts, including carts sent to remote units. Temperature test regularly.

- Make sure staff are on hand and available to pass trays in a timely manner. Staff should not be assigned meal breaks during resident meal service. All staff should be on the units to assist with meal service.

- Check diet cards to ensure they match trays.

- Make sure that all residents at a table are served before serving the next table.

- Ensure each resident receives a tray.

- When serving trays, staff should

    - inquire about need for condiments, make sure they are available or added to food

    - set up tray, if needed

    - provide a glass of water for each resident

- offer substitutes according to protocol, or if residents eat less than 50 percent of the meat or vegetable

• After trays have been served, staff should

  – encourage residents to eat, as appropriate

  – assist residents as needed

  – offer refills on beverages

  – offer to reheat or replace food items, as appropriate

  – inquire whether residents are enjoying the meal

• Monitor staff to see whether they interact with residents at meals, and provide appropriate assistance with serving trays and eating.

• Monitor residents to see whether they are receiving adequate assistance.

• Staff should report the need for mealtime changes to the nurse or dietary department, as appropriate.

• Inform the nurse of specific resident care needs.

• After meals, staff should

  – Evaluate food consumption and plate waste; document food intake and fluid intake (for residents on I & O).

  – Regularly spot-check to verify the accuracy of documented meal consumption by evaluating the plates. Several studies have been done to evaluate accuracy of meal consumption. Several of these showed that staff commonly overestimate meal intake and document it inaccurately. This leads professional nurses and physicians to make inaccurate estimates of residents' food intake. Some CNAs have great difficulty

understanding percentages. Others are busy, and may not document meal consumption until the end of the shift, or even several days later.[10]

  – Inform the nurse of meal refusals or inadequate intake

  – Follow up on needs for adaptive devices, care plan changes, dietary and nursing needs.

Quality-of-care deficiencies

Quality of care is a catchall term that means the facility has met the federal requirements for *42 CFR 483.13*, resident behavior and facility practices, *42 CFR 483.15*, quality of life, or *42 CFR 483.25*, quality of care. Most directors of nursing believe that inadequate staffing and heavy turnover result in quality-of-care problems. If substandard quality is noted during a survey, surveyors will determine whether the deficiencies constitute

• immediate jeopardy to resident health or safety;

• a pattern of widespread actual harm that is not immediate jeopardy;

• a widespread potential for more than minimal harm, but less than immediate jeopardy, with no actual harm.

The quality-of-care portions of the survey focus on outcomes, in which resident rights and quality of nursing, dietary, activities, and pharmacy services are evaluated. Surveyors employ an assortment of data collection techniques, such as direct observation of the physical facilities, resident care procedures, observation of meal service, and an evaluation of whether the dining area enhances resident independence and promotes well-being; medication pass, and group activities. Surveyors also consider information obtained during resident interviews and documentation on medical records. Surveyors evaluate dietary services for the timeliness, appearance, taste, flavor, temperature, and nutritional balance of the meals served. Sanitation in the kitchen and dining room are survey targets because of the high risk for food-borne illness. Diets of altered consistency, such as mechanical soft and pureed are also closely reviewed for nutritional value and acceptability. Surveyors will sample the food. They will monitor the mixing of thickened liquids and may question staff about how to obtain various consistencies.

During the survey, the physical environment is carefully evaluated for visual privacy, lighting, ventilation, sanitation, and overall cleanliness. Surveyors want to see odors controlled by eliminating them at the source, rather than covering them up with air freshener. A survey finding of substandard quality of care indicates the facility has one or more significant deficiencies that must be addressed and corrected rapidly to protect resident health and safety. The state agency responsible for inspecting the facility may specify a maximum time frame for correcting the deficiencies.

Quality indicators

Quality *indicators* are numeric warning signs of problems, such as a higher-than-expected incidence of pressure sores. They identify *concerns* for further investigation, but as a stand-alone measure, do not make statements about quality of care. Quality *measures* have been validation-tested to ascertain whether the indicators actually reflect the quality of care provided, taking resident- and facility-specific conditions into consideration. Measures are reliable estimates of quality.

Most facilities are familiar with the data used to evaluate quality of care. Some quality indicators (QI) come from residents' conditions based on MDS data.

Other conditions are evaluated during the facility survey. Identifying quality indicators (which are reported to the public) was a difficult job, and it continues to be a work in progress. At the time of this writing, the current set of QIs are based on MDS Version 2.0, and cover the following domains, or broad areas of care:

- Accidents
- Nutrition/Eating
- Behavior/Emotional Patterns
- Physical Functioning
- Clinical Management
- Psychotropic Drug Use
- Cognitive Patterns
- Pain/Quality of Life
- Elimination/Incontinence
- Skin Care
- Infection Control

These domains represent common conditions and aspects of life in long-term care residents. They do not represent every care category or situation that could occur in the facility. They are very closely associated with the Resident Assessment Protocols (RAPs) component of the Resident Assessment Instrument (RAI). Quality indicators and reports provide an additional source of useful information to surveyors and the facility. They are one piece of a very large puzzle, and should not be used as the only source of information about a given subject.

To do a cursory evaluation of quality of care, make rounds in the facility, try to evaluate conditions through a visitor's eyes, or a surveyor's eyes.

- What overall impression does the environment make. Is it neat, clean, and odor free?

- Does the environment appear to be organized and relatively calm?

- Do the various staff members acknowledge and greet visitors?

- Do the residents appear as if they are attended to?

- What activities are staff doing? Are they attentive or sitting around?

- Are residents well-groomed and properly dressed?

- Do staff interact with residents?

- How are residents addressed by staff?

Teach your staff how to respond to visitors and surveyors. Conduct unannounced mock surveys. Do all you can to evaluate staff performance daily. Provide positive feedback, whenever possible. Staff tend to repeat performances for which they are praised. Always remember to praise in public and criticize in private! Resident-specific full information is found in Chapter 12.

Incidents and accidents

Falls are a cause of many deficiencies, as well as many lawsuits. Falls are discussed in depth in Chapter 12. The CDC is a good source of statistical information. The CD Fact Sheet on falls is on the CD-ROM that accompanies your book. Reading this information will give you an idea of the scope and magnitude of the fall problem, as well as suggestions for prevention.

> "Failure to keep the facility free from hazards that cause accidents" is a common deficiency. The CDC Fact Sheet for Falls in the Elderly provides an excellent overview on the scope of the problem.[11]

Pressure ulcers

Pressure ulcers are declines according to the OBRA regulations. They are extremely problematic for residents and facilities. The old adage "Pressure ulcers are easier to prevent than they are to treat" is absolutely true. As with falls, many or most long-term care facility residents are at high risk of skin breakdown. Failure to prevent and properly treat pressure ulcers is a common survey deficiency, and is frequently a factor in lawsuits. However, most pressure ulcers can be prevented through a combination of risk factor identification and proper nursing care. Pressure ulcers are covered in greater detail in Chapter 11.

Risk factors for pressure ulcer development

Low-risk residents who are independent and ambulatory are usually at very high risk for skin breakdown during periods of illness. Yet these residents are thought to be at low risk, so often, no preventive plan of care is in place. If the low-risk resident becomes acutely ill, his or her risk should be promptly reassessed, and a preventive plan of care implemented.

Skin assessment should be done on admission and regularly thereafter. Many tools are available for assessing skin risk. Common sense is also necessary. Residents with fragile skin, including most elderly individuals, as well as those with a history of healed ulcers are most probably at risk. Again, common sense should prevail in risk factor identification, and a preventive plan of care can only help. Many excellent publications are available to guide you in assessing risk, preventing, staging, treating, and documenting pressure ulcers. The purpose of mentioning them here is not to guide you in their care, but to inform you of problems related to survey deficiencies and the immense legal exposure associated with pressure ulcers. Staff are responsible for the results of risk assessments. To prevent pressure ulcers and achieve successful wound healing, the nurse must carefully follow every step in wound management, including critical assessment, planning, implementation, evaluation, and documentation.[12]

Comprehensive care plans

Problems related to care planning frequently appear on lists of top ten survey deficiencies. An individualized, comprehensive care plan is developed upon facility admission, quarterly, and whenever the resident experiences a significant change in condition. The plan should be developed by an interdisciplinary team of workers, the resident, and family members of the resident's choosing. Care plan goals are to maintain or improve function, preserve autonomy, and maintain the resident's comfort and dignity. If the resident's condition is likely to deteriorate, then the care plan should be designed to slow deterioration, if possible, prevent complications, promote optimal quality of life, comfort, and dignity within the limitations of the diagnoses or disease process.

The care plan must be complete, and address all of a resident's needs, with measurable timetables and actions. The plan of care must include, as applicable, nursing and medical services, medication, dietary, treatment, and activities orders. Data elsewhere on the medical record should not contradict the care plan, and documentation should be complete, as well as reflective of the services delivered. A worker who is not familiar with the resident should be able to find everything needed to care for the resident by reviewing the plan. All caregivers should be able to find new or modified information about a resident who has experienced a change in condition and requires different care or additional monitoring.

The MDS is used to collect data that lead staff to develop a comprehensive, outcome-oriented care plan for each resident. The questions on the MDS address risk factors that place the resident at risk for adverse outcomes. The care planning process must be driven by the assessment, rather than vice versa. The resident assessment protocols, or RAPs, are analytical tools that guide the staff through problem analysis, and the utilization guidelines, which provide detailed instructions for the plan of care. The triggers and RAP summary are bridges between the assessment data and the care plan. Analyzing the RAP summary has become a priority for some surveyors, to determine whether the facility has carefully analyzed the data listed on the plan of care. Surveyors have reported finding care plans that were done prior to the assessments. The plans were not updated. Instead, they were redated the following quarter, without analysis of the assessment data. To satisfy surveyors that assessment data have been analyzed, the location of information supporting the care plan decisions should be listed on the RAP summary.

Causes of care plan problems

Legal problems and survey deficiencies often occur when facilities consider the care plan as a means of paper compliance. The plan should be developed as a "road map" to direct personnel in the care of the resident. To be effective, staff must be familiar with and follow the plan. The plan must be current, reflect problems and needs, and address risk factors. The facility "meets professional standards of quality" by developing an immediate plan on admission, even if it is not comprehensive, and updating the plan for changes in condition, even if minor. Surveyors are usually reasonable when evaluating the care plan format. They are concerned with care plan substance, and whether the plan meets the objectives of maintaining or improving the resident's condition and whether it promotes autonomy. Deficiencies are commonly written

- if the plan is not followed

- if the plan is not kept current and does not reflect care needed by the resident

- if the plan does not identify and address risk factors

- when adverse outcomes occur that were not anticipated or addressed on the care plan

The care plan is almost always an issue in lawsuits.

The problems are usually similar to those for which surveyors write deficiencies. Occasionally, the facility provides an altered plan, or a beautiful plan that was never implemented. Falsification of care plans and other documentation is discussed in Chapter 23.

Care plan standards to consider

§483.20(d) A facility must use the results of the comprehensive assessment (MDS) to develop, review, and revise the resident's comprehensive plan of care.

§483.20(k) Comprehensive care plans (1) The facility must develop a comprehensive care plan for each resident that includes measurable objectives and timetables to meet a resident's medical, nursing, and mental and psychosocial needs that are identified in the comprehensive assessment. The care plan must describe the following:

(i) The services that are to be furnished to attain or maintain the resident's highest practicable physical, mental, and psychosocial well-being as required under §483.25; and

(ii) Any services that would otherwise be required under §483.25 but are not provided due to the resident's exercise of rights under §483.10, including the right to refuse treatment under §483.10(b)(4).

Think about the standards of nursing practice described in Chapter 4. Remember that care must meet professional standards of quality. Also consider that the MDS is only one assess-

ment. Although it forms the basis for the care plan, other assessments are necessary. Facilities are responsible for assessing areas that are relevant to residents regardless of whether these areas are included in the *Resident Assessment Instrument* (RAI; MDS).

The RAI is the minimum assessment tool, not the only assessment tool. Completion of the MDS does not remove the facility's responsibility to document a more detailed assessment of particular issues of relevance for the resident. As the process of problem identification is integrated with sound clinical interventions, the care plan becomes each resident's unique path toward achieving or maintaining his or her highest practicable level of well-being.[13]

The nurse collects resident health data. Pertinent data are collected using appropriate assessment techniques and instruments. Relevant data are documented in a retrievable form. The data collection process is systematic and ongoing. Diagnoses are derived from the assessment data and are validated with other healthcare providers, when appropriate. Diagnoses are documented in a manner that facilitates the determination of expected outcomes and the plan of care. Outcomes are derived from the diagnoses.[14]

Chapter five

References

1. Nightingale F. (1859). *Notes on nursing.* London: Harrison and Sons, 1859, p. 74

2. Petty S. (2003). Quality of care under fire: Senate finance committee criticizes nursing facility deficiencies. *Caring for the Ages,* October 2003; Vol. 4, No. 10, p. 3-4. Online. *www.amda.com/caring/october2003/publicpolicy.htm.* Accessed 11/19/05.

3. Petty S. (2003). Quality of care under fire: Senate finance committee criticizes nursing facility deficiencies. *Caring for the Ages,* October 2003; Vol. 4, No. 10, p. 3-4. Online. *www.amda.com/caring/october2003/publicpolicy.htm.* Accessed 11/19/05.

4. Harrington C, Mercado-Scott C, Carrillo H. (2005). *Nursing facilities, staffing, residents, and facility deficiencies, 1998 through 2004.* Funded by the U.S. Health Care Financing Administration Cooperative Agreement #18-C-90034 and The Agency for Health Care Policy & Research #H500-97-0002.

5. Fraser MR. Nursing home civil litigation. *Nursing Home Medicine* 1995;3(4):79-82.

6. Fraser MR. Criminal liability in nursing facilities. Nursing Home Medicine 1994;2(9):197-198.

7. No. 99-0169. In the Supreme Court of Texas. (November 17, 1999). *Horizon/CMS Healthcare Corporation d/b/a Heritage Western Hills Nursing Home, Petitioner versus Lexa Auld, administratrix of the Estate of Martha Hary, deceased, Respondent. On Petitions for Review from the Court of Appeals for the Second District of Texas.*

8. No. 99-0169. In the Supreme Court of Texas. (November 17, 1999). *Horizon/CMS Healthcare Corporation d/b/a Heritage Western Hills Nursing Home, Petitioner versus Lexa Auld, administratrix of the Estate of Martha Hary, deceased, Respondent. On Petitions for Review from the Court of Appeals for the Second District of Texas.*

9. Zaleski R. (2006). Milwaukee nursing home emphasizes 'home'. *The Capital Times.* January 27, 2006. Online. *www.madison.com/tct/news/index.php?ntid=70474&ntpid=1.* Accessed 1/27/06.

10. Kayser-Jones J. (1997). Inadequate staffing at mealtime: implications for nursing and health policy. *Journal of Gerontological Nursing.* 1997, 23(8), 14–21. Accessed 11/19/05.

11. Centers for Disease Control and Prevention. *A tool kit to prevent senior falls: Falls in nursing homes.* Online. *www.cdc.gov/ncipc/factsheets/nursing.htm.* Accessed 11/19/05.

12. Hess, Cathy Thomas. (1998). *Nurse's Clinical Guide Wound Care.* Springhouse, PA. Springhouse Corporation.

13. Morris, J.N., Murphy, K., Nonemaker, S. (1996). *Long-term care facility resident assessment instrument (RAI) user's manual.* Des Moines. Briggs Corp.

14. American Nurses Association. (1998). *Standards of clinical nursing practice 2nd Edition.* Washington, D.C. American Nurses Publishing.

Survey outcomes

"The strategic planning process is valuable only if there is commitment from all levels within the organization. It can be a difficult process since it is based on open and honest communications. The honesty involves a realistic look at the individual, the organization, common goals and, most important, the changes that need to happen. It may require a "positive anger"—anger with complacence with ourselves, our organization, and our colleagues."[1]

Plan of correction

The state will notify you of its survey findings within 10 business days of the exit conference. Since notification is usually made by mail, it may take several weeks for documentation to reach you. The survey agency will send a formal written report of the survey findings. This report is commonly called "*the 2567*," referring to the form number the Centers for Medicare & Medicaid Services (CMS) uses for survey findings. The report will list the deficiencies, if any, and must be posted in a prominent location. The facility is given a designated amount of time to correct deficiencies. Administration must submit a written response, or *plan of correction* to the survey agency within 10 calendar days of receiving the 2567. The plan of correction for resident-centered deficiencies must state

- how the deficiencies identified for specific residents will be corrected

- how the facility will identify other residents having the potential to be affected by the same deficient practice

- what measures will be taken to make sure the deficient practice will not recur

- how the facility will monitor its corrective actions to ensure the deficient practice does not recur

The plan of correction for facility-centered deficiencies must state

- what will be done to correct the deficiencies

- who will make the corrections

- who will monitor the deficient area

- how similar deficiencies will be prevented in the future

Writing the plan of correction

"Once the critical issues/choices have been listed and prioritized, goals and strategies will need to be developed. Goal setting and strategy development need not be difficult and complex. Simplicity is the most effective way to keep a plan focused and on track."[2]

The *Plan of correction* is a formal statement by the long-term care facility informing the State and CMS of actions that will be taken to address deficiencies identified during a survey. The department head who is responsible for correcting the deficiencies should write the plan of correction. The deadlines for submitting an acceptable plan are tight; 10 days from the date of receipt of the statement of deficiencies. Because of this, the plan of correction should be prepared immediately. Turn the finished plan in to the facility administrator for approval and submission to the survey office. The administrator or consultant personnel will approve the plan, edit the plan for grammar and spelling, if needed, then type and submit the plan by the specified date.

The plan of correction may prove to be an important legal document. If the facility is sued for an occurrence during the survey time frames, the survey will most probably end up in evidence. The plan is also posted in the facility copy of the survey, where residents, family members, ombudsmen, members of the public, employees, and others may read it. A poorly written plan can cause an unfavorable impression of the facility and strengthen a lawsuit against the facility. A well-written plan is objective (versus defensive) and addresses each issue. When writing the plan

- A plan of correction must be written for all cited deficiencies except those at Level A. You must write a plan for each deficiency even if you plan to challenge it through the IDR or formal appeal process. Keep information for the IDR separate from the POC.

- Make sure the plan is complete, and that each response to a deficiency contains the required elements.

- If several residents are cited in a cumulative deficiency, you must identify the corrective action taken for *each resident*, in addition to the other information.

- If a single resident is listed in more than one deficiency, you must cite the corrective action taken for each finding in the respective defi-

ciencies. Do not address the first deficiency, then skip the others.

- Keep the language of the plan neutral. State the facts. Avoid comments supporting or defending the approaches used in the care or situation causing the citation.

- Avoid statements referring to "discipline," if possible. This implies guilt.

- Provide sufficient detail to prove the adequacy of your corrective action. Avoid statements, such as "will assess resident, develop, and implement a plan." State specifically what you did/are doing.

- State how the facility will identify other residents with the potential to be affected by the deficient practice. For example, you can audit medical records, interview staff, residents, or families, use direct monitoring and observation, review computer printouts, Minimum Data Sets and care plans, and so forth.

- Specifically state how the facility will make systemic changes to prevent deficiency recurrence. Be specific. For example, include policy and procedural changes, inservicing staff, competency and/or skills checklists, or initiating new programs. Specify dates for inservices, or specify when all inservices will be completed.

- Specify how the facility will monitor performance to ensure solutions are maintained. Be specific by stating who will monitor, when/how often, specifically what will be monitored, etc. (Explain how you will evaluate corrective measures for effectiveness.) Identify how you will integrate the deficiency into the quality assurance program and what the QA committee will do with the information.

- Specify the date corrective action will be

achieved for each deficiency. Make sure the time frame is acceptable in light of the magnitude of the deficiency. For example, actual or high potential harm to residents, should be corrected immediately. If the survey has specified an "opportunity to correct" date, the completion date should not exceed this date. In most cases, the completion date should be within 30-45 days after the end of the survey. All corrective actions listed on the POC for each deficiency must occur prior to the completion date specified for that deficiency.

- Write a statement of policy about the deficiency in which you outline corrective action(s) completely. For example, the care plan states resident #14 is a "one-person transfer with transfer belt." The surveyor observed nursing assistants transferring her on two occasions without a transfer belt. Your plan will say:

  - (F324) It is the policy of this facility to provide assistive devices as needed, as well as adequate supervision to reduce the risk of falls and other injuries. Other means of accomplishing this goal for resident #14 are by providing a pressure-sensitive alarm system. The resident has a bed with a low platform and a mat on the floor next to the bed. In the event he or she attempts to transfer unassisted, the monitor will alert staff and the combination bed and mat will reduce the risk of injury if a fall does occur. The resident is provided with a restorative nursing program for strengthening and contracture prevention. Her medications are regularly reviewed for potentially adverse effects that increase the risk of falls. He or she wears hip protectors. In this case, after the surveyor reported the improper trans-

fer, the care plan was reviewed with the nursing assistant, and she was reinstructed of the facility policies that state gait belts will be used for all transfers. The charge nurse has spot checked the assistant, who has complied with the policy in 10 of 10 transfers observed.

- Next, describe how the deficiency has the potential to affect other residents, and describe what is being done about it. This is another example of the same deficiency:

  - (F324) Other facility residents who transfer with assistance are potentially affected by the cited deficiency. The director of nursing reviewed the care plans and nursing assistant assignments for all residents requiring dependent transfers on (date). She re-inserviced all nursing assistant personnel on (date) and asked charge nurses to monitor for and validate transfer belt use. Staff were reminded that transfer belts are part of their mandatory uniform and must be worn to comply with the dress code. The charge nurses have verified nursing assistant transfer skills, and all residents receiving hands-on assistance were transferred with a transfer belt. No other residents were affected.

- Detail any other individual or systematic changes that have been or will be implemented to prevent reoccurrence. This is another example of the same deficiency:

  - (F324) The staff development director, under the direction of the director of nurses, will inservice all nursing personnel on (date) regarding state and federal requirements for reducing the risk of accidents, incidents, and injuries. The importance of using transfer belts, and following the plan of care and assignment sheet will be emphasized. We have ordered an additional supply of belts. One will be issued to each resident, labeled, and kept in each resident's room so it will be available when needed for transfers. To enhance currently compliant operations and reduce the risk of recurrence, all staff will be checked off on use of transfer belts and charge nurses will monitor for ongoing compliance.

- Discuss the quality assurance program. This is another example of the same deficiency:

  - Effective on (date), the facility quality review committee, under the supervision of the assistant director of nurses, will audit staff during assisted resident transfers. The assistant director of nurses or nurse member of the quality assurance committee will provide the following systemic changes:

    - Randomly audits and weekly checks of residents who require assisted transfers to ensure gait belts are being utilized.

    - Correct identified deficiencies immediately, then document and report the findings at the next quality assurance meeting for further review or corrective action.

- You have 10 calendar days to write a POC and submit it to the survey agency. Send it by certified mail, return receipt requested, or by courier with a signed receipt. Note that tracking certified mail slows it down markedly. If your time frame is tight, consider using a courier service for delivery.

The recommended frequency for random audits or quality assurance committee monitoring depends upon the severity of the deficiency cited. The committee may eliminate the audits when they determine the problem has been resolved. However, it is wise to perform periodic follow-up monitoring (such as quarterly for six months to a year) after discontinuing the original audit.

Many facilities write (or rubber stamp) a disclaimer such as those depicted in Table 6-1 on one or more pages of the survey (2567). CMS and the survey agencies do not particularly like this approach, but its use is widespread.

Table 6-1	*Example Plan of Correction Disclaimer*

Example 1

This Plan of correction constitutes our written allegation of compliance for the deficiencies cited. However, submission of this Plan of correction is not an admission that a deficiency exists or that one was cited correctly. This Plan of correction is submitted to meet requirements established by state and federal law.

Example 2

The preparation and execution of this Plan of correction does not constitute an admission or agreement by the Provider as to the truth or accuracy of the facts alleged or the conclusions set forth in the Statement of Deficiencies. This Plan of correction is prepared and executed because it is required by Federal and State law.

Discretionary remedies

Discretionary remedies may be imposed by the survey agency, based on the severity of the deficiencies identified. **The remedies are listed in the Enforcement Action Discretionary Remedies table on your CD-ROM.**

Informal dispute resolution

Facilities have a formal and an informal process for disputing deficiencies. The facility may file a formal appeal request within 60 days of receiving a formal notice of enforcement remedies resulting from survey deficiencies. A formal appeal provides the facility a structured review of disputed deficiencies by the Departmental Appeals Board of the Department of Health and Human Services. The dispute resolution process is important for facilities to use to alter survey outcomes and reduce legal exposure.

The federal government requires each state to have a written plan that the state follows for Informal Dispute Resolution (IDR). The IDR process is important because it provides facilities the opportunity to appeal

deficiencies without incurring costly legal bills. The IDR enables the facility to dispute the citation and submit documentation supporting its dispute to the state survey agency for review. If successful, the state may eliminate the deficiency entirely, or reduce the severity of the citation. One drawback is that the process can be very time consuming, and it takes facility personnel away from their responsibilities in operating the facility. However, the process is faster than moving through the court system, and the facility does not sustain costly legal fees. The IDR plan is written by each state, and there are no federal guidelines to follow, so the procedural requirements vary markedly.

After the facility has been cited for survey deficiencies, the state inspection agency must inform the facility of the IDR opportunity in writing. The facility has 10 calendar days to respond in writing and initiate the IDR process. This is the same time frame in which a plan of correction must be submitted. Some states require facilities to fax the request, whereas others prefer a mail notification. In the letter of request, the facility should state the reasons for requesting the IDR, and an explanation of the deficiencies being disputed. There is no requirement for completing the process within a specified period of time, but most state agencies report completing the process within 60 days. Survey data are posted on the CMS website, *www.medicare.gov/NHCompare/* for public information. Data are not supposed to be posted until the IDR process is complete. One study revealed that 45% of disputed deficiencies are changed by the IDR process. Of this group, 19% had modifications to the way the deficiency was written, and 19% had the citation deleted entirely.[3] Participating in the IDR process does not prevent a facility from pursuing a formal appeal later. The IDR process provides an opportunity for another review of disputed citations. The IDR process does not

- alter or delay the time frame for termination or other adverse action

- limit the legal (formal) appeal processes afforded facilities by law

- eliminate or delay the due date for the plan of correction.

The facility submits an explanation of the specific deficiencies being disputed, along with documentation supporting their position for state survey agency review. The state reviews documentation submitted by the nursing facility to dispute deficiency citations.

The IDR must not be used to delay the formal imposition of remedies or to challenge other aspects of the survey process, including

- scope and severity of cited deficiencies, except in those instances when the cited deficiency constitutes substandard quality of care or immediate jeopardy

- remedies imposed by the enforcing agency for cited deficiencies

- allegation of failure of the survey team to comply with the survey process requirements

- allegation of inconsistency of the survey team citing deficiencies among facilities

- allegation of inadequacy or inaccuracy of the IDR process

When submitting an IDR, make sure that every page from a resident's chart (even if it is a back page) has the resident's name and a date on it. Make sure the names and dates are legible. Avoid using resident (or responsible party) refusals as a defense in an IDR. Use this defense only if you can prove informed consent. Make sure documentation solidly reflects that the resident (or responsible party) was apprised of the consequences of the refusal.

Table 6-2 provides examples of when IDR may or may not be used.

Table 6-2	*IDR Examples*

Situation	Eligibility for IDR
New deficiency (i.e., new or changed facts, new tag) at revisit or as a result of an IDR	Yes
New example of deficiency (i.e., new facts, same tag) at revisit or as a result of an IDR	Yes
Different tag but same facts at revisit or as a result of an IDR	No, unless the new tag constitutes substandard quality of care

IDR Outcomes

An IDR outcome is considered successful if the disputed deficiency is deleted, reduced in severity by modifying the way the deficiency is written, or lowered in scope and severity level. A facility may not request a second review of a previous IDR decision. The dispute may be resolved at the documentation review level or may progress to an in-person interview or phone conference. Some states impose time and attendance limitations for phone and face-to-face interviews. When a final determination has been made, the facility will be notified. The federal requirements compel states to notify facilities in writing only if the IDR is unsuccessful. However, many states notify the facility of both positive and negative outcomes in writing. If the facility prevails, the disputed deficiency is removed and enforcement actions related to the disputed deficiency rescinded. CMS has the authority to reject the IDR conclusions and make a determination of noncompliance if the facility is dually participating or is certified for Medicare-only. However, this rarely occurs.

If the facility prevails at the IDR level, they may request a clean (new) copy of the survey (Form CMS-2567) for posting. However, the clean copy will be the releasable copy only when a clean (new) plan of correction is both provided and signed by the facility. The original Form CMS-2567 is disclosable when a clean plan of correction is not submitted and signed by the facility. Any survey or plan of correction that is revised as a result of the IDR process must be disclosed to the facility ombudsman. If a provider is dissatisfied with the decision at the administrative level, the facility can appeal to superior court.

Civil monetary penalties

Civil monetary penalties (CMPs) are one of eight discretionary remedies CMS may use to manage quality-of-care or safety deficiencies. The survey agency will review the facility's past compliance history and the present deficiencies when making a determination of what action(s) to take or recommend. CMS usually accepts remedies that have been endorsed by the state. However, before imposing remedies, a formal notification period must be observed and an effective date reached. The state survey office may conduct a revisit anytime during this cycle to determine if deficiencies have been corrected. During this revisit, surveyors may revise the existing deficiencies or cite new deficiencies. Enforcement action may be changed as a result of the revisit findings. CMS has the option of rescinding CMPs, imposing new actions, or adjusting time frames and due dates. Figure 6-1 provides an overview of the enforcement process.

Figure 6-1 | *Flowchart of the enforcement process*

Surveyor finds a deficiency
→ Substantial compliance — Yes → Cycle ends
No ↓
Immediate jeopardy — Yes → The state notifies the facility and CMS of recommendation to impose immediate remedies, including termination or temporary management.
No ↓
Double G rule — Yes → State notifies facility of deficiencies and mandatory remedies; requires POC
No ↓
Opportunity to correct — No → State notifies facility of deficiencies and mandatory remedies; requires POC
Yes ↓

CMS imposes remedies; notifies facility
Facility submits Plan of Correction
Revisit — Nonimmediate jeopardy deficiencies / Immediate jeopardy → Termination
Substantial compliance → Cycle ends

State notifies facility of deficiencies and mandatory remedies; requires POC
Facility submits acceptable Plan of Correction — No
Yes ↓
Revisit
Substantial compliance → Cycle ends
Nonimmediate jeopardy deficiencies
Immediate jeopardy → Remedies take effect

The state notifies CMS of recommendation to impose remedies
CMS imposes remedies; notifies facility of effective date(s).
Facility submits Plan of Correction
Revisit
Immediate jeopardy / Substantial compliance
Remedies rescinded → Cycle ends
Nonimmediate jeopardy deficiencies → Remedies take effect
If non-compliant for 3 months Denial of Payments for New Admissions goes into effect.
If non-compliant for 6 months, Medicare contract is terminated.

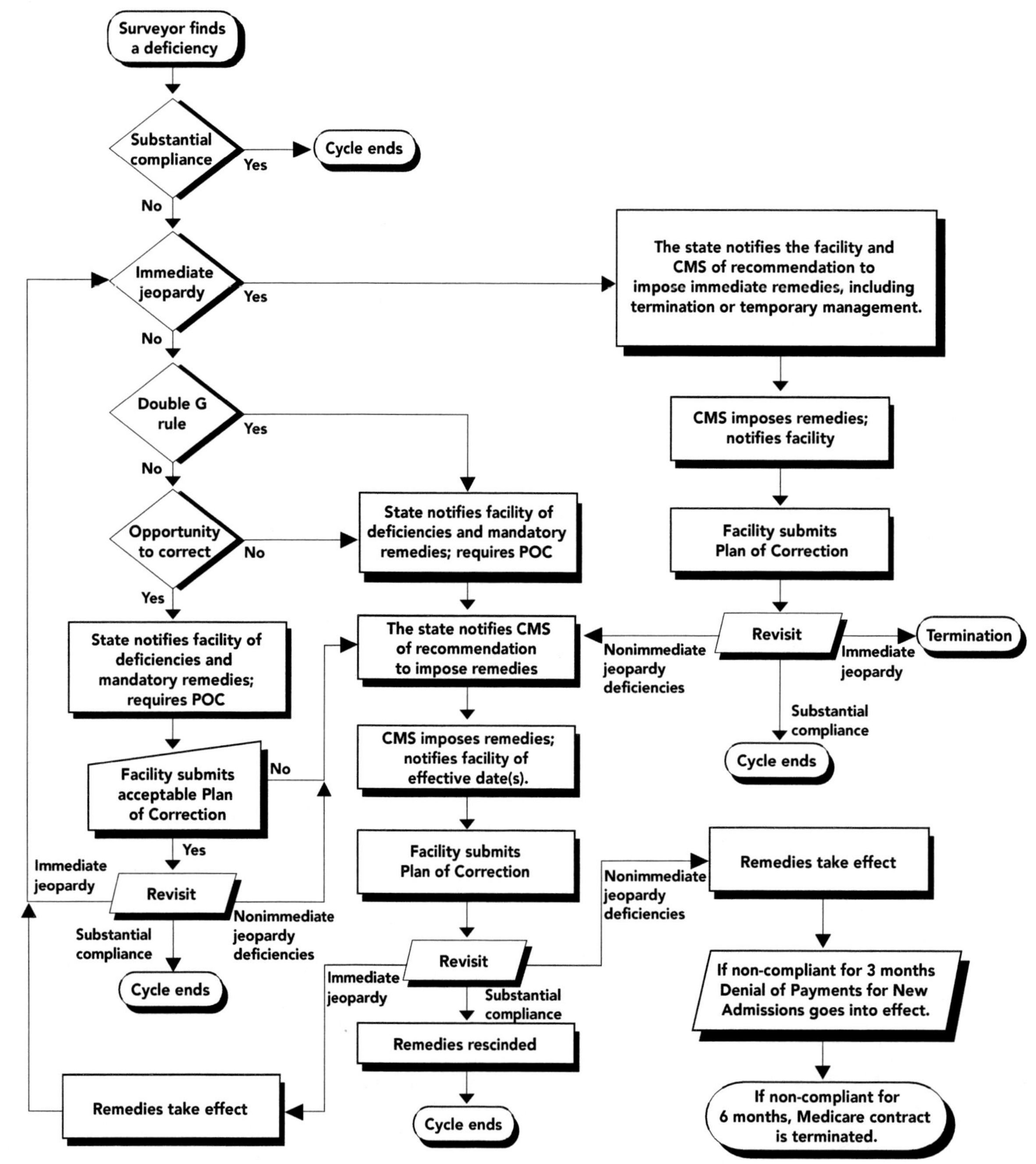

Source: Office of Inspector General Analysis of Documents, Regulations, and Interviews with CMS.

 The Long-Term Care Legal Desk Reference

The government has the option of assessing CMPs per day of noncompliance or per instance of noncompliance. The CMPs have required dollar ranges corresponding to the magnitude of harm to the resident(s). CMPs are used in approximately 51% of CMS enforcement cases.[4] However, the amounts originally imposed are often substantially reduced before payment is due. Under current regulations, systematic reductions, appeals, settlements, and bankruptcies are the main factors contributing to this decrease. Depending on the deficiency, CMPs may vary from $50 to $10,000 per day. CMS seldom assesses this amount. In fact, judgments tend to be toward the lower end of the range. The median per day for the most severe (immediate jeopardy) cases was about $4,000. The median per day imposition amount for less severe cases involving a CMP was $250. The "per instance" penalties range from $1,000 to $10,000. CMS is presently reviewing the consistency of penalties assessed and developing guidelines for streamlining collection and collecting past-due fees.

When CMS informs a facility of the CMP penalty imposed, payment must be remitted within 15 days, unless they negotiate an alternate payment schedule or file an appeal. Interest will accrue if payment is not made by the designated date. A formal appeal will stay the CMP temporarily, until an administrative decision is reached. The total amount of the CMP will be reduced by 35% if the facility waives its appeal rights. The logic for this reduction is to save both the government and the provider money that would be spent if the dispute is legally adjudicated.

The purpose of imposing remedies is to ensure prompt compliance with program requirements. Individual states may also impose remedies under their licensure authority and for Medicaid-only facilities. The per diem fines usually begin on the last day of the survey and persist until surveyors revisit and determine that substantial compliance has been achieved. *Substantial compliance* is defined as compliance with Medicare regulations or deficiencies in the A, B, or C level. Fines are usually retroactive to the last day of the survey, and there are no notification requirements. Per instance CMPs allow a set dollar amount to be imposed in relation to a particular deficiency. Per day and/or per instance CMPs were imposed in 51% of the 8,309 enforcement cases referred to CMS during the years 2000 and 2001. They were imposed almost twice as often as the second most utilized remedy, denial of payments for new admissions.[5]

Compliance dates

When the nature of the deficiencies cited warrants sanctions, CMS will notify the facility in writing. The compliance date is an issue when monetary penalties are involved. The CMS language states, *"Based on deficiencies cited during this survey and as authorized by CMS _____ Regional Office, we are giving formal notice of imposition of statutory Denial of Payment for New Admissions (DPNA) effective (insert date). This remedy will be effectuated on the stated date unless you demonstrate substantial compliance with an acceptable plan of correction and subsequent revisit. This notice in no way limits the prerogative of CMS to impose discretionary DPNA at any appropriate time. CMS Regional Office will notify your intermediary and the Medicaid Agency. If effectuated, denial of payment will continue until your facility achieves substantial compliance or your provider agreement is terminated. [Facilities are prohibited from billing those Medicare/Medicaid residents or their responsible parties during the denial period for services normally billed to Medicare or Medicaid.] The Medicare and Medicaid programs will make no payment for residents whose plans of care begin on or after the DPNA effective date."*

The compliance date is an issue unless the facility clears the deficiencies immediately. If the facility clears the cited deficiencies on the first revisit, surveyors will list the compliance date as the date submitted in the plan of correction. If the facility is in compliance with no correction or monitoring data, the correction date will be listed as the last date on the plan of correction. If the facility clears the deficiencies on the second revisit, the date of the revisit is listed as the compliance date.

However, if the facility has collected and saved data showing correction and verifying continued compliance, the compliance date is listed as the date proven by the facility's data and information.

If the facility is unable to clear the deficiencies after two revisits, CMS will list the revisit date as the date compliance was gained, regardless of data showing alleged compliance. A third revisit is granted only at the behest of the CMS Regional Administrator. The dates are very significant if CMPs are being assessed. If you have strong records of correction activities, you may be successful in gathering your proof and attempting to negotiate an earlier compliance date with CMS.

Appeals

When the state imposes sanctions, the following notification is mailed to the facility:

"Appeal Rights

*If you disagree with **the determination of noncompliance (and/or substandard quality of care, if applicable**), you or your legal representative may request a hearing before an administrative law judge of the*

*Department of Health and Human Services, Departmental Appeals Board. Procedures governing this process are set out in 42 CFR §498.40, et. seq. You may appeal the finding of noncompliance that led to an enforcement action, but not the enforcement action or remedy itself. A written request for hearing must be filed no later than (date 60 days from date of this letter) (60 days from the date of receipt of this letter via fax). Such written request should be made **directly** to:*

Departmental Appeals Board
Civil Remedies Division
Cohen Building Room G-644
200 Independence Avenue S.W.
Washington, D.C. 20201

*A request for hearing should identify the specific issues, and the findings of fact and conclusions of law with which you disagree. It should also specify the basis for contending that the findings and conclusions are incorrect. You may be represented at a hearing by counsel at your own expense. Be sure to include a copy of this letter with your request to the Departmental Appeals Board. In addition, please forward **a copy of your request** to: Attention:"*

(Insert CMS RO person assigned to your state, state/region; this example uses the address of the Dallas office):

Long-Term Care Branch
Division of Survey and Certification
Centers for Medicare & Medicaid Services
1301 Young Street Room 827
Dallas, Texas 75202

 The Long-Term Care Legal Desk Reference

References

1. Zagury CS. Making a difference: Strategic planning for the director of nursing in long term care. The Director. Online. *www.nadona.org/media_archive/media/media-238.pdf.* Accessed 08/25/04.

2. Zagury CS. Making a difference: Strategic planning for the director of nursing in long term care. The Director. Online. *www.nadona.org/media_archive/media/media-238.pdf.* Accessed 08/25/04.

3. Department of Health and Human Services Office of Inspector General. (2005). *Informal dispute resolution for nursing facilities.* Inspector General March 2005. OEI-06-02-00750. Online. *http://oig.hhs.gov.* Accessed 11/21/05.

4. Department of Health and Human Services Office of Inspector General. (2005). *Nursing home enforcement: the use of civil money penalties.* April 2005 OEI-06-02-00720. Online. *http://oig.hhs.gov.* Accessed 11/21/05.

5. Department of Health and Human Services Office of Inspector General. (2005). *Nursing home enforcement: the use of civil money penalties.* April 2005 OEI-06-02-00720. Online. *http://oig.hhs.gov.* Accessed 11/21/05.

Conflict resolution/managing complaints

Working in long-term care

Conflict is an inevitable part of working in long-term care. Staffing, stress, close environments, and rapid decision-making all set the stage for conflict on the nursing units. Since each unit is part of a larger whole and does not operate in a vacuum, conflict may occur between units, and with other departments. Conflicts may also occur with residents and family members. Instead of becoming overwhelmed by complaints and conflicts, view them as wonderful opportunities for making improvements. Doing this takes only a minor attitude adjustment and a slight change in perspective.

One study revealed that nurse managers spent 20% of their time on conflict management tasks. These managers rated conflict resolution skills as being more important than planning, motivation, communication, and decision-making.[1] Interpersonal conflict was a strong predictor of job satisfaction in several studies. Nurses who experienced more interpersonal conflict were often dissatisfied with their jobs.[2,3] Yet another study showed an inverse association between stress and job satisfaction. In this study, job satisfaction was low when stress was high. Unresolved conflict creates a stressful work environment. Stress also occurs when

the workers perceive unreasonable or inappropriate demands on their time, unfair or improper assignments, or conflicting goals and values.[4] One study seemed to suggest that there was a significant difference in the predicted and observed death rate in a facility experiencing intergroup conflict between physicians and nurses. When physicians and nurses disagree, collaboration and creativity are stifled, with an increased risk for poor patient outcomes.[5] Resolving conflict entirely is an admirable goal. If this cannot be achieved, strive for a compromise that everyone can live with, and continue to keep communication open. Properly managed conflict is helpful in improving or changing a facility, making it more efficient and competitive. Although conflict resolution does not always lead to a complete resolution of the problem, the underlying issues must be settled, or the potential for escalating future problems will always exist.

Conflict

Conflict is a normal part of working in long-term care. When issues and priorities collide, conflict usually follows. Differences of opinion are part of life, and are not necessarily bad. In fact, conflict can be healthy, such as when it exposes differences that need to be discussed and resolved. It may mean employees care deeply about an issue. Unfortunately, conflict has the potential to be very divisive. Providing a forum for open and honest conflict resolution can further employee growth. Whether the net effect of workplace conflict is positive or negative is determined by how we respond to it and how it is handled.

To a degree, identifying differences of opinion helps people develop a sense of self. Differences help people learn good communication skills. They help people take responsibility for their feelings and actions. Occasionally, conflict is a motivator, because it connects people with new ideas and other points of view and ways of thinking. However, conflict cannot be ignored. It must be managed so that workers will continue to cooperate to get things done. Handled correctly, interdepartmental conflict can enhance organizational performance and promote teamwork. It may also enhance individual performance. If unresolved conflict is ignored, it may lead to serious organizational dysfunction.

Communicating with others

Teach employees to use tact and sensitivity when communicating with others. The impression you provide can be unintentionally negative. You can be 100% right in your conclusions, reasons, beliefs, and opinions, but 100% wrong in how you express them. People who know they are right are sometimes blunt, arrogant, and offensive. You can be honest without being offensive or brutal. Always treat others, including subordinates, with dignity and respect. Attack an action, if necessary. Avoid attacking a person. Send "I" messages. Use the golden rule. A newer paradigm, the "platinum rule," implies that you should treat others how they want to be treated. The focus of relationships shifts from "This is what I want, so I'll give everyone the same thing" to "Let me first understand

what they want and then I'll give it to them."[6] Be assertive, not aggressive. The difference is that assertive individuals are respectful, whereas aggressive individuals are not. In fact, they are often abrasive.

Resolving conflict

Facility management must support conflict resolution at every level. Some facilities have trained and qualified peer mediators in place in each department. You may consider periodic inservices and role playing activities on communication, conflict management, and conflict resolution to provide staff with useful skills. These are very basic skills that are essential for all workers in the 21st century. A clear understanding of policies, procedures, and addressing conflict is necessary for all employees. The facility should have a systemic mandate and format for addressing conflict in the workplace. Likewise, assertive communication skills are a valuable, yet basic competency. Workers with good communication skills are often viewed as being very effective, compared with others in their position who are less articulate. These workers facilitate positive, respectful communication. They do not come across as being opinionated, abrasive, or offensive. Teach your staff to use "I" messages. These reflect one's own feelings, wants, and needs. On the whole, others react with much less resistance and defensiveness to "I" messages than they do to "You" messages, which are often accusatory in tone, even if that is not the speaker's intent. An "I" message has four parts:

- How I feel about this situation

- Actions of others when you _____

- Results of others' behavior on the speaker because _____

- A request for the change I would like

In addition to using "I" messages, conflict can be avoided by

- being tolerant and accepting of others

- respecting the cultural beliefs of others

- using active listening so others feel as if you understand their position (understanding does not necessarily mean you agree with it)

- using anger management techniques and positive self talk, if necessary

- being assertive

- providing psychological support to show you understand another's position (being supportive also does not mean you agree with it)

Classifying conflict

There are various descriptions of conflict in healthcare. Conflict normally falls into these categories:

- **Intrapersonal:** Having conflicting feelings about a personal course of action with a resident, family member, or another worker.

- **Interpersonal:** Having recurring differences of opinion with a peer. Occasional differences are healthy and expected. Recurring conflict between the same workers requires further investigation.

- **Intragroup:** In teams of workers on a unit, there are several parties or subgroups conflicting with each other.

- **Intergroup:** This involves an entire team opposing another, such as first-shift workers opposing second-shift workers.

Reasons for conflict

Conflict may occur between employees, between departments, or between resident family members and

staff. In long-term care, it often occurs over difference of opinion. It is also commonly caused by

- information overload

- differences in perception or understanding

- frequent changes in directions, causing confusion

- inadequate or incorrect information

- lack of information, misinformation, disagreement about what information is important or what it means

- disputes over what is needed to meet one's needs.

- poor communication, personality and behavior clashes

- stereotyping, cultural or generational differences

- differing values and ethics (these are among the most difficult to resolve)

- power struggles, feeling powerless and out of control

- unequal decision-making ability, power, and control

Other factors that increase stress and lead to conflict in long-term care workers are

- **Role conflict**—when workers have conflicting loyalties or guidelines, or are expected to do things that contradict their own ethics, values, beliefs, principles, or expectations.

- **Role ambiguity**—when workers do not clearly understand their job description or responsibilities, including what is expected, and limits on their scope of authority.

- **Work overload**—when workers perceive their workload to be too heavy, or feel they are expected to do too much work in too little time

- **Time pressures**—when workers believe they cannot complete their assigned work within the designated period of time without cutting corners, taking shortcuts, or compromising safety.

- **Low self-esteem/need for self protection**—workers are insecure and react to past or present conflict by reduced productivity, reduced risk taking to avoid criticism, and blaming others. These workers are those who are present in body, but not in spirit. They often take everything personally, and usually feel very anxious and stressed.

The factors listed above can be particularly unnerving for the workers, because, to resolve them, they probably need to meet with a supervisor, whom the worker perceives as unreceptive to the conversation.

Undoubtedly, the worker feels as if he or she is taking a risk. However, managers must be prepared to discuss and negotiate these problems, which will inevitably occur. If nothing else, the supervisor can clarify worker expectations, investigate workload problems, and make adjustments when necessary. He or she may also be able to help the worker improve his or her organizational skills. Good organization is essential in healthcare, but it must be learned in practice, not the classroom. The most successful workers are often those who are well-organized, with good time management skills.

The initial reaction to conflict is commonly influenced by emotion rather than intellect. Because managing conflict involves managing feelings and opinions, it may be difficult to resolve. Resolving conflict in a mature manner within the confines of the facility is always better than resolving it in the courtroom or through a complaint survey. Teach staff to accept conflict and complaints graciously. Avoid becoming defen-

sive because of the complaining party's tone of voice or body language. Listen carefully and respond sincerely and clearly. Monitor your own facial expression and body language. If a resident or family member complains, thank them for notifying you and assure them their concern will be addressed. (Remember to view it as an opportunity for improvement.) A charge nurse or other administrative person should follow up with them later to be sure they are satisfied with the remedy and the outcome.

Coping with conflict

Many people use a variety of coping styles and skills in conflict resolution. However, some have only one style of coping, and use nothing else. Common ways of managing conflict are

- **Competition**—Being aggressive and uncooperative. This style may be used when a person cares deeply about the problem.

- **Avoidance**—avoiding and refusing to discuss conflict because of fear of expressing it, difficulty articulating the problem, or not really caring about the person or situation.

- **Accommodation**—giving in to others because doing so is easier. People who use this style may build up anger and resentment over time.

- **Collaboration and Compromise**—This is the healthiest method of managing conflict, and people who use this style are often confident in their ability to manage it. They know that neither party will have all his or her needs met, and look for mutually beneficial solutions. This style is the most effective in major and complex conflicts in which both sides are committed to finding solutions.

- **Severe reactions**—Many healthcare workers (including nurses) have difficulty handling conflict.

Rather than face conflict, employees may call in sick, withdraw, change shifts or assigned areas, resign, or eventually leave long-term care nursing.

Collaboration

Collaboration is the most effective method of conflict resolution. Working together to solve a problem gives staff ownership, which results in a mutual commitment to working things out. To collaborate effectively, personnel meet together and agree to take an open, insightful look at the issues and available resolutions. Collaboration is a team-building skill that proves that working together helps achieve personal and departmental goals. Collaboration decreases stress and improves interpersonal (and interdepartmental) communications. Staff who participate in conflict resolution often gain a perspective of and appreciation for the big picture of facility operations.

Gathering all conflicting parties together and facilitating open communication is one of the best means of resolving the situation amicably. Ignoring conflict only allows it to fester unabated, creating potentially serious circumstances. Begin by informing all involved parties that these are important problems and that you need help and support in figuring out solutions. Before deciding how to intervene, you must identify and understand the problem as fully as possible.

To identify the problem accurately, you must use good communication skills, including active listening. Active listening shows you value the speaker's opinion. Seek to understand the speaker's message; try to understand what he or she wants you to understand. Observe the speaker's content and feeling. Try to identify the issue and restate it. For example, if someone says, "I don't think I can take any more of this," rephrase it by saying, "So you are feeling stressed and overwhelmed." Initially, your role is to listen to and interpret the data. At this juncture, don't do any

problem solving. This may be difficult because it involves temporarily giving up control. Concentrate on what is being said and what is going on with people expressing their concerns.

People are responsible and accountable for their own behavior; no one can force another person to swear, become angry, yell, pout, and so forth. Encourage each party to state their goals, feelings, opinions and beliefs without infringing on the rights of others. Set the communication ground rules:

- **Identify priorities of individuals in conflict.** What do they want to do? What is most important? What needs to be done to make this happen?

- **Develop a plan.** Set limits on manipulative behavior. This reduces hostility and stress. Reinforce positive behavior; be consistent in setting limits.

Negotiation and conflict management

Many conflicts can be readily managed when issues are accurately identified and defined, then clearly articulated so everyone is on the same page. Begin by trying to accurately identify the origin and source of the conflict. People will probably not thank you for resolving the problem with tact, skill, and diplomacy, but they will undoubtedly remember it if you ignore the problem or manage the situation badly. To solve a problem, you must understand it. Conflict resolutions can be constructive or destructive, depending on the approach. A team approach is a constructive way of resolving conflict. When the team approach is used, outcomes are often better. Poorly managed conflicts cause hurt feelings and negatively affect quality of care. By learning and using negotiation and dispute resolution techniques, your staff can probably resolve many of the interpersonal conflicts that develop each day.

Chapter seven

Negotiation is the attempt to reach an agreement or resolution through discussion. Many people view negotiation as a win/lose situation. In other words, the more you get, the less I get. Try to find a win/win, or mutually acceptable, solution. To do this, you must continue to use active listening skills. You may also have to use the skills of flexibility and persuasion. Be clear in identifying your own needs, or the speaker's needs, while remaining open to the needs of others. Try to distinguish between demands and needs. To be successful, you must

- recognize that a conflict exists; don't ignore it

- analyze and identify feelings (hurt, anger, jealousy, etc.)

- separate substantial concerns from interpersonal conflicts

- accept responsibility for your own behavior and actions

- plan your strategy

- describe how you will identify an ongoing problem, recognize it, and measure improvement

- determine what action you will take if negotiation is not successful

- set limits; avoid exceeding the limits without first stopping to think it over

The four-C structure may be useful in guiding negotiations:

- Communicate

- Clarify

- Create options

- Commit to a mutually beneficial resolution

The objective of this communication is to cultivate a stable foundation for discussing the conflict further.

Search for areas of agreement, such as identifying common goals. Begin by setting aside a mutually acceptable time and place to meet with all involved parties. Designate the time frame, such as an hour, from the outset and stay with it. Consider using a group activity:

- Have each person write down his or her description of the problem.

- Go around the room, and have each person read aloud what he or she has written.

- Next, ask each person to write down and read aloud "I" messages regarding his or her feelings about the conflict.

- Have each person write down and read aloud what he or she wants and needs and what his or her goals are in relation to the conflict.

- Now do a role reversal. Give each person a time limit to argue an opposing point of view, based on what someone else has said.

- Facilitate the meeting by writing on a flip chart or chalk board. Go around the room and ask each person to share a goal or solution, then list how various goals can be achieved, using compromise if necessary.

- Try to show participants how this is a positive situation. Show how some of each person's needs are met.

- Remain neutral. Avoid passing judgment. Keep the discussion on track and on time.

- Write down a plan of action, including what each person agrees to do, how, and when. Have participants sign at the bottom, if desired.

- The best solution is one that will satisfy the wants and needs of all involved parties. Brainstorming a list of potential solutions, then

                      The Long-Term Care Legal Desk Reference

narrowing it down to those most likely to work may help.

- After deciding on a course of action, obtain a commitment to the final solution. Ask workers if anything will keep them from fulfilling the agreement. Agree on how the plan will be implemented and set a time for a follow-up meeting to assess progress.

Managerial conflict resolution

There may be times when conflict must be resolved through managerial decision-making, or changes in policies and procedures. Regardless of whether management administers the program or peer mediators are responsible, the formal resolution process must be kept confidential. Accept that you may lose one or more workers after a serious conflict situation, even after the situation has been resolved. When feelings and emotions are involved, people do not forget, especially if they feel wronged. Anticipate that this may occur, and try to take steps to prevent similar problems in the future. When managing conflict:

- Thoroughly investigate and identify the problem.

- Avoid judging. Remain neutral.

- Identify the source of conflict by interviewing everyone who is involved separately.

- Be decisive; keep others informed of the changes to be made, and how outcomes will be measured.

- Always follow up with workers by observation and interview in a reasonable period of time so you are aware of outcomes.

Facility policies

Facility policies should promote conflict management and resolution at all levels. After policies and procedures are in place, give some thought into educating your personnel. Tim Porter-O'Grady has written some excellent articles on this subject. He suggests the following:[7,8]

- Define conflict and explain how it is a normative part of communication.

- List the elements and dynamics of conflict as part of the way humans manage their differences.

- List the basic steps of the conflict resolution process with stages and steps of conflict identified in a systematic problem-solving format.

- Describe the structure and dynamics of the facility's organized conflict resolution process, including methods of access, use, and application to the individual conflict.

- Clearly explain the systematic approaches to resolving conflict as part of the facility's commitment to doing business and resolving problematic issues.

Porter-O'Grady suggests that these elements be included in the formal conflict resolution process (shown in Figure 7-1):

Figure 7-1 *Stages of conflict resolution process*

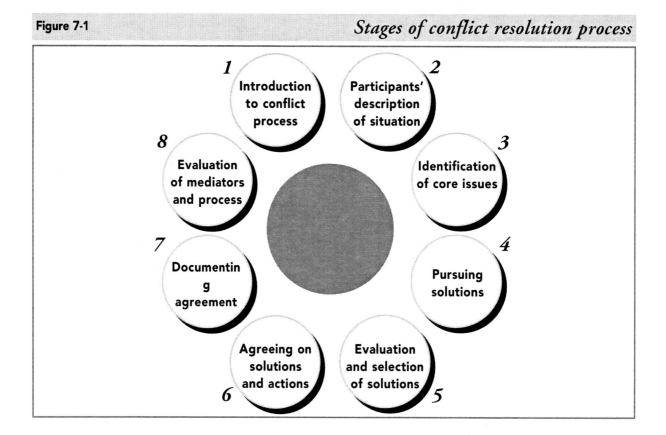

- Welcome, explanation of mediation, explanation of confidential nature of proceedings, ground rules

- Participants' description of the problem, outlining the issues

- Identifying the main concerns, restating the primary issues, writing down the specific understanding related to the issues, reordering the identified primary concerns

- Seeking solutions through participant cooperation, including presenting ideas, brainstorming, and exploration

- Evaluation and selection of ideas for resolution, including priorities of choice, discussing liability, areas of agreement, areas of emerging confluence of solutions

- Enumeration of solutions and specification of impact, response, role, and individual commitment to actions related to solutions

- Documentation of resolution, including all items, performance expectations, follow-up, and evaluation

- Evaluation of the mediation process by participants and mediator

State requirements

In some states, facilities are required to have a formal conflict resolution program for use by residents and responsible parties. Figure 7-2 is an example of the requirements for this program in Michigan facilities.

Figure 7-2   *Example requirements for conflict resolution*

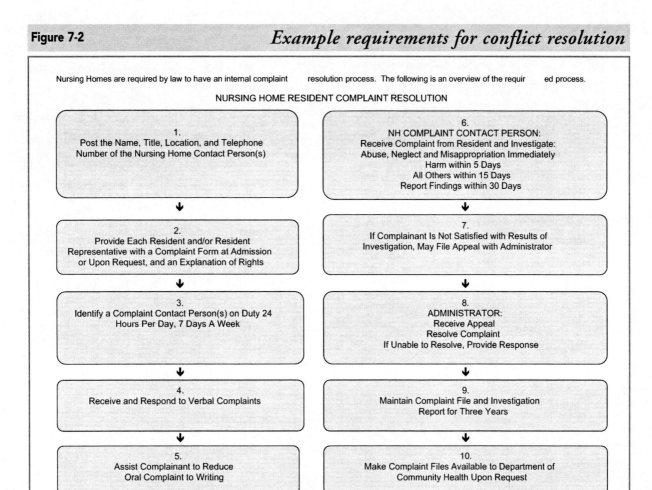

Nursing Homes are required by law to have an internal complaint   resolution process. The following is an overview of the requir   ed process.

NURSING HOME RESIDENT COMPLAINT RESOLUTION

1.
Post the Name, Title, Location, and Telephone Number of the Nursing Home Contact Person(s)

2.
Provide Each Resident and/or Resident Representative with a Complaint Form at Admission or Upon Request, and an Explanation of Rights

3.
Identify a Complaint Contact Person(s) on Duty 24 Hours Per Day, 7 Days A Week

4.
Receive and Respond to Verbal Complaints

5.
Assist Complainant to Reduce Oral Complaint to Writing

6.
NH COMPLAINT CONTACT PERSON:
Receive Complaint from Resident and Investigate:
Abuse, Neglect and Misappropriation Immediately
Harm within 5 Days
All Others within 15 Days
Report Findings within 30 Days

7.
If Complainant Is Not Satisfied with Results of Investigation, May File Appeal with Administrator

8.
ADMINISTRATOR:
Receive Appeal
Resolve Complaint
If Unable to Resolve, Provide Response

9.
Maintain Complaint File and Investigation Report for Three Years

10.
Make Complaint Files Available to Department of Community Health Upon Request

The Michigan model is an example of an excellent process to use. Regardless of the method your facility uses for managing complaints, you may want to consider keeping a complaint log listing at least the

- date of initial complaint

- summary of complaint

- name and contact information for individual making the complaint

- date complaint investigation initiated

- date and manner of resolution

You may wish to keep a separate file with private details of your investigation, depending on the circumstances of the investigation. When addressing complaints

- listen to the complaint

- repeat or paraphrase to make sure you understand the problem

- establish the real issue, if possible

- agree on a resolution

- agree on a plan of action

- follow up

References

1. McElhaney, R. (1996). Conflict management in nursing administration. *Nursing Management* 27. (1996). 49-50.

2. Cox KB. (2003). The effects of intrapersonal, intragroup, and intergroup conflict on team performance effectiveness and work satisfaction. *Nurse Admin Q* 27; (2); 153-163.

3. Irvine DM, and Evans MG. (1995). Job satisfaction and turnover among nurses: integrating research findings across studies. *Nursing Research* 44. 1995; 246-253.

4. Blegan MA. (1993). Nurses' job satisfaction: A meta-analysis of related variables. *Nursing Research* 42. (1993); 36-41.

5. Knaus WA, Wagner DP, Zimmerman JE, Draper EA. (1986). An evaluation of outcome from intensive care in major medical centers. *Annals of Internal Medicine,* 104, 110-118.

6. Allesandra T. The platinum rule. Online. *www.platinumrule.com/aboutpr.asp.* Accessed 11/27/05.

7. Porter-O'Grady, T. (2004). Constructing a conflict resolution program for health care. *Health Care Manage Rev,* 2004, 29 (4), 278-283.

8. Porter-O'Grady, T. (2004). Embracing conflict: Building a healthy community. *Health Care Manage Rev,* 2004, 29 (3), 181-187.

Risk management

Use of outside resources

If the facility does not employ a qualified professional person to furnish a specific service to be provided by the facility, the facility must have that service furnished to residents by a person or agency outside the facility under an arrangement described in section 1861(w) of the Act or an agreement described in paragraph (h)(2) of this section. Arrangements as described in section 1861(w) of the Act or agreements pertaining to services furnished by outside resources must specify in writing that the facility assumes responsibility for:

- Obtaining services that meet professional standards and principles that apply to professionals providing services in such a facility; and

- The timeliness of the services.[1]

Although 1861(w) is really not relevant to our purposes here, it is mentioned in the State Operations Manual several times, where contracts are concerned. To satisfy your intellectual curiosity, it says:

"(w)(1) The term 'arrangements' is limited to arrangements under which receipt of payment by the hospital, critical access hospital, skilled nursing facility,

home health agency, or hospice program (whether in its own right or as agent), with respect to services for which an individual is entitled to have payment made under this title, discharges the liability of such individual or any other person to pay for the services." It continues with (w)(2), which describes utilization review activities.

These services are needed (or potentially will be needed) by all residents. The facility is expected to have contracts (or letters of agreement) with an individual or company that provides these services to facility residents:

- Transfer agreement (hospital)

- Social services

- Dietitian

- Pharmacy/Pharmacist

- Medical Director

Facilities are required to provide certain services through their employees or by contracting for the services. For example, some facilities employ full-time dietitians and therapists. If they do not, they are expected to sign a contract (or letter of agreement) with an individual or company who provides these services to facility residents. Facilities are required to provide these services, *if needed* by the residents:

- Laboratory

- X-ray

- Therapy—physical (PT), occupational (OT), speech (ST), mental health/mental retardation (MHMR), respiratory (RT)

- Dentist

- Podiatrist

- Eye Care

- Hearing

If the services are not provided in the facility, the facility is expected to assist the resident in locating the necessary service, and facilitating transportation through facility van, volunteers, family members, or another acceptable method.

Other contracts and agreements

Facilities may also have contracts with other providers, such as

- Ambulance, medivan, or other form of non-emergency transportation

- Alternative housing, if evacuation of the facility is necessary

  – Transportation to alternate housing, such as city bus or school bus

- Other suppliers, such as drinking water if the water supply is interrupted

The administrator will maintain many other miscellaneous contracts, such as pest control, elevator maintenance, fire extinguisher maintenance, oxygen supplier, dialysis center, hospice, and so forth. The nature and type of these agreements vary widely, and will not be discussed here.

Quality and timeliness of service

The federal requirements make facilities responsible for quality or timeliness of service, or both. Note that for lab and x-ray services, "the facility is responsible for the quality and timeliness of the services." This is important, because it is an area in which communication commonly breaks down. If a lawsuit ensues, there is often a considerable amount of finger pointing between the facility and the outside provider regarding who is to blame. Most facilities have a contract with a lab or x-ray provider who comes to the facility. Having a method of tracking and ordering routine lab tests is essential. Once labs and x-ray have been done, there must be a system for ensuring reports are received in a timely manner, and that physician notifications and facility responses are timely.

Physician notification of abnormal values and nursing actions

Faxing a pile of normal and abnormal lab reports to the physician office may not constitute proper notification. In some situations, the facility continues to have the responsibility for identifying potential problems in the laboratory reports and notifying the physician by phone. This is especially true in coagulation tests and laboratory values suggesting dehydration, which are both commonly overlooked by nursing personnel. A nurse must review the lab reports soon after they are returned to the facility and determine whether the values warrant phone notification or further nursing action. The tracking system should make it evident if lab reports have not been returned by the lab within a reasonable period of time. Nurses should be able to tell at a glance if they are missing, then contact the lab to resolve the problem.

Additionally, nurses are responsible for recognizing conditions and risk factors for which we have nursing diagnoses. For example, these are common nursing diagnoses:

- Risk for fluid volume imbalance

- Excess fluid volume

- Deficit fluid volume

- Risk for deficient fluid volume

These conditions are readily identified through abnormal laboratory values. Dehydration is one of the most common causes of hospitalization in the over-65 age group. The resident is often in critical condition with profound hypotension before the problem is identified and treated. All long-term care nurses must be able to identify laboratory values suggesting dehydration. Blood urea nitrogen (BUN) should be measured regularly in high-risk residents. Nurses must understand the meaning of abnormal BUN values and act on them. They must be able to identify signs of possible dehydration. The nurse finding an abnormal BUN must assess the resident. Fax the laboratory values to the physician, but follow up promptly by making phone contact. Discuss the assessment findings and significance of the lab values, and ask the physician for recommendations/orders. Values of concern that warrant nursing action include

- BUN over 22 mg/dl.

- Elevated hematocrit (greater than three times the hemoglobin).

- Potassium below 3.5.

- Chloride over 107.

- Sodium over 147 (suggests severe dehydration).

- Elevated serum creatinine.

- A creatinine greater than 1.5 suggests renal disease. If elevated, determine the BUN/Creatinine ratio. Divide the BUN by the creatinine. Values over 23 suggest dehydration.

If a resident experiences any of the values listed here, direct physician notification is necessary. In addition to orders for current care, request orders for follow-up monitoring after treatment. Request a physician order for routine laboratory monitoring in high-risk residents. Update the care plan. Notify the facility dietitian on his or her next visit. Consider adding intake and output monitoring to the care plan. Carefully evaluate the resident's daily fluid intake with his or her minimum fluid requirements. Write additional nursing orders on the care plan, and pass them on in your shift report. Document the notifications, actions taken, and resident response.

As you can see, nursing responsibility to the resident does not stop with faxing an abnormal report to the physician. Your responsibility for completing the nursing process continues, even if there are no new physician orders addressing the problem. Depending on the abnormal lab value, nursing responsibility may entail a minor care plan adjustment and nothing else. Rarely does an abnormal lab value require no action at all. Grasping and acting on this simple concept will prevent many resident complications and greatly reduce the potential for legal exposure. The facility is responsible for the resident's welfare, not just passing on information to the physician.

Risk management

Your facility will have a formal or informal risk management program to reduce the risk of liability. Your insurance carrier probably has very specific policies and procedures for risk management. They can also be an invaluable source of information on reducing legal exposure. Some facilities have a formal risk manager position, whereas others have a corporate risk management office. There are no "cookbook approaches" or "quick fixes" to guarantee successful risk management. Following facility guidelines, policies, and procedures is always the best approach to take. Additionally, you and your personnel must be proactive, not reactive. Risk management and quality assurance are closely entwined. Ensuring the highest quality care for residents and protecting your facility from liability are constant concerns that parallel each other. In addition to following the formal risk-management program, some practical ways to reduce liability are

- Make customer service your first priority. Make the residents feel important and appreciated.

- Provide consistency in caregivers and in the care given.

- Ensure that direct caregivers provide input into the plan of care. Some staff resent it when the plan is devised and dictated to them by department heads who do not know the resident well. The resident will benefit because these workers have in-depth knowledge of resident needs. Staff will feel empowered and will strive to make the plan work because they have ownership in it.

- Establish solid, trusting relationships with residents and families.

- Identify dissatisfied residents and family members. Address and resolve their concerns.

- Incorporate good communication and customer relations into your ongoing staff development program.

- Strive to maintain positive relationships and keep communication open with residents and responsible parties.

- Identify potential risk factors for all residents and address them with a preventive plan of care, which is updated as often as necessary.

- Anticipate and prevent adverse occurrences whenever possible.

- Provide thorough explanations of the care plan, taking time to answer questions. Identify residents who need extra services or support and provide it.

- Use skill, tact, and sensitivity when managing adverse events. *Remain calm.*

- Document thoroughly and objectively.

- Make it a point to find out what your customers want, need, and value by asking them. In this situation, you will often get better information through regular informal meetings with residents, responsible parties, and staff than through formal meetings. Use active listening skills and compassion. Be responsive.

- Be a good employer. Make work fun for your staff. Be receptive to their suggestions.

- Ask your risk manager or legal counsel to review all contracts with outside parties.

- Verify the licensure status of all physicians, nurses, and others holding a professional license. Having a photocopy is not adequate. Check with the licensure board. You can do this online in many states. Likewise, check the nursing assistant registry. Follow state laws and facility policies for criminal history checks.

- Maintain current photographs of all residents. Keep these with the medication record, if possible. In any event, they should be accessible 24 hours a day.

- Consider using an identification band system

for residents. Color code the bands for residents in special programs, such as a red band for residents who are no code, blue band for residents who are code blue, yellow for residents at risk of falls, or green bands for residents who wander. All staff should know the meaning of the color codes; others should not.

- Keep a close eye on pressure ulcers by monitoring weekly; formally monitor them through the quality assurance program.

- Be familiar with, adhere to, and monitor standards of care. Make sure facility policies and practices reflect current standards.

- Your staff do not willfully break the law. Teach them the various laws and regulations governing long-term care, and describe how to comply with them.

- Monitor for, investigate, and analyze all incidents. Know what, how, and why they happened. Adjust care plans promptly to reduce the risk and prevent incidents from recurring.

- Study and learn from mistakes. Avoid blaming individuals. Analyze and correct systemic errors associated with increased risk and adverse outcomes.

- Develop, maintain, and promote a functional quality assurance committee. Committee members should include front line workers. Stress the important of the quality assurance program.

"The strategic planning process is not stagnant. In fact, it is fair to say that the plan is never complete. It changes continuously in order to maintain a strong presence in a complex environment. The plan becomes a blueprint and guide to move the unit, the department and/or the organization in a forward, focused and positive direction."[2]

Each insurer and underwriter is different, but to negotiate the most acceptable insurance premium, long-term care facilities should have policies, procedures, and effective programs for

- Staffing issues, including

  - orientation and initial training

  - employee background and criminal history checks

- Operations issues, including

  - medical records policies and retention practices

  - privacy and security of medical records

  - prompt reporting of potential occurrences

- Resident safety practices, including

  - fall prevention program

  - restraint reduction program

  - medication monitoring to reduce the risk of errors

  - program for residents who wander and are at risk for elopement

  - prevention of abuse, neglect, and misappropriation of property

- Resident care, including

  - pressure ulcer prevention program

  - pain management policies and procedures

  - effective program for monitoring residents and meeting nutrition and hydration needs

  - hospice or program for holistic care of residents with known terminal illness

Abuse and neglect

Many lawsuits include complaints of resident abuse and neglect, which open a gigantic can of worms, including the possibility of criminal prosecution. This is discussed in greater detail in Chapter 13. However, preventing abuse and neglect is part of your risk-management program. You should also provide ongoing orientation and inservice about abuse and neglect:

- §483.13(c), F226—The facility must develop and operationalize policies and procedures for screening and training employees, protection of residents and for the prevention, identification, investigation, and reporting of abuse, neglect, mistreatment, and misappropriation of property. The purpose is to assure that the facility is doing all that is within its control to prevent occurrences.

- Guidelines §483.13(c), F226—The facility must develop and implement policies and procedures that include the seven components: screening, training, prevention, identification, investigation, protection and reporting/response.

An example of how threads of abuse and neglect are integrated into a lawsuit is listed in Table 8-1.

Table 8-1	*Abuse and Neglect*

The ABC Nursing Home failed to protect Mary Doe from neglect. The ABC Nursing Home failed to use ordinary care, that is, failed to do that which a long-term care facility of ordinary prudence would have done under the same or similar circumstances with respect to Mary Doe's care. The ABC Nursing Home's failure to provide ordinary care demonstrates negligence with regard to its healthcare for Mary Doe. The ABC Nursing Home's healthcare for Mary Doe was a proximate cause of the injuries to Mary Doe. Concealing the true nature of these injuries from interested family members compounded the problem, adding insult to injury. Mrs. Doe was a bedfast resident who was completely dependent upon staff for her care. Personnel at this long-term care nursing facility breached the duty owed to Mrs. Doe in allowing her to develop rapid, unplanned weight loss, skin tears and bruises of unknown origin, pressure ulcers, contractures, and gangrene.

b. The ABC Nursing Home concealed their neglect of the resident by failing to inform Mrs. Doe's family members of the severity of her pressure ulcers.

c. The ABC Nursing Home failed to report resident neglect to the required state agency, as required by law.

d. The ABC Nursing Home failed to investigate the cause of abuse and neglect. They failed to ensure policies and procedures prohibiting abuse and neglect were followed.

- The ABC Nursing Home was aware that the state and federal standards for the provision of long-term care constitute the minimum acceptable standard of nursing care in a long-term health care facility. They were aware that failure to provide this mini-

Table 8-1   *Abuse and Neglect (cont.)*

mally acceptable care would result in harm to Mary Doe and other residents. Despite this knowledge, however, the ABC Nursing Home proceeded with conscious indifference and did not ensure that Mary Doe received proper nursing care and services.

- Staff in long-term care facilities are required to ensure the effective and safe delivery of resident care in accordance with professional standards and applicable statutes. Adequate and appropriate systems must be in place to ensure that quality care is delivered within facility policies, standards of care, legal requirements, and certification or regulatory requirements. The director of nursing and administrator must administer the facility in such a manner as to attain or maintain the highest practicable physical, mental, and psychosocial well-being of each resident. Effective systems must be in place to ensure that resident needs are met. This facility appeared to be without consistent nursing service administration guidance and direction. Problems such as those experienced by Mary Doe are often reflective of inadequate staffing, inadequate staff training and education, inadequate staff supervision, or a combination of all three factors. The failures listed herein, at a minimum, reveal that care rendered to Mary Doe was not in accordance with acceptable standards of long-term care facility nursing practice. The violations of the standards, whether viewed singularly or in combination constitute a significant breach of the required duty to Mary Doe.

- The ABC Nursing Home was aware of measures to provide proper services and prevent and manage complicating conditions. Sadly, this facility did neither with regards to the care delivered to Mary Doe. They did not make arrangements to transfer the resident to another facility that would provide proper nursing care to meet her needs. In my opinion, failure to use the nursing process to accurately assess and plan nursing care is a major deficiency in this client's care.

- Mary Doe suffered immensely as a result of improper nursing care, long-term care facility care, and clear violations of the state and federal long-term care facility requirements. She developed debilitation and complications from which she could not recover. Therefore, in my opinion, the ABC Nursing Home acted with conscious indifference to the rights, safety, health, and welfare of Mary Doe, resulting in serious medical complications, pain, and mental anguish.

(From an expert report of an actual lawsuit alleging progressive failures and omissions of care.)

This report builds a strong case for neglect resulting in punitive damages. These may also be called exemplary damages. Punitive damages exceed economic losses and general damages and are intended solely to punish the plaintiff because of reckless or malicious acts. The award is also intended to deter others from committing a similar act. Typically, punitive damages are awarded when the plaintiff's conduct is viewed as willful, wanton, malicious, or outrageous. (Remember the legal definition of malice in Chapter 3.)

Punitive damages sometimes exceed the amount of actual damages by a factor of two or three. In states in which medical malpractice awards are capped at a certain dollar amount, punitive damages will be limited to the capped amount. Because of this, plaintiffs often name many individuals and companies (such as the facility parent company, management company, governing body, and owners) so they can receive punitive damages from each party. As you can see from the details, the facility administrator and director of nursing are named in this report, and adding charge nurses and others would not be difficult. The risks for abuse and neglect are great. Make prevention an active part of your risk management program and avoid charges such as these at all costs.

Managing cardiac emergencies

The standards of care hold nurses accountable for maintaining competence needed to perform procedures that are part of the job responsibility. Cardiopulmonary resuscitation (CPR) is a procedure that is occasionally needed in the care of the residents. The American Heart Association and American Red Cross offer classes for health professionals to teach cardiopulmonary resuscitation and other emergency procedures. The procedures taught by these agencies constitute the standard of care for emergencies in

which the resident is choking on food or a foreign body, or if respirations and/or circulation have ceased.

Brain death begins within four minutes of the time of cardiac or respiratory arrest, or occlusion of the airway. Because of the narrow time frame, nurses must begin emergency resuscitation procedures while awaiting the arrival of an ambulance. Nurses are expected to maintain proficiency in the skills needed to manage the resident pending ambulance arrival, and for complete and accurate documentation of the event. This means accepting the professional responsibility for keeping CPR certification current. Although this is the nurse's professional responsibility, the facility may also be liable under the respondeat superior doctrine if the nurses mismanage an emergency. This is an unnecessary, avoidable risk.

Nursing responsibilities

The information below is based on a state board of nursing position paper on nursing management of emergencies in long-term care facilities:[3]

- Whether CPR is initiated or not, the nurse may be held accountable if the nurse failed to meet standards of care to assure the safety of the resident, prior to a cardiac or respiratory arrest such as

    - Failure to monitor the resident's physiologic status

    - Failure to document changes in the resident's status and to adjust the plan of care based on the resident assessment

    - Failure to implement appropriate interventions that might be required to stabilize a client's condition, such as reporting changes in the resident's status to the resident's primary care provider and obtaining appropriate orders

– Failure to implement procedures or protocols that could reasonably be expected to improve the resident's outcome

Documentation

- After assessment of the resident is completed and appropriate interventions taken, the nurse must accurately document the circumstances and the assessment of the resident in the medical record. Important documentation elements include

  – Description of the discovery of the resident.

  – Any treatment of the resident that was undertaken.

  – The findings for each of the assessment elements outlined in the standards.

  – All individuals notified of the resident's status (e.g., 911, the healthcare provider, the administrator of the facility, family, coroner, etc.).

  – Any directions that were provided to staff or others during the assessment/treatment of the resident.

  – The results of any communications.

  – Presence or absence of witnesses.

  – Documentation should be adequate to give a clear picture of the situation and all of the actions taken or not taken on behalf of the resident.

  – Even if a decision not to initiate CPR was appropriate, failure to document can result in an action against a nurse's license by the board of nursing. Furthermore, lack of documentation places the nurse at a

disadvantage should the nurse be required to explain the circumstances of the resident's death.

  – Nurses should be aware that actions documented at the time of death provide a much more credible defense than needing to prove actions not appropriately documented were actually taken.

Equipment malfunction

Emergency equipment is not used regularly. It tends to disappear. Parts become separated. Supplies such as portable oxygen and suction are not always properly maintained. Because of this, facilities should consider a checklist system for regularly monitoring the emergency box (or crash cart) and supplies. The contents of your emergency box are recommended by the quality assurance committee. List each item on a checklist and designate a time (every shift, every day, every week, etc.) for personnel to check the emergency box against the list. Make sure equipment with moving parts (such as oxygen and suction) are properly assembled and in working order. Check to be sure the portable oxygen source contains sufficient oxygen. Drugs are maintained separately, and are usually kept in a locked medication room. At a minimum, your emergency box should contain

- gloves and other personal protective equipment (PPE)

- pocket mask with oxygen inlet and antireflux valves (extra valves should be stocked elsewhere in the facility; the valve is discarded and replaced after each use)

- extension tubing for oxygen (connect pocket mask to tank)

- portable suction machine

- variety of suction catheters

- oral airways

- backboard/CPR board

- tape

- assortment of dressings and bandages

- automatic defibrillator, with pads and supplies, if available

- portable oxygen source

- assortment of oxygen masks (face and tracheostomy) and oxygen tubing

- oxygen precautions sign(s)

Use of oxygen in an emergency

Oxygen is necessary for life. Some diseases and conditions prevent enough oxygen from nourishing the body's tissues, so supplemental oxygen is administered. Oxygen is a basic need at the lowest level of Maslow's hierarchy of needs. Needs at the lower levels must be fulfilled before needs at the higher levels become important. Since the need for oxygen is a low-level need, the resident who is having trouble breathing cannot focus on much else. Oxygen is a prescription item, and a physician's order is necessary to administer it to a resident. Your facility policies may permit nurses to administer oxygen in an emergency, but if a general standing order is eventually implemented for a resident, physician notification and a proper order are necessary.

Oxygen delivery devices

Many different types of oxygen administration devices are used. The *nasal cannula* is most commonly used in long-term care facilities to provide oxygen at low-liter flows. In a cardiac emergency, high-liter flows are necessary. Because of this, oxygen masks are used in emergencies. A *mask should never be used with liter flows below five* because it may cause rebreathing of the resident's exhaled carbon dioxide, and has a smothering effect, which is very frightening to the resident who is struggling to breathe.

The *nonrebreathing mask* is a modification of the *simple oxygen mask*. The nonrebreathing mask is used for residents with severe hypoxemia. The mask has one way plastic flaps on the sides. Exhaled air escapes through the flaps, but outside air cannot enter. A reservoir bag is connected to the bottom of the mask. The combination of bag and mask increase the amount of oxygen delivered to the resident. If the system is working properly, the bag will be inflated at all times. It should not collapse more than halfway during inhalation.

Oxygen delivery systems

In some facilities, oxygen is piped in through an internal system in the walls. The flow meter is connected to a wall adapter. Oxygen is delivered when the flow meter is turned on. Some units have more than one adapter. Oxygen is always color coded with a green label in the United States. Read carefully when initiating oxygen through a piped-in system. Make sure you are using the correct adapter and plug. In facilities with piped in oxygen systems, small portable oxygen cylinders are used for transporting residents from one area to another, and may be used in emergencies in hallways or other areas without a piped-in source.

Most long-term care facilities use oxygen cylinders or concentrators. The oxygen concentrator converts room air to oxygen and delivers it to the resident. Oxygen also comes in a liquid canister. The canister delivers a higher concentration of oxygen than a concentrator, but is portable and convenient. It does not require electricity to operate. It is quiet compared with a concentrator, which has an electric motor and makes a humming noise. Liquid and cylinder oxygen is more expensive than using a concentrator. Generally speaking, a concentrator will not convert room air to oxygen in liter flows over five. Therefore, use a portable tank or liquid canister in an emergency. Do not use a concentrator.

Flow meters

The flow of oxygen to the resident is regulated by a flow meter that shows how many liters of oxygen are being delivered each minute. Increase the flow by turning the knob clockwise, and decrease the flow by turning it counterclockwise. Flow meters come in various sizes and shapes, but all work the same way. However, the various size cylinders use different gauges. If you are setting up a cylinder, make sure the gauges fit. Read the label on the flow meter to ensure it is for use on oxygen tanks. In this case, *you cannot depend on color coding*. Colors are not always consistent with flow meters, as they are for oxygen cylinders and other parts.

Oxygen regulator fires

In 2006, the FDA issued a warning about safety hazards associated with the washers and gaskets used in oxygen regulators. FDA has received reports in which regulators used with oxygen cylinders have burned or exploded, in some cases injuring personnel. Some of the incidents occurred during emergency medical use or during routine equipment checks. FDA and NIOSH believe that improper use of gaskets/washers in these regulators was a major factor in both the ignition and severity of the fires, although there are likely other contributing factors.

Two types of washers, referred to as *CGA 870 seals*, are commonly used to create the seal at the juncture of the cylinder valve and regulator interface: The type recommended by many regulator manufacturers is a metal-bound elastomeric *sealing washer* that is

designed for multiple use applications. The other common type, often supplied free-of-charge with refilled oxygen cylinders, is a plastic (usually Nylon®) *crush gasket* suitable for single use applications. When used more than once, the nylon crush gaskets require increased pressure to tighten the unit at each use. (The unit is assembled and tightened by hand.) As the wear on the gasket increases, a wrench is necessary to obtain a proper seal. Unfortunately, the pressure from the wrench increases the risk of damage to both the gasket and the regulator. Leakage of oxygen across the surface of the gasket increases the risk of spontaneous ignition. To prevent injury, FDA and NIOSH recommend:

- Using crush gaskets one time only, then replacing them.

- Cracking cylinder valves to allow the escape of oxygen before attaching a regulator to the cylinder.

- Using the sealing gasket recommended by the manufacturer.

- Inspecting the regulator and CGA 870 seal before attaching it to the valve to ensure the correct gasket is used and it is in good condition.

- Make sure the gasket, valve, and regulator are free from grease and oil.

- Tighten the T-handle firmly by hand; avoid wrenches and tools.

- Open the post valve slowly. If gas escapes at the juncture of the regulator and valve, quickly close the valve. Verify the regulator is properly attached and the gasket is properly placed and in good condition.

For additional information and FDA medical device notifications, go to *www.fda.gov/cdrh/safety.html.*

Pressure gauge

The pressure gauge shows how much oxygen is in the cylinder. It is connected to the flow meter on an oxygen cylinder. Oxygen is measured in pounds. Check the gauge regularly and make sure another unit is available before the cylinder is empty. Most facilities consider cylinders empty when the pressure reaches 500 pounds. You may have to estimate how long a cylinder will last based on the cylinder size and the number of liters per minute of oxygen use.

The formula for calculating the duration of oxygen cylinder use is listed in Table 8-2.

Table 8-2	*Simple Formula for Determining Duration of Oxygen Cylinder Use*

Number of minutes the cylinder will last = Gauge pressure in pounds per square inch (psi) minus 200 (which is the safe residual pressure) times the cylinder constant (see below) divided by the liter flow per minute.

Cylinder Constants
D = 0.16
E = 0.28
G = 2.41
H = 3.14
K = 3.14
M = 1.56

Example:
Determine the life of an E cylinder that has a pressure of 2000 psi on the pressure gauge. The flow rate is 10 liters per minute.

$$\frac{(2000-200) \times 0.28}{10} = \frac{504}{10} = 50.4 \text{ minutes}$$

If the number of minutes exceeds 60, you can convert to hours by dividing by 60. For example, you determine that a cylinder will last 135 minutes. $135 \div 60 = 2$ hours and 15 minutes.

Humidifiers

Some facilities attach humidifiers to the oxygen equipment. *Humidification is not necessary in liter flows below five. Do not delay emergency oxygen to look for a humidifier.* Over a prolonged period of time, dry oxygen may become uncomfortable at high-liter flows, but this is not an issue in the early stages of an emergency when seconds count. Use of oxygen humidifiers is a controversial subject, and some facilities have eliminated them entirely.

The humidifier moistens the oxygen for comfort and prevents drying of the mucous membranes in the nose, mouth, and lungs. The humidifier bottle screws into a male adapter on the flow meter. Oxygen passes through the water in the humidifier to collect moisture before it reaches the resident. The cannula or mask plugs into a male adapter on the side of the humidifier. *Never use tap water to fill a humidifier.* Inhalation of tap water is associated with an increased incidence of Legionnaire's disease. Sterile distilled water should always be used. Keep the water level in the humidifier at or above the "minimum fill" line on the bottle.

When the system is functioning correctly, water in the humidifier will bubble. Oxygen will not exit the tubing into the mask or cannula if the tubing is kinked or obstructed. If this occurs, pressure builds up in the unit and discharges through a pressure relief valve. When setting up a humidifier, check the valve to make sure it works by turning the oxygen on and pinching the connecting tubing.

Preparing the oxygen cylinder

Supplies needed:

- Oxygen cylinder
- Wrench, depending on type of flow meter used
- Handle or wrench for opening the cylinder valve
- Flow meter to fit the cylinder
- Sterile humidifier bottle, if used
- Sterile distilled water for humidifier (or use sterile prefilled humidifier)
- Tubing and delivery device

1. Obtain the cylinder. Check the color and read the label to verify the contents.

2. Transport the cylinder chained to a wheeled dolly.

3. Position the cylinder upright on the dolly, upright in a base, or chained to the wall.

4. Stand to the side. Remove the metal or plastic cap, or wrapper protecting the outlet.

5. Attach the handle to the cylinder. Crack the main valve for one second. Close the valve.

6. Position the cylinder valve gasket on the regulator port.

7. Check the regulator. Turn the knob to make sure the regulator port is closed.

8. Align the two holes in the outlet with the two pins in the regulator, or thread the nut onto the male adapter on the outlet. Tighten the T-screw for the pin yolk, or use a wrench to tighten the threaded outlet. If you are using a small cylinder-type regulator, a Teflon "O" ring must be in place or the connection will leak.

9. Turn the cylinder on and check the pressure gauge. The cylinder should be full. Listen for air leaks. If you hear a leak, turn the cylinder off, remove the regulator, then reapply.

10. Attach the humidifier filled with sterile distilled water, tubing, and delivery device, if used.

11. Post the oxygen precautions sign(s) according to facility policy.

Discontinuing an oxygen cylinder

Your facility will have policies and procedures for cleaning and storing oxygen cylinders after they are used. A portable emergency cylinder or transport cylinder may be used for a brief time, then returned to the storage area for reuse. Before storing an oxygen cylinder, *you must turn the oxygen off.* When this is done, a certain amount of oxygen remains in the gauges. Bleeding the cylinder is a simple, yet essential procedure that ensures no oxygen remains in the gauges. Bleed the gauge by turning the oxygen supply from the cylinder to the flow meter off (by turning the valve on top). Next, turn the flow meter on. Although the cylinder is turned off, the flow meter will rise momentarily, then the liter flow will drop to zero. This removes the remaining free oxygen from the gauges so the tank is safe to store.

Liquid oxygen

Many long-term care facilities use liquid oxygen, which is created by cooling the oxygen gas. Oxygen gas is compressed and stored in steel or aluminum cylinders. The cylinders are available in many sizes. As a rule, larger ones are usually left in the resident's room, and smaller ones are used for leaving the room or facility, and for emergencies. One advantage to this system is that large amounts of liquid oxygen can be stored in small, convenient containers which can be filled from a larger unit.

However, transferring liquid oxygen from one container to another must be done in an area specifically designated for the transferring. Liquid oxygen cannot be stored for a long period of time, because it will evaporate. The canister delivers higher oxygen concentrations than a concentrator, and is portable and convenient.

Safety precautions for liquid oxygen

- Do not transfer liquid oxygen from one vessel to another unless you are properly trained in this procedure and safety precautions.

- Never transfer oxygen from one container to another in a resident's room. Transferring must take place only in rooms that are properly protected, sprinklered, and ventilated. A room in which liquid oxygen is transferred from one container to another must be

  - separated from any portion of the facility where residents are housed, examined, or treated, by a separation of a fire barrier of one-hour fire-resistive construction;

  - at least eight feet (or more) away from sources of ignition and electrical appliances;

  - mechanically ventilated, sprinklered, and has ceramic or concrete flooring; and

  - posted with signs indicating that transferring is occurring, and that smoking in the immediate area is prohibited.

- Wear full protective equipment, including a face shield when transferring liquid oxygen from one container to another.

- Avoid opening, touching, or spilling the liquid oxygen container. The oxygen is nontoxic, but will cause severe burns upon direct contact.

- Liquid oxygen is stored in a container that is similar to a thermos bottle. Never transfer it into another type of container. Use only a container manufactured and labeled for liquid oxygen use.

- If your skin or clothing accidentally contacts liquid oxygen, flush the area immediately with a large amount of water.

- High concentrations of oxygen build up very quickly when liquid oxygen is used. Some materials are very flammable when saturated with oxygen. Follow all safety precautions for preventing sparks and fires.

- Never seal the cap or vent port on the liquid oxygen. Doing so will increase pressure within the system, creating a potentially dangerous situation.

- Keep the liquid oxygen container away from sources of heat.

- Keep the liquid oxygen canister upright at all times.

- If a bottle falls or tips, evacuate yourself and the resident from the room immediately and close the door. Do not reenter the room.

  The Long-Term Care Legal Desk Reference

Follow facility policies for getting assistance in this type of emergency.

- Review the material safety data sheet (MSDS) before using liquid oxygen.

- Store liquid oxygen in a well-ventilated area. Never store it in a confined space, behind curtains, or in a closet.

- Keep flammable chemicals and cleaning products away from the liquid oxygen cylinder.

General standards of care for administering oxygen in an emergency

Do not delay mouth to pocket mask resuscitation while waiting for portable oxygen to arrive. Initiate mouth to mask ventilation immediately. Connect the oxygen to the inlet on the side of the face mask when it arrives, using an extension tubing. Run the oxygen at high liter flows, usually 12 to 15 liters per minute, or according to facility policy.

To meet the standard of care for administering oxygen safely

- Follow facility policies for administering oxygen by standing order; notify the physician of the change in the resident's condition as soon as possible. Prepare to transfer the resident to the emergency department according to facility policy.

- Notify the physician immediately of deterioration in condition, or follow facility policy for transporting the resident to the emergency department via 911 ambulance.

- Before initiating oxygen therapy, check the resident's room to make sure it is safe for oxygen delivery.

- *Oxygen is always color coded with a green label or*

green tank in the United States. Never use a tank or wall inlet with a different color. Read carefully.

- *The parts for an oxygen system fit together readily. If they do not fit, double check the system to ensure you are using oxygen and that the parts are for oxygen therapy. Make sure you are using the correct adapter and plug.* Never attempt to modify an oxygen apparatus to fit a tank or wall outlet. If the connectors do not fit, the device is not intended for use. Never bypass or modify parts to make them fit together.

- Never force the flow meter into the wall or cylinder when assembling an oxygen unit. Forcing the flow meter may cause a valve to stick in an open position, causing oxygen to leak out.

- Obtain an oxygen cylinder or canister for emergencies. Never use a concentrator.

  - Never use an oxygen mask with a concentrator.

  - Never use an oxygen cannula in an emergency. Use a mask with high-liter flows.

  - Never use grease or oil on oxygen cylinder connections.

  - Transport oxygen cylinders carefully. They should be chained to a carrier during transport. Avoid dropping them.

  - Secure oxygen cylinders or canisters in a base or chain them to a carrier or the wall. Avoid dropping the tank. By itself, oxygen is not highly explosive. However, cylinders can explode if the unit is dropped and the valve is damaged.

- Post "Oxygen in Use" signs over the bed and on the door of the room, or according to facility policy. The sign should list warnings, such as not smoking.

- Remove all sources of ignition from the room, including matches and lighters, cigarettes, and some electrical appliances.

- Assess the resident's vital signs every 15 minutes, or according to need.

- Assess and document capillary refill and pulse oximeter readings upon initiation of oxygen therapy. Continue to check these periodically while oxygen is being used.

- If using piped-in oxygen, gently pull the flow meter to ensure it will not fall out. If the humidifier is not used, screw the triangular adapter ("Christmas tree") to the bottom of the flow meter. Connect the tubing to the point of the triangle.

- Turn the oxygen on; set at the designated flow rate by adjusting the knob on the flow meter.

- Check the flow of oxygen by placing your hand in front of inlet and feeling for the flow of oxygen.

- Position the mask over the resident's nose, mouth, and chin. Mold the metal band at the top of the mask to the resident's nose.

- Slip the elastic strap behind the resident's head. Tighten the adjustment so the strap is secure, but not too tight.

- Elevate the head of the bed when the resident is receiving oxygen.

- Dress the resident in a cotton gown and cover him or her with a cotton blanket. Avoid using wool and synthetic blankets and clothing. The resident's gown and linen on the bed absorb extra oxygen from the air. Extra oxygen may

cause objects to burn much faster than they normally would.

- Some facilities remove the call signal and replace it with a bell that is used manually. The call signal may cause a spark.

- If oxygen equipment makes an unusual noise, take corrective action or notify the appropriate person immediately. If you suspect a cylinder or wall outlet is leaking, remove the resident from the room and close the door.

Other considerations for oxygen use

Learn how to turn off oxygen in case of a fire emergency. Piped-in oxygen may be turned off at a zone valve in the hallway. Cylinders, canisters, and concentrators must be turned off at the unit. Facility personnel must learn and follow facility policies and procedures for transporting and evacuating residents needing continuous oxygen in an emergency. Follow infection control precautions when caring for residents using oxygen, such as keeping the tubing, mask, or cannula covered when not in use. Keep the tubing and delivery system off the floor. Follow all other facility policies and procedures for oxygen safety.

Managing non-cardiac emergencies

The facility must have detailed written plans, policies, and procedures for managing all potential emergencies and disasters. In some states, an emergency manual is required, listing state-specified emergency procedures and inservice requirements. The facility must make provisions for teaching employees their role and responsibility in various emergencies. Review and update all policies and procedures at least annually. Consider using "mock codes" and similar hands-on training, by implementing unannounced staff drills to familiarize personnel with emergency procedures.

The physician should be notified immediately if the resident's condition shows signs of significant deterioration, respiratory distress, or abnormal vital signs. If one nurse is on duty, notify the physician as soon as you can safely do so. Follow his or her orders for treatment. Notify the nearest relative or responsible party when you can safely do so. Many facilities have policies permitting nurses to call 911 for immediate hospital transport, bypassing the need for physician orders. If this is the case, concentrate on getting the resident to the hospital, then notify the physician and responsible party. Use a 911 ambulance in a life or death emergency, not a transfer service. If the resident is not transferred to the hospital, continue monitoring for at least 24 hours or until the emergency is completely resolved and the resident is stable.

Document the entire situation carefully and completely, including exact times for changes in condition, observations, notifications, vital signs, and emergency diagnostic tests and care provided. Document the resident's response. Complete a separate incident report, if appropriate, and according to facility policy. If an incident is of a serious nature, it should be investigated by or under the direction of the director of nurses or quality assurance committee. Some incidents also must be reported to state authorities. Follow facility policies and state law.

Incident reports

An *incident* is an unusual occurrence or event that interrupts normal procedures or causes a crisis. It may or may not result in an injury to a resident or worker. An *incident report* is a form that is completed for each accident or unusual event or occurrence in a long-term care facility. The incident report describes what happened and contains other important information. Each facility has policies, procedures, and forms for incident reporting. Some facilities use a separate form for medication-related incidents. Each state also has requirements for reporting incidents to the regulatory body. Reportable incidents usually include those in which a resident is seriously injured or dies. The definition of what constitutes "serious" also varies. In some states, fractures are considered serious, whereas in others they are not. Know and follow your facility policies and state laws for incident reports.

The ultimate goal of incident and adverse event reports is to use them for root cause analysis. This process is used to answer questions such as

- What happened?

- Why did it happen?

- What can be done so it does not happen again?

Nursing responsibilities

Nurses are accountable for

- being familiar with facility policies and procedures for incidents, accidents, and emergencies

- being familiar with and implementing the applicable standards of care for emergencies

- maintaining competence in emergency procedures

- being familiar with each resident's code or advance directive status, knowing where to find this information quickly in an emergency, and knowing how to interpret and when to apply the information

- monitoring the resident's physiologic status

- documenting changes in the resident's status

- adjusting the plan of care based on changes in resident status and assessment

- implementing appropriate interventions to stabilize a resident's condition

- reporting changes in the resident's status to the primary care provider, obtaining, and following appropriate orders

- reporting changes in the resident's status to the responsible party

- implementing procedures or protocols that could reasonably be expected to improve the resident's outcome

- following facility policies and procedures for immediate 911 transport in the event of a life-threatening emergency

Take incident reporting seriously. Completing an incident report and documenting on the medical record may seem redundant. However, do not cut corners. Be thorough and concise. The incident report for an accident or injury such as a fall should include

- circumstances of the incident

- date, time, location, shift, unit

- witnesses, staff and resident accounts of the incident

- interventions taken to care for the resident immediately after the incident

- notifications made as a result of an incident

- resident symptoms prior to the incident

- vital signs and observations made after the incident

- resident activity at the time of the incident

- injuries/medical problems associated with the incident

- environmental hazards or faulty equipment contributing to the incident

- presence of any new incident risk factors

- corrective actions taken to reduce the likelihood of another incident

Nursing actions to take if an incident occurs:

- Immediately after the incident, the nurse should

  - Get help (if needed)

  - Provide emergency care to stabilize the resident; take the appropriate action

- Notify the appropriate individuals:

  - Facility administrative personnel, such as director of nursing and administrator (follow facility policy for notification)

  - Physician

  - Resident's family or responsible party

  - State agency, if incident falls within mandatory reporting guidelines

If the incident involves a piece of medical equipment, know your reporting responsibilities under the Safe Medical Devices Act of 1990. Each healthcare facility is required to have a designated individual to report to FDA, using a special form. This is discussed in Chapter 9 of your book.

- Complete an incident report:

  - The incident report is used to alert administrative personnel to problems, to gather data, and to provide quality assurance information for studies and statistics designed to reduce incidents and injuries. Avoid referring to the incident report elsewhere in your documentation. Referring to it makes it part of the medical record.

- Make sure all information on the incident report is legible.

– Avoid referring to incident reports to visitors, family members, and non-employees.

– Avoid documenting your opinions or assumptions on the incident report. Document only facts.

– Avoid mentioning action to prevent recurrence in the incident report, such as having a piece of equipment repaired. However, if a single piece of potentially faulty equipment is mentioned in the incident report, it is appropriate to note immediate action taken. For example, you suspect a bed rail is not holding securely. Note that the resident was placed in another bed until the bed rails can be inspected by maintenance.

– Never refer to an investigation or report to an insurance company on the incident report or medical record.

– Avoid making statements that place blame. This is a personal judgment. State the facts objectively.

– Complete the entire incident report during the shift on which the incident occurred.

– Use black ink.

– Document the particulars of the incident, including date, time, and notifications. Make sure the times are accurate.

– Avoid leaving blanks in data that may be questioned later. Be objective and avoid speculation. Describe what you saw or were told by the resident and witnesses.

– State the names of witnesses. Some facilities do not want addresses and phone numbers recorded, feeling that this provides helpful information to plaintiff attorneys. Follow your facility policy.

– Never ask a family member or visitor to complete or sign an incident report. Doing this entitles them to a copy of the report. If they insist on completing an incident report, do not provide a facility form. Have them write a statement on a piece of paper and sign it. Forward it to the appropriate administrative person.

– Never alter or falsify a medical record. Complete your documentation on incidents and injuries during the shift in which they occurred. Avoid late entry charting, if possible.

• Initiate ongoing monitoring and plan for aftercare:

– Update the care plan

– Pass the information on in your shift report

– Provide follow-up monitoring and care

– Initiate the proper forms for monitoring vital signs, neurological checks, etc.

– Document post-injury assessment, intervention, and monitoring

– Document notifications

– Include your signature and title.

– Monitor the resident every shift, or more often if necessary, until the incident is resolved and the resident has been stable for more than 24 hours. Follow facility policy for vital signs and neurological checks. When the incident is resolved, make a notation in the nurses' notes describing the resident's condition related to injuries incurred in the incident.

- Initiate an investigation (This investigation is initiated/completed by nurses on the unit, according to facility policy. Investigating incidents is a learning experience for staff and charge nurses and the results are very useful to resident care and services):

  – Identify the incident or adverse event

  – Determine priorities for investigation and time frame; emergencies or environmental problems may require immediate investigation

  – Determine who will investigate the incident

  – Gather information

  – Determine the chronology of the incident; investigate the time line and potential precipitating and contributory factors

  – Determine whether a pattern exists

  – Analyze the data; turn raw data into information, information into knowledge, and knowledge into an action plan

  – Document your findings and maintain a record of the investigation and outcome

  – Implement the plan

  – Keep a quality assurance log or other record to look for trends in accidents that can be anticipated and avoided.

Documentation

In most facilities you will chronicle the incident in the nurses' notes without mentioning the incident report. Some facilities do not want facts of an incident stated on the medical record. The theory is that the medical record is for resident injury and care issues. The incident report focuses on other details and circumstances. Assuming your facility requires documentation of the incident in the nursing notes, do so after assessment of the resident is completed, appropriate interventions taken, and the resident stabilized. Important elements of this documentation are

- Description of discovery of the resident

- Treatment provided

- Assessment findings

- Notifications (e.g., 911, the healthcare provider, the administrator or director of nursing, family, coroner, etc.)

- Results of communications

- Explanation of directions provided to staff or others during the assessment/treatment of the resident

- Presence or absence of witnesses; witness statements

- Documentation should provide an articulate picture of the situation and actions taken on behalf of the resident

Potential personal legal exposure

Even if nursing decisions and actions are appropriate, failure to document can result in untoward actions by the state health department, by the board of nursing, or in a civil lawsuit. Absence of documentation places the nurse and facility at a disadvantage if they are required to describe the circumstances of a serious injury or death. Documentation from the time of the event is often viewed as much more credible than late entry charting (which may be viewed as self-serving), verbal statements, or testimony at a trial or hearing.

If you are involved in an incident in which you believe you have personal liability, you may wish to notify your malpractice insurer of the event. Remember that accurate and concise incident reporting offers a measure of protection as well as a means for analyzing trends to reduce incidents and injuries in the future. Providing the data on incidents provides an opportunity for teamwork and commitment. As you can see, the report has many useful purposes and completing it is much more than an exercise in paper compliance!

Follow up on adverse events or incidents

A successful nurse manager must know what is happening on the resident care units from day to day. Being aware of incidents and adverse events and taking the appropriate action is critical to reducing legal exposure. The primary purpose of the incident report is to communicate this information in one succinct document that can be reviewed by many individuals.

The details of an incident are recorded in the resident's medical record. Medication errors may require a special type of incident report. Although falls are the most common adverse events, an incident report should be completed for any abnormal occurrence. Studying the incident reports each day will help you

- discover the cause of the fall or other event

- identify circumstances surrounding the fall, as well as potential contributing causes

- identify methods of preventing another incident from occurring

- employing measures to protect staff and the facility against legal action

Incident investigation

All incidents should be reviewed, investigated, and analyzed in a timely manner. Astute managers will use the data on incident reports to track, trend, and profile incidents on the unit. At a minimum, review and look at incident reports cumulatively to see whether you can identify preventable patterns in the:

- **Time of Day**

  – Analyzing trends for the time when most incidents occur causes the manager to look at staffing and other factors (such as whether more incidents occur at mealtime, when staff are occupied or off the unit), leading to changes in numbers of staff and other routines.

- **Day of Week**

  – Some days are perpetually short staffed. Knowing that shortage of staff increases incidents on certain days may effect positive changes in staffing.

- **Nature of Incident**

  – Managers look for patterns in the nature and type of incident. For example, if there are patterns of incidents involving transfers or wet floors, the astute manager will institute changes in procedure to reduce injury.

- **Type of Incident**

  – Does the incident involve an employee, resident, or both? The manager will investigate methods to reduce incidents in this population. If a certain employee is repeatedly involved in incidents, he or she should receive remediation or additional education to prevent future events.

- **Environmental Factors**

  – Reviewing environmental factors may surprise you. Although most incidents occur indoors, in a temperature controlled environment, you may find confounding factors. For example, on a carpeted floor surface, non-slip soles may cause residents to stumble. A shiny floor may reflect light, causing a glare and making it difficult for residents to see. Alternating light and dark tiles may alter the residents' perception. One facility discovered that some residents perceived dark tiles to be holes. The residents tried to step over the holes, resulting in loss of balance and falls.

- **Notifications**

  – Typically the incident report will list notifications made as a result of the incident. The manager will audit this area to ensure that the physician, responsible party, or other notifications are made consistently. Failure to communicate is enormously problematic.

- **Follow-up**

  – The perceptive manager will use the incident reports as a means of following up on staff investigation and post-incident monitoring. Monitoring continues until resolution of the incident. For example, an unwitnessed fall or known head injury is followed on all shifts for at least 72 hours to rule out subdural hematoma.

Quality assurance is given various titles within the healthcare facility. Regardless of the title, the quality assurance committee should take an active interest in incident reduction. If a unit or facility has a pattern of incidents, the committee will review potential contributing factors and act on them through education or other methods of risk reduction. Most nursing personnel view completion of incident reports as "paper compliance." All papers generated by facility staff are tools for communication, and incident reports are no

exception. The quality assurance committee will take them very seriously.

Witness statements

Getting eyewitness and staff information is an important part of your investigation. However, in some situations employees make incorrect assumptions, such as believing that talking loudly to a hearing-impaired resident constitutes verbal abuse. Grammatical errors, misspellings, and incomplete sentence structure usually do not project a positive or professional image of facility personnel. In a court of law the defense attorney must try to defend the employee statements. Statements regarding "short staffing" can be particularly damaging. If documentation of these interviews or written witness statements are subjective or point blame at someone or something, you may find the investigation information used against you. Verbal and written statements may contain indefensible or irrelevant information.

Because of the potential problems with taking written employee statements, you may wish to consider verbal employee interviews. Although interviewing is more time consuming, it enables you to obtain accurate information. Write a summary of the relevant information, then ask the employee to review it and sign it to verify its accuracy. Once an employee statement has been written, avoid asking the individual to rewrite it. Rewriting suggests the investigator was attempting to get the employee to change his or her story, or was trying to influence the documented information. If it is necessary to add information, do so by using an addendum page. Written statements must never be destroyed. Destruction of records and statements suggests a cover-up or wrongdoing.

Check with your risk-management department or legal counsel regarding a format to use to document the investigation. Written information and documentation are usually considered permanent. The rules of discovery in your state may permit opposing counsel to obtain all documentation and incident investigation information. Typically, employee statements are not protected.

Risk-reduction programs

Facilities should consider investigating all incidents, even if there are no injuries. Develop or test recognized resident risk-assessment tools that meet the needs of your facility population when developing effective systemwide side rail and restraint reduction programs. No single assessment tool is appropriate for all facilities. Several different assessment tools may be needed to meet the needs of your resident population. However, you should limit the number of assessments for a singular purpose (such as fall risk or restraint reduction) as much as possible to avoid confusing staff.

All healthcare facilities have a risk-management process. Incident reports with injuries involving potential liability or those with high risk of legal exposure must be referred to the risk-management department immediately. Expect the risk manager to interview witnesses and gather additional information.

This is done to protect all parties involved. It should not be perceived as a punitive process done for the purpose of "getting" the involved employee. In fact, studies have revealed that many incidents are caused by systematic errors instead of employee negligence. However, reporting all incidents and accidents is essential despite the potential for personal consequences. The root cause analysis will reveal whether an organization or systemic failure or breakdown caused or contributed to the incident.

Need for individualized care

One reason that formal incident and fall-prevention programs are unsuccessful is that they take a "one "size fits all" approach. Individualize incident and fall prevention measures to the residents' problems and needs. It goes without saying that no two residents are exactly alike. Certain approaches are generic to all residents, and should not be considered part of the individualized plan. When every fall-prevention care plan says, "call light in reach," and "remind resident to call for help," your plan is not individualized. A review of the MDSs may reveal that the residents at greatest risk have short- and long-term memory loss. An individualized approach that says, "Remind the resident to use the call signal" is likely to be forgotten by the resident, and the MDS verifies this fact. When a resident falls, nurse managers say, "But we had a fall prevention plan in place." Did you, really? Was it generic or individualized? A generic plan may be the problem. Evaluate your plans before serious injury occurs.

For success, the fall and incident prevention plan must be personalized to each resident's individual problems and needs. This seems obvious, but in the real world it does not always happen. Review the residents' incident prevention plans. See whether they are generic (such as listing the approaches above) or individualized. Then check to see whether the planned approaches have been implemented. Look for proof of that implementation. This is exactly the type of audit that a medical-legal reviewer will do if your chart is involved in litigation. You will be either surprised or pleased at the results. (Surprise occurs if you find generic, "one size fits all" plans. You will be pleased if you find individualized plans. You will be surprised if you find no documentation that fall prevention has been implemented, and pleased if you do.) In any event, this review is an excellent way to evaluate and improve the effectiveness of your fall prevention program, and gives you one perspective on the medical-legal review.

The next step in evaluating your program is to look at the risk-assessment tool you are using. *Make sure the assessment means more than paper compliance.*

Then

- Ask the nurses for their interpretation of the residents' risk status, and how their care changes when a resident's risk increases.

- Compare the questions on the tool with the needs of the residents. Do the questions identify specific medical problems that increase fall risk? Residents have a variety of problems and needs.

- Make sure the tool you use is appropriate for your facility population. If a tool identifies a resident as being at high risk, make sure the interventions implemented (and listed on the care plan) are aggressive and match the degree of risk.

- Avoid using routine, low-risk interventions for a high-risk resident. The monitoring and protection to the resident should increase proportionately with the degree of risk.

- Implement interventions as soon as the risk factor is known. Do not wait until an incident or untoward event occurs!

To err is human

In 1999, the Institute of Medicine (IOM) Committee on Quality of Care in America released a report called, *To Err Is Human*.[4] The report identifies major areas of patient injury and death. Common errors are:[5]

- Diagnostic
  - Error or delay in diagnosis
  - Failure to employ indicated tests

- Use of outmoded tests or therapy
  - Failure to act on results of monitoring or testing

- Treatment
  - Error in the performance of an operation, procedure, or test
  - Error in administering the treatment
  - Error in the dose or method of using a drug
  - Avoidable delay in treatment or in responding to an abnormal test
  - Inappropriate (not indicated) care

- Preventive
  - Failure to provide prophylactic treatment
  - Inadequate monitoring or follow-up of treatment

- Other
  - Failure of communication
  - Equipment failure
  - Other system failure

One of the report's main conclusions (and one that must be learned in long-term care) is that most errors are not the result of individual recklessness. Most often, errors result from faulty systems, processes, and conditions that cause employees to make mistakes or fail to prevent them. The report contends that it is best to prevent mistakes by designing the health system to make it safer; and to make it easier to do a job right and more difficult to do something wrong. They note that when an error occurs, blaming an individual does little to make the system safer and prevent someone else from committing the same error.

A commentary about the IOM report in the Harvard Healthcare Review describes how one physician risk manager contacted NASA to learn how to improve quality in his hospital.[6] The following is excerpted from this story, but take the time to read and motivate yourself by this powerful safety message:

"In response to the question, "How do you get good enough to get to the moon?" Guy Cohen had no one-liners to offer me. He didn't say, 'Report Cards,' or 'Market Forces,' or 'Incentive Pay,' or even 'Accountability.' In fact, as I recall it, not one of those words came up in the time we spent together. His views of human nature, organizations, systems, and change would not permit one-line answers." The writer makes an analogy between a serious rocket problem that was almost overlooked and a medication error with the potential for patient injury or death. When asked how the hospital would handle a similar incident, he explains that they would discipline or fire a nurse. The NASA administrator's response was, *"Then you will never be safe."* The risk manager concludes, *"I think the point is clear. You have to be very smart to design a rocket right, and even smarter to figure out what happened and correct it when something goes wrong. However, you have to be even smarter still to design and lead the supra-ordinate system—not the system of work, but the system of leadership and management in which the work system will thrive or wither."[7]*

The IOM report emphasizes that the healthcare system must learn from mistakes. Think of how this applies to residents with a history of falls. Most residents who fall have a history of recurrent falls before a fracture or other serious injury occurs. Your actions immediately after a resident falls have the potential to mitigate the fall risk. Immediately after a fall, you will assess, stabilize, and treat the resident, make notifications, document the incident, and complete reports. Next, you will establish a monitoring system for vital signs, neurological checks, and other data as appropri-

ate. This is where nursing action commonly ends. Do not stop here! The actions you take from here on out will probably affect the likelihood that the resident will fall again.

Based on the present fall, the resident's fall risk has just increased. Completing your documentation and returning to your other responsibilities will not affect this resident's risk of future falls. You may need to request assistance in caring for other residents so you can complete the fall-related care. Doing so will reduce the risk of personal liability, as well as reducing the facility's legal exposure. Now you must investigate the incident and take steps to reduce future fall risk. This cannot wait until the next care conference. It must be done now.

Most falls occur as the result of multiple factors. Some are environmental, but others are intrinsic (medical, personal). Identify and mitigate as many risk factors as possible. Consider conditions such as osteoporosis or history of previous fracture, use of anticoagulant drugs, or problems that will worsen a potential fall. Social factors are probably not significant, but may be worth considering. For example, knowing the type and size of the bed the resident formerly slept in, and patterns of social behavior (such as noncompliance or need for independence) may give you insight into fall risks and behaviors. Consider the activity the resident was engaged in at the time of the fall. Reevaluate the risk factors. Complete another fall risk-assessment tool after each fall. If the resident was found on the floor after an unknown period of time, determine why he or she was not found sooner. Determine whether unmet needs contributed to the fall. This is commonly true in residents who cannot communicate their needs.

Evaluate the orthostatic blood pressure.[8] This is an

important, and often omitted, step. Evaluate the medication regimen. Research has shown that fall risk increases when residents take four or more medications.[9] Assess the resident for signs and symptoms of acute illness, which accounts for almost 25% of falls.[10] Many falls occur during the first few days of admission, when the resident is new and unfamiliar with the environment. Likewise, staff are not familiar with the resident's problems and needs. Identify as many risks as possible. Ask for ideas from nursing assistants on strategies for reducing risk. Determine what care plan changes need to be implemented. Notify the resident and responsible party of the results of the risk assessment. Collaborate on prevention strategies. Be candid when discussing quality of life versus risks of preventive care, such as restraints, alternatives, and assistive mobility devices.

Note that all falls cannot be prevented, but the facility will do all they can to reduce the risk of fall-related injuries. Determine whether fear of falling will affect the resident's future behavior, activities, mobility, or family attitudes. If so, address the fears in the plan of care. Develop and implement a plan that modifies as many risk factors as possible, based on your analysis of the incident. Implement multiple risk-reduction strategies, and modify the environment to further reduce the risk. Communicate with other staff and keep them apprised of approaches to use in care of the resident.

Individualize the plan to your assessment data. Generic approaches that are used regularly in the care of all residents are probably not appropriate, and need not be listed. List approaches that are assessment-based and likely to be effective. Whenever possible, initiate a system of documentation that reflects use of the nursing process[11] and is individualized to the resident's needs. Develop, maintain, and evaluate a format for documentation that facilitates desired outcomes. Documentation should reflect proactive care. Surprisingly, fall documentation is often reactive. Proactive care recognizes that the resident is at risk for certain complications, so preventive care is provided. Documentation may be done by means of a flow sheet or checklist. It need not be lengthy or narrative. Succinct, focused statements showing individualized care are very effective. Reactive approaches to falls defy nursing ethics and the principles upon which nursing practice is based.[12]

Regularly evaluate the effectiveness of the fall prevention plan, and document the results. Although some falls cannot be prevented, immediate post-fall assessment, regular evaluation and individualized risk reduction strategies will most likely reduce the total number of falls and risk of serious injuries.

Learning from errors

Study and learn from incidents and injuries. Instead of automatically blaming individuals, evaluate the system to determine whether it promoted the problem. Determine whether a voluntary reporting system will enhance facility data collection and risk reduction. This type of system focuses on errors that do no or minimal harm. This type of quality assurance program will help identify and correct system weaknesses before serious injury occurs. The IOM also recommends implementing safety systems and promoting a "culture of safety" that focuses on improving reliability and safe care.

Safety should be an explicit organizational goal that is demonstrated by strong leadership. This means incorporating a variety of well-understood safety principles, such as designing jobs and working conditions for safety; standardizing and simplifying equipment, supplies, and processes; and enabling care providers to avoid reliance on memory. Systems for continuously monitoring resident safety must also be created and supported.

Public image when an accident occurs

Facilities are sometimes inclined to cover things up, or to squarely point fingers of blame if an accident or injury occurs. Because of this, the incident is not adequately investigated through root cause analysis, and the accident is repeated! If a serious accident occurs

- Notify the risk manager/legal counsel.

- Formulate a public relations plan for dealing with potentially adverse publicity in advance; follow the plan.

- Begin an investigation immediately; your initial priority is to interview all involved staff and witnesses.

- Avoid pointing fingers or placing blame.

- In the initial stages of the investigation, avoid making assumptions before all facts are in and analyzed.

- Avoid making promises or accepting blame.

- Apologize, if appropriate. Several states have passed laws stating that apologies cannot be used as the basis for a subsequent lawsuit.[13]

Anecdotal evidence has revealed that an apology can persuade a patient or resident not to sue.[14]

- Avoid the appearance of impropriety by withholding information from the resident and family. One person should act as spokesperson. Likewise, information should be given to one family member who can advise the others. Avoid communicating through and with multiple individuals, who each may tell a slightly different story.

- If mechanical or electrical equipment is involved, remove it from service and promptly have it checked by an *independent*, knowledgeable person. The maintenance workers and manufacturers' representatives are *not independent sources*.

- If a resident or staff member is seriously injured, make arrangements with social services, pastoral care, mental health, or others to debrief workers and assist them in managing their feelings of pain and loss. Be careful in discussions with counselors and avoid giving out confidential information. Medical and clinical information about the event is probably appropriate only for the quality assurance committee. The counselors may be required to testify in a lawsuit later.

Chapter eight

References

1. §483.75(h). *State Operations Manual.*

2. Zagury CS. Making a difference: Strategic planning for the director of nursing in long term care. The Director. Online. *www.nadona.org/media_archive/ media/media-238.pdf.* Accessed 08/25/04.

3. Texas Board of Nurse Examiners. (2003). Position statements. 15.20 nurses in the management of an unwitnessed arrest in a resident in a long-term care facility. Online. *www.bne.state.tx.us/position.htm#15.20*

4. Institute of Medicine. (1999). To Err Is Human. Online. *www.nap.edu/books/0309068371/html/.* Accessed 12/3/05.

5. Leape, Lucian; Lawthers, Ann G.; Brennan, Troyen A., et al. (1993). Preventing Medical Injury. Qual Rev Bull. 19(5):144–149, 1993.

6. Berwick, D. (2000). Improving patient safety. *Harvard Health Policy Review.* Fall 2000; Volume 1, Number 1. Online. *http://hcs.harvard.edu/~epihc/ currentissue/fall2000/berwick.html*

7. Berwick, D. (2000). Improving patient safety. *Harvard Health Policy Review.* Fall 2000; Volume 1, Number 1. Online. *http://hcs.harvard.edu/~epihc/ currentissue/fall2000/berwick.html*

8. Orthostatic hypotension is the most common cardiovascular risk factor for falls, and the risk increases in persons over age 70. This problem involves a transient systolic blood pressure reduction of at least 20mmHg when the resident assumes an upright position. Volume depletion, bleeding, diarrhea, and certain medications commonly cause orthostasis, although many other factors may induce the problem. The drop in blood pressure reduces blood flow to the brain, precipitating dizziness, loss of balance, or fainting that results in a fall. (Colgan J. Syncope: A fall from grace. *Prog Cardiovasc Nurs.* 2001;17(2):66-71.)

9. A toolkit of best practices for care of the elderly. Presentation. Ontario Hospital Association Conference. 2001. Online. *www.joannabriggs.edu.au.* Accessed 12/22/02.

10. Kuehm AF, Sendelweck S. Acute health status and its relationship to falls in the nursing home. *J Gerontol Nurs.* 1995;21(7):41-49.

11. American Nurses Association (ANA) standards of nursing practice require that documentation be based on the nursing process and that it should be ongoing and accessible to all members of the health care team. (Better Documentation. (1992). Springhouse, Pa.: Springhouse Corp., 39.)

12. Nursing encompasses the prevention of illness, the alleviation of suffering, and the protection, promotion, and restoration of health in the care of individuals, families, groups, and communities. Nurses act to change those aspects of social structures that detract from health and well-being. *The Code for Nurses* is the standard by which ethical conduct is guided and evaluated. It provides a framework within which nurses can make ethical decisions and discharge their professional responsibilities to the public, to other members of the health team, and to the profession. *The Code for Nurses* is not open to negotiation in employment settings, nor is it permissible for individuals, groups of nurses, or interested parties to adapt or change the language of this code. *The Code for Nurses* encompasses all nursing activities and may supersede specific policies of institutions, of employers, or of practices. Therefore, the content of the *Code for Nurses with Interpretive Statements* is nonnegotiable. *Code for Nurses.* (1985, 2001). Washington, D.C. American Nurses Publishing).

13. Oklahoma — You can't use the doc's apology against him. (2004). *Nursing Home and Law Litigation Report.* Vol. 4, No. 8. August 2004. Page 251.

14. The 'I'm sorry' movement is gaining momentum, unfortunately. (2004). *Nursing Home and Law Litigation Report.* Vol. 4, No. 8. August 2004. Page 251.

The facility environment

> *"Unnecessary noise is the most cruel abuse of care which can be inflicted on either the sick or the well."*[1]
>
> —*Florence Nightingale, 1859*

Importance of the environment

Discussing the environment could fill an entire book. Many environmental factors will affect the facility's legal exposure. Those related to falls and infection control are discussed elsewhere in this book. This chapter will focus on many miscellaneous environmental factors that increase liability.

In addition to being homelike, the facility must be safe, clean, comfortable, and relatively fireproof. It must comply with the *Life Safety Code*. It must promote resident autonomy and individuality, and be flexible enough to accommodate resident needs. It must provide and promote links to the residents' pasts. Residents' rooms may be cluttered, as long as they are safe and sanitary. The facility environment must promote resident independence, self-control, and the highest personal level of well-being. It must have adequate windows to help residents maintain orientation to day, night, weather, and season. The environment must provide structure, for residents who need structure. These tags from the *State Operations Manual* cover the primary environmental requirements:

- §483.15—A facility must care for its residents in a manner and in an environment that promotes maintenance or enhancement of each resident's quality of life.

- §483.15(h)—The facility must provide— §483.15(h)(1) A safe, clean, comfortable and homelike environment, allowing the resident to use his or her personal belongings to the extent possible.

- §483.25(h)—The facility must ensure that— §483.25(h)(1) The resident environment remains as free of accident hazards as is possible.

- §483.25(h)(2)—Each resident receives adequate supervision and assistance devices to prevent accidents.

- §483.65—The facility must establish and maintain an infection control program designed to provide a safe, sanitary, and comfortable environment and to help prevent the development and transmission of disease and infection.

- §483.70—The facility must be designed, constructed, equipped, and maintained to protect the health and safety of residents, personnel and the public.

Chapter nine

Fire, disaster, and life safety

F517 §483.75(m)(1) notes that the facility must have detailed written plans and procedures to meet all potential emergencies and disasters, such as fire, severe weather, and missing residents. §483.75(m)(2) requires each facility to teach employees emergency procedures when they begin to work in the facility. Periodically review the procedures, and carry out unannounced staff drills using those procedures. The Interpretive Guidelines §483.75(m) note:

- The facility should tailor its disaster plan to its geographic location and the types of residents it serves. "Periodic review" is a judgment made by the facility based on its unique circumstances. Changes in physical plant or changes external to the facility can cause a review of the disaster review plan. The purpose of a "staff drill" is to test the efficiency, knowledge, and response of institutional personnel in the event of an emergency. Unannounced staff drills are directed at the responsiveness of staff, and care should be taken not to disturb or excite residents.

- Review disaster and emergency preparedness plan, including plans for natural or manmade disasters.

- NOTE: Also, construct probes relevant to geographically specific natural emergencies (e.g., for areas prone to hurricanes, tornadoes, earthquakes, or floods, each of which may require a different response).

Developing facility-specific disaster plans

When developing a facility-specific disaster plan:[2]

- Describe all events covered by the plan.

- Include facility floor plans.

- Outline all staff members and their responsibilities.

- Identify action to take if advance warning is available.

- List first-responder procedures, including who should be contacted for each type of emergency.

- Identify immediate steps to take.

- Describe what will be done during the event.

- Describe actions to take once the initial evacuation has been made.

- List plans for returning the facility to normal.

Appendices and ancillary information may include

- evacuation/floor plans

- emergency services

- emergency response team members, contact information, and their responsibilities

- location of keys

- fire/intrusion alarm procedures

- facility volunteer list

- facility prevention checklist

- how needed supplies such as batteries, oxygen, and necessary medical items will be moved or obtained

- how medical records and medications will be protected

- recordkeeping forms for objects moved in salvage efforts

- detailed salvage procedures

- insurance information

- in-house supplies

- suppliers and services

Facilities should also consider

- The frail conditions of many residents, including

their increased vulnerability to injury and illness during evacuation conditions.

- Time constraints related to evacuation. Moving dependent residents is very time consuming. However, residents who ambulate independently with walkers and mobility aids also move slowly.

- Handicapped-accessible vehicles should be available to transport residents to safety.

- Residents are at high risk of malnutrition and dehydration without accessible food and water.

- Residents will require medications; some of these may need to be administered during transport, such as insulin and pain medications.

- Plans for mutual aid agreements with other facilities in the area for select disasters.

- How the facility will handle an influx of unexpected residents from other facilities or locations during a widespread disaster.

- The confusion that will ensue among residents when their regular routines and environment are disrupted. Posttraumatic stress disorder is relatively common among survivors of disasters, but is significantly worse for the elderly.[3]

Fire emergencies

Facilities are expected to meet local, state, and federal fire safety codes. Many safety factors are built into facility design, and features such as flame retardant floor covering and fire doors will slow the spread of a fire. Unfortunately, smoke kills more people than flames, and it is virtually impossible to control the spread of smoke. Smoke dampers are useful in areas with common ventilation systems, but these were also not commonly used in older construction. All health-care facilities are subdivided into separate smoke compartments. This facilitates moving residents without going outside or changing floors. It is estimated that

20%–30% of the long-term care facilities in the United States have no sprinkler system because the facilities were built before sprinklers became mandatory.[4]

Several states have changed their rules and now require all facilities to have a sprinkler system. At the time of this writing, legislation has been prepared to require sprinklers in all facilities. This was done in response to long-term care facility fires in which there were a high number of fatalities. *Retrofitting* involves modifying an existing structure to incorporate changes not available at time of original construction. Retrofitting an existing facility is often more costly than installing a sprinkler system into a new structure. A large Illinois hospital was retrofitted with a sprinkler system. Shortly after the sprinklers were installed, a fire began in a basement storage area. Apparently, someone discarded a cigarette, which caused wooden pallets and boxes of toilet tissue to catch fire. The five-story building was occupied and in full operation at the time of the fire. Although some smoke escaped and patients were moved temporarily to another area, a single sprinkler in the storage room contained the fire, and damage was minimal. This success story shows that the investment in the sprinkler system likely saved many lives.[5]

Facility units should have a means of egress, or escape from each area. Two unobstructed, marked, unlocked exits are required. Locks on exit doors must be approved for this purpose, and staff must be able to open them quickly. Additionally, the pathway should not be obstructed by equipment or other items. In most states, fire inspectors tolerate (wheeled, not stationary) linen carts and hampers in the hallway, but storing broken equipment or permanent items is strictly prohibited. Each unit should have a manual fire alarm, and one or more extinguishers. Fire extinguishers must be regularly inspected, maintained, and dated.

The fire-safety portion of the state survey may be done separately from the quality-of-care survey. Many state survey agencies have surveyors who are qualified to perform the fire inspection, but some contract with the state fire marshal's office for survey purposes. If a deficiency is received, the facility must determine the best way to correct it. Structural deficiencies are more difficult and expensive to correct than many other types of deficiencies. The facility may request a waiver of the requirements if the change required is cost prohibitive. Generally speaking, waivers are granted only when cited for "less than actual harm." Compensating requirements, such as barrier doors, are also considered when a waiver is granted. Although a temporary waiver may be granted, the facility may be required to develop a long-term strategy to correct the problem. Another alternative to receiving a deficiency is to undergo a Fire Safety Evaluation System (FSES) assessment.[6] The facility may also use a combination of waiver and FSES assessment to meet the requirements. FSES uses a grading system to compare the facility with a hypothetical facility that meets each of the fire standards. To pass, the facility must meet or exceed the score of the hypothetical facility.

Safe practices

Nursing facility fire requirements are based on a combination of engineering controls and staff response. Evacuation can be particularly problematic in multistory buildings. Because some residents are mentally or physically unable to evacuate, the current life safety codes are designed to keep the fire away from the residents rather than to move the residents away from the fire. Because of this, facilities must have provisions for detecting a fire early, containing it, and extinguishing it rapidly. This requires careful planning and coordination. The time to evaluate the effectiveness of your fire plan is under normal (nonfire) conditions. The purpose of fire drills is to practice and critique the plan. Facili-

ties are expected to teach staff how to respond in a fire emergency, and to conduct regular, unannounced fire drills. Teach staff how to read evacuation maps and understand the various fire zones in the facility.

The initial response to a fire is geared toward moving residents to a safe area (behind a fire barrier) rather than total evacuation. This type of response is practiced during the fire drill. After residents are moved to a safe area, staff remove potentially combustible materials from the hallways, and close all open doors to resident rooms. Sadly, failure to conduct regular fire drills is a common survey deficiency. This is easily prevented. Holding unannounced fire drills is important so staff react on automatic pilot in a real fire situation. Pulling the fire alarm is important. Some facilities hesitate to do this on the midnight shift for fear of disrupting the residents. If you do not pull the alarm, your staff may not be able to identify the sound in a real fire emergency! Try to select a time that is least disruptive to the residents, such as very early or very late in the shift, when many are out of bed. Follow your state inservice requirements for fire safety.

At a minimum, conduct a fire drill once each quarter on every shift, and two or more disaster drills annually. Make sure your personnel know procedures to follow during a fire emergency. Consider an inservice on how to use a fire extinguisher. It is not as simple as it looks! See whether the fire department will assist with a hands-on inservice, such as in the parking lot during warm weather. Light an old mattress on fire, and have staff use an extinguisher to put it out. Fire extinguishers have an expiration date by which they must be recharged. Rather than wasting the charge in the extinguisher, this is an excellent time to practice fire fighting. Teach staff to use the PASS method:

- **P** Pull the pin out of the upper extinguisher handle

- **A** Aim the extinguisher at the base of the fire

- **S** Squeeze the handle to discharge the contents of the extinguisher

- **S** Sweep the extinguisher from side to side while keeping it aimed at the base of the fire

Cigarette smoking

Kitchen and laundry dryers are leading cause of facility fires. Resident deaths are most commonly associated with cigarette smoking. Because of this, each facility should have policies and procedures for retaining smoking materials and supervising smoking. Many facilities are now smoke free and will no longer accept residents who smoke, but most have grandfathered in residents who were known smokers when the facility policies changed. Every year, a number of lawsuits are filed related to resident injuries and deaths as a result of unsupervised or unsafe smoking habits. Some of these are settled with contributory negligence findings (Chapter 3), but in a surprising number, the facility is found to be at fault. Consider the following procedures for residents who smoke:

- Retain smoking materials and sources of ignition, even for competent residents.

- Monitor visitors; make sure they do not provide smoking material or lighters to the residents.

- Assess (and document) resident dexterity, skills, and abilities to use smoking materials, and for unsafe smoking behavior.

- Designate a smoking area. Post a sign on the door. Consider also posting a schedule for when the room is open, such as every two hours. Post the specific times, such as 8:15 to 8:30 a.m., 10:15 to 10:30 a.m., etc., if possible. Have staff document supervision of resident smoking on a sign-in sheet.

- Keep a fire extinguisher in the smoking area and be sure that staff know how to use it.

- Make sure the smoking area is equipped with a call system, even though staff are present. In a resident emergency, staff may not be able to leave to summon help.

- Maintain a supply of large, deep ashtrays. Each state seems to interpret the ashtray requirement differently. Check with your surveyors before purchasing ashtrays to ensure they meet the necessary requirements.

- Make sure the smoking area is equipped with a metal can with a lid for discarding cigarettes.

- Maintain a supply of smoking aprons.

- Plan smoking times carefully for residents who use oxygen. The resident's clothing will absorb extra oxygen. Avoid smoking for 30 minutes after oxygen is administered. A resident died in 2006 when he went outside to smoke with his oxygen tank turned on.[7]

- Maintain a log for documenting unsafe smoking behavior, such as smoking in the resident room or bathroom, hoarding matches, etc.

- Inform the responsible party (or appropriate family member) if the resident is noted to have unsafe smoking practices.

- Have the QA and A Committee formulate policies, procedures, and rules for safe smoking. Distribute these to all smokers and their responsible parties. Consider also posting the rules in the smoking area.

- Have the QA and A Committee define violations of the safe smoking policy, and list penalties for non-compliance. These should be similar to the progressive discipline system used for employees in which the penalties increase with each violation. Realistically, you cannot punish a resident beyond giving an oral or written warning. However, a specific number of smoking policy violations may ultimately result in giving the resident a thirty-day notice stating your intention to transfer or discharge the resident.

- Have the QA and A Committee formulate a job description, policies, procedures, and rules for individuals who monitor resident smoking. Include information such as how many cigarettes to distribute, lighting cigarettes, discarding lit cigarettes, when to use a smoking apron or other safety device, how to manage and report unsafe smoking behavior, how to extinguish a fire, using the fire extinguisher, etc. When formulating the job description, consider who may monitor resident smoking. For example, one resident may not supervise another resident. However, an adult family member of Resident A may be permitted to supervise Resident A and his friend Resident B while smoking. (You may wish to ask family members who supervise smoking to sign an acknowledgment that they have read and understand the smoking policies.) If a family member leaves residents alone, even momentarily, he or she will have his or her supervisory privileges revoked, although the family member may be welcome to accompany the resident while a staff member supervises smoking activity.

- Keep the door to the designated smoking room locked during times when no supervision is available.

- Make a "quit smoking" class available to residents and staff. If residents express a desire to stop smoking, consult the physician to see if a nicotine patch or other alternative is available to ease withdrawal symptoms.

Restraints

Another very real consideration for fire injuries is residents who are cognitively impaired and are restrained in the bed or chair. Their propensity to obtain matches and lighters from visitors and other residents should also be assessed and monitored. Some residents have obtained incendiary devices to burn through the restraints, only to burn themselves instead. These have resulted in resident deaths and heavy facility liability.

Fires in resident rooms

Fires occasionally start in resident rooms as a result of unsafe smoking, or heating/cooling unit malfunctions. Items in resident rooms, such as draperies, privacy curtains, furnishings, and decorations must be flame resistant. Doors are fire rated. However, there are no restrictions on clothing and bedding. Many pajamas sold in the United States are flame resistant. Hospital gowns are not. Institutional deaths caused by fire or burns are usually the result of fires that begin on the clothing, mattress, bedding, or upholstered furniture. Consider fire-retardant properties when purchasing resident-care materials, such as mattress overlays. Many of these have fire retardant protection when they are new. However, one washing will remove the fire retardant, rendering the overlay unsafe. Before purchasing overlays, find out about the fire retardant properties. Maintain a file of the details for using and caring for the overlays to preserve their fire retardant properties.

Hospital bed fires have been the subject of a number of news headlines over the past few years. Fires caused by hospital beds must be reported to the FDA under the Safe Medical Device Act. Approximately 100 bed fires were reported in the past decade. The FDA assumes that normal facility fire precautions are in place. They make the following recommendations for clinical staff related to hospital beds:

- Connect the bed's power source directly to the wall. Make sure it fits securely and that the pin has not been removed from the three-prong plug.

- Avoid extension cords, plugs, or multi-outlet strips.

- Regularly inspect the power cord for damage (this is a visual check).

- Avoid covering the bed's power cord with a rug, carpet, or other object.

- Monitor furniture placement; make sure furnishings are not placed on top of the power cord.

- Check the insulation on the power cord to ensure it is intact and not cracked.

- Keep the bed clean; regularly monitor the motor and moving parts for buildup of dust.

- Keep the area below the bed clean; avoid dust buildup on the mattress, frame, and other hardware.

- Make sure the bed's hand control cable and all other power cords are not threaded through mechanical parts of the bed or bed rails where normal bed movement may damage or cut the cable.

- Test the bed to ensure it moves freely to its full limit in both directions. In many facilities, wall-mounted outlets are located directly behind the hospital bed. Check to be sure that the vertical motion of the bed does not interfere with the bed's power cord or plug.

- Test the bed's hand and panel control, including the resident lockout features, to ensure that the bed is working properly.

- Inspect the covering of the bed's control panel and the resident control panel to ensure that the covering is not cracked or damaged. Cracked or damaged covers can allow liquids or other conductive material to penetrate to the switches.

- Check bed occupancy monitors and other equipment in the room with plug-in power supplies for indications of overheating or physical damage. Make sure that the power supplies are plugged into a wall socket where they cannot be contacted by bed clothes, bedding, etc.

- Report any unusual sounds, odors, or movement deviations in the controls, motors, or the limits-switch functions.

- Follow manufacturers' directions for bed use, recalls, and urgent safety notices.

- If a replacement mattress is needed, obtain a mattress of the proper size. This is discussed further in Chapter 11.

To read more about the FDA's recommendation, read the article on your CD-ROM.

Disaster preparedness

In addition to having a fire disaster plan, your facility should have policies and procedures for natural disasters that are likely in your area, such as tornadoes, hurricanes, floods, and earthquakes. Other policies and procedures should include

- severe weather, including disruption of services due to winter storms

- water shortage or disruption

- power outage

- chemical spills

- bomb threat

- radiological accident

- bioterrorism, contamination of food/water

- call system failure

- heat and humidity problems, including loss of heating or air conditioning

- loss of telephone system

- elevator breakdown, if relevant

- environmental emergencies related to leaving residents in heat or cold in the facility van

Sample evacuation disaster policy and procedure

Purpose:

A disaster may be a fire, tornado strike, gas leak, flood, phone or electrical power outage, heating failure, explosion, bomb threat, or any other situation that warrants action in order to protect the lives and safety of the facility's staff and residents. This policy and procedure will inform employees of the basic steps that should be taken in the event of a disaster. However, keep in mind that each situation will be different, and modifying the sequence for the procedures may be necessary.

Procedures:

1. The charge nurse will immediately contact the administrator, maintenance director, and director of nursing by phone.

2. Call 911 to report the situation, if required.

3. The administrator or director of nursing will determine whether the situation requires evacuation, and implement the facility call tree to obtain available persons to evacuate the residents to safety.

   - Administrator contacts medical records and business office personnel

   - Director of nursing contacts social worker and activity director

   - Maintenance director contacts housekeeping/laundry supervisor and dietary manager

   - When business office and medical records personnel arrive, they will contact other off-duty personnel to come and assist with the evacuation.

4. A command center will be established at the administrator's direction. The center will be in a convenient location outside the area of danger.

   - The administrator, or highest-ranking person at scene, is the "commander" who coordinates and directs the evacuation.

5. Alternate placement for residents must be arranged. The administrator, or highest-ranking person at scene, will designate someone to coordinate a shelter.

6. The administrator, or highest-ranking person on scene, will assign a second person to coordinate transportation.

7. Once a shelter is arranged, the commander designates a meeting spot outside the facility. Begin evacuating residents in an orderly fashion.

8. All departmental personnel will report to the designated location with the supplies they are assigned to gather.

9. Medical records personnel are responsible for tagging and identifying all residents upon evacuation. They must ensure that the residents' medical records (or a summary of medical information, such as a transfer form) are transported with the resident.

10. Nursing personnel are responsible for caring for residents. The charge nurse is responsible for taking the medication cart to the meeting spot.

11. Housekeeping and laundry personnel are responsible for gathering linens and supplies needed for

resident care. If possible, attempts should be made to gather resident clothing.

12. Dietary personnel are responsible for gathering food, beverages, and dietary supplies.

13. The social worker is responsible for contacting family members to notify them of the disaster and where residents are being transported.

    • The social worker will reassure and supervise family members and on-lookers who arrive on the scene.

14. Activities personnel are responsible for the facility pets, and will assist wherever needed.

15. The business office manager gathers all departmental employee schedules and the employee roster, as well as other pertinent business office supplies and records.

16. The administrator, or designated person, will check all rooms before leaving the grounds. Mark an "X" on each door to verify that the room has been checked and is empty.

    • Designated staff members will assist with a last walk through of the building to ensure that no residents, staff, or pets are left behind.

17. After everyone has been evacuated and supplies gathered, boarding of residents and supplies for relocation begins in an orderly fashion.

18. The social worker will keep an official roster with names of residents, staff, board members, and volunteers present at the time of disaster and during the evacuation.

    • Information to be recorded shall include name of resident and next of kin/responsible party; shelter transferred to and person accompanying resident; medications, med

sheet, and chart sent with resident to location of transfer.

Sound judgment and common sense are the best practices in an emergency. Remember that you may have minimal staff on duty (such as during the middle of the night) when the need to evacuate occurs. Develop an alternate plan to ensure that personnel have been assigned to cover all essential tasks. Personnel are expected to use good judgment and make the best decisions possible, depending on the circumstances.

Storm evacuations

The hurricane season of 2005 showed us that disaster and evacuation plans for long-term care facilities require regular review. Agencies that regulate and license facilities check to see that a plan exists, but do not review the plans for realism or efficacy. Realistically, the licensure agencies may not have the manpower or expertise to advise facilities on how to correct flawed plans.

In some communities in 2005, the evacuations became almost as life-threatening as the storms.[8] One nursing home failed to evacuate and 35 dependent residents drowned in post-hurricane flooding. The Houston Chronicle revealed that hundreds of Texas and Louisiana facilities had no evacuation plans. Of those who did, many plans were outdated and ineffective. Some families inquired about nursing home evacuation plans, were satisfied with the response, and began their own evacuation. By the time family members learned the nursing home was having evacuation problems, they were miles away, often stuck in traffic jams themselves. They were unable to return. Problems encountered in Houston and New Orleans should be considered when reviewing evacuation plans:

• Facility personnel were not familiar with their evacuation plans, which were outdated. Some of the hospitals and long-term care facilities designated as shelters for their residents had subsequently closed, but no one was aware of it. Although other facilities were operational, they were also in hurricane zones and flood plains, so were also in a position in which they had to evacuate. Some residents ended up in churches and auditoriums, with no beds, food, water, power, sanitation, or other provisions.

- Local emergency managers did not have lists of the most vulnerable facilities, and did not prioritize or consider their need for help. Emergency agencies did not know how to help them. There were no plans or provisions for evacuating special-needs patients, including those in hospitals who were unstable and critically ill.

- Facilities housing evacuees did not have enough staff, equipment, or supplies to care for the increased resident load.

- Many facilities said they would use school buses for evacuation. The buses are not wheelchair-accessible, and some residents could not climb into them. Several bus companies stipulated they would not be responsible for resident injuries. The school districts were not involved in any evacuation planning. An evacuee was struck and killed by a car after getting off the bus. The school district is being sued for damages.[9] Facilities did not consider that a Chauffer License was needed for individuals serving as drivers, and did not have personnel with the proper licensure. One administrator recounted how the bus company had called to inform her that the drivers had "bailed out" and they would not be able to transport her 120 residents. Fortunately, the police responded to the administrator's call for help. Within 30 minutes of her call, local police and correc-

tions officers arrived to evacuate the residents. Some were loaded into the back of an open-ended truck with nothing but a tarp draped over them to keep the elements out. Some residents cursed and refused, some were fearful, and others cried, recognizing the good will of strangers. All were eventually evacuated safely. They spent a week in the high school gymnasium before returning to the facility.[10]

- All the facilities contracted with the same bus companies and transportation providers. The overcommitted transportation providers caused shortages and panic. Some did not notify the facilities of vehicle shortages. They simply failed to respond when called. These businesses quickly ran out of vehicles, leaving some residents stranded. More than half of the homes surveyed by the *Houston Chronicle* scrambled at the last minute to find alternate transportation.

- There were major traffic jams during the evacuation. The six-hour drive from Houston to Dallas took 24 to 36 hours. Gas stations ran out of gas. The fragile residents lacked the stamina for the long trip. Bathroom facilities were limited to nonexistent. Many residents went without food, water, and medications.

- Many of the buses used to transport residents were not air conditioned. The daytime temperatures were in the 90s. The fragile residents experienced heat-related complications. Some died of dehydration and other medical problems during the trip.

- One bus transported multiple unsecured oxygen cylinders in the cargo bay. The bus experienced a brake and axle problem and caught fire. The fire was fueled by oxygen. Twenty-three residents died.

- Residents were transported without records or

caregivers. Some were sent out of state. Many were temporarily lost to their families.

- Airport triage areas lacked necessary medical supplies, oxygen, dressings, and medications. Workers did not bring supplies because they thought patients would be flown out quickly. Instead, they waited for hours to be evacuated. One situation became so desperate that several police officers and medical workers planned to go to a pharmacy and break in to obtain pain medicine.[11]

- Financial costs for the evacuation were staggering: Many paid $10,000 to $30,000 for transportation alone, and even those who evacuated for a week or less reported losses of more than $100,000.[12]

In response to the Gulf Coast evacuation problems of 2005, JCAHO published *Surge Hospitals: Providing Safe Care in Emergencies*. Surge hospitals are defined as facilities that assist the community in absorbing an overwhelming number of patients seeking care during emergencies, such as mass-casualty events or infectious disease outbreaks. They will provide care when permanent facilities exhaust their capacity or cannot operate because of damage or other conditions. This publication is available for download on the Joint Commission Web site.

Fire safety and alcohol-based hand cleansers

In October 2002, the CDC published new guidelines for hand cleansing to reduce the risk of infection. The guidelines were based on studies which showed a lower risk of infection and improved worker compliance when alcohol-based hand cleansers were used instead of washing hands at the sink. Although there are times when hand washing with soap and water is necessary, the CDC recommended using an alcohol-based hand cleaner during most routine care.

Healthcare facilities embraced the new guidelines, and quickly began mounting alcohol hand cleaners in patient/resident rooms, service areas, and in hallways. Most were delighted to see how quickly the staff complied with using the products. Their happiness was short-lived. Fire marshals quickly began citing facilities for having alcohol products, which are flammable, in the corridors and other areas. Infection control professionals protested, correctly stating that the "risk of dying from infection is greater than the risk of dying in a fire." The fire marshals were not convinced, and persisted in writing deficiencies. Their concerns were justified, however. Alcohol-based hand-rubs are a Class I Flammable Liquid, with a flash-point of approximately 75° F. Although there were several hospital and long-term care facility fires in 2002 and 2003, none was reported as being related to the use of alcohol hand-cleansing products.

The conflict between facilities and fire marshals continued to escalate. Representatives from more than 20 organizations met in Washington, DC, in July 2003 to discuss patient and fire safety issues associated with the use of alcohol-based hand cleaners in healthcare facilities. The meeting participants represented hospitals, infection control, fire safety, public health, government agencies, accrediting bodies, professional societies, unions, and long-term care facilities.

The National Association of State Fire Marshals representatives distributed their report *Alcohol-Based Waterless Hand Sanitizers Assessment and Recommendations*. This report includes the statement: "We have absolutely no doubt that alcohol-based waterless hand sanitizers will save lives. Tens of thousands of patients die each year from cross-infections, and these cleansers are regarded as a critical hygiene tool. The issue is not whether these products should be used, but how they can be used safely." The fire marshals also noted

- There is no universal fire code. National, state, and local authorities each have independent jurisdiction. Which national code is enforced, or if a state or municipal code is created and enforced, is the decision of each jurisdiction.

- Fire marshals have a legal responsibility to enforce the fire codes as they currently exist. The only way to alleviate existing restrictions on alcohol-based hand-rub placement is by modifying the current fire codes. Appropriate modifications to the codes should be crafted, taking into consideration ways to manage the fire risks (as discussed during the fire modeling study presentation).

Because of this meeting, CDC recommend that when using alcohol-based hand-rubs:

- Personnel should rub their hands until the alcohol has evaporated (i.e., hands are dry).

- Alcohol-based hand-rubs should be stored away from high temperatures or flames, according to CDC and National Fire Protection Agency recommendations.

- Supplies of alcohol-based hand-rubs should be stored in cabinets or areas approved for flammable materials.

A report was commissioned by the American Hospital Association[13] to further study the issue. Some recommendations were subsequently adopted by The American Society for Healthcare Engineering (ASHE). The results of the study indicate that installing hand-rub dispensers is acceptable in both corridor and suite locations. The results also showed the spacing of dispensers at or near each patient room entrance not to be a significant risk for additional ignition and involvement of more than one dispenser. Based on these results, ASHE recommends the following for the use and storage of the alcohol-based hand rub solutions:

- Single containers installed in an egress corridor should not exceed a maximum capacity of 1.2 liters for alcohol-based hand-rub solutions in gel/liquid form. Single containers installed in a suite should not exceed a maximum capacity of 2 liters for alcohol-based hand-rub solutions in gel/liquid form.

- Dispensers should not be installed over electrical receptacles or near other potential sources of ignition.

- Dispensers that project more than 3 inches (4 inches if a proposed edition of the *Life Safety Code* is adopted) into the corridors should be noted in the facility fire plan and training program.

- All storage of replacement alcohol-based hand-rub containers on patient floors, whatever the quantity, should be within an approved flammable liquid storage cabinet.

- The quantity of replacement alcohol-based hand-rub containers stored and used on any floor, including bulk storage in central supply rooms, should not exceed the maximum quantity permitted by the local prevailing building and fire codes.

Although the issue is not completely resolved, the fire professionals subsequently issued additional stipulations, which are summarized below. See the full text for complete requirements:

- Alcohol hand cleanser dispensers may be installed in corridors that are at least 72 inches wide.

- The dispensers must be at least 48 inches from each other.

- The dispensers must not be placed over or adjacent to a light switch or electrical outlet.

- On carpeted surfaces, the dispensers must be mounted in sprinklered areas.

- No more than an aggregate 10 gallons of alcohol-based hand-rub solution will be in use in a single smoke compartment outside a storage cabinet.

- Storage of quantities greater than five gallons in a single smoke compartment must meet the requirements of NFPA.

- Any required aisle, corridor, or ramp will not be less than 96 inches in clear and unobstructed width where serving as means of egress from patient sleeping rooms, unless otherwise permitted by the following:

  - Aisles, corridors, and ramps in adjunct areas not intended for the housing, treatment, or use of inpatients will not be less than 44 inches in clear and unobstructed width.

  - Where minimum corridor width is 72 inches, projections of maximum six inches from the corridor wall, above the handrail height, will be permitted for the installation of hand-rub dispensing units.

  - Exit access within a room or suite of rooms complying with the requirements of NFPA fire code 19.2.5 will be permitted.

  - Corridors will be permitted to have projections of less than six inches on both sides. Projections must be less than three feet in length. Each projection will be positioned a minimum of 40 inches above the floor. Substantiation: There are numerous existing projections into the required corridor width. Projects vary from pictures and wall hangings to manual fire alarm stations to fire extinguishers. This encroachment on the corridor width will not reduce the level of life safety in new or existing facilities. There is adequate width for the normal

function of a healthcare occupancy and emergency egress or emergency response.

Additional rules were issued concerning psychiatric hospitals and "limited care" facilities. This type of facility is not defined. A hospital fire occurred in summer 2004, reportedly because of mounting an alcohol gel dispenser over a light switch (source of ignition). The dispenser was known to drip. Fortunately, the fire was quickly contained and there were no injuries. Another problem was reported in the June 2002 issue of the *American Journal of Infection Control*. After putting alcohol hand gel in her palm, a worker removed a 100% polyester gown, placed it on a metal sink, and began rubbing the gel with her hands. Next, she touched a metal sliding door, causing a static spark. Flames briefly shot out from her hand, the Journal reports. The worker apparently didn't allow enough time for the hand gel to dry before touching the door.

Oxygen/medical gas mixups

In 2000, three long-term care facility residents died and seven others were hospitalized as a result of a mixup with an oxygen tank. The medical gas supplier accidentally included a cylinder of nitrogen in with the regular oxygen delivery. Nitrogen displaces oxygen and will cause asphyxia. The nitrogen tank had an oxygen label, which had been partially covered by a "nitrogen" label. Apparently, no one noticed the difference. The facility was running low on oxygen, and a maintenance worker was asked to connect a new cylinder to the piped-in system. The fitting to the nitrogen bottle was not compatible with the oxygen fitting. This is a safety feature to prevent accidental mixups. However, the employee was not aware of this feature, and switched the fitting, connecting the nitrogen bottle to the oxygen delivery system.

The long-term care facility was not the only agency in which human error has occurred with medical gases. Several hospitals had similar problems. The FDA studied the issue and discovered several commonalities in the facilities in which medical gas mixups occurred:

- The person connecting the vessel to the oxygen system was unaware that connection incompatibility is a built-in safeguard.

- The person making the connection did not examine the label on the cylinder to ensure that the product was medical oxygen.

Several other problems were identified that resulted in delivery of the wrong vessels to healthcare facilities, and poorly trained personnel connected the wrong cylinder to oxygen delivery systems, despite built-in incompatibilities. All of the incidents described above could have been avoided if a few simple safety procedures had been followed. It is important that all employees handling a medical gas be alerted to and reminded of the possible hazards associated with using medical gas. The FDA recommends implementing the following:[14]

- Store medical-grade products separately from industrial-grade products. The storage area for medical-grade products should be well defined. One area should be used for receiving full vessels and another area for storing empty vessels.

- Personnel who will be handling medical gases should be trained to recognize the medical gas labels and examine them carefully before connecting them.

- If the supplier uses 360-degree wraparound labels to designate medical-grade oxygen, personnel must be taught to make sure each vessel they connect to the oxygen system bears such a label.

- All personnel who are responsible for changing or installing cryogenic vessels must be taught to connect medical gas vessels properly. Personnel should understand how vessels are connected to the oxygen supply system and be alerted to the serious consequences of changing connections and fittings.

- Emphasize repeatedly that the fittings on these vessels should not be changed under any circumstances. If a cryogenic vessel fitting does not seem to connect to the oxygen supply system fitting, the supplier should be contacted immediately. The vessel should be returned to the supplier to determine the fitting or connection problem.

- Once a cryogenic vessel is connected to the oxygen supply system, but prior to introducing the product into the system, a knowledgeable person should ensure that the correct vessel has been properly connected.

Environmental safety and security

In addition to your responsibilities for protecting residents from fire and disaster, other environmental problems affect the facility's ability to provide quality care and increase legal exposure. Remember that the general public cannot evaluate the services the facility provides in the same manner as a health professional. Because of this, they tend to evaluate the facility by using their senses. They make decisions and pass judgment based on what they see, hear, smell, and feel. Because of this, strive to ensure the facility is respectable in appearance. Having a policy requiring beds to be made by 10:00 a.m. each day is reasonable. Odor control is essential. Odors should be situational, not permeating. They should be eliminated at the source, and not masked. Cleaning incontinence promptly, maintaining a continence management program, and keeping soiled linens in soiled containers are essential. Hidden sources may include mattresses which are cracked, absorbing urine into the foam, and floor tiles surrounding toilets. Over time, the grout becomes worn and urine leaks under the tiles.

Noise control

Environmental noise may be called the "invisible pollutant." Noise control is essential in long-term care. Surveyors will cite facilities for excessive noise. §483.15(h)(7) notes: "For the maintenance of comfortable sound levels. 'Comfortable' sound levels do not interfere with residents' hearing and enhance privacy when privacy is desired, and encourage interaction when social participation is desired. Of particular concern to comfortable sound levels is the resident's control over unwanted noise." The *State Operations Manual* also mentions excessive noise in the behavior management and chemical restraint standards.

In 2002, several RNs conducted a nursing research study in which they were hospitalized as patients.[15] The staff were unaware that they had been admitted for study purposes. The researchers measured noise levels with special instruments. The nurses who acted as patients reported that the normal unit noise prevented them from falling asleep. Once asleep, noise from equipment alarms, phones, carts, x-ray machines, opening and closing doors, using the paging and intercom system, roommates, and nursing personnel interrupted their sleep. Other sounds that may disrupt residents are door and wandering alarms, call bells, telephone systems, vacuum cleaners, floor buffers, steam cleaners, church groups visiting, and noise from televisions and radios of other residents. Staff tend to incrementally speak more loudly to be heard as the noise level in the vicinity increases. Some noises are tolerable during waking hours, but the nurses reported they were intolerable during the night. A Houston-area study was done in 13 long-term care facilities in 2004. This study provided addi-

tional information, because it included written surveys completed by staff members to gain subjective information on individual perceptions of noise and its physiological and psychological effects.[16]

The findings that resulted from the 2002 study garnered a great deal of media attention, and called attention to the need for noise reduction in healthcare facilities. Comfort, rest, and sleep are important for well-being. Excessive noise impairs oxygen consumption, disrupts immune system function, causes feelings of stress and irritability, increases heart rate, blood pressure, and overall metabolism, and delays healing. It causes agitation, worsens confusion, and may trigger wandering in residents with cognitive impairment. Residents who do not sleep well at night may be dissatisfied with the facility and the care provided. Some will be unable to stay awake during the day for meals and therapy.

The volume of sound is measured in *decibels* (db). The Occupational Safety and Health Administration (OSHA) has published noise standards for employee safety. Workers must not be exposed to 90 decibels of sound for more than eight hours. Average noise levels are listed in the Noise Levels table on your CD-ROM. The Environmental Protection Agency (EPA) recommends that noise levels in hospitals and healthcare facilities should not exceed 45 decibels during daytime hours. The nursing study revealed decibel levels as high as 113 during the night. Shift change was the noisiest time, when visitors, physicians, and nursing staff were entering and leaving the unit.

A Johns Hopkins study revealed that the average noise level of hospitals was 57 decibels in 1960, and is 72 today, an increase of 15 decibels.[17] The Johns Hopkins researchers analyzed previous research on the subject and found that in 1995 the World Health Organization had issued noise guidelines for hospitals that put the preferable noise levels in patients' rooms at 35 decibels. The study also revealed that few, if any, hospitals achieve this level of peace.[18] In the 2004 Houston study, noise levels in several facilities averaged 70 to 101 decibels. Seventy percent of the nurses (135 nurses in 13 facilities) reported feeling agitated or irritable when the environment was noisy. They concurred that staff are prone to errors in a noisy atmosphere. The most common noise-related physiological problems reported by staff were irritability, agitation, difficulty concentrating on work, anxiety, and headaches. Fewer felt physiological responses such as a faster heartbeat or flushing.

It is unrealistic to think that noise is easily reduced. However, the administration should do as much as possible to decrease noise. Suggestions for reducing noise from the Houston study include

- administrative control (of employees)
  - restricting shouting and loud talking by staff
  - limiting staff conversation
- turning down or eliminating the intercom system
- purchasing silent pill crushers
- lowering ceilings
- applying carpeting, including on walls
- central vacuum system
- separate visiting rooms (such as a sunroom where residents can visit with family and friends)
- consider noise when purchasing equipment

Suggestions from other studies include:

- put padding in chart holders

- replacing noisy roll-type paper towel dispensers with silent folded dispensers
- keep doors closed; use door closers that are quiet
- quieter toilets
- quieter ice machine (or place behind a closed door, in a non-patient care area)
- repair wheels on devices that clatter, such as some carts and IV poles
- evaluate noises from alarms; consider lowering the volume on alarms on warning devices in resident rooms while adding redundant alarms at the nurses' station
- reduce noise emitted from the air handling, heating-cooling system
- set pagers, phones, and personal communication devices to vibrate instead of ring
- limit use of overhead paging to emergencies only; equip staff with personal communication devices
- post large, brightly colored signs that say "Quiet Please, Healing in Progress" or a similar message
- dim lights and keep hallways quiet at night
- turning down televisions and radios, moving speakers to head of bed, or providing individual headsets
- identifying residents who do not need nighttime care, leaving those rooms quieter
- using enclosed rooms (rather than the nursing station) for report and conversations
- anticipating completion of IVs and tube feedings and making changes before the pump alarm sounds
- using a personnel locator system in which staff wear badges that transmit their location

- arrange for linens, supplies, and other deliveries during waking hours

- post signs over hall phones noting, "Do not use between 10:00 p.m. and 6:00 a.m."

- place foam padding in pneumatic tube holders to prevent banging when tubes arrive

Staff resistance to noise reduction may be an obstacle. In addition to providing education for all staff members, include staff from various disciplines to make suggestions and contribute to policy and procedure development.

Residents have little control over the facility environment. Healthcare workers are also adversely affected by excessive noise. Taking measures to reduce or eliminate noise improves the working environment for staff, and quality of life for residents. A quiet environment promotes a favorable image to visitors. The effects of noise and sleep deprivation are areas in which additional study is needed. The process improvement efforts from these studies benefited many facilities, and called attention to the need for ongoing nursing research. It is safe to say that the study proves that nighttime noise is disruptive. In keeping with your facility policies, do all that you can to reduce noise. Consider studying and addressing noise levels through the quality assurance committee.

Burn risk

Many physical and cognitive changes increase the risk of burns in older adults. Changes in motor and sensory perception reduce reaction time. Elderly individuals also experience diminished visual acuity, depth perception, hearing, and sense of smell, as well as deficits in mobility and balance. Individuals with cognitive impairment have reduced awareness of safety risks. Typically, elderly individuals also have very thin skin. This may result in a much more serious burn, compared with a younger individual exposed to the same agent. Some have chron-

ic diseases and conditions such as paralysis and other neuromuscular disorders, which further increase the risk. Any one of these aging changes can make an individual more vulnerable to a burn injury.

In 1981, one study revealed that 81% of injuries treated in burn centers were due in part to carelessness.[19] Another study suggests that 75% of all fires and burns are preventable.[20] Another study revealed that approximately 30% of elderly fire victims were intimately involved with the ignition of the fires that caused their deaths.[21]

Electrical burns

Review facility policies for items such as heating pads, electric blankets, and individual electric heaters. Some facilities allow these items if they are Underwriter's Laboratories (UL) approved, and if the maintenance department checks the item for safety before use. The resident or responsible party may be asked to sign a waiver releasing the facility from liability for injury. Some facilities do not allow these items at all. Follow your facility policies and state laws. If electronic heating devices are permitted, make sure residents and staff are familiar with safety precautions and safeguards for their use. Maintain a master listing of where these items are in the facility. Inspect them regularly for safety and document your findings.

Use grounded (three-prong) plugs, whenever possible. Never bend or break a three-prong plug so it fits in a two-slot outlet or extension cord. In general, avoid extension cords and plug extenders. Do not place furniture on top of electrical cords or roll carts over them. Electrical burns may be caused by electrical current, power lines, appliances, certain batteries or lightning. Other considerations are

- Personnel on each shift should know the location of the main power grid. Label all valves, panels, boxes, and doors to rooms containing electrical panels, sprinklers, water, and gas shut-offs. If these areas are locked, make sure the keys are available 24 hours a day.

- Assign a worker to check cords and appliances in resident rooms periodically. Monitor for cracked, frayed, or split cords and for loose or damaged plugs. If found, repair or replace these items immediately.

- Make sure that cords are not pulled tight or wrapped around themselves. This causes damage and overheating.

- Monitor for and repair nonworking outlets. Also be alert to light switches that are hot to the touch, and lights that flicker or spark.

- Use bulbs that are the appropriate wattage for the size of the fixture. Over-bed lights are sometimes a problem. The fixtures melt if the wattage is too high. Appliances are usually labeled with the correct wattage. If you are unsure, do not exceed 60 watts.

If a resident or employee has received an electrical shock, avoid going near or touching the victim until you are sure the power has been disconnected, the plug has been disconnected from the source, or the victim is free from the electricity. Once he or she is removed from the source, treat injuries, such as burns. Electric shock can cause respiratory and cardiac arrest, so be prepared to provide resuscitation and defibrillation.

Burns from hot water

In addition to the risk of burns from fire, careless smoking, and burning through restraints, residents are also at risk for burns from hot water and other hot liquids. Your facility should have policies for food temperature. In most facilities, coffee and other hot liquids should be served at 140° F to 150° F. Follow your state laws and dietitian's recommendations. Regularly use a food thermometer in a test tray to check food temperature at point of service.

All states have laws governing water temperature in resident care areas. Areas such as the laundry and dietary department may have water as hot as 185° F, but in most states, water on resident units and in bathing areas should not exceed 120° F. Learn what your state's maximum stipulation is. The maintenance worker or other designated person should check water temperature at random faucets at least once a week, or more often. Keep a log listing the date, location, and temperature. Most adults will experience a third-degree (full thickness) burn if exposed to water at

- 155° F for one second

- 140° F for five seconds

- 133° F for fifteen seconds

- 120° F for five minutes

However, because the skin in elderly residents is thinner than younger adults, a shorter exposure time may result in more serious burns. Residents with altered peripheral circulatory disorders such as diabetes are at increased risk for scald injuries, as well as for increased complications if a burn injury occurs.[22] Red and blue faucet handles may be purchased for about $10 each as a warning to residents who care for themselves. Use the red for the hot water and blue for cold. Colored duct tape may be used temporarily, but over time, tape on faucets presents a host of infection control problems. A better solution may be to apply the tape to the wall behind the faucet.

Keep a supply of thermometers available for checking food and beverage temperature and water temperature. Use utility thermometers for these tasks, not clinical thermometers. Make sure staff know when and how to use these thermometers to check items such as food and bath water, and stress the importance of using them. If no thermometer is available, instruct staff to use common sense. For example, check food temperature by dropping a few drops onto the inner forearm with a spoon. If bath water is steaming, check the temperature with your own elbow. Likewise, check water temperature on the forearm. Although regulators are required to maintain safe water temperature, these devices sometime fail. Impress the need for double checking temperatures of all hot items before exposing a resident to a potential burn risk.

Sometimes we correct one problem, then cause another. Legionnaires' disease is known to develop in the water supply system. It has been spread by aerosolized water, including decorative fountains and hot tubs. The bacteria that cause Legionnaires' disease

- are dormant in water that is 68° F

- can live in water at 122° F, but cannot multiply at this temperature

- will die in five to six hours in water that is 131° F

- will die within 32 minutes in water that is 140° F

- will die within two minutes in water that is 151° F

- will die immediately in water that is 158° F

Legionnaires' disease can and does occur in long-term care facilities. There were outbreaks in facilities in both the US and Canada in 2004 and 2005. Because of this, the hot water in the water heater should be 140° F to 180° F. Water this hot may be necessary in the laundry and dietary departments. A valve called a *master tempering valve* should be used for water going to resident care areas. This type of valve reduces water temperature to within safe limits and reduces the growth of bacteria. However, valves are mechanical devices that some-

times fail, so routine temperature checks and logs are necessary. This safeguard will reduce the risk of burns and scalds, while inhibiting bacterial growth.

For additional guidance on water temperature and environmental infection control, see *Morbidity and Mortality Weekly Report,* June 6, 2003/Vol. 52/No. RR-10, "Guidelines for Environmental Infection Control in Health-Care Facilities: Recommendations of CDC and the Healthcare Infection Control Practices Advisory Committee (HICPAC)."

Chemical burns

Chemical burns may be caused by ingestion of, or contact with, many disinfectant and cleaning products, lawn and garden products, or other chemicals. Even personal hygiene and cosmetic items such as nail polish remover and denture cleaning tablets have the potential to harm a cognitively impaired person if ingested. When facilities stock cleaners and other chemicals, the manufacturer or supplier must provide a material safety data sheet (MSDS) for each. Make sure to keep these in an organized file in an accessible area. Other safety precautions include:

- Some products come in large containers that are cumbersome, difficult to handle and dispense, and prone to spills. Ask the distributor to provide smaller, properly labeled containers for the product. Never repackage them into another type of container.

- Keep dangerous products such as denture cleaner and nail polish remover in a locked cupboard for resident use. Provide the item promptly upon request.

- Keep chemicals and cleaning products in locked cupboards when not in use. When these products are used in resident care areas, they should be under visual control of the employee.

This means the employee must never turn his or her back on the product.

- Never mix chemicals. For example, bleach and ammonia are common chemicals found in a laundry. One would think that mixing them together would create a super cleaner. Instead, the resulting product becomes a toxic gas, called a chloramine, that may be fatal upon inhalation. At the very leasy, chloramines burn the mucous membranes and are very painful when inhaled. A combination of bleach and ammonia was used in varying concentrations during World Wars I and II to create weapons using toxic fumes. You may have heard about "mustard gas." This is the nickname used for the chloramine product. Depending on the concentration of the mixture, a combination of these two products can cause:

  - *Chlorine* gas, which is harmful or fatal if inhaled; it causes a very painful death

  - *Nitrogen trichloride*, which is toxic and explosive

  - *Hydrazine*, which is a component of rocket fuel; the heat is so great that the mixture is unstable and prone to explosion

(Bleach and ammonia in combination is used as an example here. Bleach also reacts violently with a number of acids. In any event, this common household product should never be mixed with anything other than water. However, facilities must avoid mixing all chemicals randomly. Bleach will also react with hydrogen peroxide, oven cleaners, and some insecticides. Pool chemicals may contain calcium hypochlorite or sodium hypochlorite [active ingredients in bleach] and should not be mixed with other cleaning products.)

- Wear utility gloves when using chemicals. Make sure goggles, masks, and other protective items are available, if needed.

- Store chemicals and flammable liquids in a cool, dry area. Avoid sources of heat.

- Do not use flammable products in areas where oxygen is stored or in use.

Emergency burn care

Burns are among the most complex injuries seen in the emergency department. Rapid evaluation and management are essential to preventing complications. Assess the resident. The ABC's are your first priority. Document vital signs and monitor for signs and symptoms of shock. Treat the burn with first aid measures, depending on the cause. Identify and consider underlying problems, such as diabetes or heart disease. Monitor for complications of these chronic conditions. You should also:

- Stop the burning process by pouring clean, cool water over the burn, or hold the area under cool running water for a minimum of 10 minutes up to a maximum of 20 minutes. Do not use ice or any method that will cause frostbite or freezing of the skin. Monitor for signs and symptoms of hypothermia.

- Assess the extent of the injury. If widespread or complex, facilitate immediate transfer to the emergency department.

Thermal and chemical burns:

- Apply personal protective equipment (gloves, eye protection), if necessary, and gently brush any dry chemicals off the skin.

- Water can be safely used for chemical burns, unless the burn is caused by products containing metallic sodium, potassium, or calcium. These items react violently on contact with any aqueous solution, resulting in the production and release of heat, noxious solutions, and hydrogen. Because of this, these chemicals are normally available as an oil-based solution, which should be wiped off with a clean, dry cloth or dressing. Check the product MSDS, which should be readily available in your facility.

- If the eyes are involved, continue flushing with water until an ambulance arrives.

- Remove jewelry and other sources of metal, such as zippers or fasteners. Remove clothing, if necessary, but avoid pulling clothing that has adhered to the skin, causing further tissue damage. Remove any contaminated clothing. Be careful not to expose uninjured body parts or yourself to the chemical.

- Do not apply creams, ointments, or other topical products.

- Cover the area with a suitable dressing. Select a dressing that will not adhere to the wound. Some specialists recommend covering the skin with a clear film food wrap, such as Saran Wrap®. If this product is used, unroll the outside of the film roll and discard it. Apply the film in small, overlapping sections. Make sure it is not too tight. The film may be covered with a dressing or bandage.

- If the resident will not be transferring to the hospital, assess his or her need for tetanus prophylaxis.

- Assess and document the depth, size and location of the injury.

- Take appropriate measures to relieve pain and edema; avoid ice.

- Take measures to reduce the risk of infection.

- Protect the wound from further trauma.

- Assess for and manage pain.

Medical intervention

The physician and responsible party must always be notified if a resident is burned. In some situations, the resident may remain in the facility, whereas others require prompt, acute care intervention. As a general rule, burns that should be seen in the emergency department are those that:

- are larger than the size of the palm of the resident's hand

- are circumferential, such as wrapping around a body part or extremity

- involve the face, airway, hands, feet, major joints, or genital area

- are of chemical or electrical origin, because damage may not be immediately obvious

- occurred in a small, enclosed space, because of the risk of smoke inhalation

- are white, gray, leathery, or painless

- result in complications related to underlying chronic illness, unstable vital signs, or shock

Lockout/tagout

Lockout/tagout is an OSHA-required procedure for deactivating electrical, mechanical, hydraulic, and pneumatic equipment until it can be serviced. A locking device is placed on the equipment in a location or manner that prevents the equipment from being turned on or used. The lock should be positioned to hold an energy-isolating device in a safe position. A tag notes the equipment is broken and warns others not to use it. If a piece of equipment is locked and tagged, do not attempt to use it. Locks and tags must be removed only by the person who applied them, after the device is repaired.

Generally speaking, the maintenance department will lock and tag items for repair. However, all other personnel must understand the meanings of the locks and tags and actions to take if a piece of equipment is locked out. Equipment that is locked and tagged increases the risk of injury and death if it is used improperly. OSHA has inservice requirements for this program. Make sure employees have been oriented and inserviced on lockout/tagout policies and procedures.

Intruders

Employees usually feel safe at work, and may not consider the safety risks to residents and staff associated with intruders. Facilities should have security policies and procedures, and employees must be prepared to handle potentially violent situations, including drug holdups, personal threats, sexual assault, and potential injuries to residents. Employees must be aware of who is wandering the hallways, and be prepared to call law enforcement to have unauthorized individuals removed. Remember, the facility and its employees are responsible for resident safety. Lock doors in the late evening, and take safety and security issues seriously.

Handguns

Each year, a number of resident and employee shootings are reported in long-term care facilities. In some states, it is legal for residents to carry concealed weapons. However, healthcare facilities may put a sign on the entrance noting that guns are not permitted in the facility. If the signs are posted at the entrance, only law enforcement personnel may carry guns in the facility. All facilities should have policies and procedures advising staff on actions to take if a handgun is noted.

Visitor safety

The long-term care facility is a public area, and has a duty to use reasonable care to keep the property, parking lot, and premises in a reasonably safe condition. Visitors are considered invited guests, so the facility bears some responsibility for their safety. Facilities should be reasonably safe and not expose visitors to unnecessary danger. At the very least, post signs or warn visitors of dangerous areas. Although the facility is not directly responsible for visitor safety, anyone can bring a civil claim for "premises liability." This means that an unsafe condition caused injury. The injured party would bring a claim, alleging that improper maintenance or other negligence resulted in an injury. Areas and problems that commonly result in claims caused by injuries outside the facility are

- improper removal of ice and snow; sidewalks and parking lot slippery

- poorly maintained walking surfaces outside, such as holes, cracked or uneven cement

- poor or inadequate lighting, including bulbs burned out in parking lots

The entrance to the facility is a common area for falls to occur, especially when the outside conditions are wet. The individual enters the facility with wet footwear, and slips on the tile floor. Wrinkled or wadded floor mats inside the doorway have also been implicated in falls. The entry area should have a safety mat. **A pattern for keeping the floor mat smooth is on your CD-ROM.** However, make sure that the height is not significantly different from (elevated above) the primary flooring. Falls may also occur if the carpeting is wet. The shoes pick up moisture, causing the individual to slip and fall when he or she reaches the tile. Cordon off and clearly mark wet areas on all floor surfaces. Mop spills immediately and place a "wet floor" sign.

The facility should also take care to avoid an obstacle

course in the hallway. Place all equipment on one side, leaving the handrail on the opposite side free for use by residents and visitors. Make sure that unused equipment is removed from resident rooms. Never obstruct exits and fire doors.

The facility should have policies and procedures for visitor injuries. At the very least, a nurse should assess an injured visitor and complete an incident report. Inform the facility administrator, risk-management department, and insurance carrier if an injury to a visitor occurs.

Remember, unsafe conditions in the facility may also cause injury to a resident or employee. Facilities are not insurers of resident safety, but owe them the duty of ordinary care to protect them from danger or injury which can reasonably be anticipated from unsafe conditions or acts of others. The major legal issue is foreseeing potentially unsafe conditions. In recent court decisions, the courts have recognized that facilities are businesses, and the facility cannot accommodate the needs of each employee, resident, and visitor to the degree that protection and accommodation disrupt the normal operations of the facility.

Environmental rounds

The administrator should assign all department heads, as well as selected staff employees, to perform random environmental rounds in their departments on a regular basis. Forms should be available for employees to rate conditions in their assigned areas. These should be objective, although a space should be available for comments and remarks. Your facility may have quality assurance audit forms available. **Additional forms are available on the CD-ROM accompanying this book.** If no checklist is available, develop one! The forms on your CD-ROM entitled, "QA & A Audit" and "Environmental Audit" may be used as a template to personalize to meet your facility's specific needs.

General environmental safety

Environmental safety is a broad topic, and sometimes environmental challenges become so overwhelming to residents that they develop irrational fears and maladaptive behaviors that increase the risk of injury. Rather than focusing on specific environmental changes, first focus on the individual resident's problems and needs. When evaluating a resident and his or her circumstances, consider issues that increase the risk of falls. To some extent, these are personal issues, so the list below is not necessarily all inclusive. Common risk factors that should be considered include

- Unfamiliar surroundings (such as new admissions, when a resident will be discharging to the hospital, an adult child's home, or another facility)

- History of falls within the previous year

- Dizziness, unsteady gait, or other balance problems

- Cardiovascular disease

- Neurological disease

- Postural hypotension

- Slow reflexes

- Edema

- Recent surgery

- Paresis or paralysis

- Lower extremity injury, presence of a bandage, splint, or cast

- Use of a walker, cane, crutches, or wheelchair

- Weakness

- Seizure disorder

- Impaired vision

- Hearing impairment

- Stiffness or immobility in joints caused by arthritis or an injury

- Cognitive impairment

- Inability to understand or follow directions

- Impaired judgment (besides being caused by cognitive impairment, judgment can also be affected by denial of illness or disability, or embarrassment over limitations)

- Urgency or incontinence

- Episodes of diarrhea

- Drugs:

  – with the potential to affect thought processes and mental clarity

  – laxative and diuretics

  – polypharmacy or use of multiple medications

  – other drugs, such as antihypertensives

  – drug-drug, food-drug, or supplement-drug interactions

  – can the resident take his or her medications correctly and as ordered

- Inappropriate footwear, including stocking feet

- Clothing of appropriate length; pants, nightgowns and robes are not too long so as to cause tripping

- Wandering behavior

Determine whether preventive maintenance is needed. Ask the physical and occupational therapists to assist with environmental safety evaluations whenever possible. They can also make recommendations for maintaining self-care and promoting safety.

Primary goals for environmental safety involve a variety of factors, level of resident independence, knowledge, and learning needs. Being independent should not be so exhausting that it increases the risk of falls. If this is the case, assist the resident in learning modified independence, such as using a wheelchair for long distances instead of a cane or walker. (However, discourage wheelchair use for short distances if the resident can ambulate safely.) Remember that the wheelchair is a mobility device, and not a transportation device. The resident will weaken and eventually become non-ambulatory if he or she unnecessarily rides in a chair all the time. Other goals and considerations for environmental safety include

- Promoting general safety, including but not limited to falls

- Facilitating independence as much as possible, but avoiding overwhelming, tiring, or otherwise endangering the resident

- Ensuring that needed equipment and adaptive devices are available

- Need for a gait belt and one or two assists to transfer and ambulate

- Counseling the resident if denial or embarrassment are safety risks for the resident

- Negotiating and communicating changes with the resident and gaining his or her acceptance and cooperation

- Ensuring the resident's security in making environmental modifications and making sure nursing assistants understand changes for providing care, if applicable

Specific safety factors are usually covered by institutional building codes and governmental regulations. However, if the resident will be discharging to a private home, additional teaching is necessary. **A list of safety factors for the home setting is on your CD-ROM.**

Quality assurance

§483.75(o) Quality Assessment and Assurance

(1) A facility must maintain a quality assessment and assurance committee consisting of—

    (i)   The director of nursing services;

    (ii) A physician designated by the facility; and

    (iii) At least 3 other members of the facility's staff.

Intent §483.75(o)

The intent of this regulation is to ensure the facility has an established quality assurance committee in the facility which identifies and addresses quality issues, and implements corrective action plans as necessary.

Interpretive Guidelines §483.75(o)

The quality assessment and assurance committee is responsible for identifying issues that necessitate action of the committee, such as issues which negatively affect quality of care and services provided to residents. In addition, the committee develops and implements plans of action to correct identified quality deficiencies. The medical director may be the designated physician who serves on this committee pursuant to §483.75(o)(1)(ii).

The quality assurance committee is discussed in detail in Chapter 21. This committee, or other designated committee should review the results of the audits and take the appropriate action. Remember to give employees ownership in plans for corrective action. This will increase the likelihood of success!

Safe Medical Devices Act of 1990

The Safe Medical Devices Act of 1990 became effective November 28, 1991. The reporting requirements were modified slightly in 1996. The act requires all healthcare facilities to report to the Food and Drug Administration (FDA) any deaths in which a medical device was a causative or contributing factor. This reporting is mandatory under federal law. Facilities are also required to notify the manufacturer of the device if a serious injury or illness occurs. These reports are sent to the FDA only if the manufacturer is unknown. Deaths must be reported to both the FDA and the device manufacturer. Reports must be submitted within 10 working days. All resident information reported to the FDA is kept confidential.

An *adverse event* is a serious, undesirable event that results from using a medical product. This includes reporting related to user error associated with the device. The event must be reported if the resident dies, is at substantial risk of death, or the facility suspects that continued use of the product increases the risk of death. A *serious injury* or *serious illness* is life threatening, results in permanent impairment of a body function or permanent damage to the body, or necessitates immediate medical or surgical intervention to preclude permanent impairment of a body function or permanent damage to a body structure. Examples of deaths and serious injuries include the following:

- A resident is trapped between the side rail, headboard, or footboard and mattress and asphyxiates.

- A resident in a vest restraint attempts to climb over the rails, and is suspended by the restraint. She dies of strangulation.

- An intravenous pump malfunctions, resulting in a liter of fluid infusing rapidly. The resident dies of fluid overload. A serious injury occurs if the resident is injured from excessive dosing of a medication as a result of pump failure, or develops a condition such as congestive heart failure as a result of excessive fluid.

- An oxygen concentrator fails to convert room

air into oxygen. The resident's condition worsens as a result, and he is hospitalized.

Other situations that should be reported include those that

- result in hospital admission

- prolong the resident's stay in the facility

- result in a significant, persistent, or permanent change or impairment to the resident's body structure, function, or activities, or quality of life

- cause a congenital anomaly because of exposure to a product prior to or after conception

- require medical or surgical treatment to prevent permanent impairment or damage

Problems must also be reported if there is a concern about quality, performance, or safety. However, this reporting is covered by the voluntary reporting program (see below). Problems in this category may occur during manufacturing, storage, or shipping.

For example:

- product contamination

- defective components

- poor packaging or product mix-up

- questionable stability

- device malfunctions

- labeling concerns

Reporting adverse events and problems related to nutritional supplements and medications is important, but *voluntary*. The FDA uses these reports to investigate and identify problems. They will determine the severity of the hazard, if any, and inform the healthcare community if corrective action is necessary. The FDA enters the reported information into their database. Part of their evaluation involves comparing

the product or device with other, similar reports. This process helps them correct and repair risks associated with using the device. If the risk is identified as high, the FDA may issue a product safety alert or product recall. This was done for Vail beds in 2005, and the manufacturer subsequently went of out business, because it could not comply with the FDA's ongoing requirements. Vail bed systems are padded beds covered with nylon netting that is zipped to enclose the resident. They are an alternative to physical or drug restraint to reduce falls or other injuries. Although this action was considered a recall, the manufacturer went out of business and did not take the beds back. The FDA advised that if the Vail bed was the only option, users should follow new safety precautions. They specified that the beds should not be used for residents who are less than 45 inches in height or weigh less than 46 pounds. This is an example of a useful, well-known product with unsafe components that increased the risk of strangulation and suffocation in certain circumstances.

Nurses are usually the first to recognize medical device problems. Pharmacists are often the first to identify and report drug-related problems. The identities of voluntary reporters are confidential unless the reporter authorizes the FDA to release their identity. This is sometimes done so the reporter can work with the device manufacturer for further follow-up.

If this is the case, his or her identity is concealed from the public. However, in the recent past, identities of both residents and voluntary reporters were disclosed in lawsuit discovery motions. The FDA believes that concealing the identity of voluntary reporters is key to encouraging professionals to report. Because of this, a 1995 law extended protection against disclosure to voluntary reporters by preempting state discovery laws.[23]

Changes resulting from the reporting system include label changes and changes in instructions for use. Boxed warnings are used on the label for the most serious notices for safe product use. Recalls and complete product withdrawals are also some of the most serious actions that the FDA undertakes. Products may be removed from the market temporarily or permanently, depending on the problem and degree of risk. In some cases, product availability is restricted to certain highly controlled circumstances.

Facilities must also provide the FDA with a summary of all reporting events annually by July 1. The report for the second half of the year must be submitted by January 1. Reports must be submitted even if no adverse events have occurred. Facilities must maintain records of adverse events for at least two years. This is the information pertaining to the incident and reported to the FDA. It is not a copy of the entire medical record.

Before the Safe Medical Devices Act of 1990 was enacted, manufacturers and importers were required to report injuries and deaths to the FDA. Unfortunately, facilities were not reporting problems to manufacturers, so many incidents were unreported. Although the act has been in place since 1991, many nurses are unaware of the requirements, and some reportable incidents and deaths continue to be unreported. Restraints, wheelchairs, side rails, and other equipment used daily in facilities are covered by the reporting act.

The facility must have written policies and procedures related to the reporting process. Facilities should develop written procedures for identification, evaluation, and timely submission of reports and compliance with recordkeeping requirements. Each facility is required to designate an individual to report to the FDA. In long-term care facilities, this is usually the administrator or his or her designee. A special form is used for written

reports. Information and forms for reporting ate available at *www.fda.gov/medwatch/getforms.htm*. Nurses must be alert to reporting requirements, including potential relationships between an injury or death and medical devices. All professionals have an important responsibility in the reporting process. The report from your facility may be the only notification the FDA receives. Reporting has the potential to protect many residents from future harm. Reporting forms and guidelines are available from

Food and Drug Administration
5600 Fisher's Lane (HFZ-240)
Rockville, MD 28057

To subscribe to email alerts, use the link at *www.fda.gov/medwatch/elist.htm*. Additional information, tools, instructions, and forms for mandatory and voluntary reporting are online at *www.fda.gov/medwatch/* and *www.fda.gov/cdrh/mdr/* and *www.regsource.com/*.

Additional information and tools for reporting are online at *www.fda.gov/medwatch/* and *www.fda.gov/cdrh/mdr.html* and *www.regsource.com/*

Grannycams/hidden cameras

Some states have enacted laws addressing the use of hidden cameras, or "grannycams." These have been widely used by resident families throughout the United States. No law expressly prohibits the use of cameras, but their use is accompanied by a host of barriers, potential residents' rights violations and strong opposition of the long-term care industry. In 2006, the Office of the New York Attorney General worked with family members who planted hidden cameras in a long-term care facility for surveillance purposes. The investigation led to the arrests of 14 employees and a civil action against the owner of the facility. The cameras allegedly revealed employees napping, leaving the facility, and watching movies instead of caring for the residents. One man was allegedly not given incontinent care or repositioned for 76 hours. Staff also allegedly took call signals away from residents and falsified documentation.[24] The Attorney General's report on video surveillance activities urges consumers to visit facilities, actively monitoring the care, speaking with other family members or friends in the home, and consulting knowledgeable professionals to ensure proper care is being given.

Hidden cameras raise a number of resident rights, privacy, and legal issues that have not been resolved by the courts. Some facilities welcome hidden cameras, believing that staff respond to the threat of being watched. With competent staff, cameras provide visual evidence of staff doing good work. They are just another tool to ensure quality care. Critics say cameras make it difficult for facilities to attract and retain qualified staff in an industry that is plagued with turnover, where the work is demanding and pay is low. They also believe their care will be evaluated by uninformed, uneducated family members who will misconstrue their actions. Some fear the videotape will make them the target of aggressive attorneys. On the opposite side of this argument, employees are sometimes wrongly accused of neglect, theft, abuse, and other actions. The cameras protect them by providing a record of their actions.

Many employees, such as bank tellers and cashiers at convenience stores work under constant electronic surveillance. Employees have no right to privacy on the job. However, there are various laws covering illegal covert surveillance. A few facilities are equipped with web cams in external and internal public areas, so family members can log onto the Internet and check on loved ones. Families may pay a nominal fee to cover the cost of this convenience. Some of these facilities have experienced substantial reductions in their insurance premiums as a result of the camera monitoring system.

Facility policies and procedures should address the use of hidden cameras. Privacy during personal care procedures is a major issue. Although family members may think nothing of viewing their loved one in a compromised position, the resident may mind. Your first concern is protection of the residents' dignity and privacy. Another concern is the roommate. A roommate should never be subjected to video surveillance and monitoring without explicit consent.

The issues surrounding the use of grannycams are not likely to be resolved soon. If you suspect there are hidden cameras in the facility, inform your staff, even if you do not know or cannot disclose the location of the surveillance equipment. Staff will be much more likely to be guarded if they suspect they are being recorded. Handle this potentially thorny issue by being proactive, developing policies and procedures, promoting and providing quality care, and providing resident, family, and staff education.

References

1. Nightingale F. (1859). Notes on nursing. London: Harrison and Sons, 1859.

2. HCPro. (2000). Disasters: Are you ready? *Briefings on Long-Term Care Regulations.* Published October 2000. Online. *www.hcpro.com/content/10440.cfm?.* Accessed 12/15/05.

3. HCPro. (2000). Disasters: Are you ready? *Briefings on Long-Term Care Regulations.* Published October 2000. Online. *www.hcpro.com/content/10440.cfm?.* Accessed 12/15/05.

4. General Accounting Office. (2004). Nursing home fire safety: Nursing home fires highlight weaknesses in federal standards and oversight. Washington, DC: General Accounting Office.

5. Fire Watch (1998). *NFPA Journal*, January/February, 1998.

6. Centers for Medicare and Medicaid Services. (2003). Memorandum to survey and certification regional office management, state survey agency directors, and state fire authorities from Steven A. Pelovitz, Director, US Department of Health and Human Services, Centers for Medicare and Medicaid Services: Adoption of new fire safety requirements for long-term care facilities, et al, No. S&C 03-21. May 8, 2003.

7. Associated Press. (2006). SOCAL nursing home patient with oxygen tank ignites while smoking. *San Jose Mercury News.* Online. *www.mercurynews.com/mld/mercurynews/news/breaking_news/13619043.htm.* Accessed 01/13/06.

8. Khanna R, Olsen L, Hassan A. (2005). Storm evacuations: Elderly were left with weak safety net. Houston Chronicle. Online. *www.chron.com/disp/story.mpl/metropolitan/3516805.html.* Accessed 12/10/05.

9. Hanson E. (2005). Rita's Aftermath; Red tape could be deadly next time: Special-needs patients were at serious risk, judge tells Perry's panel. *Houston Chronicle.* Dec. 13, 2005. *www.chron.com/disp/story.mpl/metropolitan/3523627.html.* Accessed 12/13/05.

10. Penix M. (2006). Nursing home grateful to police. Slidell Sentry February 1, 2006. Online. *www.slidellsentry.com/articles/2006/02/01/news/news04.txt.* Accessed 2/1/06.

11. Hanson E. (2005). Rita's Aftermath; Red tape could be deadly next time: Special-needs patients were at serious risk, judge tells Perry's panel. *Houston Chronicle.* Dec. 13, 2005. *www.chron.com/disp/story.mpl/metropolitan/3523627.html.* Accessed 12/13/05.

12. Khanna R, Olsen L, Hassan A. (2005). Storm evacuations: Elderly were left with weak safety net. *Houston Chronicle.* Online. *www.chron.com/disp/story.mpl/metropolitan/3516805.html.* Accessed 12/10/05.

13. Jaeger, T; Leaver, CM; Glenn, R. (2003). Alcohol-based hand rub solution fire modeling analysis report. Illinois, Oak Brook. Gage-Babcock & Associates, Inc.

14. U.S. Department of Health and Human Services Food and Drug Administration Center for Drug Evaluation and Research (CDER). (2001). Guidance for Hospitals, Nursing Homes, and Other Health Care Facilities FDA Public Health Advisory. March 2001 Compliance. Online. *www.fda.gov/cder/guidance/4341fnl.htm.* Accessed 12/01/05.

15. Cmiel CA, Karr DM, Gasser DM, Oliphant LM, Neveau AJ. (2003). Noise control: A nursing team's approach to sleep promotion. AJN 2004; 104(2):40-48.

16. McClaugherty L, Valibhai F, Womack, S. (2005). Physiological and psychological effects of noise on healthcare professionals and residents in long-term care facilities and enhancing quality of life. The Director Volume 13,2. Online. *www.nadona.org/noise.htm.* Accessed 8/30/05.

17. Britt RR. (2005). Hospitals getting noisier, threatening patient safety. LiveScience. Online. *www.livescience.com/othernews/051121_noisy_hospitals.html.* Accessed 11/22/05.

18. Szegedy-Maszak M. (2005). As noise rises, so do the dangers. *Los Angeles Times.* November 28, 2005. Online. *www.latimes.com/.* Accessed 11/28/05.

19. Feller, I., James, M.H., & Jones, C. A., Burn epidemiology: Focus on youngsters and the aged, Journal of Burn Care and Rehabilitation, 3, 285-288,1982.

20. Victor, J., Lawrence, P., Munster, A., & Horn, S.D., A Statewide Targeted Burn Prevention Program, *Journal of Burn Care and Rehabilitation, 9,* 425–429, 1988.

21. Petraglia, J.S., Fire and the Aging of America, National Fire Protection Association Journal, 85, 36-46, 1991.

22. American Burn Association. (2003). Campaign kit for burn awareness week 2003 – senior safety. Chicago. American Burn Association. Online. *www.ameriburn. org/Preven/2003Prevention/2003BurnAwarenessKit.pdf.* Accessed 12/14/03.

23. *Federal Register.* April 3, 1995; 60:16962 - 16968.

24. Office of the New York Attorney General. (2006). Hidden cameras reveal neglect at nursing homes. Online. *www.oag.state.ny.us/press/2006/jan/ jan05a_06.html.* Accessed 01/05/06.

Change in condition

The nurse administrator develops, maintains, and evaluates patient/client and staff data collection systems and processes to support the practice of nursing and delivery of patient care. The nurse administrator develops, maintains, and evaluates an environment that supports the nurse in analysis of assessment data and in decisions to determine relevant diagnoses. The nurse administrator develops, maintains, and evaluates organizational systems that support implementation of the plan for effective nursing care. The nurse administrator develops, maintains, and evaluates information processes that promote desired, client-centered outcomes. The nurse administrator evaluates the plan and its progress in relation to the attainment of outcomes. The nurse administrator develops, maintains, and evaluates organizational planning systems to facilitate the delivery of nursing care. The nurse administrator systematically evaluates the quality and effectiveness of nursing practice and nursing services administration.[1]

Recognizing changes in condition

Nurses are responsible for identifying and acting upon changes in condition. In fact, recognizing a change in condition and acting on it by using the nursing process is the best method of providing quality of care and preventing litigation. Another factor to consider is that family members often note subtle changes before a problem is apparent to facility personnel. This is not a negative. Take their concerns seriously. Family members know the resident intimately, much better than you do. They will appreciate you for welcoming their observations, and including them in the care process. Being attentive to their concerns goes a long way in helping to avoid future litigation.

Because of normal aging changes, a change in condition can be very subtle and difficult to identify. Try to learn all you can about the residents. If they act differently from normal, this is a clue to a change in condition. Likewise, impress upon the nursing assistants the importance of reporting, even if a problem seems minor. Review laboratory reports and other diagnostic tests. These are often a key to recognizing changes in condition. For example, Mrs. Rabb has seemed more confused than usual for the past few days. As you are scanning the routine labs the courier just delivered, you note that her blood urea nitrogen (BUN) is 26. All her other chemistries are normal. This suggests that the increased confusion is related to dehydration. Act on this information! Write nursing orders to increase fluids and monitor intake and output. Notify the physician. Pass the information along in report so the resident is monitored more closely until the situation is resolved. Failure to identify, monitor, and act on changes in condition in a timely manner is a common component of many lawsuits.

The practice of nursing

The practice of nursing involves assisting individuals to attain or maintain optimal health, implementing a strategy of care to accomplish defined goals, and evaluating responses to nursing care and treatment. Nursing practice includes

- basic healthcare that helps persons cope with difficulties in daily living associated with their actual or potential health or illness status

- those nursing activities that require a substantial amount of scientific knowledge or technical skill.

Nursing practice includes, but is not limited to

- Providing comfort and caring.

- Providing attentive surveillance to monitor resident conditions and needs.

- Promoting an environment conducive to well-being.

- Planning and implementing independent nursing strategies and prescribed treatment in the prevention and management of illness, injury, disability, or achievement of a dignified death.

- Promoting and supporting human functions and responses.

- Providing health counseling and teaching.

- Collaborating on aspects of the health regimen.

- Advocating for the resident.

Nursing is both an art and a scientific process founded on a professional body of knowledge; it is a learned profession based on an understanding of the human condition across the lifespan and the relationship of a resident with others and within the environment.

Nursing is a dynamic discipline that is continually evolving to include more sophisticated knowledge, technologies, and resident care activities.[2]

Assessing individual risk factors, developing, and implementing a resident-specific plan of care is what providing professional long-term care is all about. (An excellent definition of professional nursing further explores this concept at *www.rcn.org.uk/downloads/definingnursing/definingnursing-a5.pdf*). The residents we care for are individuals who don't fit a single mold, nor should they be expected to fit. Nurses (and other licensed professionals) employ critical thinking skills and the nursing process in meeting the human needs of the residents. In doing so, we look at the whole person with many strengths and needs. This forms the basis for our plan of care. Successfully and systematically providing holistic care in meeting the residents' individual needs is what our jobs (and professions) are all about. The "return to basics" approach may be the key to safety success in the high-tech world of the 21st century.

Standard of care for monitoring residents with acute illness or infection

Nurses and paraprofessional nursing personnel are responsible for regular, ongoing monitoring of residents who have experienced an acute illness, infection, incident, or other event. Any change in condition, no matter how minor, falls into this category. The resident must be monitored for as long as necessary to ensure that the event is resolved and the resident's condition has been stabilized. Most facilities monitor the resident for the abnormal condition every shift until 24 hours after he or she is stabilized and the illness or event resolved. If abnormal observations are noted, the licensed nurse must take the appropriate nursing action, providing the necessary interventions and notifications. You will find additional information about documenting changes in condition in Chapter 23. If a resident experiences a change in condition, nursing personnel should

1. Monitor the resident regularly on all shifts until at least 24 hours after the acute event is completely resolved. Monitoring may continue for days or weeks, depending on the nature of the precipitating occurrence, and resident's response.

2. Monitor vital signs (temperature, pulse, respirations, and blood pressure) at least once every eight-hour shift. Check vital signs more frequently if one or more of the values is abnormal, or the resident's condition warrants.

3. Conduct a focused assessment of resident systems, based on the nature of the resident's problem, at least once each shift. For example, for a resident with upper respiratory infection, the nurse should assess and document

   - Auscultation of lung sounds; assess the nature of sounds and adequacy of chest expansion, rate, rhythm, depth of respirations, and use of accessory respiratory muscles

   - Color of the resident's skin, lips, and fingernail beds

   - Change in mental status or level of consciousness

   - Increased restlessness

   - Shortness of breath or other difficulty breathing

   - Presence or absence of cough; if present, note if productive or non-productive, with color, character, and amount of secretions

   - Presence or absence of signs and symptoms related to the specific infection; for example, presence or absence of nasal drainage

4. Report results of monitoring to the oncoming nurse in the change-of-shift report.

5. Notify the physician immediately if abnormalities are noted.

6. Inform the responsible party of the change and action taken.

7. Update the care plan to reflect the additional observations, monitoring, and care required because of the acute illness, infection, change in condition, or abnormal observation.

8. Document the results of monitoring, observations, nursing interventions, notifications, and the resident's response in the nurses' notes. If the resident is on antibiotics or other therapy, document the condition for which the antibiotics are being given. Avoid entries such as "no side effects to antibiotics." This is an appropriate entry in addition to other information, but absence of side effects can be easily noted on the medication record or flow sheet. Your nursing notes should address your assessment of the acute medical problem or injury and actions taken, as noted above.

9. If the resident is not responding to treatment for an acute medical problem, contact the physician.

Legal protection by applying ANA standards

To protect yourself and your facility legally, apply the standards established by the American Nurses Association:

- Nurses must deliver competent care as demonstrated by the nursing process, including assessment, diagnosis, outcome identification, planning, implementation, and evaluation. The nursing process encompasses all significant actions taken by nurses in providing care to all residents, and forms the foundation of clinical decision-making.[3]

- When making clinical judgments, nurses must base their decisions on consideration of consequences, which prescribe and justify nursing actions. The recipients of professional nursing services are entitled to high-quality nursing care.[4]

- The nurse assumes responsibility and accountability for individual nursing judgments and actions.[5] The recipients of professional nursing services are entitled to high-quality nursing care.[6]

- The gerontological nurse collects data through assessment, analyzes the data, plans nursing care, implements the Plan, and evaluates the effectiveness of the Plan of Care. The process is fluid and ongoing to ensure quality nursing care.[7]

- The nurse exercises informed judgment and uses individual competence and qualifications as criteria in seeking consultation, accepting responsibilities, and delegating nursing activities to others. The nurse collaborates with members of the health professions to meet the health needs of the public.[8]

- The nurse acts to safeguard the resident and the public when healthcare and safety are affected by the incompetent, unethical, or illegal practice of any person.[9]

- The nurse is responsible and accountable for individual nursing practice and determines the appropriate delegation of tasks consistent with the nurse's obligation to provide optimum patient care.[10]

- The gerontological nurse considers factors related to safety and effectiveness in planning and delivering resident care.[11]

- The gerontological nurse systematically evaluates the quality of care and effectiveness of nursing practice.[12]

Illness, ongoing monitoring

- *The purpose of monitoring a resident with an acute illness who is receiving antibiotic therapy is to monitor the condition.* Avoid writing notes that state, "no adverse reaction to antibiotic." Making a statement such as this is acceptable, but only as part of a more comprehensive entry. You must also document vital signs, focused system assessment, and other nursing observations related to the condition for which the resident is receiving the antibiotic. This shows you are aware of and are monitoring the problem. For example, write, "Urine clear amber. Resident denies pain and burning on urination."

- Document any change in condition, the resident's vital signs, neurological checks, your actions, and notifications of physician, family, or others.

  – Remember that documentation alone is not a resolution to the problem, and you are responsible for the resident's well-being. For example, documenting you faxed the physician non-emergent information and received no response is not the end of the matter. The fax machine on the other end may not be working, the physician's office may be closed at that time, or the fax is simply engulfed in a pyramid of other information and the message is not transmitted or is buried in a pile of other papers. Your priority is ensuring the physician has been notified of the change in condition, and you should receive a response. Do not stop short of ensuring the resident has been properly cared for.

– If the resident remains unstable as a result of the change in condition, ongoing assessment and documentation are necessary. Regularly monitor vital signs, neurological checks, and other observations of the resident's condition.

– If a resident has experienced a fall, has a fever, or has had any change in condition, monitor every shift until 24 hours after the abnormality is resolved. Do focused assessments of the affected body systems. Take vital signs every shift, and more often, if abnormal.

– Start intake and output monitoring as a nursing measure, if indicated. However, make sure you do more than record meaningless numbers. To be meaningful, fluid intake and output should be evaluated for adequacy. If it is not adequate, initiate corrective action!

Incidents and accidents

• Document all unusual occurrences, such as falls, wandering away, drug reactions, or change in condition. Document notifications of physician, family, and others related to the change in condition. Document nursing actions and the resident's response.

• Follow facility policies for completing an incident report. Regardless of whether incident reports are used, nurses are responsible for documenting the details of all unusual incidents and events in the residents' medical records. This documentation should include the nature of the event, accident, or incident, including focused (systemic) assessment, care, notifications, and follow-up monitoring. Be honest and objective about the incident. Avoid making entries that are untrue or give the reader the wrong impression of the cause of the incident. There is a difference between defensive documentation and dishonest documentation. Although health professionals can be expected to practice defensive documentation, dishonest charting is unethical at best and illegal at worst. For example, if a resident fell, state this in your documentation. Do not say, "NA eased resident to the floor" if this is not true. The practice of documenting falls in this manner is sadly common. The next greatest problem is omission of documentation entirely. This may be done because the nurse does not know how to document a problem without implicating or placing blame on someone or something. Suddenly, the nurses' notes reflect monitoring that is not routine for the resident. Documentation does not provide an indication as to why the monitoring is suddenly necessary.

• If the resident experiences an incident, such as a fall, review the plan of care immediately and update it to prevent further incidents and injuries. If the resident has a fall-prevention plan, it is either ineffective or is not being implemented. Correct the problem immediately. Do not wait until the next care plan review.

• If part of your safety plan for a confused resident includes reminding the resident to use call signal, make sure you document other safety precautions as well. Because of the resident's mental status, you cannot depend on occasional safety reminders to protect you or the facility if the resident does not use the call signal, falls, and sustains an injury. The legal reviewer will check the resident's short-term memory against the MDS. If the MDS notes memory problems, reminding the resident to use the call signal will most likely be considered an ineffective approach.

- Review the old care plans to ensure an ineffective intervention that was used previously is not repeated. Facilities are often cited for implementing repeat interventions that have previously failed to keep the resident safe.

- Consult with your risk management department or legal counsel regarding a format to use to document an incident investigation. Asking employees to write statements or opinions may not be a good idea.

Communication

- Document communication with others regarding the resident.

- If a change in a resident's condition warrants physician notification, you must communicate essential information in a clear and logical manner that expedites understanding and intervention. Have all essential data available before making the call. Be direct and paint a word picture for the physician. Document his or her response. Some facilities have a form to complete with all relevant information before contacting the physician. This is a good idea, in that it keeps the nurse focused and ensures the needed information is conveyed to the physician.

- On weekends or during second and third shifts, you may communicate with an on-call physician instead of the attending. He or she is probably not familiar with the resident. Clearly summarize the resident's background before describing the problem. Document his or her response.

- Document all attempts to reach the physician. If you observe significant or serious changes in a resident's condition, do not just chart them—notify the physician. If he or she does not respond, notify the alternate physician, on-call physician, or medical director. If the situation appears emergent, consider sending the resident to the emergency department by using facility standing orders, as permitted.

- Inform the responsible party of the initial change and keep him or her updated on resident response to treatment.

- Document notifications and referrals, such as notifying the social worker of the need for behavioral intervention, or the dietitian of a pressure ulcer, weight loss, or abnormal lab values.

- When obtaining physician orders for medications, you must also obtain a diagnosis to correspond with the medication. State the reason the medication is being given. Many medications have multiple uses.

- If the physician orders subsequent laboratory monitoring, make sure the lab is scheduled for the correct day and time.

- Reservations about physicians' orders, and action taken: Legally, you must advocate for the residents. If, in your professional judgment, you believe the physician orders place a resident in jeopardy, you must intervene and clarify the treatment plan. If the physician is non-responsive, contact your supervisor and go up the chain of command from there. Document the actions taken to advocate for the resident.

References

1. American Nurses Association (eds). (1995). *Scope and Standards for Nurse Administrators.* Washington, D.C. American Nurses Publishing.

2. Modified from: National Council of State Boards of Nursing. (Eds.) (2002.) Model Nursing Practice Act. Chicago. National Council of State Boards of Nursing. Online. *www.ncsbn.org.* Accessed 7/20/04.

3. American Nurses Association (eds) (1998) *Standards of Clinical Nursing Practice.* Washington, D.C. American Nurses Publishing.

4. American Nurses Association (eds.). *Code for Nurses.* (1985). Washington, D.C. American Nurses Publishing.

5. American Nurses Association (eds.). *Code for Nurses.* (1985). Washington, D.C. American Nurses Publishing.

6. American Nurses Association (eds.). *Code for Nurses.* (1985). Washington, D.C. American Nurses Publishing.

7. American Nurses Association (eds.). *Scope and Standards of Gerontological Nursing Practice.* (1995). Washington, D.C. American Nurses Publishing.

8. American Nurses Association (eds.). *Code for Nurses.* (1985). Washington, D.C. American Nurses Publishing.

9. American Nurses Association (eds) (1985, 1999). *Code for Nurses with Interpretive Statements.* Washington. American Nurses Publishing.

10. American Nurses Association (eds). (2001). *Code for Nurses with Interpretive Statements.* Washington. American Nurses Publishing.

11. American Nurses Association (eds). (1995). *Scope and Standards of Gerontological Nursing Practice.* Washington, D.C. American Nurses Publishing.

12. American Nurses Association (eds). (1995). *Scope and Standards of Gerontological Nursing Practice.* Washington, D.C. American Nurses Publishing.

Leading causes of lawsuits: Pressure ulcers

Lady Justice

Lady Justice is the name given to the representation of justice in which a blindfolded woman is holding a set of scales. The origin of this figure goes back to the ancient Egyptians, at which time she assisted in meting out justice in the judgment of the dead by weighing their hearts. The figure was also found in ancient Greece, where the woman was known as Themis. Themis was known as the organizer of the communal affairs of humans, particularly assemblies. Ancient interpretations of the figure evolved, and it is believed the sword was not added until the 15th century. The blindfolded lady was first used when there were few books, and many people were unable to read. It has been a powerful and enduring statement of the importance of law and justice in every society. Today, the name given to the blindfolded lady is Justicia.

A common representation of Justice is a blindfolded woman holding a set of scales. The sword in the other hand signifies power, implying swift and powerful enforcement of the law. The figure implies that the onus of justice will not be affected by race, religion, social class, or gender. The blindfold is an assurance of impartiality. In some statues, Justicia is tying the blindfold on herself, suggesting she voluntarily assumes a mantle of objectivity and impartiality. Although there are many different interpretations, Lady Justice symbolizes the fair and equal administration of the law, without prejudice or favor. It is evident that the scales are intended to depict the fact that justice requires a consideration and careful weighing of both sides of a legal case. The facts for each side are placed on a scale.

There is disagreement about what is to be weighed. Some believe the current interpretation of the figure is a reference to the Old Testament (Job 31:6). Others believe the scales represent weighing as a symbol of judgment in the Koran. The most commonly accepted theory for the scales is that "each person receives his or her due; no more and no less." The information presented in the courtroom is the basis for the information. Jurors should not do independent research into the situation or facts (beyond their existing knowledge when they are selected for the jury). They must rely on the information given to them. In a 2004 murder trial, a juror measured her own queen size bed and reported her findings to the jury. The information was used to estimate distance after a blood spatter expert testified. Jurors cannot conduct independent research or experiments, so the judge declared a mistrial.[1] In a 2001 trial, a new trial was granted because a juror used calipers to measure his own body to determine the depth of the victim's wounds. He drew certain conclusions from this information, and reported his findings to other jurors.[2] Many mistrials have been declared because jurors independently visited crime scenes.

Pressure ulcers: The leading cause of lawsuits

The most common cause of lawsuits against long-term care facilities is skin breakdown. This includes pressure ulcers and related skin problems, such as venous, arterial, or diabetic ulcers. Skin tears are often listed as a secondary injury especially if the resident has experienced many falls, but the magnitude of the injury does not warrant the filing of a lawsuit as a distinguishing factor.

Most lawsuits have many peripheral and contributing factors, including development of contractures, malnutrition, dehydration, infection, and sepsis. The plaintiff usually alleges that negligence, short staffing, and related factors led to ulceration and eventual gangrene and amputation, pain, and suffering. The typical defense position is to argue the ulcer was unavoidable, or was due to a preexisting condition, whereas the plaintiff will argue that the ulcer was preventable despite the presence of underlying chronic diseases and risk factors. The jury is asked to sort it out, based only on evidence presented in the courtroom. Lawsuits involving details of this nature are often gruesome for the general public, who are not exposed to medical care daily. They often invoke strong emotions and feelings of sympathy, especially if the medical record chronicles large and deep pressure ulcers with color photos.

Risk factors for pressure ulcer development

Pressure ulcers are declines according to the OBRA regulations. They can be prevented in most residents through a combination of risk factor identification and proper nursing care. Avoid thinking that *the presence of one or more risk factors equals inevitability of an untoward condition or event. Risk factor management is the essence of nursing practice and reflects the essence and focus of the OBRA legislation!* High risk conditions are identified in many different ways. Once the risk of developing a complication is known, nursing personnel plan care designed to reduce, minimize, or eliminate the risk, thus preventing the complication. A plan of care is always needed to address high risk conditions. The plan of care is designed to prevent or delay the development of a high risk condition. If the problem is present, the care plan is designed to stabilize (maintain) the condition and prevent it from worsening. The care plan also focuses on approaches that prevent additional complications from developing. Planning, implementing, and evaluating resident response to preventive care is an important nursing function that must not be overlooked if a positive outcome is to be achieved. You may want to view the situation in this manner: The facility becomes at-risk when its own assessment shows a resident is at-risk for pressure ulcers and no specific interventions are implemented. Causative factors of skin ulcers include

- pressure
- arterial insufficiency
- venous stasis
- burns
- diabetes (ischemic and neuropathic)
- trauma

Remember, very few pressure ulcers are truly unavoidable. If a defendant facility alleges that skin breakdown was unavoidable, the plaintiff attorney will ask a legal nurse consultant or medical-legal reviewer to look for the qualifying factors signaling inevitability:

- The resident has been accurately assessed

- The problem, based on analysis of assessment findings, is adequately care planned

- The care plan is actually implemented

- The interventions are evaluated periodically and modified according to the resident's responses to interventions

Medical-legal reviewers seldom, if ever find all four factors on the charts of residents with pressure ulcers for whom the lawsuits are filed.

Identification of risk factors and implementation of a preventive plan of care are among the most important nursing functions. In the event of pressure ulcers, the standard is for all "at-risk" residents to have a systematic skin inspection at least once a day. In most cases, this can be done by a nursing assistant, who reports his or her findings to the nurse. If the assistant reports a red or open area (or other skin problem), the nurse should assess the area promptly. Licensed nurses should check high-risk residents' skin weekly, or according to facility policy. Keep in mind that the conditions of residents are not static, so pressure ulcer risk requires routine reexamination.[3]

Low-risk residents who are independent and ambulatory are usually at very high risk for skin breakdown during periods of illness. Because these residents are at low risk under normal circumstances, a preventive plan of care is seldom, if ever, in place. If a resident becomes acutely ill, his or her risk should be promptly reassessed, and a preventive plan of care implemented.

Do not omit this important step in your change of condition assessment! These residents are particularly vulnerable, because staff do not regularly assist them with turning, repositioning, and other measures. The heels are a very susceptible area of the body.

Other residents at high risk for pressure ulcers are those who are tube fed, those with chronic lung disease, and those who are largely dependent and bedfast. The care of these residents involves elevating the head of the bed into the semi-Fowler's or Fowler's position. Elevating the head of the bed greatly increases the risk of skin breakdown on the hips, buttocks, and coccyx area. Anticipate this and plan your care to position the residents frequently and correctly.

Newly admitted residents are also at high risk because staff are not familiar with them, and there may be no care plan to guide their care. Common pressure ulcer risk factors are listed in the "Pressure ulcer risk factors" table on your CD-ROM. However, use common sense when evaluating risk. A resident with an existing pressure ulcer or healed ulcer is always at greater risk than residents with no history of skin problems. If he or she has an ulcer, preventive measures must be employed to prevent additional (further) breakdown. Do not depend on pressure-reducing surfaces. These are good adjuncts, but do not replace hands-on nursing care. Residents can and do develop pressure ulcers on therapeutic beds and overlays if they are not regularly repositioned.

This is often a source of confusion for nursing assistants, so staff teaching my be in order.

Pressure ulcer prevention measures

1. Systematically inspect skin daily. Closely observe skin folds and bony prominences. If skin is clear

and intact, documentation of the daily skin inspection may be done by initiating a flow sheet.

2. Cleanse the skin with mild soap and water or a facility-approved product after each incontinence, and at routine intervals. Avoid very hot water. Use a pH-balanced product.

   - Initiate an incontinence management or retraining program. Many residents are *environmentally incontinent*. This means they know they need to use the bathroom, but either cannot communicate the need, or physically cannot get to the toilet. This type of incontinence is 100% reversible. Make sure your staff are sensitive to communication problems and physical barriers!

   - Consider absorbent briefs or pads; use a good product that wicks moisture away from skin.

   - Use an external catheter, if necessary.

   - Use an indwelling catheter only as a last resort.

3. Use moisturizers regularly to keep skin supple. Apply moisturizers after bathing to trap water in the upper layers of the skin, reducing dryness and itching. Select products containing petrolatum, mineral oil, linoleum, ceramides, dimethicone, or glycerin. (However, use caution if these products contact bed linen; the flash point is low and a large amount of product increases the risk of dryer fires. Hot water and adequate detergent in the washer may correct the problem, but these products do not predictably wash out.) Some facilities have discovered that vegetable shortening is miraculous for dry skin and minor injuries. Unfortunately, use of this produce (which has a low flashpoint), is a leading cause of dryer fires. Avoid products containing alcohol, which is drying and irritating. Individualize the plan of care to the resident's needs.

4. *Avoid massage over bony prominences and reddened areas*. This is an old treatment that is no longer recommended, because it increases tissue destruction.[4]

5. Apply barrier products to reduce skin exposure due to incontinence, perspiration, or wound drainage. Avoid powder or cornstarch, which can be irritating.

6. Avoid friction and shearing by using proper positioning, transferring, and turning techniques.

   - *Friction* is rubbing the skin against a sheet or other surface.

   - *Shearing* is moving the resident so the skin is stretched between the bone inside and the sheet (or other surface) outside, causing skin damage. The bone moves in one direction, but the skin remains stationary or moves in the opposite direction.

7. Provide adequate intake of fluid, protein, and calories. Monitor and *evaluate* intake and output for adequacy.

8. Improve the resident's mobility status, if appropriate, and as indicated.

9. Reposition residents every two hours, or more often if indicated. Some residents may require positioning every 60 to 90 minutes.

10. Use props and positioning devices to keep bony prominences and skin folds from rubbing or contacting one another. If residents are positioned in bed with knees, ankles, and other bony areas touching each other, place bath blanket, pillow, or other positioning device between legs.

11. Keep heels elevated off the bed, or hanging over the end of the mattress in bedfast residents. Note: *Use of heel protectors reduces friction and shearing, but does not relieve pressure*. Avoid doughnut-type devices[5], which increase pressure.

12. Avoid positioning directly on the trochanter. Use the semisupine and semiprone positions whenever possible. These are comfortable positions that relieve pressure on all major bony prominences. Make sure staff know how to differentiate the semiprone and semisupine positions from the lateral position.

13. Use lifting devices to move residents in bed whenever possible. If a lifting sheet is used, avoid dragging the heels on the surface of the sheet.

14. Maintain the head of the bed at the lowest degree of elevation possible, (consistent with the resident's medical condition, physician orders, need for tube feeding, and other restrictions). Avoid elevations over 45 degrees as much as possible. Elevating the head of the bed increases pressure on the sacrum, coccyx, and buttocks. If the head of the bed must be elevated for any reason, encourage or help the resident to reposition frequently. Avoid prolonged periods of elevation.

15. Apply pressure-reducing mattresses and pads to bed and chair. The most common pressure-relieving devices are made of foam. Sheepskin prevents friction and shearing, but does not relieve pressure. Most foam overlays have been treated with fire-retardant chemicals during the manufacturing process. However, washing the overlay removes the fire-retardant. For this reason, many facilities discard and replace the overlay each time it becomes soiled. This can be an expensive proposition, yet it may be necessary

for resident safety. However, using heavy padding on the overlay to protect the surface may defeat the purpose of using the device. Before purchasing pressure-relieving mattresses and overlays, check the fire-retardant properties. Next, check with your surveyors to learn their requirements and procedures for evaluating these devices for potential survey deficiencies.

16. Keep the bed crumb and wrinkle free. In addition to contributing to skin breakdown, crumbs and wrinkles can be surprisingly painful on sensitive skin.

17. Reposition chair-bound residents at least hourly. Teach residents to shift their weight every 15 minutes.

18. Provide education to residents, family, and staff caregivers on the prevention of pressure ulcers. Teach preventive care for residents with risk factors for diabetic, vascular, and arterial ulcers.

19. Provide adequate calories and protein to meet the resident's needs. Increase fluid intake. Provide supplements and snacks as ordered. Ask the dietitian to evaluate the resident related to skin risk. Follow his or her recommendations. Nutritional assessment and management are keys to successful pressure ulcer prevention and treatment programs. Vitamin and mineral supplements may be necessary. Positive nitrogen balance and protein intake are important as well. Studies have demonstrated an association between malnutrition and the development of new pressure ulcers. If dietary intake remains inadequate, nutritional support (such as tube feeding) should be provided if this is consistent with the goals of care. Approximately 30 to 35 calories/kg/day and 1.25 to 1.50 grams of protein/kg/day are recommended to place the resi-

dent in positive nitrogen balance. Monitor intake and output, meal and supplement intake, when indicated.[6]

20. Involve the resident in restorative nursing programs to maintain or improve his or her mobility and activity.

21. Monitor and document all interventions and outcomes.

22. Apply the principles of standard precautions if contact with blood, body fluids, secretions, excretions, mucous membranes, or nonintact skin is likely.

23. Institute an aggressive contracture-prevention program. Involve other professionals (physical, occupational therapy, and restorative nursing), as appropriate. Be aware that there is a close relationship between contractures and pressure ulcers. Contractures cause capillary occlusion in bony prominences. It is estimated that 60% of all wounds involve some sort of unattended contracture. Contractures can begin within four days of immobility and inactivity. After 15 days, the resident begins to lose range of motion.[7]

24. Weigh the resident. Monitor for significant weight loss (5% in 30 days; 10% in six months).

25. Monitor lab values for nutritional deficits:

    Hemoglobin <12mg/dl

    Total Lymphocyte Count <1800mm3

    Serum Albumin <3.5 mg/dl

    Total Protein <6.0 mg/dl

26. Assess the need for vitamin/mineral supplements, such as Multivitamin with Minerals, Vitamin C, and Zinc, or as recommended by dietitian.

27. Educate the staff! Most resident care is provided by nursing assistants. Make sure they understand aging changes to the skin, principles of geriatric skin care, safe transfer and repositioning techniques, methods of preventing and reducing friction and shearing, correct use of protective supplies (e.g., Geri gloves and sleeves, extremity stockinette, long sleeves, etc.) and equipment (e.g., mattress overlays, heel protectors, padded side rails and wheelchair arms, footrests, seats in good repair, etc.), how and when to report skin conditions to a nurse, signs and symptoms of infection, and expected wound appearance during the healing process.

Pressure ulcer care plan management

Reassess pressure ulcers frequently. If the condition of the resident or wound deteriorates, reevaluate the treatment plan as soon as any evidence of deterioration is noted.[8] The nurse documents the results of this assessment and uses it to evaluate the effectiveness of the treatment plan. The plan is modified based on the resident's response to care. Generally speaking, if there is no progress in healing in two weeks, the wound should be reevaluated and consideration given to changing the treatment. The physician is contacted for treatment orders to promote healing. No single treatment will provide a panacea for all wounds. Nurses like hydrocolloids and transparent film dressings because they require infrequent changes. However, they can worsen infected wounds, and their use is contraindicated in some types of wounds. Individualizing the treatment to the wound characteristics is always best. Other treatment and care plan approaches are:

1. Assessment is always the starting point for ulcer treatment. Assess the resident completely, not just the ulcer. In many cases, other healthcare professionals, such as the physical therapist should also assess the resident and make recommendations.

2. Measure the size (diameter or length and width), depth, necrotic tissue, presence or absence of odor, drainage, and appearance of wound periphery/surrounding skin. Also consider and document the location, stage, and presence or absence of sinus tracts, undermining, tunneling, exudate, granulation tissue and epithelialization.

3. Reassess and measure at least weekly or sooner if deterioration of the ulcer is noted. Always document your findings in detail. If a formal risk-assessment scale is used by the facility, promptly complete a new risk-assessment tool. The resident's risk increases when breakdown is present.

4. Promptly inform the physician (and responsible party, as appropriate) of new pressure ulcers. Obtain and initiate treatment orders. Report all of the following to the physician:

   • Vital signs

   • Anatomical location of wound

   • Wound measurements (in centimeters, proximal to distal, medial to lateral)

   • Condition of the periphery (surrounding tissue)

   • Condition of the wound base (e.g., beefy red, fibrotic, necrotic)

   • Signs and symptoms of infection

   • Overall appearance (new, healing, worsening, unchanged)

   • Current treatment and a review of the past treatment, as appropriate

5. Update the care plan to reflect the change in condition and new treatment goals and approaches. Develop an effective plan of care consistent with resident goals and wishes.

6. Implement a preventive program to prevent additional (new) ulcers from developing. The presence of one ulcer means the resident is at risk for additional ulcers. Ensure that all new preventive measures are listed on the care plan and flow sheets.

7. Initial ulcer care involves debridement, wound cleansing, dressing application, and possible adjunctive therapy.

   • Note: Never debride eschar on stable heel ulcers for residents with arterial or vascular conditions or diabetes. Edema, erythema, fluctuance, or drainage would necessitate eschar debridement.

8. Eliminate infection, if present. An infected wound will not heal.

9. Use normal saline for wound cleansing at a pressure between four and 15 pounds per square inch (psi). Avoid products such as povidone iodine, iodophor, Dakin's solution, sodium hypochlorite solution, hydrogen peroxide, and acetic acid as they destroy granulation tissue and may be cytotoxic. If these products are essential, make sure they are well diluted and thoroughly rinsed. Additionally, many of these products will dry the wound bed, and your objective is to maintain a moist healing environment.

10. Protect the wound with dressings. Apply a petroleum gauze prior to the cover dressings, as appropriate. Remember to keep the wound bed moist, but not wet. An ideal dressing should protect the wound, be biocompatible, and provide ideal hydration. The cardinal rule is to keep the ulcer tissue moist and the surrounding intact skin dry to prevent maceration.

11. Wound drainage is not necessarily a sign of infection. Normal exudate in a wound stimulates

healing. Carefully evaluate both wound drainage and the resident's total condition to identify signs and symptoms of infection.

12. All stage II, III, and IV ulcers are colonized with bacteria. Regular wound cleansing should prevent colonization from proceeding to infection. A contaminated wound will heal, but an infected wound will not. Topical antibiotics may be appropriate. Watch for response and sensitivity. Avoid unnecessary systemic antibiotics. However, systemic antibiotic therapy is appropriate for residents with bacteremia, sepsis, advancing cellulites, or osteomyelitis.

13. Avoid swab cultures, which only show surface contaminants. Use needle aspiration, if possible, to obtain fluid or soft tissue biopsy for culture and sensitivity testing.

14. Use sterile instruments and clean or sterile dressings during wound care. Treat the most contaminated ulcer last in residents with multiple wounds. Change gloves and wash hands between each ulcer.

15. Discuss treatment options with residents and their families. Do resident and family teaching, as appropriate.

16. Encourage residents to actively participate in their care. Create an environment conducive to resident adherence to the treatment plan.

17. Avoid positioning residents directly on a pressure ulcer. Avoid donut-type-devices, which increase pressure. Reposition bedfast residents every two hours or more often. Reposition chairfast residents at least hourly. Teach chair-bound residents to shift their weight every 15 minutes.

18. Regularly assess the resident for pain related to the ulcer or its treatment.

19. Promptly notify the physician if the wound does not respond to treatment. A clean pressure ulcer with adequate blood flow should show some improvement in two weeks. Reassess your plan of care. Make sure it is being implemented. Modify the plan as needed.

20. Continue using the steps of the nursing process to promote wound healing and modify the plan of care.

Wound documentation

Accurate and complete documentation of all risk assessments ensures continuity of care and may be used as a foundation for the skin care plan. Avoid subjective comments, such as "healing well" in pressure ulcer documentation. Document what you see! Assess and document the following information:

- Measure (and document) length, width, and depth in centimeters. Use a head-to-toe axis for length and a hip-to-hip axis for width. If the wound is large or irregularly shaped, document that the measurements were taken at the longest and widest parts of the wound. Draw a picture of the wound and mark its features and measurements in your notes. Measure depth at the deepest point in the wound bed. Stage the wound based on size and characteristics.

- Assess (and document) the appearance of the wound. Begin at the center and work outward. If the wound is various colors, describe them by using percentages, such as 80% red, 20% black. This is helpful if you cannot identify the red tissue. Granulation tissue is usually beefy red, granular, and bubbly in appearance. Exposed muscle has a smooth surface, and is pink to red. Slough is usually lighter in color, and has a thin, stringy consistency. It is commonly yellow, tan, or gray in color. Eschar is black or dark-brown, but is occasionally deep red. It is often thick and leathery in appearance. Also, identify tunnels and sinus tracts within the wound bed. Tunnels are larger and easily observed; sinus tracts are small, with a narrower opening.

- Assess (and document) the edges of the wound. Note whether they are well-defined or diffuse, if the edges have rolled under, if there is new skin growth, or undermining. Check for scarring, callus formation (hyperkeratosis), and dry scaling.

- Assess (and document) the color, odor, amount, consistency, and nature of wound drainage (exudate).

- Note (and document) the appearance and temperature of the periwound skin. Monitor for signs of infection, such as erythema, edema, induration, warmth, cellulitis, crepitus, maceration, and damage such as skin tears or abrasions from previous dressings.

Monitoring systems

Many long-term care facilities lack systems for monitoring and managing pressure ulcers. Each facility should have one or more nurses who have been educated in wound assessment. This individual should conduct weekly (or more often, if needed) assessments of all pressure ulcers. He or she should furnish a log to the director of nursing with information on each ulcer and how it is progressing. When facilities have a formal system for monitoring and managing pressure ulcers, survey deficiencies and lawsuits decrease in frequency and are more defensible. Resident outcomes are better when nursing administration is attentive to pressure ulcers. Additional benefits are reduced costs for the resident and facility, and improved quality of life for the resident.

Leg ulcer comparison

Leg and foot ulcers are commonly mistaken for pressure ulcers. In some cases, ulcers on the lower legs are caused by pressure, such as when the resident maintains a cross-legged position. However, nurses must be careful in assessment and documentation to differentiate vascular and arterial ulcers. Resident and family teaching is also very important where arterial and vascular ulcers are concerned. Many of these result in eventual amputation, and the resident's first inclination is to file a lawsuit to compensate for the loss. **The "Leg ulcer comparison" table on your CD-ROM describes ulcers whose origins are arterial, vascular, and venous.**

Identifying residents who are at risk of pressure ulcers on the feet

Pressure ulcers on the feet often have devastating consequences for elderly adults, including pain, loss of mobility, gangrene, and lower-extremity amputation. The heel is exposed to high pressure when it rests on the bed or other surface. The capacity of the heel to absorb and reduce shock declines with age, further increasing the risk for skin breakdown.[9] Tightly tucked upper bed linen may increase pressure and reduce mobility. Many support surfaces (overlays and mattresses) provide pressure relief to the torso, but few relieve pressure to the heels and feet. Heel protectors effectively prevent friction and shearing, but most do not eliminate pressure. Appliances, casts, splints and orthotics, and other devices attached to the feet may also increase pressure. Likewise, tight shoes create blisters and pressure areas, especially on the toes. Proper fitting and padding will decrease, but not eliminate the risk. If a pressure-relieving device is applied to the feet, it must be monitored regularly. Residents may accidentally or deliberately remove or dislodge the device.

Many excellent pressure-reducing devices are available. Fortunately, the heels are the easiest bony prominence from which to relieve pressure. Pressure-reducing devices should transfer pressure off the heels and onto the calves. Elevating the resident's calves on pillows will suspend the heels over the surface of the bed, eliminating pressure. In fact, several studies suggest that using a pillow in this manner is more effective than many specialty products.[10,11,12] This method is also useful when the resident is in the lateral position, to relieve pressure on the bunion area and sides of feet. Loosening the upper bed linen will also prevent downward pressure on the feet.

Medical conditions that increase the risk of foot and heel ulceration

The Braden Scale is an excellent tool for predicting pressure ulcers on the heel. Residents with a Braden score of 15 or less are at high risk for pressure ulcer development. Residents with hip and pelvic fractures also seem particularly vulnerable. However, residents with certain chronic diseases, and those who have experienced recent trauma or surgery, are also at particularly high risk by virtue of their underlying medical problems. Regardless of the Braden score, maintain a high degree of awareness that residents with the conditions listed below are at high risk for skin breakdown (and other complications) on the feet. Develop a preventive plan of care on admission, and use the nursing process to maintain the plan for residents who are bedfast, who need physical assistance for bed mobility and transfers, and those with

- Recent hip fracture or hip surgery, such as joint replacement (pain and immobility may also be contributing factors)

- Cerebrovascular accident (CVA)

- Recent major surgery

- Poor or very limited mobility

- Poor quality popliteal, ankle, or foot pulses

- Absence of foot/ankle pulses (the posterior tibial and dorsalis pedis should be palpable manually)

- Doppler/ultrasound test results on the chart indicating narrowed blood vessels and reduced blood flow to the feet

- Diabetes mellitus

- Neuropathy (loss of sensation in feet)

- Peripheral Vascular Disease (PVD)

- Peripheral Arterial Disease (PAD), arterial occlusive disease

- Paralysis, including hemiplegia, diplegia, paraplegia, and tetraplegia (quadriplegia)

- Unconsciousness

- Past history of pressure ulcers anywhere on the body

- Malnutrition or at high nutritional risk

- Dehydration

- Spasticity

- Multiple Sclerosis, post polio syndrome, Huntington's disease, Lou Gehrig's disease, or any other progressive neurological disease

- Contractures or other deformities of the feet or lower legs

- Agitation

- History of thrombophlebitis in the lower extremity

- Acute exacerbation or unstable Congestive Heart Failure (CHF)

- Edema of lower extremities

- Improper fitting antiembolism hosiery, socks, or shoes

- History of prior amputation

- Charcot joint deformity or equinus deformity of the ankle

- Feet/legs always cool to touch; color abnormal

Antiembolism hosiery

Antiembolism hosiery may also be called graduated compression hosiery (GCS), or by the brand name, such as TED® hose or Jobst® hose. They are applied upon physician order to prevent deep venous thrombosis and leg ulcers. The stockings used in healthcare facilities have a hole at the toe end (called an "inspection toe") for circulation checks.

Residents with diabetes, neuropathy, connective tissue diseases, signs of clinical infection in the extremity, and peripheral arterial disease have an increased risk of complications. Contraindications for hosiery use are

- Severe arteriosclerosis or other ischemic vascular disease

- Pulmonary edema, congestive heart failure

- Massive leg edema

- Local conditions such as dermatitis, postoperative vein ligation, recent skin graft, and gangrene

- Deformity of leg

- Circumference greater than 25 inches (63.5cm) at the gluteal fold, if thigh-high hose are ordered

Potentially serious complications resulting from hosiery use include

- reduced blood flow and tissue oxygenation

- pressure ulcers

- arterial occlusion

- thrombosis

- gangrene

Complications are usually associated with improper fitting hosiery, failure to remove the hose for skin and circulation checks, folding and bunching up of hosiery, causing a tourniquet effect to the skin. Ill-fitting and twisted hosiery that have not been regularly removed have been implicated in lawsuits related to pressure ulcers of the toes, feet, and heels. Ill-fitting or twisted above-the-knee type hosiery have been implicated in serious breakdown behind the knee.

Before applying the compression hosiery initially, consider these safeguards:

- Review the physician order and clarify hosiery length, if necessary.

- Hosiery are available in light compression, moderate compression, and firm compression. Clarify the compression strength with the physician.

- Systematically inspect the resident's skin and each lower extremity for appropriate use of compression.

- Check the skin condition for potential pressure points, fragile skin, open areas, rashes, signs of infection, healed ulcerations, and areas of possible vulnerability.

- Review contraindications; ensure the hose are not contraindicated for the resident.

- Assess the peripheral circulation, popliteal, posterior tibial, and dorsalis pedis pulses and document.

- Check the resident's allergies. Although the incidence of allergic reaction is low, some brands contain latex, nylon, Lycra, and other potential allergens.

- Proper fit is essential to produce the required therapeutic benefits. Avoid guessing at the size. Measure both legs. A slight difference in leg size is normal. Some residents have legs of vastly different size, such as those with post polio syndrome and other neuromuscular diseases. If this is the case, two different sizes may be necessary.

- Obtain measurements after the resident has been in bed, with legs elevated, when edema is least.

- Document leg measurements and stocking size as a baseline for future assessment. If the resident's condition or leg size subsequently changes, measure again to ensure that the size has not changed. If edema is present, measure the legs periodically to determine whether a larger size stocking is needed. Remeasure if the resident gains or loses weight. An increase in leg circumference of 5cm doubles the pressure being applied by the stockings.[13]

- Follow the manufacturer's directions for measuring the legs. The tape measure should be snug, but not tight. Mark the leg, if necessary to provide reference points.

For knee-high stockings, measure

- The narrowest part of the ankle, about 2.5cm above the medial malleolus

- The base of the heel to just below the knee

- The widest part of the calf

For thigh-high stockings, measure

- The narrowest part of the ankle, above the ankle bone

- The base of the heel to just below the knee

- The widest part of the calf

- The widest part of the thigh

- The distance between the base of the heel and the gluteal fold

- Review facility policies and procedures for fitting, application, and circulation checks, and follow them; add the hosiery to the plan of care

Medical-grade stockings have a hole in the toe end. Look through the hole to monitor circulation in the toes every four hours, or according to facility policy. Document circulation checks. If edema is present, more frequent monitoring will be necessary. Normal checks may be documented on a flow sheet. However, if abnormalities are noted, document in the narrative notes and list corrective actions taken. Document color, sensation, swelling, temperature, and ability to move. Although residents may wear the hosiery continuously, they should be removed daily for bathing and skin care. Some physicians order hosiery to be worn during the day and removed at bedtime. Assess the skin condition carefully upon application and removal.

Make sure the nursing procedure manual has information for measuring and fitting size, applying the hose, and circulation checks. Avoid referring the reader to "follow manufacturer's directions" for hosiery use. The manufacturer's directions provide some information, such as where to purchase and how to launder the hosiery. They do not provide information that is essential to nurses, such as frequency of application, removal, or observations to make during circulation checks. Make sure nursing assistants are familiar with the instructions and know to remove the hose each day for bathing and skin care. Surprisingly, nurse researchers found that only 33% of nurses did circulation checks, and did not know if nursing assistants were aware that the hose could or should be removed at bath time.[14] It is conceivable that some may bathe the resident with the hosiery in place (by covering with a plastic bag, as you would a cast).

Preventive measures for the feet and legs

The first step in pressure ulcer prevention is a complete nursing assessment at the time of admission. Evaluate pressure ulcer risk using a validated measure, such as the Braden scale. Use common sense and identify other factors, such as those listed above, that increase the risk of lower-extremity ulcers. Immediately develop and implement a preventive plan of care. Do not wait for MDS completion. Remember, this assessment is being done for a specific purpose. It is not strictly paper compliance! An experienced facility administrator puts it this way. "Prevention makes the difference between the dog wagging the tail or the tail wagging the dog."

Individualize preventive measures to meet the resident's needs, and note them on the plan of care. Use the nursing process to evaluate their effectiveness quarterly, and more often if there is a change in condition. Suggested care plan approaches include

- Careful attention to foot care, including regular washing with mild soap

- Teach nursing assistants the importance of drying well between toes

- Applying moisturizers to feet to manage dry skin and cracking (Avoid area between toes)

- Daily foot inspection by nursing assistant

- Weekly foot inspection by licensed nurse during routine check

- Podiatrist care, according to resident needs

- Well fitting shoes with round or box toes; avoid pointed toes

- Check shoes for fit and pressure

- Special orthopedic/custom/diabetic shoes, as needed and ordered

- Clean, absorbent socks that fit properly

  - Teach nursing assistants and resident the importance of changing daily

  - White cotton socks if fungal infection (athletes' foot) is a problem

- Ensure properly fitting antiembolism hose according to actual measurements, as specified by manufacturer. Avoid guessing on size. Measure for accuracy.

  - Check the antiembolism stockings periodically to be sure the tops have not rolled or turned down. Keep the fabric straight.

  - Apply antiembolism hose correctly. Most have a hole in the toe end to allow access for circulation checks. In some hosiery, the hole is on the top of the foot, and on others it is on the bottom. As long as the heel is centered, the hole will be in the correct place.

  - List the wearing schedule for the antiembolism hose on the care plan, according to physician orders and facility policies. For most residents, the hosiery is applied during the day and removed at bedtime. Avoid assuming that nursing assistants will remove the hosiery for bathing. Specify times when the hose should be removed.[15]

  - Make sure the resident has two pairs of antiembolism hose available. Hand wash the hose in mild soap when they are removed and hang them to dry. Never send them through the facility washer and dryer.

- If diabetic, maintain blood sugar control (Hb A1C of <7%)

- Protect feet and legs from injury

  – Keep covered with pants, socks, stockings, etc. Consider using skin sleeves or covering with stockinette.

  – Always wear shoes when out of bed; never get up in stocking feet or barefoot

  – Room free from obstacles

  – Trim toenails regularly (clip straight across, check for sharp edges)

  – Pad side rails, if needed

  – Pad wheelchair leg rests, if needed

  – Position the resident correctly in the chair or wheelchair

  – Support feet when the wheelchair is moving; never allow them to drag on the floor

  – If the legs are too short to reach the footrests of the wheelchair, ask therapy or maintenance to shorten the leg rests or add a commercial foot elevator

  – Support feet on footrests, floor, or stool when the wheelchair is parked; legs should never dangle

  – Push the wheelchair from behind, by guiding it with the handgrips. Avoid walking too fast. Slow down and look before turning corners.

  – Approach swinging doors with caution. Prop the door open before entering, if possible. If not, back the wheelchair through the doorway.

  – Always back the wheelchair over the thresholds in doorways.

- Turn and regularly reposition immobile residents

- Palpate pedal and posterior tibial pulses during weekly skin check; document results on a flow sheet

- Elevate heels from surface of bed

- Support the sole of the foot to prevent foot drop

- Avoid tucking upper bed linen in tightly over the feet

- Reduce sources of friction and shearing to feet

  – Teach nursing assistants to move resident without dragging heels on bed

- Monitor foot appliances one or more times each shift for proper placement and adequacy of circulation to foot

- For residents with unilateral lower extremity amputation, position the remaining joints and extremity in extension. Avoid elevating the stump on pillows. These residents are at high risk for contracture development. Contractures further increase the risk of pressure ulcers. Specify positioning instructions on the care plan.

Other considerations in special circumstances

In certain circumstances, more intense monitoring and aggressive preventive measures may be necessary. Aggressive interventions include

- At the end of each shift, the off-going nurse checks the resident's feet and opens or loosens any pressure-relieving devices. Doing this enables the leg to rest while the skin cools and dries.

- At the beginning of each shift, the oncoming nurse monitors, observes and palpates the resident's heels, checks lower extremity pulses, and replaces/fastens the pressure-relieving device.

- Monitor circulation in the resident's feet and toes every four hours, or as specified on the care plan. Note color, sensation, swelling, temperature, and ability to move. Report abnormalities.

- Check the circulation in the toes of residents

wearing antiembolism hose (TED hose, compression hose, graduated-pressure hosiery) one or more times each shift by looking through the hole in the toe end of the stocking. Document this monitoring on the flow sheet. Antiembolism hose are difficult and time consuming to remove for inspection, palpation, or visualization of the heels. Making a vertical split across the heels of antiembolism hosiery enables you to retract the stocking to inspect or palpate the heel and relieves pressure.

Myths and facts

There are many myths and facts surrounding preventive foot care. Nurses should review current literature and bring their practices into line. Professional literature is replete with examples that show that certain practices thought to aid in prevention of heel ulcers may actually contribute to their development. For example, many nurses fill a latex glove with water and prop the heel on it to relieve pressure. This creates a higher pressure than if the heel is resting on the bed. Interface pressure between the heel and the water-filled glove in 40 residents averaged 144.6 mm Hg, while interface pressures between the heel and the bed averaged 126.5 mm Hg.[16] Suspending the heels off the surface of the bed is a much more effective strategy. Remember the pressure that causes most ulcerations is between the bone and the skin, not the skin and other surfaces.

Many commercial heel protectors increase pressure. The seams may also irritate or damage the skin. Select a heel protector to meet the resident's needs, but do not depend on this measure alone for preventive care. Remember that there is no single panacea for prevention of foot and heel pressure ulcers. The solution lies with initial and ongoing nursing and risk assessment, an individualized plan of care, and diligent positioning of the resident.

Wound pain

Pressure ulcers and superficial skin wounds are painful! One old health care myth notes that Stage IV ulcers are below the nerve endings, and thus are no longer painful. The myth fails to consider that the resident experiences a great deal of pain as the ulcer progresses from Stage I through Stage IV. It also does not take into consideration that the edges of the wound are not always as deep as the center, and nerves are often exposed. The standard of care is to regularly assess for and manage pressure ulcer pain. Because short-acting analgesics are usually used in long-term care, pain assessment should be frequent. Once daily is usually not adequate.

The standard of care in long-term care facilities is to relieve pain and ensure each resident's quality of life is as high as possible:

- A nursing facility must be administered in a manner that enables it to use its resources effectively and efficiently to attain or maintain the highest practicable physical, mental, and psychosocial well-being of each resident.[17]

- Every resident should be assessed for pain systematically and regularly. Treat chronic pain, even when a specific cause for the pain cannot be identified. Individualize the administration of medications to meet residents' needs. Such a flexible regimen may place more demands on caregiving staff but is likely to result in more effective pain management.[18]

- The goal of pain management in the resident with pressure ulcers is to eliminate the cause of the pain, to provide analgesia, or both. Assess all residents for pain related to the pressure ulcer or its treatment. Caregivers should not assume that, because a resident cannot express or respond to pain, it does not exist. In this situation, it may be best to assume pain is present unless otherwise proven. Manage pain by eliminating or controlling the source of pain. Because pain may be evoked or may be especially acute during dressing changes and debridement, anticipate and prevent this discomfort. Provide analgesia as needed and appropriate.[19]

Assessment and management of wound pain

Many elderly residents have at least one painful, chronic medical condition. Immobility, improper moving, friction, and shearing often increase pain. Sixty to 80 percent of residents with chronic wounds experience some pain, and 50% of residents with pressure ulcers have pain, especially those with Stages III and IV ulcers.[20] Residents with paralysis and spinal cord injury may experience persistent pain in areas that otherwise have no sensation. Open areas on the skin can be excruciatingly painful. Ineffective pain management results in delayed healing, lack of compliance, and prolonged care. Blood flow to the wound can be decreased during episodes of pain. Pain subsides with healing in acute wounds. However, the protracted inflammatory response seen in chronic wounds may cause an increased sensitivity in the wound (*primary hyperalgesia*) and surrounding skin (*secondary hyperalgesia*). If the resident experiences additional pain during debridement, dressing changes, movement, etc., this may trigger allodynia, a condition in which ordinarily nonpainful stimuli cause pain. Since wounds damage nerves, some residents may develop *neuropathic pain*, a condition in which the pain response is exaggerated. Minor sensations, such as air on a wound, light touch, or change in temperature will evoke intense pain. Other complications such as infection and ischemia may also contribute to the resident's pain response. Inadequate wound management contributes to wound pain.

The European Wound Management Association (EWMA) published a position statement in 2002 with recommendations for managing pain during the dressing change.[21] Consider premedicating the resident and using the newer (advanced) dressings to decrease frequency of dressing changes. Avoid assuming that wound size affects pain. A small wound can be very painful, whereas a large wound in a different resident is described as mildly uncomfortable. There is no proven relationship between the intensity of pain and the type or size of the wound. This factor is highly variable and individualized.[22] The results of one study revealed that the degree of pain is related to the stage of the pressure ulcer. This dispels the belief that Stage IV pressure ulcers are painless.[23]

Regularly assess residents with open wounds and pressure ulcers for pain using a validated pain scale, if possible. (You will find additional pain assessment information in Chapter 16 of your book.) If the pain is frequent or constant, consider giving a scheduled pain medication. If the resident has an order for PRN analgesics, give them at the earliest sign of pain. Do not wait for pain to get out of control. Always evaluate the resident's response to pain-relieving medication. Strategies for pain relief at dressing change are

- Offer analgesics when pain is anticipated. Premedicate the resident at least one hour before dressing change or debridement. Evaluate the resident's response by assessing the effectiveness of the medication during the procedure. If the procedure is exceedingly painful, a stronger premedication may be needed. Another option is to use a topical product, such as those containing lidocaine. These are highly effective, but take approximately two hours to work.

- Dispel myths and teach the resident facts about pain and pain management. For example, the old adage "no pain, no gain" is a myth. Teach the resident that less pain means more gain in wound healing. Another common myth is that responsiveness to pain decreases with age. Many nurses believe that pain tolerance decreases, and elderly residents increase their complaints. Sensory processing of painful stimuli *does not change* with age. Older adults experience many painful chronic diseases. They may experience more pain than younger adults, yet complain less.

- Involve the resident in decision-making and give him or her a sense of personal control over the pain.

- Provide anti-anxiety medications, if requested by the resident.

- During the dressing change, monitor the resident's body language and nonverbal cues carefully for signs of pain.

- Avoid unnecessary manipulation of the wound. Protect it from sources of irritation, including air flow from a fan or window.

- Warm the cleansing solution prior to cleansing the wound, if possible.

Pay attention to wounds!

I try to avoid using first person when I write my various missives. I also try to avoid telling war stories, although much of what I write was learned in the school of hard knocks, or by personal experience. This is the only place in this book where I will digress to first person and war stories, but it is a subject that is very important to me. I also believe that sometimes simple methods of managing complications are the most effective.

When I was a director of nursing of a large SNF, I conducted various wound product studies, looking for the panacea to quickly heal all the pressure ulcers. I finally concluded that no panacea existed, and I learned to match the treatment product to the wound characteristics. This was effective, and a good learning experience. However, the most important lesson I learned was that I had fewer wounds if I paid a great deal of attention to the numbers. My staff did not want me on their units checking behind them, monitoring and adjusting care plans, or generally ranting and raving about the evils associated with in-house pressure ulcers, and did all they could to prevent them. If a minor area developed, they usually identified and healed it quickly. If I got busy or distracted for a few weeks, the numbers seemed to find a way of increasing. Because of this, I encourage you to make your dislike of pressure ulcers very clear.

Although they are not 100 percent preventable, most can be prevented with aggressive nursing care. Develop a weekly tracking and reporting system. If a new ulcer develops or an existing ulcer is non-healing, make it your business to investigate the situation. I think you will be surprised and pleased, just as I was when I learned that simply paying close attention to pressure ulcers had a dramatic effect on resident care in the facility!

- Use only normal saline or pH-neutral wound cleansers. Be gentle when cleaning the wound.

- Allow the resident to stop and rest during a painful procedure, such as a dressing change. Agree on a signal in advance.

- Match the dressing and treatment product to the wound. Use dressings that are non-adherent and reduce pain. Avoid woven, cotton gauze, which is highly irritating to sensitive skin.

- Select wound products that maintain a moist environment in the wound bed. Do not allow the wound to become desiccated.

- Select treatments that can remain in place for a prolonged period of time. Avoid frequent dressing changes by using advanced products, if possible.

- Consider contact layer dressings that remain in place, decreasing the need to manipulate the tender wound bed and increasing pain.

- Use compression bandages, if needed, to reduce edema, relieving pain.

- Apply barrier products to protect the wound margins, preventing maceration and further breakdown. This is particularly important if chemical debriding agents are being used.

- Many residents complain that pain is intense during dressing removal. Allow the resident to remove his or her own dressing, if desired.

- Remove tape and dressings carefully and gently. If the dressing or tape sticks to the skin during dressing removal, apply normal saline, then wait a few minutes.

- If the resident's skin is sensitive, or if he or she is at risk for skin tears, minimize the use of tape. Use bandage, Montgomery straps, Coban®, etc. to cover the dressings.

- Follow manufacturers' instructions for removal of hydrocolloids and transparent films. To remove a transparent film or hydrocolloid dressing, maintain gentle traction on the skin, pressing down. Loosen the adhesive in one corner of the dressing, peeling it back slightly. Now go to the opposite corner. Loosen the adhesive and peel the dressing back slightly. Stretch the dressing horizontally, gently lifting it over the open area. The stretching helps to break the adhesive bond. Always remove the dressing by pulling in the direction of hair growth. If the skin is not hairy, the corners on opposite sides of the dressing can be lifted. Stretch the dressing from the edges toward the center and lift off.

- Avoid treatments that increase unpleasant or painful sensory stimulation, such as wet-to-dry dressings.

- Splint or immobilize the wound during movement and treatment, if possible.

- Teach residents to use relaxation and distraction techniques, such as guided imagery, slow, deep breathing, biofeedback, and listening to music through a headset.

- Your bandage scissors are a potential source of cross contamination. Wash them with soap and water and dry well after each use. Also consider the treatment cart and plastic bags used for dressing trash as potential sources of cross contamination. Keep clean and soiled items separate. Infection control is discussed in greater detail in Chapter 14.

References

1. Hammock v. State, 592 S.E.2d 415 (Ga. 2004).

2. State v. Chervenell, 2001 Wash. App. LEXIS 1764 (July 30, 2001).

3. U.S. Department of Health and Human Services (Eds). (1992). *Pressure Ulcers in Adults: Prediction and Prevention.* Rockville, MD. Agency for Health Care Policy and Research.

4. U.S. Department of Health and Human Services. (1992). *Pressure Ulcers in Adults: Prediction and Prevention.* Rockville, MD. Agency for Health Care Policy and Research.

5. U.S. Department of Health and Human Services. (1992). *Pressure Ulcers in Adults: Prediction and Prevention.* Rockville, MD. Agency for Health Care Policy and Research.

6. U.S. Department of Health and Human Services. (1994). *Pressure ulcer treatment.* Rockville, MD. Agency for Health Care Policy and Research.

7. Anderson, Peter. (1998). Contracture care management: an emerging healthcare field. (1998). *Medtrade News.*

8. U.S. Department of Health and Human Services. (1994). *Pressure ulcer treatment.* Rockville, MD. Agency for Health Care Policy and Research.

9. Smith I. Two heel aids. *Nursing Times* 1984; 80:35-39.

10. De Keyser G. Dejaeger H. De Meyst H. Evers G. *Pressure reducing effects of heel protectors.* Advances in Wound Care 1994; 4:30-32. 5.

11. Tymec AC, Vollman K, Pieper B. *A comparison of two pressure-relieving devices on the prevention of heel pressure ulcers.* Advances in Wound Care 1997; 10:39-44.

12. Smith I. Two heel aids. Nursing Times 1984; 80:35-39. 6. Williams C. Using water filled gloves for pressure relief on heels. *Journal of Wound Care* 1993; 2:345-348. *Return to Cover of Wound Care Institute* Newsletter Vol. 4. No.1, Jan/Feb 1999

13. Agu O, Hamilton G, Baker D. (1999). Graduated compression stockings in the prevention of venous thromboembolism. *Br J Surg* 1999;86:992-1004.

14. Hayes JM; Lehman CA; Castonguay P. (2002). Graduated compression stockings: updating practice, improving compliance. *Medical-Surgical Nursing Journal.* Online. *www.ajj.com/.* Accessed 12/20/03.

15. Hayes JM; Lehman CA; Castonguay P. (2002). Graduated compression stockings: updating practice, improving compliance. *Medical-Surgical Nursing Journal.* Online. *www.ajj.com/.* Accessed 12/20/03.

16. Williams C. Using water filled gloves for pressure relief on heels. *Journal of Wound Care* 1993; 2:345-348.

17. Centers for Medicare and Medicaid Services. State Operations Manual. Appendix PP. Guidance to Surveyors for Long-term Care Facilities. (Rev. 1, 05-21-04). F250 §483.15(g)(1).

18. American Medical Directors' Association (AMDA). (Eds). (1999). *Chronic pain management in the long-term care setting.* Columbia MD. American Medical Directors' Association.

19. U.S. Department of Health and Human Services (Eds). (1994). *Pressure Ulcer Treatment.* Rockville, MD. Agency for Health Care Policy and Research.

20. Langemo D, Bates-Jensen B, Hanson D. Pressure Ulcers in Individuals at the End of Life: Palliative Care and Hospice, Pressure Ulcers in America: Prevalence, Incidence and Implications for the Future, NPUAP Monograph 2001:145.

21. European Wound Management Society. (2002). Position Document: Pain at Wound Dressing Changes. London, UK: Medical Education Partnership Ltd., 2002:2, 8.

22. European Wound Management Society. (2002). Position Document: Pain at Wound Dressing Changes. London, UK: Medical Education Partnership Ltd., 2002:2, 8.

23. Szor JK, Bourguignon C. Description of pressure ulcer pain at rest and at dressing change. *J Wound Ostomy Continence Nurs* 1999;26:115-20.

Leading causes of lawsuits: Falls

"Sarah Stone was admitted to the BMJ Nursing and Rehabilitation Center on or about June 14, 2001. Previously, she had been a resident of another long term care facility. She was diagnosed with Alzheimer's disease and required the services of a secured unit. She was also diagnosed with atherosclerotic cardiovascular disease (ASCVD) and degenerative joint disease (DJD). She had a history of falls at the previous facility. This was a major concern to her son, who informed the BMJ nurses of her high fall risk and history on admission.

Mrs. Stone was unsteady on her feet and began experiencing skin injuries and falls shortly after admission. She was placed in an adult walker (Merry Walker; similar to an infant walker), but she promptly tipped it. Restraining the resident in a wheelchair was ineffective. She required a vest restraint when she was in bed. Despite the restraint, she was agitated and managed to get out of bed a number of times. The resident's agitation worsened in August and September 2001. She was found to have a urinary tract infection. After treatment for infection, the agitation subsided to the resident's normal level.

Mrs. Stone's pattern of falls with skin injuries persisted until May 1, 2002, when she was found on the floor with signs and symptoms of a hip fracture. She was sent to the hospital, where she was diagnosed with an intertrochanteric fracture of the hip. She was treated surgically and returned to the long term care facility on May 7, 2002. Upon return, the resident was less agitated than usual. On May 25, 2002, she was very lethargic. She developed respiratory distress and was found to have a fever during the late afternoon. She was sent to the hospital, where she expired soon after admission.

The BMJ Nursing and Rehabilitation Center failed to develop, maintain, implement, and evaluate a proper plan of care using the nursing process to meet the needs of Mrs. Stone. They failed to observe or assess the resident, failed to plan her care based on that assessment, and failed to intervene on her behalf. They failed to initiate the plan on admission, leaving this high risk resident with no care plan direction to staff until June 27, 2001. During this period of time, she had at least two fall incidents. Subsequently, several different injury prevention approaches were tried but were ineffective.

The plan was not updated. Geri hips were ordered in July 2001 and were added to the plan at some point as a handwritten entry, but the entry is not dated, so there is no way of knowing when the information was added. There is no documentation showing the hip protectors were used.

The admission nursing note indicates the resident had a history of falls and required monitoring every 15 to 20 minutes. This information would also have been appropriate for an initial (interim, temporary, or admission) plan of care, as well as for the permanent plan. Unfortunately, no initial plan was done and it is not listed on the plan of care or flow sheets. There is no evidence it was ever done. Despite the resident's recurrent falls and injuries, there were no changes to the approaches used for injury/fall prevention after July 2001, and the plan of care was not updated in any way. Padded side rails were ordered in September 2001, but this does not constitute a change, in that the rails had been used previously without an order. The padded side rails were never listed on the care plan.

Personnel were aware that the plan was not working and the resident continued to sustain falls and other injuries, but the incidents were not investigated, the resident was not reassessed, and the ineffective plan was not updated. The plan did not list methodologies to keep the resident in bed and prevent injuries when it became evident that the vest restraint was not working.

The plan did not include other important information about the resident, such as the need to evaluate for urinary infection and illness if the resident's agitation worsened. The plan did not describe the resident's high risk for dehydration, and did not list preventive care. A nurse reviewed the laboratory values in January 2002 and knew the abnormal values were an indication of dehydration. She increased fluids on her shift, as did the oncoming nurse. Unfortunately, after this no special measures were taken and the hydration information was not added to the plan of care. No further labs were done in the facility, but the lab values continued to be abnormal on May 1, 2002 when the resident was admitted to the hospital for the hip fracture."

The resident experienced 38 fall events between June 2001 and the hip fracture in May 2002.

"The plan did not adequately describe care for changes in the resident's condition during periods of acute illness. Although the nursing process remains the same, the nurses failed to include new information that would dictate a new approach. It did not adequately describe moving the resident and hip precautions to take following the hip fracture surgery. In fact, the plan was not started until a week after the resident's return to the facility, leaving personnel without instructions in postoperative care. Important data were not listed on the plan from the physician orders, so all personnel were not informed of approaches to implement for the resident's safety and postoperative care. The plan did not adequately describe the resident's special positioning needs, aside from placing an abduction pillow. The plan did not specify when the pillow should be used. It did not list observations to make and report regarding complications of hip surgery. The antiembolism hosiery (TED hose) and non-slip socks ordered by the doctor were not added to the plan, nor were they issued or applied to the resident, depriving the resident of medically necessary care and increasing her risk of complications."

(From an expert report of an actual lawsuit alleging progressive failures and omissions of care.)

Falls and fractures

Pressure ulcers are the leading cause of lawsuits against long-term care facilities. Next in line, falls and fractures are a close second. More than 50% of all nursing facility residents fall each year. Of these, approximately 40% experience repeated falls. Of these, approximately 11% experience significant injuries associated with the fall.[1] Common injuries include hip fracture, which increases mortality. Pelvic fractures and other long bone fractures, as well as subdural hematoma and other head injuries are common causes of lawsuits associated with falls. Although no studies have been published related to mortality of head injuries in the long-term care population, they are often devastating to the elderly, and many suffer irreversible declines after a fall resulting in injuries to the face and head. Family members often view the injury as being much worse than it is because of the vascularity of the head and face. Injuries to this area often result in profuse bleeding and extensive bruising because of the high number of blood vessels in the area.

Assessment

Preventive care begins with an assessment of each resident's fall risk. Since most facility residents are at risk for falls, the emphasis of assessment is identifying individual risk factors, and the focus of care planning is mitigating risk factors. All residents should have a fall risk assessment on admission. An effective "best practice" is to consider all newly admitted residents at high risk for the first 72 hours (or a designated time frame, such as 21 days) after admission. Include multiple, high-risk resident interventions. After the resident has been more fully assessed, remove those that are unnecessary.

Successful fall prevention requires a thorough clinical assessment of residents who fall (or have a history of falls) and their environment. The care plan should list risk factors. This list is a combination of the resident's personal problems (intrinsic factors) and environmental (extrinsic) factors that contribute to fall risk. Intrinsic risk factors include normal aging changes, acute and chronic conditions, and medications. Extrinsic risk factors are risks that are most common in bedrooms, bathrooms, dining rooms and hallways.[2] Safe equipment, such as wheelchairs that fit the resident properly with working brakes, are also a consideration.

Defining falls

Make sure that nursing personnel are familiar with the current MDS fall definitions, including the "near miss" definition, such as when staff intervene to prevent a fall from occurring. *Complete an incident report for each fall or near miss.* Near misses identify potential problems that always warrant further investigation. Acting on a near miss may prevent an injury in the future. For example, staff intervene when a resident becomes dizzy and unstable. An investigation into the cause of the dizziness reveals the resident is mildly dehydrated. Treating this condition eliminates the dizziness. By completing an incident report on all defined falls, your statistics may increase over the short term. However, over the long term, acting on these data will reduce the severity of injuries associated with falls. An example of the MDS definitions for falls is given in Table 12-1.

Table 12-1	*Fall definitions*

Type of fall	Definition and commentary
Unwitnessed Fall	The resident is found on the floor. The facility is obligated to investigate and try to determine how he or she got there, and to put an intervention into place to prevent this from happening again. Unless there is evidence suggesting otherwise, the most logical conclusion is that a fall has occurred.
Near Miss	An episode in which a resident lost his or her balance and would have fallen, were it not for staff intervention, is a fall. An intercepted fall is still a fall.
Fall	The resident moves from a higher place to a lower surface, such as from the standing position to the floor. The distance to the next lower surface (in this case, the floor) is not a factor in determining whether or not a fall occurred. If a resident rolled off a low bed or mattress that was close to the floor, this is a fall. The presence or absence of a resultant injury is not a factor in the definition of a fall. A fall without injury is still a fall.

Risk factors and fall injuries

The high incidence of mortality associated with falls in the elderly is due to underlying medical problems, and not the fall incident.[3] The statistics listed here are somewhat conservative. Other studies have shown a much higher morbidity and mortality related to falls in the elderly. The cliché "Old age starts with the first fall and death comes with the second"[4] is certainly an exaggeration, but sadly, it has a familiar ring of truth to it.

Fall prevention programs are wonderful if they are implemented. Unfortunately, many facilities have assessment tools for identifying fall risk. They complete the fall assessments, and perhaps even write a fall prevention care plan. However, they fail to implement the plan, so the resident falls (or continues to fall). Remember that all healthcare professionals are responsible for acting on the results of the assessment

data. Completing fall risk questionnaires is not an exercise in paper compliance, and is certainly not done for personal edification!

The long-term care facility has a duty to prevent injuries. When a facility accepts a resident, it has a duty to care for the resident. Many residents are admitted because of a history of falls at home, and the facility is usually aware of this problem at the time of admission. If we know of a fall history, or independently identify a fall risk, we have a duty to take active steps to prevent falls and keep the resident safe. The facility's duty is heightened by the reality that the facility and its staff accepted the obligation to take active measures to ensure the safety of the residents entrusted to their care. *A facility has the duty to take every reasonable action within its power to minimize falls and injuries.* Identifying fall risk and implementing fall policies and procedures works if you implement them! A fall prevention care plan offers a measure of protection. However, the plan must be current and personalized to the resident. Avoid generic, computer-generated plans describing routine care given to all residents, such as ensuring the call signal is within reach. For cognitively impaired residents, avoid meaningless approaches such as "remind resident to use call signal." If the MDS reveals the resident has short-term memory loss, and he or she seldom uses the call signal, this approach will be ineffective. Aside from that, it is a routine measure used for all residents that does not need to be listed on the care plan.

Terminology used for describing transfers on care plans should be very specific. For example, the term "two-person lift" can be used to designate at least three distinctly different techniques. Make sure to specify which technique should be used. Listing the many personal and environmental factors that could appear on a fall prevention care plan would take an entire book. Consider all relevant factors for each resident, develop realistic approaches, and list them on the care plan or critical pathway. Communicate the fall prevention plan to all direct care staff. Avoid using the same, computer-generated approaches for all residents in the facility. Personalize them! Avoid duplicating an old approach that was previously found to be ineffective.

After an individualized plan has been developed, staff must follow the plan. Having a plan that staff do not read or follow is as bad or worse than having no plan at all. Many facilities have been successful in involving all employees, including maintenance and housekeeping in the fall prevention program.

For example, a housekeeper finds a resident climbing through the side rails. Rather than ignoring the situa-

tion, he or she should remain in the room and try to calm the resident, while using the call signal, phone, or calling out for nursing assistance.

The care plan requires thorough fall risk assessment and development of resident-centered interventions for fall prevention. Evaluate the effectiveness of fall risk reduction interventions, and document the results so care plan adjustments can be made based on effectiveness.[5] If a fall occurs, your individualized care plan is not working and should be revised promptly. When a fall occurs

- Assess the resident promptly to identify and treat injuries. If the resident has been on the floor for an unknown period of time, determine why it was not noticed earlier.

- Identify what the resident was doing when the fall occurred, by interviewing the resident and witnesses.

- Question staff to determine whether other factors may have contributed to the fall. For example, determine whether the resident was more confused than usual at the time of the fall. If so, try to determine why. Mild, asymptomatic dehydration is a common cause of worsening confusion in residents with cognitive impairment.

- Repeat the initial fall risk assessment, including intrinsic and extrinsic factors listed in this chapter.

- Check orthostatic blood pressure. This is an important and commonly overlooked part of your evaluation.

- Identify intrinsic and extrinsic factors associated with this fall.

- Assess the resident's medical conditions (e.g., prior stroke, other neurological illness, osteoporosis) to determine whether they contributed to the fall.

- Evaluate the resident's problems to determine whether they are being managed in a manner that decreases fall risk. If not, ask yourself whether improved management could help prevent future falls.

- Determine whether the resident had unmet needs that contributed to the fall; if so, develop a plan to meet the needs and reduce fall risk.

- Evaluate the total medication regimen. Residents taking more than five medications daily have a greater risk for falls.[6,7]

- Determine whether antidepressants, hypnotics, anxiolytics, antipsychotics, antihypertensives, or diuretics are being used. If so, assess each specific drug for side effects.

- Consult the pharmacist and physician to determine whether the medication regimen can be modified (e.g., lowering doses, drug interactions) or medications associated with fall risk eliminated.

- Modify staff and facility safety practices to prevent falls and to detect them quickly when they do occur.

- Evaluate gait and balance by watching the resident stand and walk. Note the gait. Instruct the resident to turn around and return to the chair. Based on this part of the assessment, identify and address

    – Lower extremity weakness

    – Gait abnormalities

    – Balance abnormalities

    – Need for (or appropriateness of) assistive devices

    – Need for (or appropriateness of) personal assistance

    – Need for (or appropriateness of) restraints or alternatives

    – If the resident uses a wheelchair, assistive device or restraint, determine whether the selection of the device is optimal for the resident, it fits properly, and is used correctly

    – Determine whether environmental modifications are needed.

- Assess the resident's level of ADL dependence to ensure he or she is receiving the needed assistance.

- Assess the resident's mental status and level of cognitive impairment.

- Document the results of the fall investigation, note whether intrinsic, extrinsic, or other factors, such as obstacles or being pushed down by another resident, contributed to the fall.[8]

- Evaluate the knowledge and attitudes of the resident, responsible party, and staff pertaining to the importance of resident autonomy and fall prevention. Educate them about fall risk management and interventions that reduce fall risk. Teach staff skills and strategies to reduce fall risk, improve residents' gait, balance, and strength.[9]

- Evaluate the effectiveness of each fall risk reduction intervention listed on the care plan and modify the plan to enhance effectiveness.

- Determine whether the fall affected the resident's confidence in his or her ability to transfer or ambulate; fear of future falls can lead to inactivity, loss of muscle strength, and other complications.

- Discuss falls with residents, families, and staff. Ask them to verbalize their expectations. Not every fall is preventable, but some falls have no injuries. The goal is to reduce falls as much as possible, and to reduce the risk of serious injuries.

Less-common problems to assess

The problems in this section are sometimes overlooked during fall risk assessment. Aging and diseases often erode the nervous system and sensations. Impaired sensation can occur in any age group, but is most common in the elderly. Sensory loss may be mistaken for memory loss and disorientation. Sensory loss causes reduced orientation to the environment. Residents who cannot see or hear well may appear confused, not understand safety instructions, and not use environmental safety features. They are often more dependent on staff. Diminishing sensation can cause everyday tasks to become very hazardous. We worry about elderly drivers being able to see, hear, and react quickly when driving a car. Correcting vision and hearing problems improves safety and increases independence and safety in driving. They also improve safety for residents in a facility, and should be included in your fall risk assessment and plan of care.

Loss of sensation occurs in many chronic conditions, such as diabetes, peripheral neuropathy, and stroke. Since neurological problems develop slowly, the resident may not know that his or her sense of position is impaired. Partial and complete sensory loss affect fall risk. Humans gather information about location, position, and balance from the hands, legs, and feet. Residents may not know where their feet are or how they are positioned. Assess all residents for impaired sensation. You may be unaware of the problem in residents who seem otherwise healthy.

Balance problems are very real for residents who have had a stroke. Reduced, abnormal, or absent sensation in the feet is especially important. Delayed reaction time compounds the problem. Proper sensory feedback is critical to the resident's reaction when he or she starts to fall. Researchers in one small study theorize that loss of sensation in the feet results in the need to take more steps (baby steps) than individuals with normal sensation.[10] When a sensory-impaired individual begins to fall, he or she must take more steps to maintain balance. Because falls are so unpredictable, the resident is unable to move the feet quickly or to take a step, and falls to the floor. Planning and preparing a proper response is impossible. Research is being done to study various shoes and orthotic devices to identify ways of compensating for sensation loss, but this will take years. Meanwhile, protect the residents' feet, and make sure the shoes are appropriate to the floor surface. Provide ambulation devices, such as canes and walkers. Consider a therapy or restorative program that develops balance and strength by assisting the resident to stand on one leg, and other activities that increase balance, grip and upper-body strength.

When a resident has sensory losses that increase fall risk, he will probably use other senses to compensate. For example, a resident with sensation impairment in the legs may use the eyes to help compensate. Knowing this, you can assist by maximizing visual function. Ensure there is enough light in the area. If the resident wears glasses, make sure they are clean and in place. Identify the resident's compensatory mechanisms and use them as strengths when planning care. Understand why you are doing this. These are not generic approaches. They are individualized to the resident and use strengths to overcome needs.

Consider pain a fall risk factor. Residents who are in pain are less active and sometimes assume peculiar positions when ambulating and transferring to compensate for the pain. Movement may be stilted or rigid. If this is the case, include corrective approaches in your plan of care. Acute pain is easier to identify and treat than chronic pain. Quarterly pain assessments are not sufficient. Evaluate cognitively impaired residents regularly for presence of pain. Behavior problems often reflect pain or another discomfort, such as needing to use the bathroom. Frequent pain assessment is necessary, encompassing all shifts and various activities and behaviors. Review the American Geriatrics Society pain guidelines to ensure residents are not using analgesics that are not recommended for elderly persons or those that markedly increase fall risk. (In a fall risk situation, these are often the first drugs targeted for elimination. Assess the residents' response to the drugs; do not eliminate them unnecessarily.) In any event, always consider pain when developing a fall prevention plan.

Review the medication regimen as part of the fall assessment. Polypharmacy and drug incompatibility have been implicated in increased fall risk. Delirium caused by new drugs or a combination of drugs also increases fall risk. Psychotropic drugs have been implicated in increased risk of falls and fractures. A pharmacist is a valuable team member when planning care for persons with complex drug regimens.

Remember to assess the resident's fear of falling, which is problematic for some residents. They tend to be afraid to move, or are dependent on staff because of their fear. Assess the "fear factor" as part of the fall assessment, and address it in the fall prevention plan, if necessary.

Orthostatic hypotension is a transient reduction in blood pressure identified as the most common cardiovascular risk factor for falls. Some medications, conditions that cause volume depletion such as dehydration and diarrhea, and medical problems that cause reduced blood flow to the brain have been implicated. Orthostatic hypotension presents a real

problem for many residents taking psychotropic drugs. Decreased blood pressure contributes to dizziness and syncope. Unusual conditions, such as chronic bronchitis, paroxysmal coughing, and post voiding reactions in males can trigger dizziness and syncope.[11] Conditions such as bearing down to have a bowel movement slow the vagus nerve, potentially causing loss of consciousness. Orthostatic blood pressure values are frequently overlooked. Because of the magnitude and variety of problems associated with orthostatic hypotension, do not omit this important part of fall assessment.

Fall history is another important consideration. A single fall within the past year increases the annual fall risk. Identify the resident's fall history, circumstances, and causative factors and include them in the plan of care. Consider pain, orthostasis, and other problems listed here. Ask your therapists for suggestions and individual approaches. Therapists are invaluable resources for planning fall prevention and restraint reduction. Do not overlook them or devalue the importance of their participation when planning safety and fall prevention programs. Some facilities feel so strongly about this that they have therapists review all falls for causation and preventive care.

As you can see, most of these conditions are not included in the standard fall assessment tools. This in no way devalues the tools that are available. Some are excellent, and if they work for your facility, please continue to use them! However, use common sense and consider individual problems that are not on the printed form. Considering that many individuals do not fit the "one size fits all" mold is often the key to success when planning fall prevention and safety. Remember these principles from the MDS instructions:

- Facilities are responsible for assessing areas that are relevant to residents, regardless of whether these areas are included in the Resident Assessment Instrument (RAI; MDS). The RAI is the minimum assessment tool, not the only assessment tool.[12]

- The care plan is a dynamic document that needs to be continually evaluated and appropriately modified based on measurable outcomes. This continual evaluation takes into consideration resident change relative to the initial baseline—in other words, if the resident has declined, stayed the same, or improved at a lesser rate than expected, then a modification in the care plan may be necessary.[13]

- As the process of problem identification is integrated with sound clinical interventions, the care plan becomes each resident's unique path toward achieving or maintaining his or her highest practicable level of well-being.[14]

- When the care plan is implemented in accordance with the standards of good clinical practice, then the care plan becomes powerful and practical, and represents the best approach to providing for the quality of care and quality of life needs of an individual resident.[15]

Behavior management and fall risk

Behavior problems are common in long-term care facility residents. All behavior has a meaning, although the meaning may not be apparent to you. Sometimes "behavioral" problems are not problems at all. They are cultural variations that residents may not consider problematic. Always consider cultural influences on behavior. All behavior patterns develop across the lifespan and are affected by heredity, culture, environment, and lifetime experiences.

Defense (coping) mechanisms are tools for managing stress and compensating for losses. Defense mechanisms protect self-esteem. Everyone begins developing coping mechanisms early in life, although they become more pronounced, sophisticated, and refined with age. Once we have developed them, we use the same basic methods of coping with stress throughout our lifetime. Common coping/defense mechanisms are:

- **Denial**—refusing to admit that a problem exists

- **Projection**—blaming someone or something else for the problem

- **Compensation**—using strength, overcompensating, or overachieving in one area to overcome weakness in another

- **Rationalization**—providing an acceptable but untrue explanation for a problem

All residents use coping mechanisms in response to stress. Confused residents also use their well-defined coping mechanisms. Anger is a common defense mechanism. Although many caregivers take resident anger personally, this is seldom the case. Most commonly, the resident is angry with loss of control, and not the workers. Understanding this and using positive self-talk helps workers cope with their own frustration. Evaluating and identifying the underlying cause of the problem may help the resident. If the underlying problem can be eliminated, the resident's behavior will change. Another key is to modify your approach to the resident in response to the behavior. Modern behavior management focuses on staff reaction. Older behavior management techniques (such as reality orientation) have been proven ineffective with residents suffering from dementia. Be empathetic and try to assist the resident in understanding what is happening. He or she may feel out of control, empty, or powerless to do anything about it.

The ABCs of behavior management

The ABC plan is a very effective method for managing behavior problems. It may be used for both alert and cognitively impaired residents. The plan evolves from identifying and modifying the *antecedent* or *consequences* of the behavior. If one or both are eliminated or modified, the behavior will cease. When using the ABC method

> A = antecedent (the cause or trigger of the behavior)
>
> B = the behavior itself
>
> C = consequences (reward or outcome of the behavior)

Using the three-step behavior management plan

* **Step 1**—Attempt to identify the cause (trigger or antecedent) of the behavior. Determine whether the behavior occurs in specific environmental conditions, at a certain time of day, during a certain activity, in the presence (or absence) of certain other persons such as family, visitors, other residents, or staff. Is the resident feeling lack of control or out of control? Is he or she having pain or unmet physical needs?

Identifying the antecedent is almost always done through trial and error. Residents with communication problems can be especially frustrating for staff. Many confused residents display negative behavior in response to unmet physical needs, such as pain, hunger, thirst, too much or too little environmental stimulation, uncomfortable environmental temperature, or need to use the bathroom. Alert residents commonly display negative behavior in response to pain or unmet psychosocial needs. Common causes are feelings of loss of control over their bodies, family situations, finances, or the environment.

* **Step 2**—Eliminate the cause of the behavior. Identifying and eliminating the cause will change or stop the behavior.

If the cause of the behavior is known, eliminate it. If you are using trial and error, try, for example, giving the resident a drink. Take him or her to the bathroom. Don't forget that unrelieved pain is often a common cause of behavior problems in residents with dementia or communication deficits. Giving the resident a dose of acetaminophen will not hurt. Researchers found that residents with moderate to severe dementia had positive behavioral changes after being given acetaminophen. The findings suggest that unrecognized, untreated pain keeps them from being as active as they can be.[16]

* **Step 3**—Explore the consequences of the behavior. It may be necessary to modify the consequences in order to change the behavior. This takes practice, and the resident may need reinforcement. For example, a confused resident can't find her room. She wanders about the hallway crying. Staff give her a hug, take her by the hand, and lead her to her room. The hug is a reward for the behavior. Try to modify her behavior by giving her hugs periodically before she becomes lost. Sitting and holding her hand, or paying attention to her, may, over time, modify the behavior. The extra attention she receives for becoming lost may be reinforcing the behavior problem. Here, modifying the consequences changes the behavior. However, keep in mind that the resident's behavior will not change overnight if it has been rewarded for a long period of time. Be patient and persistent. All healthcare providers must pay regular attention to the resident and follow a single plan of care before results are apparent consistently. In this case

A = the resident's perceived need for love and attention. (Other factors may also trigger the wandering and getting lost, but these are unknown without further investigation.)

B = getting lost and crying

C = hugs and attention serve as a reward

Modifying the consequences of behavior is an effective method of eliminating behavior problems. Staff become frustrated with the inability to identify the trigger (cause) of the behavior. This may be because the consequences require modification. If the resident responds well to a certain method of stopping behavior, implement this approach routinely, before the behavior starts, and see if it is successful.

Residents who use the call signal frequently for problems considered minor are distressing and annoying to staff. Minutes after you leave the room, the resident signals again. This is often caused by feeling fearful or lonely, although the resident may not be willing to admit it. The call signal is a means of getting attention. When you leave the room, inform the resident when you will return. Keep your word and return at that time. Stop to check on the resident between times, as often as possible. This requires a team approach. As the resident gets more attention, unnecessary use of the call signal decreases. In this case

A = the resident's loneliness and fear

B = using the call signal for minor requests

C = attention and companionship when you are in the room

Checking on the resident frequently and keeping promises shows that staff are dependable, changing the consequences of the behavior. The resident gets regular companionship and attention, which calms

her fear and loneliness. She does not use the call signal as often, because she has no reason to continue.

In these examples, the consequences were modified to change the behavior. Sometimes, the antecedent must be changed. For example, a confused resident is fine during the day, but yells, cries, or screams each night at bedtime when you leave the room. When staff return and turn on the light, the behavior stops. The resident may be afraid of the dark. Through trial and error, you discover that she stops screaming if you leave a light on in the bathroom at night. In this case, the antecedent caused the problem.

A = the resident's fear of the dark.

B = screaming when she is alone in a dark room.

C = the bathroom light is turned on, eliminating her fear and enabling her to sleep.

A team approach to behavior management works best. Team members must communicate well with each other. The care plan is essential for this approach to be effective, and it must be kept current. An effective behavior management plan is based on the resident's strength and needs. If you discover an effective approach, update the plan of care and communicate the new information to others. Repeat this process until success is achieved. Staff consistency is a key factor in achieving your goal. Make sure to include front line caregivers in planning.

For example, one resident with a behavior problem never exhibited the behavior when a certain nursing assistant was on duty. Through investigation, the facility learned that the assistant brought the resident a sandwich each day when she came on duty. The resident had no behavioral issues during her shift.

Implementing the behavior management plan

List approaches on the care plan in the order in which they should be implemented. Initiate the plan, using the steps in the order listed immediately when the behavior begins. Never wait until the resident loses control. Modifying your behavior in response to the resident's behavior is often successful. Control your responses and reactions to the resident. Monitor your body language. Eliminate triggers to the behavior, if known. Other methods that are helpful in reducing or eliminating negative behaviors are

- Discuss family, friends, or other pleasant information.

- Meet the resident's physical needs.

- Allow residents as much control over care and routines as possible. Allow physically dependent residents to direct their own care. Give residents choices whenever possible, but limit choices to one or two for residents who are cognitively impaired. Many choices may be overwhelming.

- Be patient.

- Control your own reactions; make sure your body language does not betray you.

- Be happy and smile often; make small talk with the resident.

If psychotropic drugs (chemical restraints) are ordered, use them as a last resort, or the last approach listed on the plan of care. Try other, nonchemical approaches first. Remember that chemical restraints may cause balance problems and increase fall risk. Note this on the care plan.

Rewarding residents for positive behavior is also helpful. Behavior that is rewarded is usually repeated.

(This is a lesson to remember when dealing with staff, as well.) With residents, using hugs, smiles, verbal praise, positive feedback, and other signs of approval are often effective. Some residents respond well to treats of food or beverages. Your goal is to show the resident healthy ways of directing his or her energy.

Teamwork, good communication, good listening skills, and practicing empathy are important when working with residents with behavior problems. The ABC plan is a simple, effective method of directing your own energy, as well as the energy of the residents in achieving positive outcomes.

Personality issues affecting fall risk

When developing a fall prevention plan, consider personality issues. Some residents will be in denial. They understand fall prevention teaching, but will not admit they need help, so will not ask for it. Remember that many of today's residents were raised during a time when great value was placed upon self-reliance and autonomy. Many are fiercely independent. Asking for assistance devalues the resident's perception of him- or herself. Suddenly, the resident is no longer independent and self-reliant. Viewing him- or herself as dependent on others is a negative trait, which affects self-esteem.

Some residents will reject the use of assistive devices because they are only for the "handicapped." Residents who have cared for a spouse or other relative at home often see themselves as caregivers, and have difficulty accepting care. This is especially true if the resident also happens to be a nurse, physician, or other healthcare worker. Most residents with self-esteem issues do not deliberately place themselves at risk of falls. They know they need help, but their self-esteem needs and denial are so strong that they cannot bring themselves to ask. The key to planning care involves reframing their thinking. Help them understand that asking for help and using assistive devices will maintain their independence over the long term.

Some residents have basic trust and mistrust issues. These problems may be more pronounced when their assigned caregiver is young. The residents have their own, well-established way of doing things and believe they know best. Although the worker's method may be safest, the resident refuses to cooperate. Avoid telling the resident he or she is wrong. If possible, find a compromise by incorporating the resident's method into a safer way of accomplishing the task. This may take the expertise of the entire care planning team.

Medical problems

Residents who have had a cerebrovascular accident (CVA) are often impulsive. Some have spatial-perceptual deficits. Many have difficulty sequencing tasks and performing the steps in the correct order. The care plan should teach awareness of the problem and measures for controlling it. For example, a resident with spatial-perceptual deficits may misjudge the distance from the bed to the wheelchair. He or she attempts to transfer without assistance, then falls to the floor. The care plan goal is to teach the resident that he or she is misjudging the distance because of the residual effect of the CVA. Teach other means of compensating. Help impulsive residents to learn methods of slowing down or pacing themselves.

Cognitive impairment

Teaching safety to confused residents can be exasperating. Although the resident can safely perform a procedure when you are in the room, he or she cannot be trusted when alone. A plan of care that says, "Keep call signal within reach, remind resident to call for help" is probably an exercise in futility for residents with short-term memory loss. Instead, try a variety of

approaches to reach the resident, including verbal, visual, written, and demonstration. Break the task down into small, manageable steps. Practice the steps with the resident frequently until he or she can verbalize the instructions and return demonstrate safe practices. After that, repeat and reinforce your teaching daily to promote retention. Move to the next small step.

Try a sign in the line of vision to remind the resident of the desired action, such as "Call for help to get out of bed." (Test the resident's ability to read first; some residents lose the ability to read and are reluctant to admit it. If this is the case, a picture sign may work.) Remind the resident of the sign each time you are in the room. If this is ineffective, try a gentle reminder, such as a lap buddy. The most important issue in planning care is to identify the reason(s) for the resident's problems and counteract them with your approaches. Cognitive impairment by itself is not a reason for falls. Short-term memory loss is the reason in most of these residents. Your approaches should address the short-term memory loss. Do not give up because of the cognitive impairment. Your persistence will pay dividends over the long term. Avoid developing a plan that is more appropriate for an alert resident. This is a common problem in long-term care. In general, individualized fall prevention programs involve the following steps:

- Assess the resident for underlying causes and reversible contributing factors for falls, such as chronically poor fluid intake as revealed by a consistently elevated BUN. Involve appropriate long-term care professionals, such as physical and occupational therapists, in the assessment process.

- Evaluate the medication regimen for drugs with the potential for side effects such as motor or mental agitation, confusion, and gait disturbance.

- Evaluate patterns of problem behavior. Note the time of day and relationship to other precipitating factors, such as the need to eliminate, hunger, thirst, pain, or presence of other conditions. Develop a plan to address or minimize these patterns, thereby eliminating the problem.

- Assess for impaired communications, i.e., the inability to make needs and wants known. This can be caused by many different factors, including chronic disease, cerebrovascular accident, or dementia.

- Evaluate the resident's vision, and correct if necessary.

- Assess for unmet psychosocial needs, such as the need for diversional activity or social interaction.

- Assess for spatial-perceptual deficits, self-esteem needs, and impulsiveness. Design the plan to address and counteract these issues.

- Assess the resident for alternatives to restraints and side rails. Document the results of this assessment on the medical record.

- Establish a routine for addressing unmet functional and psychosocial needs. Document the routine on the plan of care. Communicate the routine to all staff on the unit, including housekeepers and others who interact with the resident.

- Eliminate identified causes of falls and risk factors, such as obstacles on the floor.

- Keep the environment free from hazards and obstacles.

- Provide adequate lighting.

- Teach residents to use grab bars.

- Make sure wires and cords are behind furniture.

- Promptly meet resident needs. Anticipate needs in cognitively impaired residents and those with communication problems.

- Make certain the resident has a call signal within reach at all times. Explain how to use it. If he or she cannot use a regular call signal, try a different type of device, such as a hand bell or jingle bells. Answer promptly when the resident signals. (You can remind the resident to call for help, but do not depend on his or her memory.)

- Supervise ambulation and assist if the resident is weak or unsteady. Provide regular exercise.

- Provide assistive devices for ambulation, if necessary for safety.

- Use a transfer belt for all transfers. Issuing a permanent belt to each resident may be more effective than issuing belts to staff.

- Try hip protectors for residents with osteoporosis and those at high risk for hip fracture.

- Elbow protectors may also be a viable alternative for some residents.

- Use hard pads, such as helmets, shin, and wrist pads (similar to those used by children in athletics) only if necessary; many residents are embarrassed to wear them. Some surveyors consider this equipment demeaning and will cite the facility for resident rights and dignity violations when these items are used. If they are essential to resident safety, be sure you have strong justification on the medical record for using them. A mere physician order is probably not adequate justification. If in doubt, check with your survey office to learn what documentation is acceptable.

©2006 HCPro, Inc.

- Try pressure-sensitive pads and alarms that sound when the resident attempts to stand. (Be cautious when using alarms. Numerous alarms on a hall limit effectiveness and cause staff to become insensitive to the sound of alarms. They may assume it is another false alarm, and not respond appropriately. If alarms are used, enforce a strict policy that alarms must never be turned off. This is a common problem in many fall-related lawsuits.)

- Document the resident's response to care.

- If, after attempting to use restraint alternatives, the resident continues with unsafe behavior or is at high risk for injury, assess him or her for use of physical restraints. Consider the least restrictive device necessary to keep the resident safe. Document the results of the assessment on the medical record. The record should reflect an escalating pattern of devices. In other words, restraints should not be the initial approach to unsafe behavior, except in an emergency.

- Assess the need for side rails. Avoid rails whenever possible. Try half rails first.

- Develop an individualized, written, goal-oriented plan of care that takes into account the resident's clinical condition, cognitive status, as well as individual aging changes in hearing, vision, and mobility. Communicate the identified risk of falls and plan of care to all members of the interdisciplinary team. Develop a routine to ensure that all team members check on the resident frequently. Supervising a resident who is at high risk of falls may be overwhelming for the primary caregiver who has others to care for.

- Implement the individual, assessment-based plan of care.

- Communicate the resident's response to the plan of care to other members of the interdisciplinary team verbally and in writing. Evaluate the resident's response.

- Faithfully implement the plan of care based on the resident's individualized pattern, and ongoing evaluation of the resident's responses to the approaches listed. Reevaluate the plan if a fall occurs or if observation/assessment reveals that the plan is ineffective.

Fall prevention is an attainable goal with most residents, including those with cognitive impairment. The key to success is an individualized plan that takes all of the residents intrinsic and extrinsic factors into consideration. Be persistent. Work with the resident and other team members, and use the nursing process to continually evaluate the resident and the effectiveness of the plan. Modify the plan as often as necessary until success is achieved.

Hip fracture

A hip fracture is a break of the proximal femur at the connection, where it angles into the hip socket. Most hip fractures occur in the femoral neck, 1–2 inches from the joint. An intertrochanteric fracture is another common injury that occurs when the break is 3–4 inches from the joint. The incidence of hip fractures increases with age, doubling for each decade beyond age 50.[17] In the United States, one of every three adults over age 65 falls each year. Approximately 350,000 individuals are hospitalized for hip fracture annually in the United States. By the year 2050, there will be an estimated 650,000 hip fractures annually; or nearly 1,800 hip fractures a day. Ninety percent of these are the result of falls.[18] Hip fracture is a devastating injury for persons of all ages, particularly the elderly. Only one in four patients recovers completely,

40% will require nursing facility care, 50% will need a cane or walker, and 24% of those over age 50 will die within 12 months of complications.[19] Falls are the leading cause of injury-related deaths in the elderly. Of all fall deaths, at least 60% involve individuals over age 73. Of all fractures from falls, hip fractures cause the greatest number of deaths and lead to the most severe health problems. Women sustain 75% to 80% of all hip fractures. However, fall-related deaths are higher in men than women, and differ by race. Caucasian males have the highest death rate, followed by Caucasian females. African-American males have the third highest death rate, followed by African-American females.[20]

Risk factors

Risk factors for hip fractures also include

- advancing age

- inadequate nutrition

- immobility

- weakness

- gait and balance problems

- dependence in bathing and dressing

- having one or more chronic diseases

- neurological and musculoskeletal disorders

- osteoporosis

- psychoactive medication use

- dementia

- history of previous falls

- cigarette smoking

- lower extremity disability or foot problems

- visual impairment

- height (females over 5'8" have twice the risk of females under 5'2")

Women who have broken an arm in the past have an increased risk of hip fracture.[21] Environmental risk factors include slippery surfaces, uneven floors, loose rugs, poor lighting, unstable furniture, and objects on the floor. Residents who climb over side rails or the foot of the bed are particularly susceptible to hip fractures because of the height from which the fall occurs. Another concern is having footwear appropriate to the floor surface. Non-slip footwear is appropriate for tile floors. However, shoes with thick, soft soles increase the risk of falls if the facility is carpeted. These shoes may cause the resident to stumble and can affect balance or become a fall hazard by catching in carpeting. In carpeted facilities, leather-bottom shoes often work best.

Risk reduction

Because of the magnitude of hip fracture injuries, long-term care facilities have a vested interest in doing all they can to prevent falls and fractures. Identifying the reason for unsafe behavior and falls, then implementing an individualized plan based on that reason is often the key to success. Residents in long-term care facilities commonly experience several falls before finally sustaining a hip fracture. Many of these have a history of 12 to 30 falls before a serious injury occurs. A legal reviewer takes the number of falls and the time frame into consideration when reviewing the medical record to determine whether a prospective lawsuit has merit. Although allowing the resident to fall repeatedly is less than desirable, the falls should alert you to the resident's ongoing high risk and the ineffectiveness of the fall prevention care plan (or need for a fall prevention care plan). Do not ignore this warning! As with all other falls, evaluating patterns of falls and modifying the plan of care each time is an important consideration. If the resident falls, the plan is probably not working and needs to be tweaked. Build your plan based on the resident's individual needs and your assessment of the cause of lack of safety awareness or other reason for falls. Remember to avoid generic safety/fall prevention plans.

In addition to general risk reduction and environmental measures, residents should eat a diet rich in calcium to strengthen long bones. Foods that are rich in calcium include dairy products, cheese, milk, yogurt, and dark green, leafy vegetables such as broccoli. Vitamin D is also necessary to enable the body to absorb calcium. Some residents may take calcium supplements or multiple vitamins containing calcium. The dietitian will make these recommendations during his or her chart review.

Standing to bear weight, exercising, ambulating, or doing weight-bearing exercises also helps minimize bone loss. Some physicians recommend hormone replacement therapy (HRT) for females, but this has proven controversial because of increased risk of cardiovascular and cerebrovascular complications. At the time of this writing, articles are being published noting that previous studies and conclusions about hormone replacement therapy may have been flawed.[22] This is an area in which much additional study is needed, and it may take years for physicians to definitively reach a consensus.

Only a very small percentage of fractures are thought to occur spontaneously. Because spontaneous hip fractures (without a fall) are so rare, many gerontologists recommend applying padded protectors to absorb the impact of the fall and reduce the risk for hip fracture. The jury is still out on the effectiveness of this approach, but it is worth consideration in high-risk individuals. Hip protectors are similar to panty girdles that have extra padding around the trochanters to absorb energy from falls. Some studies have shown that the use of hip protectors can decrease the incidence of hip fractures of frequent fallers by up to 50%.[23,24,25]

Symptoms of hip fracture

The most common symptoms of hip fracture are severe pain in the hip or lower groin, and shortening and external rotation of the affected leg. The shortening occurs because the muscles in this area are among the strongest in the body. When the continuity of the femur is disrupted, the muscles contract, shortening the leg. The resident will experience limited range of motion, particularly internal rotation. Attempting range of motion may cause extreme pain. If this is the case, stop the procedure. Heel percussion may also produce pain, as will deep palpation in the inguinal area. The resident complains of tenderness with palpation over the femoral neck. Swelling and ecchymosis may also be present. The femur is very vascular, and an ecchymosis the size of an adult fist represents the equivalent of a one-pint blood loss. Most residents with hip fracture will be unable to stand or use the leg normally. Occasionally, a resident with a fracture will be able to walk with difficulty, but most are unable to ambulate after a fall and hip fracture.

Most hip fractures are the result of falls, although occasionally the femur will break as a result of severe osteoporosis. This type of fracture is considered a *stress fracture*. The resident may hear a pop in the bone. The resident may or may not fall. A resident with a stress fracture may have subtle symptoms, such as pain in the groin or thigh. The pain increases with activity and may persist for hours afterward. It will eventually become constant, even without activity. This pain is generally in the groin; however, it can also be referred to the knee. The resident may walk with a limp.

Chapter twelve

"Emergency care and monitoring following a fall" can be found on your CD-ROM

Diagnosis of hip fracture

Diagnosis of a hip fracture is usually made by x-ray. Occasionally, a fracture is not seen on the initial x-ray (called an occult fracture), but a hip fracture should always be suspected if the resident has sudden onset or worsening hip pain or a recent fall. An MRI scan is used to provide better images of bone and soft tissues, or a bone scan (which involves injecting a dye, then taking images that show slight fractures) may be done. Fractures that were not clearly visible on an x-ray generally show up on an MRI or bone scan.

The portable X-ray that is used in the facility may miss a hip fracture. For a more accurate study, send the resident to the hospital. Do not forget that obtaining an X-ray and having the film read will take several hours. Hip fractures are very painful. Make sure to assess the intensity of the resident's pain and administer analgesic medications while waiting for the film interpretation. In this situation, mild analgesics such as aspirin or acetaminophen will probably not be adequate to control the pain.

Treatment overview

The goal of treatment for hip fractures is to return the resident to his or her previous level of function whenever possible. Surgical treatment is the most common and effective, but occasionally it is not done if the individual has serious underlying health problems, or is already bedfast. The type of surgery is determined by the resident's age, health, activity level, degree of osteoporosis, and the type of fracture. An open reduction, internal fixation (ORIF) is commonly done, but total joint replacement may be a better alternative in some residents. If the resident is a high surgical risk, Buck's traction may be used on a short-

or long-term basis to align the bone ends, but this is the least desirable method of treatment.

Rapidly mobilizing the resident after surgery is often the key to successful recovery. Older adults may need extensive therapy. A common problem is that therapy mobilizes the resident, but nursing personnel are afraid the individual will sustain another fall, so apply restraints. Avoid falling into this trap. Work with the resident, therapist, and other personnel to find approaches that do not involve the use of restraints. When the resident is in bed, an abduction pillow and hip precautions may be necessary.

Information and a list of hip precautions can be found on your CD-ROM

Complications of hip surgery

Complications after hip surgery can be very serious. These include infection, thrombus or pulmonary embolism, pneumonia, and pressure ulcers. Most complications result from bed rest and immobility. Complications become more serious when other factors are involved, such as advancing age and underlying health problems or chronic disease. Pressure ulcers on the heels develop rapidly in many residents after hip surgery. Remember, heel protectors prevent friction and shearing. They do not relieve pressure. Elevating the heels from the surface of the bed is the best approach.

Summary

As you can see, hip fracture can be a very serious injury that is exquisitely painful, with high mortality in the elderly. Never take chances where resident welfare is concerned! Be proactive by applying risk reduction and fall prevention programs. Osteoporosis is the single most important contributing factor to hip fractures. For nonwitnessed falls, defense attorneys commonly take the position that a spontaneous hip fracture occurred as a result of osteoporosis. Thus, the fracture resulted in a fall, and not vice versa. Although this is certainly possible, it is improbable. Femoral neck fractures comprise 5–10% of all stress fractures.[26] A stress fracture of the femur almost always occurs in the femoral neck, so stress fractures in the shaft are most unlikely. Interestingly, spontaneous fractures are more common in athletes than in elderly persons. Stress fractures are more common in women than in men.

Head injuries

Falls are a leading predictor of morbidity and mortality in the elderly, accounting for more than two-thirds of all accidents in this age group. Elderly individuals have a high incidence of subdural hematoma. These commonly occur when the head strikes a broad, hard object, such as the floor, causing internal bleeding. Bleeding into the subdural space may be either arterial or venous. It is this constant leaking that causes a condition called subdural hematoma:

- **Acute subdural hematoma**—The onset of symptoms is rapid. Mortality is approximately 50%. Survivors often have neurological deficits.

- **Subacute subdural hematoma**—Has gradual onset of symptoms, with progressive neurological decline occurring over 24 to 36 hours.

- **Chronic subdural hematoma**—Produces neurological signs and symptoms up to six weeks after the initial injury. Because of the prolonged period between the initial injury and manifestation of signs and symptoms, the resident and caregivers have usually forgotten about the causative injury. They may not associate the current problem with a head injury from the recent past. This lesion can grow quite large before becoming symptomatic. The

mortality rate for a chronic subdural hematoma is approximately 10% in the elderly.

Signs and symptoms of subdural hematoma may be insidious and often mimic those of a stroke or dementia, so accurate, repeated assessment is necessary. The prognosis for the resident is determined by the length of time between injury and surgery, how quickly intracranial pressure increases, and any associated intracerebral damage. Complications include seizures, brain stem herniation, and death. Because subdural hematoma is a fairly common injury in the elderly with potential for serious complications, including death, careful nursing assessment, monitoring, and intervention are required for residents with known head injury and unwitnessed falls.

The standard of long-term care nursing practice is to monitor vital signs and neurological checks for at least 72 hours, and longer if symptoms are present. The frequency of monitoring is intense. Most facilities have policies and procedures requiring intensive monitoring, such as every 15 minutes, immediately after the fall. Over a 24-hour period, the frequency of monitoring decreases to every four or eight hours, depending on resident condition, physician orders, and facility policy.

Purpose of neurological assessment

The neurological assessment is performed on residents with suspected neurological conditions or disorders. The most common of these are head injury and stroke. If a resident experiences a change in mental status or neurological signs, reassess the resident and notify the physician immediately.

Resident evaluation

The resident's level of consciousness and mental orientation are important indicators of neurological status. A change in level of consciousness is the most important sign of neurological deterioration. To assess level of consciousness and orientation:

- Ask the resident his or her name. If he or she responds correctly, evaluate response to date/time, place, and situation. If response is appropriate, ask about season and year.

- Disorientation commonly affects the resident's knowledge of date first, followed by time, place, caregiver, and self.

- Assess the quality of the verbal response. Evaluate the clarity of the resident's speech. Assess the resident's ability to make him- or herself understood. Rambling responses suggest the resident is having problems with thought processes and organization.

- Assess the resident's ability to follow directions. Determine whether he or she can follow a simple command. Evaluate the resident's ability to remain focused on the task.

- If the resident does not respond to verbal stimuli, try painful stimuli. Assess for a response on both sides of the body to rule out monoplegia (paralysis of one limb).

To evaluate motor function:

- Test the resident's grip strength using both hands simultaneously. Instruct the resident to squeeze your fingers as hard as possible. Compare the grip strength in both hands. The dominant hand may be slightly stronger.

- Instruct the resident to close his or her eyes and extend the arms forward. Position the palms facing upward. Determine whether either arm falls downward or pronates, indicating muscle weakness.

- Apply gentle downward pressure to the resident's leg. Instruct the resident to raise the leg while you press gently downward. Press gently on the mid-thigh to evaluate muscle strength.

- To assess an unconscious resident, apply painful stimulus. Press on the fingernail bed. If the resident withdraws, compare the strength of each arm.

  Note: If decorticate or decerebrate posturing develops in response to painful stimuli, discontinue the assessment and immediately notify the physician. If the physician does not respond immediately, send the resident to the emergency department using an emergency (911) ambulance. Do not call a transfer service.

- Manually flex and extend the extremities to evaluate muscle tone.

- Stroke the lateral foot with your thumbnail to evaluate the plantar reflex. The toes should flex. Observe for a positive Babinski sign, suggesting an upper motor neuron lesion. (A positive Babinski sign is extension of the great toe and abduction of the other toes instead of the normal flexion reflex).

- Complete the neurological assessment by checking vital signs, pupils, and completing the Glasgow coma scale.

Neurological checks

Neurological (neuro) checks are performed when a neurological disorder or injury is suspected. Neuro checks are normally documented on a flow sheet. The following points are essential to a thorough assessment. Avoid documenting, "neuro's negative." List each component of the assessment individually and note the results.

Level of consciousness

The level of consciousness is always the most important indicator of cerebral injury or other neurological problem. Apply the following definitions consistently when describing the resident:

- **Alert**—The resident is awake and responds appropriately.

- **Lethargic**—The resident is very sleepy, but arouses to stimulation.

- **Obtunded**—The resident is difficult to arouse, but responds appropriately.

- **Stuporous**—The resident is not completely alert, but responds to pain.

- **Semicomatose**—The resident has reflex movements and responds to pain.

- **Comatose**—The resident is completely unresponsive to stimuli.

Orientation

Orientation is a measurement of the resident's awareness to:

- Person

- Place

- Time

- Situation

Judgment

Judgment is the ability to discern, evaluate, and form opinions. Evaluate whether the resident:

- Expresses coherent thoughts

- Expresses distorted thoughts

- Formulates an appropriate verbal response

Memory

Memory is the ability to recall what is experienced, learned, or retained. Evaluate the resident's ability to remember:

- **Short term**—Short-term memory is the primary or active memory. It stores a limited amount of information for a limited amount of time. Some experts state that no more than seven items can be stored in the short-term memory.

- **Past**—The past memory is the result of recent mental processing. It may be called the working memory.

- **Long-term**—Long-term memory stores an unlimited amount of information indefinitely. It can be described as the capacity (or capacities) to retain information in an active, highly available state.

Affect

Affect is the emotional tone, feeling, or mood attached to a thought, including its external manifestations. During neurological evaluation, affect may be described as being:

- Alert

- Pleasant

- Restricted

- Dull or blunt

Speech

The resident's ability to speak at will is described as:

- **Aphasia**—inability to speak

- **Dysphasia**—difficulty speaking

- **Articulate**—speaks fluently

- **Appropriate/inappropriate**

Pain

The response to pain is a measure of the resident's response to external stimulation.

- **Reaction to stimulation**—note the reaction to verbal stimuli, touch, smell, or other stimuli

- **Reaction to painful stimulation**—the resident's reaction to painful stimuli, such as a sternal rub or pressing on the nail bed with a pen.

Pupil assessment

Early assessment of pupil size and response to light is critical to establish a baseline measurement. Continue to monitor and compare the pupil response during subsequent neurological checks. Increased intracranial pressure or temporal lobe herniation will cause pupil dilation. This almost always develops on the side of increased pressure. Initially, the pupil on the same side is reactive to light. It subsequently becomes sluggish, then fails to respond to light at all. As the intracranial pressure increases, the pupil on the opposite side is similarly affected. Determine whether pupils are

- Equal

- Reactive/nonreactive

- Sluggish

Motor response

This is the best response to motor stimulation. Examine all four extremities. Inform the physician immediately if the resident becomes:

- **Decorticate**—A unilateral or bilateral postural change; arms are flexed and adducted and legs are involuntarily positioned in rigid extension. (Also refer to Figure 12-1A.)

- **Decerebrate**—A postural change consisting of episodes of opisthotonos (spasticity in which the spine and extremities are bent forward, the body resting on the head and the heels), rigid extension of the arms and legs, with internal rotation of the arms, and marked plantar flexion of the feet. (Also refer to Figure 12-1B.)

Figure 12-1A and 12-1B   *Decorticate and decerebrate*

Decorticate   **Decerebrate**

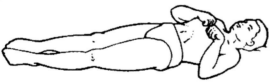 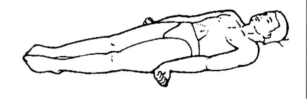

Decorticate rigidity and decerebrate rigidity are signs of serious neurological injury

---

Signs and symptoms of subdural hematoma

Onset of signs and symptoms may be insidious. Suspect a subdural hematoma if the resident shows:

- Confusion, memory loss

- Weakness in one or more extremities

- Ataxia, gait, or balance disturbances

- Difficulty speaking, aphasia

- A visible injury, such as an old bruise or scab over the site of a previous head injury

- Pupil size or reaction unequal

- Vision deterioration (in acute subdural hematoma)

- Intense headache in acute subdural hematoma

- Recurrent, chronic headache in subacute and chronic hematomas

- Changes in level of consciousness

  - May be rapid in acute subdural hematoma.

  - Decline in level of consciousness slower in subacute subdural hematoma.

  - In chronic subdural hematoma, the resident may alternate between periods of alertness, lethargy and confusion.

Assessment and intervention for subdural hematoma and head injury

Glasgow coma scale

The Glasgow coma scale is used to monitoring neurological dysfunction after trauma, stroke, and other neurological illnesses and injuries. The nurse determines the best response the resident can make to stimuli. Higher point values are assigned to responses that indicate increased awareness and arousal. The tool is simple, but effective. It is an excellent, standardized tool that provides the physician with objective, concrete information with which to evaluate the magnitude of the resident's injury.

The Glasgow coma scale and a policy and procedure for neurological checks can be found on your CD-ROM.

Wheelchair-related safety issues

Although addressing wheelchair safety may seem peculiar in a chapter about falls, wheelchair safety is an important consideration when addressing fall risk. Transfers into and out of the wheelchair constitute a fall risk. Since many long-term care facility residents use wheelchairs when they are out of bed, it is appropriate to discuss wheelchair size in a chapter about falls. Wheelchairs are also discussed in Chapter 13.

This information is important for enhancing function and quality of life and preventing many different negative outcomes. Unfortunately, it is not well known, and the information in this section may be new to many readers.

The wheelchair is a mobility device, not a transportation device. Sadly, the wheelchair is commonly used for transportation in long-term care facilities, particularly at mealtimes. Staff push residents in wheelchairs because doing so is faster, and it is easier than allowing residents to propel the chairs themselves. However, residents who have the ability to walk should be encouraged to do so, even if a staff person is required to assist with a gait belt. Residents who can propel their wheelchairs independently, albeit slowly, should also be encouraged to do so. Propelling the chair is a form of exercise and helps with cardiovascular fitness in non-ambulatory residents. Using wheelchairs for transportation instead of mobility causes residents to lose their existing abilities. Although we may increase facility efficiency, we are not doing the residents any favors by pushing them! Propelling a proper-fitting chair is not difficult for most residents.

In long-term care, residents in restraints sometimes tip their wheelchairs, resulting in falls. This is particularly problematic with very tall men. Tipping the wheelchair is a serious issue. However, the risk of tipping can be remedied by paying close attention to the position of the small caster wheels at the front of the wheelchair. Lock the brakes when the chair is parked. *The large part of the small front wheels should face forward when the chair is parked.* Survey the chairs in your facility as you walk by them. You will probably find the wheels facing sideways or backward on the majority of chairs. Positioning the small front wheel sideways or backward completely changes the center of gravity of the chair, making tipping a very real possibility if the resident bends over to reach something on the floor, or is restless and rocks or slides forward. Positioning the large part of the front wheel facing forward and locking the brakes stabilizes the chair, making it much more difficult to tip. Using this approach usually solves tipping problems, but for residents who rock violently, anti-tipping and anti-roll back devices are available from medical suppliers, and should be used when appropriate.

Another common wheelchair problem is that residents who sit in wheelchairs for meals often have problems eating. Transferring the resident into a regular dining chair with arms is much better, for a number of reasons. The arms of the wheelchair prevent the resident from sitting close to the table. Thus, he or she must extend the arms and may struggle to reach for the food. Depending on the resident's height, the wheelchair seat may be too low, or the table height too high. This forces the resident to lift the shoulders and raise the elbows to reach the food. After several minutes, this activity becomes too tiring and frustrating, and may be painful. Some residents give up and simply do not eat their meals, resulting in weight loss. The problem is easily remedied by using regular dining chairs. If this is not possible, grouping several residents together and using trays that fasten to the chair with Velcro® may be a better alternative.

Wheelchair size

Contrary to popular myth, there is no "one-size-fits-all" wheelchair. However, in most facilities, a purchasing agent, corporate office, or non-licensed individual purchases the durable medical equipment, including wheelchairs. The selection of the model and brand is often based on cost. All standard wheelchairs are the same size. Because the wheelchairs do not "fit" the residents properly, some will require restraints to prevent falls. The residents will have difficulty pro-

pelling an improper fitting wheelchair. Now that someone has called your attention to the problem, chances are you can envision someone in your facility right now with an improper fitting wheelchair. The resident may also have significant pain if the chair does not fit correctly. Positioning problems are common. Residents lean to the side, slide forward, or sit slumped in the chair. The risk of skin breakdown is increased. To correct positioning problems and prevent falls, nurses apply restraints unnecessarily. However, even with restraints, using pillows, props, foam bolsters, or additional positioning aids may also be necessary. For many residents a proper fitting wheelchair solves the problem! In extreme cases, staff seat the resident in a reclining chair. This is a situation in which solving one problem (reducing restraints), causes another. Reclining chairs can cause very serious physical and mental declines. Residents stare at the ceiling all day. The lights bother them and they tend to lose contact with their surroundings. This creates or increases confusion. The resident cannot participate in activities because he or she cannot see well enough in the reclined position. They cannot feed themselves or drink unassisted because of their position, so they commonly develop nutrition and hydration problems. Their muscles weaken, and they lose upper-body strength, including head and neck control. Because of this, recliner use should be reserved for only extreme cases. If recliners are used, head rests are available to position the head forward and promote eye contact. As you can see, attention to wheelchair fit is very important, and using reclining geriatric chairs or lounge chairs as a restraint alternative must be seriously considered.

Many types of wheelchairs are available. The physical/occupational therapist can assist you in doing a seating evaluation and recommending the correct type of chair, plus modifications to meet individual resident needs. For example, a resident may need an accessory such as an extension for locking the brakes. Always select the wheelchair to meet the resident's size and physical needs. Various additional accessories are also available to enable the resident to perform certain functions. **Common wheelchair measurements are listed in the "Standard wheelchair sizes" table on your CD-ROM.**

The wheelchair selected is determined by:

- an assessment of the resident's physical condition

- the resident's size

- the resident's special needs

- the needs of caregivers

- the environment in which the chair will be used

If a resident will be purchasing a wheelchair, or using a wheelchair for a prolonged period, the best way to ensure proper fit is to take measurements. Seat the resident on a firm surface with a solid back. Measure with a tape measure.

Conclusion

When reducing restraints in the long-term care facility, assess residents while seated in their wheelchairs. Physical and occupational therapists are qualified to assist in determining proper wheelchair type and fit. If the resident looks uncomfortable, is difficult to position, or has difficulty propelling the chair, request a therapist assessment to determine the size and type of chair to use. Unfortunately, Medicare does not pay for wheelchairs in the long-term care facility. This is an item the facility is expected to provide. However, purchasing a variety of sizes saves money in the long run by reducing accidents and restraints. More important, it increases resident quality of life, improves mobility and the ability to move about at will, and

decreases pain. These factors serve to increase resident satisfaction! Medicare Part B will pay for wheelchairs for residents living in the home or in an assisted living facility. Discharge planning begins on admission to the long-term care facility. If you are evaluating the resident at home or in an assisted living facility, consider the need to purchase a wheelchair before admission. In any event, after the resident has been admitted, you should facilitate the purchase of a wheelchair of the proper size and type! Also, include the need for a wheelchair and accessories at home in the discharge plan.

An overview and summary of resident safety and legal liability can be found on your CD-ROM.

Fall prevention policies and procedures

The long-term care facility has a duty to prevent injuries. When a long-term care facility accepts a resident, its staff have a duty to care for the resident. If nursing personnel assess for and identify a fall risk, we have a duty to develop a viable, reasonable plan to prevent falls and keep the resident safe. The facility has the duty to take every reasonable action possible to reduce the risk of falls and injuries. Identifying fall risk and implementing fall policies and procedures works, but all staff must share a commitment to safety and implement the plan!

Falls with serious injuries are a leading cause of lawsuits against long-term care facilities. Although it is certainly possible, serious injuries seldom occur with the first fall. Usually, the resident has a history or pattern of falling that has not been adequately addressed. A fall in an elderly person always signals a need to reevaluate the individual's physical and environmental conditions.

Beyond the liability issues, falls have the significant

potential to alter an elderly individual's lifestyle and reduce quality of life. Even if the resident isn't injured, a single fall may set in motion a downward spiral of events, both physical and emotional, from which the resident will never recover. He or she may stop certain activities, for fear of falling. The fear can be powerful and overwhelming. The resident becomes socially isolated and depressed. Before you know it, he or she sits in a chair all day. The inactivity and lack of exercise cause various physical ailments. This sequence of events is very real, with many variables.

Evaluating fall prevention program effectiveness

Quality assurance is a continuous process, and fall prevention is an area that requires frequent oversight and evaluation.

The obvious goal of the fall prevention policies, procedures, and programs is to eliminate falls. However, falls are sometimes inevitable. Long-term care providers have a duty to minimize the frequency as much as possible and limit the impact of injuries. The long-term care facility administrator, director of nursing, and supervisors have a duty to ensure that an adequate fall information and reporting system exists. They also have the obligation to actively oversee the safety program, rather than acting as passive recipients of the information. Review the policies and proce-

dures to ensure they were followed accurately and completely for each incident. Ask questions to determine whether staff have followed the program and have not bypassed one or more steps. Managers have a duty to exercise the proper amount of care in decision-making. Examine all falls in detail. Avoid writing them off as being unavoidable.

If a resident falls repeatedly, the medical record should show abundant evidence of assessment and problem analysis, resulting in care plan modification. The record will verify these modifications have been implemented. Despite all this, falls persist.

If you find a breakdown in one or more of the five elements listed above, analyze where the system breakdown has occurred and correct the problem. Analyzing falls from this perspective will reveal weaknesses and measures to take to improve or enhance your fall prevention program. With some residents, the best you can hope for is to decrease the number and frequency of falls, but with many, falls can be prevented completely. Remember that fall prevention involves much more than simply having written policies and procedures in place. Effective fall prevention involves following the policies and procedures. A managerial commitment and analysis of fall incidents enhances the program and helps ensure success.

References

1. Braun J and Capezuti E. (2000). The legal and medical aspects of physical restraints and bed siderails and their relationship to falls and fall-related injuries in nursing homes. *DePaul Journal of Health Care Law*, 4(1), 1-72.

2. Texas Department of Human Services. *Problem-oriented best practices: Managing fall risk*. Online. *http://mqa. dhs.state.tx.us/*. Accessed 7/19/03.

3. Steinweg, KK. (1997). The changing approach to falls in the elderly. American Family Physician 1997;56(7): 1815–23

4. Baraff, L, Della Penna R, Williams N, Sanders A. (1997). Practice guidelines for the ED management of falls in community dwelling elderly persons. *Annals of Emergency Medicine* 1997;30(4):480–92.

5. Texas Department of Human Services. *Problem-oriented best practices: Managing fall risk*. Online. *http://mqa. dhs.state.tx.us/*. Accessed 7/19/03.

6. Neutel CI, Perry S, Maxwell C. (2002). Medication use and risk of falls. Pharmacoepidemiology and Drug Safety 2002;11(2):97 104.

7. Svensson ML, Rundgren A, Larsson M, Oden A, Sund V, Landahl S. (1991). Accidents in the institutionalized elderly: a risk analysis. Aging [Milano] 1991; 3:181 92.

8. Texas Department of Human Services. *Problem-oriented best practices: Managing fall risk*. Online. *http://mqa.dhs.state.tx.us/*. Accessed 7/19/03.

9. Texas Department of Human Services. *Problem-oriented best practices: Managing fall risk*. Online. *http://mqa.dhs.state.tx.us/*. Accessed 7/19/03.

10. Perry S, Edmondstone M, McIlroy W, Maki B. (1998). *Sensory correlates of impaired compensatory stepping performance in healthy older adults*. Online. *http://asb-biomech.org/onlineabs/NACOB98/110/*. Accessed 12/15/05.

11. Colgan J. Syncope: A fall from grace. *Prog Cardiovasc Nurs*. 2001;17(2):66 71.

12. Morris, J.N., Murphy, K., Nonemaker, S. (1996). *Long Term Care Facility Resident Assessment Instrument (RAI) User's Manual*. DesMoines. Briggs Corp.

13. Morris, J.N., Murphy, K., Nonemaker, S. (1996). *Long Term Care Facility Resident Assessment Instrument (RAI) User's Manual*. DesMoines. Briggs Corp.

14. Morris, J.N., Murphy, K., Nonemaker, S. (1996). *Long Term Care Facility Resident Assessment Instrument (RAI) User's Manual*. DesMoines. Briggs Corp.

15. Morris, J.N., Murphy, K., Nonemaker, S. (1996). *Long Term Care Facility Resident Assessment Instrument (RAI) User's Manual*. Des Moines. Briggs Corp.

16. Pain masked by dementia may be eased with tylenol. (2005). *Caregiver's Home Companion*. November 2005. Online. *www.caregivershome.com/news/article.cfm?UID=765&TargetURL=VGFyZ2V0VVJM*. Accessed 11/29/05.

17. Ellis TJ (2003). Hip fractures in the elderly. *Current Women's Health Reports* 2003, 3:75-80.

18. AAOS Fact Sheet. *Falls and hip fractures*. Online. *http://orthoinfo.aaos.org/fact/thr_report.cfm?Thread_ID=77&topcategory=Hip*. Accessed 7/08/02.

19. AAOS Fact Sheet. *Hip fracture*. Online. *http://orthoinfo.aaos.org/fact/thr_report.cfm?Thread_ID=229&topcategory=Hip*. Accessed 7/08/02.

20. Centers for Disease Control and Prevention Fact Sheet. *Falls and hip fracture among the elderly*. Online. *www.cdc.gov/ncipc/factsheets/falls.htm*. Accessed 7/08/02.

21. AAOS Fact Sheet. *Falls and hip fractures*. Online. *http://orthoinfo.aaos.org/fact/thr_report.cfm?Thread_ID=77&topcategory=Hip*. Accessed 7/08/02.

22. *Study: Key hormone therapy trial was flawed*. (12/16/05). Reuters. Online. *www.msnbc.msn.com/id/10491951/*. Accessed 12/16/05.

23. Kumar BA, Parker MJ. (2000). Are hip protectors cost effective. *Injury 2000*, 31:693-695.

24. Lauritzen JB, Peterson MM, Lund B. (1993). Effect of external hip protection on hip fractures. *Lancet* 1993, 341:11-13.

25. Kannus P, Parkkari J, Niemi S, et al. (2000). Prevention of hip fractures in elderly people with use of a hip protector. *N Engl J Med* 2000, 343:1506-1513.

26. Markey KL. (1987). Stress fractures. *Clin Sports Med.* Apr 1987;6(2):405 25.

Common singular event problems

The Nightingale Pledge

"I solemnly pledge myself before God and in the presence of this assembly, to pass my life in purity and to practice my profession faithfully. I will abstain from whatever is deleterious and mischievous, and will not take or knowingly administer any harmful drug. I will do all in my power to maintain and elevate the standard of my profession, and will hold in confidence all personal matters committed to my keeping and all family affairs coming to my knowledge in the practice of my calling. With loyalty will I endeavor to aid the physician in his work, and devote myself to the welfare of those committed to my care."[1]

Identifying and acting on risk factors

Solid, consistent use of the nursing process reduces your legal exposure. Remember, identifying and acting on residents' risk factors is a primary nursing responsibility in long-term care. Many injuries and other events that end up in the courtroom could be identified and prevented or mitigated by nursing action, intervention, good communication, and developing solid nurse-resident relationships. Begin by ensuring that staff caring for residents are consistent and know resident needs. Residents and families feel more secure with consistent caregivers. After identifying risk factors (or a new risk factor/change in risk status), involve the resident and appropriate family members in making decisions and planning care. Document all discussions and risk factor teaching carefully.

Some of the injuries in this chapter occur as a result of inattention to risk factors. However, many of these

are singular-event injuries that are common causes of lawsuits. In these cases, the cause is said to be "efficient." The time that elapses between the negligent conduct and the appearance of an injury is minimal. Compare this with the progressive injuries in other chapters. Progressive injuries evolve gradually and a specific time of occurrence cannot be identified. For injuries resulting from singular events, the defense will usually state that the facility was not responsible, because the resident's behavior was so psychologically dysfunctional that the resident was impossible to monitor and control.

Injuries to residents

Preventing a long-term care facility lawsuit from being filed by providing safe, effective care is far less costly than defending one.[2] Many of the lawsuits filed against long-term care facilities are the direct result of

- inadequate staffing

- heavy staff turnover

In addition to these problems, some lawsuits specifically allege that the injuries sustained by the resident were the result of

- inadequate staff training and education

- inadequate staff supervision; or

- a combination of all four factors

Staff in long-term care facilities are required to ensure the effective and safe delivery of resident care in accordance with professional standards and applicable statutes. Adequate and appropriate systems must be in place to ensure that quality care is delivered within facility policies, standards of care, legal requirements, and certification or regulatory requirements. The director of nursing and administrator must administer the facility in such a manner as to attain or maintain the highest practicable physical, mental, and psychosocial well-being of each resident.

Effective systems must be in place to ensure that resident needs are met. Although any nursing service turnover is detrimental, facilities with turnover in the director of nursing position seem to have many problems related to lack of consistent nursing service administration guidance and direction. Because turnover has a pronounced effect on legal exposure, facilities should do everything possible to stabilize staff. Many nurses complain that they need more staff to improve efficiency and care. This may or may not be the case, and nursing requests for additional staff require careful study and analysis. Some facilities are adequately staffed, but staff are not well-supervised or well-organized. The results of inadequate organization and supervision can be just as devastating as short staffing. However, the cumulative anticipated nursing workload should not exceed the physical capacity and available time of the staff on duty at any given time.

Hiring staff without conducting criminal background checks

A court can find a healthcare facility negligent for hiring or retaining an employee who has a violent or criminal propensity. It is necessary to prove that the facility knew or should have known of the employee's prior record or dangerous characteristics prior to an assault being committed upon a resident. If the facility knows or suspects the employee may pose a danger to the residents, facility management has an ethical duty to act on it, by imposing adequate supervision (or eliminating the employee) to prevent harm to the residents.[3]

Two Michigan studies conducted in 2005 by the office of the Michigan Attorney General revealed that almost 10% of the employees caring for the state's vulnerable adults have criminal backgrounds that include homicide, criminal sexual conduct, weapon charges, and drug offenses. In both studies, the criminal histories included homicides, armed robberies, criminal sexual conduct, weapons violations, drug charges, and retail fraud. As a result of the study findings, the Attorney General's office proposes tighter controls on hiring, and has submitted a comprehensive proposal to the Legislature to enhance Michigan's existing criminal background statutes.

Many states require long-term care facilities to complete criminal background checks on certain categories of employees at the time of hire. Because of heavy staff turnover and other priorities, some facilities fail to complete these checks in a timely manner. Another problem is the lack of resources with which to run a criminal background check. Paper checks are very slow. All long-term care facilities have Internet access. Thousands of web sites are available for investigating criminal history for free or a nominal fee. A simple search will bring these up. Regardless of your state laws, this is an area in which you should not develop a casual attitude. Investigate the criminal background of all prospective and existing employees. Rechecking annually is also a good idea, since some may have been convicted of crimes you are not aware of. Avoid those specified by your state laws, as well as employees in any department with felony records for injuries to adults or children, theft, and other convictions that place the elderly residents at risk.

Identity theft has become a serious problem in healthcare facilities. Prospective employees with a history of fraud and financial abuse should not be hired for positions in which sensitive information, such as social security numbers or resident financial data are accessible.

Another concern is rehiring of nursing assistants who previously resigned or were discharged for unacceptable behavior or inadequate care. Do all that you can to check employee references, and avoid becoming so desperate that you must turn to rehiring someone who presents a known risk to the residents.

Failing to protect residents from mistreatment

The long-term care facility has a duty to protect residents from abuse and neglect. Failure to protect the residents is a common factor of lawsuits. Most commonly, the facility is charged with neglect, resulting from conditions such as pressure ulcers, malnutrition, and dehydration. Neglect is the failure to provide goods and services necessary to avoid physical harm, mental anguish, or mental illness. Neglect occurs on an individual basis when a resident does not receive care in one or more activities of daily living (e.g., fail-

ure to bathe residents regularly, or failure to frequently monitor a resident known to be incontinent, resulting in being left to lie in urine or feces). Failure of the facility to report neglect of this type is a common peripheral element in lawsuits. Although the lawsuit typically lists one major factor, such as a pressure ulcer, detailing and enumerating many lesser peripheral offenses is believed to strengthen the case by proving an ongoing pattern of poor care. In addition to having a duty to protect the resident, the facility also has a

- *Duty to report:* A facility must ensure that all alleged violations involving mistreatment, neglect, or abuse (including injuries of unknown source), and misappropriation of resident property are reported immediately to the administrator of the facility and to other officials in accordance with state law through established procedures (including to the state survey and certification agency). (42 C.F.R. § 483.13(c)(2).)

- *Duty to investigate:* The facility must have evidence that all alleged violations are thoroughly investigated, and must protect the resident to prevent further potential abuse while the investigation is in progress. (42 C.F.R. § 483.13(c)(3).)

- *Timing of report to state licensing agency:* Results of all investigations must be reported to the administrator and the Division of Licensure and Certification within five working days of the incident. (42 C.F.R. § 483.13(c)(4).)

Abuse and neglect

Abuse and neglect of dependent elderly individuals is considered a crime. In most facilities, abuse and neglect are reported to law enforcement authorities for prosecution. Because abuse and neglect allegations are considered criminal offenses, the statute of limitations may differ from medical negligence lawsuits. Some lawsuits alleging abuse and neglect have been filed as civil rights violations. Some lawsuits alleging long-term care facility abuse or neglect are filed as "breach of contract" lawsuits. The reason may be that in many states, the statute of limitations for breach of contract is considerably longer than the statute for personal injury. For example, in Louisiana, the statute of limitations is 10 years for breach of contract, and one year for personal injury lawsuits. They note, "If entrusting one's money to an investment company creates a business relationship of trust and accountability, one would hope, at least in principle, that entrusting a valued family member to the care of a business entity such as a nursing home would carry similar responsibilities."[4]

All facilities have policies and procedures expressly forbidding abuse and neglect of the residents. To reduce legal exposure, facility management should

- Make clear that the abuse and neglect policies allow for zero tolerance.

- Implement policies and procedures for education, prevention, reporting, investigation, documentation, and response to reports of abuse and neglect.

- Complete criminal history checks for every employee.

- Check references, state registries, and licensure boards carefully when hiring new staff. Maintain records of these checks.

- Perform drug and alcohol tests upon employment; do random tests on current employees.

- Make sure staffing is adequate.

- Teach staff how to identify and manage stress and burnout.

- Provide resources for employees to use if needed for stress or anger management.

- Teach staff how to manage residents with aggressive or combative behavior, verbal aggressiveness, and catastrophic reaction.

- Evaluate employee discipline situations, incident reports, and other problematic matters to determine whether the matter could be misconstrued or interpreted as neglect.

- Immediately investigate reported or suspected abuse and neglect. Report to the state survey agency as required by law.

Sexual assault

The facility is expected to protect residents from sexual assault. This may be caused by an attack by an employee, family member, another resident, or an intruder in the facility. Sexual assault complaints commonly have many components, including:

- alleged negligence

- violation of the residents' bill of rights

- inadequate staffing and failure to provide safe minimum levels of care

- recklessness and indifference

- negligent infliction of emotional distress, pain, and mental anguish

In 2004 and 2005, an organization released several abysmal reports documenting widespread sexual abuse, assaults, and other criminal offenses in which long-term care facility residents were victims.[5] The reports also document more than 20 recent cases of rape, assault, and murder committed by residents of long-term care facilities with criminal records. The study does not include assisted-living facilities. Although ongoing studies are not yet complete, this group has located 800 registered sex offenders in long-term care facilities in 36 states. States that do not have online sex offender registries were not included in the study. Many of the offenders were not physically debilitated, and 45% were under the age of 65. This study found residents in long-term care facilities who were

- Registered sex offenders
- Sex offenders who were not required to register
- Parolees
- Violent offenders who were believed incompetent to stand trial
- Felons
- Prisoners and county jail inmates

Many of the individuals identified by the study had their placement facilitated by

- Department of Corrections
- Department of Human Services
- District Court Judges
- County Sheriffs
- County District Attorneys

In response to the identified problem, the State of Illinois passed a law called the Vulnerable Adults Protection Act, requiring the identification and management of convicted felons residing in long-term care facilities, and provide for notification to other residents of the facilities. The long-term care industry has expressed grave concerns about this legislation because of the excessive implementation costs to facilities, and inability of the state agency to reimburse the costs.

Signs and symptoms of sexual abuse in the elderly

- Signs of trauma (bruising, lacerations, bleeding) on the inner thighs, vaginal, or anal area

Common singular event problems

- Difficulty standing or walking
- Sexually transmitted diseases
- Pain/itching in the genital area
- Exacerbation of existing illness, worsening of mental confusion
- Scared or timid behavior
- Depressed, withdrawn behavior, crying for no apparent reason
- Sudden changes in personality
- Odd, misplaced comments about sex or sexual behavior
- Fear of certain people or of physical characteristics

Whistleblowers

Employees are often reluctant to report abuse and neglect. Many states have whistleblower laws that protect individuals who report abuse and neglect to the authorities. For example, the Iowa law states: "A person participating in good faith in reporting or cooperating with or assisting the department in evaluating a case of dependent adult abuse has immunity from liability, civil or criminal, which might otherwise be incurred or imposed based upon the act of making the report or giving the assistance. The person has the same immunity with respect to participating in good faith in a judicial proceeding resulting from the report or cooperation or assistance or relating to the subject matter of the report, cooperation, or assistance." The Iowa law further states, "It shall be unlawful for any person or employer to discharge, suspend, or otherwise discipline a person required to report or voluntarily reporting an instance of suspected dependent adult abuse." It follows with, "A person required by this section to report a suspected case of dependent adult abuse who knowingly and willfully fails to do so commits a simple misdemeanor. A person required by this section to report a suspected case of dependent adult abuse who knowingly fails to do so or who knowingly interferes with the making of a dependent adult abuse report or applies a requirement that results in a failure to make a report, is civilly liable for the damages proximately caused by the failure."

However, despite whistleblower protection and the risk of prosecution for not reporting, many employees refuse to become involved and turn a blind eye to blatantly obvious abuse and neglect. Elizabeth Morris, executive director of the Alabama Nursing Association, wrote an editorial in the Montgomery Advertiser, which supports her belief that the unspoken medical code of silence threatens the lives of residents in Alabama. She notes, *"Whistleblowers—who more times than not are whispering, not whistling—are not welcome in the health care institutions of Alabama. An attempt to report a mistake in such an institution is tantamount to resignation. There is no protection for the nurse, physician or health care employee who tells the truth about patient care."* She further noted that shortcuts routinely place patients in harm's way. However, there is no mechanism to ensure that healthcare whistleblowers are protected. Ms. Morris refers to the Nightingale pledge, which suggests the nurse will do all within her power to preserve the health of her patients. Ms. Morris called for a public policy exception to Alabama's at-will employment rule to protect a nurse or other healthcare provider who reports inappropriate healthcare practices from being terminated for doing so.[6]

Studies have revealed that physicians are less effective than some other professionals in identifying cases of elder abuse, and are overall unfamiliar with mandatory reporting laws for suspected abuse and neglect.[7] Patterns of long-term care facility neglect result from a systematic breakdown in fundamental procedures that were designed to ensure delivery of care to residents. One law firm reveals that physicians seldom use differential reasoning to rule out neglect as a cause of resident injury. In more than 100 death cases involving injuries recognized by the Institute of Medicine as prima facie indicators of long-term care facility neglect, this law firm reports they have seen fewer than five cases in which the attending physician considered neglect as a possible cause.[8]

In one Florida lawsuit, a resident of the facility for one year developed severe pressure ulcers, malnutrition, and dehydration. During the trial, the plaintiff offered extensive evidence of understaffing, falsification of records, and employee incompetence. The jury awarded punitive and compensatory damages. The court wrote: *"The nursing home cannot escape responsibility by managing its facility with managers who close their eyes, refuse to hear, and dull their sense of smell. Certainly, the managing agents should not be charged with knowing every isolated event that occurs, but the events surrounding decedent were not isolated. . . . It is difficult to imagine that an employee with managerial responsibilities either knew of this resident's plight and failed to take any action to assist this totally dependent human being or so totally ignored the operation of the nursing facility that the resident's plight went unnoticed. Either situation exhibits a reckless disregard for human life or of the safety of persons exposed to its dangerous effects, or reckless indifference to the rights of this resident for whom the nursing home was being compensated for every detail of sustaining his life in the most dignified and comfortable way possible."*[9]

Some employees frequently call the state reporting hotline as a means of retaliating against their employer for perceived injustices. They subsequently claim whistleblower protection when they are terminated or disciplined. The reports to the state may or may not be factual (they often are not). However, these individuals do not usually qualify for whistleblower protections. To qualify for legal protection from retaliatory action for reporting abuse or neglect, the individual must usually file a formal report with appropriate officials. The individual must report in good faith, based on a belief that abuse or neglect (or other covered offense), as defined by law, has occurred. Personal or professional differences of opinion over resident care issues, and complaints about policies, procedures, and facility management do not constitute formal reports of neglect or abuse, and are not given any special protection under the law.[10]

Wanderers

Residents who wander are those who walk about or propel their wheelchairs about the facility aimlessly, without direction. Several types of wanderers have been identified:

- **Exit Seeking Wanderer**

  The *exit seeking wanderer* is looking for a way to leave the premises. He may not know where he is, but knows he does not want to be there. This wanderer is very persistent in finding a way to leave, and may sneak out. He may be mistaken for a visitor and assisted out by staff or visitors. He looks for opportunities to exit, and quickly seizes them if the opportunity presents itself.

- **Critical (Precarious) Wanderer**

  The *critical (precarious) wanderer* wanders for self-stimulation. She is usually disoriented and easily bored. If the resident turns a door knob by happenstance, expect her to exit. This wanderer has very poor safety judgment and is at great risk of injury. Providing diversion through

the activities program, exercise, and walking may reduce the behavior by replacing the seemingly endless need for stimulation.

- **Purposeful Wanderer**

  The *purposeful wanderer* has an agenda to fulfill. The resident will probably be unable to communicate the agenda or his needs to you. Identifying the agenda or needs is often simple, and is done through trial and error. Begin with logical things, such as hunger, thirst, pain, or wandering in search of the bathroom. Distracting this wanderer with activities or exercise may exacerbate the behavior. Begin by meeting physical needs, such as hunger, thirst, elimination, and pain. If the wandering persists, progress to more complex psychosocial needs to see if this solves the problem.

- **Aimless (Indiscriminate) Wanderer**

  The *aimless (indiscriminate) wanderer* is completely disoriented. He will wander aimlessly, believing he is in his own home. He rummages through closets or drawers, and is at serious risk of injury if he encounters chemicals, sharps, or other harmful items. The pillaging and ransacking are often very stressful to the caregivers, although the behavior is generally harmless. This resident is in danger of being harmed by other residents who believe he is stealing from them. Providing a chest of drawers, box, basket, or suitcase in the hallway to search through may reduce the behavior. This wanderer may respond to paper streamers strung across the doorway, with or without a sign that prohibits entry (such as a stop sign, danger sign, construction sign, etc.).

- **Modeling Wanderer**

  Most long-term care facilities have at least one set of *modeling wanderers*. The residents may be either ambulatory or confined to wheelchairs, or one of each. One resident wanders and the other follows. If the first wanderer exits the building, both will leave. Finding the first wanderer's agenda and fulfilling it will usually stop the behavior.

- **Akathisia Wanderer**

  Akathisia is a syndrome in which the resident has motor restlessness and quivering, causing constant movement. The movement seems to relieve the muscular discomfort. Akathisia is caused by long-term use of neuroleptic or psychotropic medications, and is generally irreversible. Symptoms may develop within several weeks of modifying (usually starting or raising) the dose of the older neuroleptic medications (such as *Thorazine*®) or reducing the dose to treat extra pyramidal symptoms. *Akathisia wanderers* pace the hallways continuously. Many have been in mental institutions and may pace with their arms crossed over the abdomen, holding the waist area. Some have a mask-like appearance and tardive dyskinesia as a result of years of psychotropic drug use.

Definitions

Elopement and wandering are two distinctly different behaviors. Documentation should reflect which behavior is present. The two terms should not be used interchangeably. Wandering is aimless, purposeless walking or meandering about in a wheelchair. Eloping is an attempt to leave the facility. It is usually purposeful behavior, and the resident has a plan to go to a specific place. He or she recognizes that windows and doors are a means of egress.

Eloping behavior

No one can accurately predict who will begin wandering as a result of Alzheimer's disease. Likewise, we cannot predict when wandering will begin in residents with other diagnoses. The most common pattern is for wandering to begin in the late first stage of Alzheimer's, peak in the middle stage, then diminish. It usually stops entirely in the third stage of the disease, but since each resident is an individual, these patterns are not set in stone.

Incidents of elopement occur in every state and in all levels of care. Here are some alarming statistics:

- Ten percent of all long-term care lawsuits involve elopements

  - Of these, 70% involve the death of a resident.

- The primary causes of death in residents who elope are:

  - being hit by a vehicle.

  - exposure to temperature extremes

  - drowning

  - physical and/or sexual abuse

- In 80% of these cases, the residents were known to be wanderers with a past history of eloping

- In 45% of these cases, the resident eloped during the first 48 hours of admission

In 2006, a resident was noted missing from her room in a North Carolina long-term care facility. She was found under a table inside an unlocked storage room at the facility four days later. Staff reported completely searching the 289-bed facility at least six times. A search dog was unable to pick up the resident's scent outside, and staff were instructed to search the premises further, but they did not find the resident. A police investigation was initiated to determine why the storeroom was unlocked and why the resident was not found during facility searches. The resident was dehydrated and was transferred to a hospital, where she subsequently died.[12] When a resident begins wandering, he or she is not safe inside or outside. Dangers inside the facility include sharps, medications and chemicals (including grooming and cosmetic products), hazardous appliances and electrical devices, and other items. It goes without saying that the facility should anticipate these risks and make the environment as safe as possible. Outside the facility, the unsupervised, confused resident is in great danger.

Common hazards include exposure to temperature extremes, falls resulting in fractures, and being hit by a vehicle. Some residents have wandered away while being cared for by family members at home. It is often fear of wandering that precipitates the decision to admit the resident to the facility. Avoid restraints, if possible. If essential to resident safety, try combinations of restraint alternatives and nursing measures first. Residents who wander may not be restrained for nursing convenience, which means staff do not have (or do not take) the time to monitor the resident. Determining whether a restraint is applied for nursing convenience or resident protection may be difficult. You may want to consider keeping a wandering log verifying the resident's location has been checked periodically. **A form for 15 minute/hourly checks is on your CD-ROM.** Also document what he or she is wearing. This documentation can be informal, such as on the assignment sheet.

In addition to the obvious safety risks, excessive wandering has the potential for causing many other physical problems. Continuous or frequent wandering increases caloric needs, resulting in significant weight loss if nutritional intake is not maintained. The resident may be so obsessed with wandering that he or she cannot remain at the table long enough to finish a meal. Elderly residents normally have a diminished sense of thirst, and a confused resident may misinterpret or ignore the limited signals to drink fluids, leading to dehydration, especially in hot weather. He or she may misinterpret or ignore feelings of fatigue, leading to exhaustion from constant movement, and increasing the risk of falls. Blistering of the feet can lead to ulcerations, infection, and other serious complications, particularly in diabetics and residents with peripheral vascular disease. We cannot depend on a resident with Alzheimer's to put on socks when he or she dresses, further increasing the risk of injury to the feet. The discomfort from ill-fitting shoes may be obvious in an alert resident, but is less evident in a resident with Alzheimer's. Even if the resident is uncomfortable, he or she may be unable to identify and communicate the problem. An ulcer, infection, or other serious injury may be present before the injury becomes apparent to the staff.

The plan of care: Management goals and objectives

Identify wanderers, as well as those who are at risk for wandering. Make sure to have a current photograph available. A digital or instant (Polaroid®) is best because the photo can be accessed quickly if the resident elopes. Take photos at least annually or any time the resident's appearance changes. If the resident normally does not wear makeup or has an unkempt appearance, take a photo this way. Your objective is to have a photograph that looks like the resident does most of the time.

Teach responsible family members about wandering. If the behavior is new, reassure them that nothing is medically wrong. Teach the family that wandering is part of the disease process, and that he or she must avoid taking the behavior personally. Discuss care plan objectives with the responsible party. Be sensitive and ask his or her opinion about care plan approaches. When meeting with the responsible party, you should find out, and document in a prominent, easy to find location, the answers to the following:

- If the resident wanders (or insists on leaving the facility), where does he or she "need" to go?

- Find out the resident's nicknames and spouse's name.

- What are the resident's former occupation, hobbies, habits, and patterns, such as bedtime, rising time, nocturnal confusion, wandering?

- In prior episodes of wandering (if any), where did the resident say he or she was going?

- What is/was the name of the resident's spouse?

Since safety is paramount, your overall objective is to prevent injury. Other important goals are

- Prevent physical and mental declines

- Prevent a deterioration of the resident's symptoms

- Preserve and promote dignity

- Promote the highest level of independent function possible

- Reduce or eliminate environmental (or other) stressors

- Provide consistent routines, predictability, structure, and repetition in care and the environment

- Provide safety within the facility

- Prevent the resident from eloping

- Identify, decrease or eliminate stressors that trigger wandering

- Preserve family support and unity as much as possible

- Ask the pharmacist to review the drug regimen to determine whether the drugs may trigger wandering. **A list of drugs with the potential to exacerbate wandering is on your CD-ROM.**

- Healthcare professionals should:

  – Develop a therapeutic relationship with the resident

  – Involve the resident and family caregiver(s) in planning care as much as possible

Care plan implementation/intervention

- Consider a photo identification card, as well as fingerprinting the resident.

- Alert your local police department that some residents have the propensity to wander and ask them to watch the neighborhood when they are on patrol.

- Review the Alzheimer's Association "Safe Return" program to determine whether it meets facility needs. Although a registration fee is required for each resident, this program has shown remarkable results in finding lost individuals, and the services provided are well worth the nominal investment. Additional information can be obtained at *www.alz.org* or from your local Alzheimer's chapter.

Suggestions that should be implemented for all wandering residents include

- Make sure the resident wears glasses and hearing aid, as appropriate.

- Maintain a comfortable environment; adjust the temperature for comfort. Keep noise and confusion low.

- Avoid clutter in the environment, which tends to make the resident feel nervous, trapped, or closed in.

- Provide a night light. If it causes shadows (which may frighten the resident), leave a bathroom or hallway light on at night.

- Sit and talk several times a day. A volunteer or activities staff member may be able to assist with this.

- Ensure that physical needs are met, including hunger, thirst, and elimination.

- Assess the resident for pain and medicate as needed.

- Frequently remind the resident that he or she is in the right place; communicate regularly.

- Make sure that the resident wears some type of identification bracelet (Identiband®), identification jewelry (Medic Alert®), and has identification in his or her clothing.

- Have identifying information, such as fingerprints and a description of clothing, available for the police in the event the resident wanders off.

- Remove hats, coats, purses, and other triggers to going outside.

- Purchase brightly colored or reflective outer clothing. Reflective tape can be purchased and sewn to coats and outerwear.

- Apply a shirt or sweater to the wandering resident for 6–8 hours. Remove it and seal it tightly in a plastic bag. Place the bag in a closet. Keep the garment available in case the resident wanders off. This will provide the resident's scent for a tracking dog. If a garment is unavailable, another alternative is to use the resident's pillow. If the resident wanders away, make a specific request for a tracking dog from your local law enforcement agency. Dogs are trained for different purposes, and a drug dog, for example, may not be able to track a missing person. Requesting a search dog early is best, as the dog and handler may need to be brought in from outside the community. The law enforcement agency should be involved with a network that can make these arrangements. Modern technology and global positioning system (GPS) devices may soon make the need for search dogs obsolete. Devices are now available to track the location of wandering residents, although they are expensive and not commonly used.

- When redirection is necessary, keep it simple and positive. This may sound elementary, but it is particularly important and effective. For example, avoid saying, *"Don't go outside."* Following this direction involves a multi-step, complex thought process. The resident must first think about going outside, then "unthink" it. Giving this complex type of direction may actually worsen the behavior. A more effective, less complex direction is, *"Stay inside."*

- Individual interventions are listed in Table 13-1. Use trial and error approaches based on your assessment of the resident's wandering pattern and category/type of wandering to determine those interventions that have the greatest chance of success, and implement these first.

| Table 13-1 | *Wandering Interventions* |

Type of Wanderer	Nursing interventions
Exit-seeking	• Restore the state of mind the resident is looking for; he or she is looking for a state of mind, not a physical location (e.g., Resident, "I am going home to cook dinner for the children." Nurse: "What do you like to cook? How do you prepare that?" Resident: "I must hurry or I will be late to work." Nurse: "What kind of work do you do? Tell me about it. This is very interesting.") • Requires a high degree of supervision • Distraction • Validation therapy • Reminiscence • Avoid reality orientation; may increase resident's agitation • Avoid arguing with the resident; he has lost the ability to reason • Reduce noise and confusion in the environment • Try childproof door handles or handles with an unusual texture, such as those that feel soft and furry or harsh, like sandpaper. • Check with the fire marshal. See if you can camouflage exit doors (another option is full-length mirrors on doors) • Identify and follow the resident's agenda • Find ways to make the resident feel wanted, loved, and busy. Give the female resident a dust cloth, or stack of towels to fold. Give the male resident a task such as setting tables (wash hands first). • Personalize the resident's activities to previous life experiences, as much as possible
Critical/Precarious	• Requires a high degree of supervision • Exercise • Diversion • Responds well to repetition, structure, consistency, and predictability in routines
Purposeful	• Determining his agenda will help you meet his needs and plan care. Use trial and error. Begin with simple physical needs, such as regular toileting, food, and beverages. Regularly assess the resident for pain. • Monitor resident's response to noise and temperature in the environment. Wandering may be a means of escaping uncomfortable temperature, or loud noise. • Exercise and diversional activities may agitate this resident. Instead, focus on identifying and meeting his needs.

The Long-Term Care Legal Desk Reference

Table 13-1	*Wandering Interventions (cont.)*
Type of Wanderer	**Nursing interventions**
Aimless/ Indiscriminate	• Paper streamers across doorways • Signs that say "stop," "do not enter," or "construction zone." • A radio with headphones may calm the resident • Frequent reassurance that he is safe. • Provide a dresser or night stand in the hallway with items that he can safely rummage through. • Give the resident junk mail, linen, or other items to sort, coupons to clip, etc. • Try jingle bells over the door, infrared beams, door alarms, or pull-apart personal alarms (inexpensive at commercial electronics stores).
Akathisia	• Management is by trial and error. Any approach that relieves muscular sensation may be effective. • May respond to exercise, or walking in a group with others.
Modeling	• Identify the leader's agenda and fulfill it.

Additional physical considerations needing regular assessment that should be listed on the care plan include

- ensuring the resident's food and fluid intake are adequate; offer extra snacks and drinks

- monitoring the weight frequently (weekly)

- checking the feet for blisters or injury daily by nursing assistant, weekly by nurse

- evaluating elimination daily to ensure that constipation is not causing discomfort; keeping a written record of the resident's elimination pattern

Additional interventions

Additional interventions that may be useful (use trial and error to determine which are appropriate for the resident):

- Avoid startling the resident. Speak when approaching, and approach from the front whenever possible. When walking, fall into step with the resident, then circle back.

- Provide signs and other visual reminders of person, place, and time as appropriate. Make sure they are large enough for the resident to read.

- Distract the resident with food, drink, or conversation.

- Reminisce with the resident using photo albums, travel brochures, etc., to restore the state of mind the resident is seeking. (The Briggs Corporation has excellent books available with catalog photos of clothing and age-appropriate items for reminiscence and conversation.)

- If the resident "wants to go home," taking him for a short walk or drive may be effective. Upon returning, he may recognize the facility.

However, avoid this approach if it increases the risk of worsening agitation. Never take the resident out alone. Two people should accompany the resident in a car.

- Play the resident's favorite music. A radio or cassette with earphones is calming for some residents.

- Place an identifying object where the resident can find it; when she asks you where she should go, direct her to the "blue bow," "dried flowers on the table," etc.

- Assign repetitive tasks, such as adding numbers on an adding machine, folding laundry, sorting coins, folding napkins, wrapping silverware, etc.

- Consider seating the wanderer in a beanbag chair to promote rest. They are comfortable and promote rest, yet make rising difficult.

- Provide regular, planned exercise each day. Walking is a good activity for the caregiver to perform with the resident, such as walking in an enclosed area.

- Respond to emotions the resident is expressing. Make appropriate statements, such as "I know you are feeling lonely" or "Are you feeling scared?"

- Provide frequent, calm reassurance.

- Try humor or cajoling the resident.

- Try written reassurance such as "Dinner will be at 5:00."

- Limit the number of persons redirecting the wanderer to avoid overwhelming her.

Additional suggestions for managing residents with sundowning and night time wandering include

- Avoiding long naps during the day.

- Try warm milk and honey at bedtime. Calcium is nature's tranquilizer, and this may help the resident sleep. This beverage provides comfort and may remind the resident of something he or she drank as a child.

- Plan periodic activities intermittently during the day to combat boredom and promote exercise.

- Avoid arguing with the resident about the time of day. Tell him the time. Providing a digital clock that is marked "AM" and "PM" may be useful.

- Determine whether physical problems, pain, or incontinence are interfering with sleep.

- Allow the resident to sleep in a recliner, beanbag, or wherever is most comfortable.

- Try a different bedroom, or rearrange the furniture to see if this reduces night time wandering.

- If the resident wakes at night, make sure his or her physical needs are met.

- Avoid confronting the resident about being awake; don't demand an explanation. If the resident awakens, reassess physical needs of hunger, pain, thirst, and elimination.

- Reassure the resident that others are safe and everything is fine.

Monitoring wanderers

In 2006, a nursing assistant from an assisted living facility was charged with reckless conduct for not responding to a window alarm. A resident with dementia climbed out the window, disappearing entirely. Searches with dogs and helicopters were unsuccessful. Police were not involved in a search until an hour after the resident was first reported missing, because the facility personnel searched for the resident first. The resident had a history of wandering away, but had been found unharmed in the past.[13] Unfortunately, turning off or not responding to exit alarms is a common scenario, because the alarms are annoying to staff and some residents.

Develop policies and procedures for door alarms and electronic monitoring alarms, and make sure all staff are familiar with them. Check alarms regularly, and keep a log. Door alarms and electronic monitoring bracelets must never be turned off. If an exit door alarm or monitoring bracelet sounds, staff must investigate thoroughly, even if they suspect it is a false alarm. You must be firm with this policy, disciplining staff for infractions.

Intermittent monitoring is *not* an adequate intervention for residents who wander continuously and have known risks for elopement. Electronic bracelet systems are excellent adjuncts, but one-on-one supervision may be necessary. Monitoring a wanderer adequately and carrying a full resident care assignment may not be humanly possible for the nursing assistants. Sharing the responsibility and accountability with all staff on the floor is safer for the resident and less stressful for staff. Anyone can monitor the resident's whereabouts. The monitor does not have to be a licensed nurse or nursing assistant. Housekeepers, activities, unit secretaries, and others on the unit for all or part of a shift can supervise the resident. To be successful, a team effort is necessary. Getting the cooperation of staff from other departments may take gentle persuasion from the administrator, who must support nursing efforts to ensure resident safety and reduce the risk of liability.

At the beginning of the shift, the charge nurse assigns all personnel on the unit to one or more 15-to-30-minute "shifts," during which time each person is responsible for supervising the wanderer. The nurse or medication aide should not be assigned during med pass times. Staff are responsible for their designated

time(s), and must find a replacement if they cannot fulfill their responsibility. For the system to be effective, you must physically find your relief and "tag off" with him or her at the end of your "shift." Your relief may be occupied or have forgotten it is time to monitor the resident. If this is the case, you must continue supervising the resident until the relief person is free. Communicate the plan to all staff. Document the monitoring to protect the staff and facility. A flow sheet can be modified for this purpose. Write "Verified location of resident this 30 (or 15) minutes" on the flow sheet. Each person monitoring the resident initials the flow sheet at the end of each 30-minute shift. Consult your facility's legal counsel for specific language.

Some facilities use distinct color identification bracelets to identify wanderers. Some place colored self-adhesive dots on the back of the resident's robe, clothing, or wheelchair to provide a visual clue to all staff that the resident is a wanderer. These methods of identification must be fairly inconspicuous, and the key to the facility's system known only to staff. In some states, visual identification of any type is not acceptable. Follow your facility policies and surveyor guidelines.

Other recommendations

- Do not rely solely on electronic alarms and other devices to manage wandering or elopement behavior. If an alarm sounds, make sure staff respond promptly.

- Never turn alarms off, even if they are annoying.

- Regularly monitor documentation on flow sheets for accuracy, consistency and meaningfulness.

- Keep an elopement record (or book) with details about each resident at risk for elopement. Include the items listed above, known destination, etc.

- Do not be tempted to admit residents you cannot safely care for.

- Review policies and procedures annually or more often to ensure they are current and consistent with current standards of care for managing wanderers.

When admitting residents with a history of wandering, carefully assess the resident's needs and facility resources to determine whether you have the resources to monitor the resident adequately. For example, determine whether you have enough staff to monitor the resident. Determine whether this monitoring will take care away from the other residents. Make sure you can meet the wandering resident's needs, and remember, you are responsible for that resident's care from the time he or she enters until the time he or she is discharged. Some facilities use an elopement risk assessment tool at the time of admission to identify risk factors for leaving the facility.

Consider the wandering resident's needs first and be proactive in planning his or her care. Communicate with other staff to develop a workable plan. Caring for wanderers requires patience, cooperation, teamwork, flexibility, and resourcefulness. Wanderers can be managed without restraints if the facility has a plan, and staff work as a team!

Example missing resident policy and procedure

Purpose: To ensure the resident's safety utilizing the least restrictive means available. The purpose of this policy and procedure is to ensure that all necessary steps are taken in the event that a resident is missing or wanders away from the facility.

Procedures:

- Obtain information during pre-admission

or admission care conferences regarding any history of wandering or the potential for wandering and eloping.

- Document all instances of wandering or attempted elopement in the medical record.

- Develop and implement a plan of care with specific approaches and goals for the wanderer.

- Orient new staff to the policies and procedures for identifying and managing at risk residents.

- The facility will conduct a missing resident drill at least once each quarter on every shift.

If monitoring devices are used:

- A monitoring device will be placed on the high-risk resident according to manufacturer's directions. (Placing it on the wrist of the dominant hand makes it more difficult to remove.) Exit monitoring system will be kept operational 24 hours a day.

- Maintenance personnel are responsible for ensuring that alarms are operational for 24-hour service and are checked routinely. Maintain documentation of these checks in the preventive maintenance log book.

- Nursing personnel are not permitted to turn alarms off.

- In the event of an alarm malfunction, notify maintenance immediately. In the event of the inability to locate maintenance personnel, contact the administrator or alarm company.

Missing resident activities

- Any staff member observing a resident attempting to leave the facility will attempt to prevent such departure. Never leave the resident alone outside, even briefly.

- If a resident is found to be missing, personnel should

  – Notify the charge nurse.

  – Notify the supervisor or administrator on duty.

  – Assign staff on each unit to systematically search the entire facility, both inside and outside, including resident rooms, under beds, closets, bathroom, shower and tub rooms, utility rooms, and service areas. Assign two persons to check each hallway, one on each side.

  – Assign two personnel to check the area immediately outside the facility. Outside personnel should work their way around the facility in opposite directions. When they meet in the middle, they should return inside for reassignment.

  – Assign two personnel to check the kitchen, basement, lobby, activity room, chapel, elevator, stairwells, offices, and any other ancillary, utility, or service areas.

  – Assign available staff to begin a search of the neighborhood. (Some staff members should always remain in the building with residents.)

  – Contact the Administrator and Director of Nursing, if not on duty at the facility.

  – If the resident has not been found within 15 minutes, or after a search of the facility and immediately outside the building, the person in charge will carry out these steps:

    - Notify the police or local law enforcement agency.

    - Notify the family or responsible party.

    Explain what is being done to find the resident.

    - Notify other regulatory agencies, as required by law.

- When law enforcement arrives, give them

  – Resident's name, nickname, gender, age, height, weight, race, hair and eye color, mental condition, language spoken

  – Description of clothing

  – Picture of the resident

  – Former address, or possible location, if known

  – Other information that will assist in determining the resident's whereabouts.

  – The authorities may assume command and direction of the search from this point.

Upon return of the resident to the facility, the charge nurse or director of nursing will

- Completely assess the resident for injuries, and contact the attending physician and report findings and condition of the resident.

- Inform the responsible party immediately of the resident's return.

- Notify all previously contacted persons and organizations of the return of the resident.

- Complete an incident report detailing the incident in its entirety.

- Document the incident in the nursing resident's chart. Documentation should be objective, concise and reflect the actual facts as they relate to the incident including

  – times

  – persons contacted

– physical, mental and emotional status prior to the event

– times and details—last seen, staff actions, status of how, when and where found, condition

– assessment, injuries, condition of resident upon return to the facility, clothing, temperature outside, areas of skin exposed, etc.

– physician notification

– physicians' orders

– treatment given, if any

– responsible party notification

– other pertinent information

• Review and revise/update the care plan to reflect the incident and modify approaches to prevent recurrence. Consider whether a significant change MDS should be done.

Quality assurance

The JCAHO considers eloping a sentinel event, for which the facility is required to complete a root cause analysis. The results of the root cause analysis must be submitted to JCAHO. Accredited facilities are required to describe their analysis in the form of a policy, and list accountability factors in a procedure. However, regardless of accreditation status, this is a serious event. All facilities should perform a thorough and comprehensive root cause analysis of the elopement. Review policies, procedures, and systems to ensure they are effective, and sufficient to protect all residents who wander. Questions that need to be asked may include

• Were the alarm systems working properly?

• Were all internal and external doors visually checked?

• Were there any deficient practices or system failures?

• What is being done to prevent recurrence?

Summarize and discuss the root cause analysis information at the next Quality Assurance meeting. Keep records of all incidents so that trends and risks can be identified and reduced. Other QA functions include:

• Randomly testing door and personal alarm systems.

• Staging quarterly mock drills on each shift to test compliance of the plan.

• Reviewing policies and procedures, making recommendations for updates.

• Randomly questioning staff about routine wandering procedures and emergency procedures to follow if a resident elopes.

• Reviewing wandering documentation and flow sheets verifying resident location.

In most states, elopement is included in the mandatory reporting requirements, and surveyors will investigate each incident, especially if the resident is injured or cannot be located. The immediate jeopardy guidelines define neglect as the lack of supervision of residents with known elopement risk. If the resident's risk of eloping was known by facility staff, surveyors almost always cite the facility for immediate jeopardy with a G or J-level deficiency. In general, judges and juries have imposed extremely harsh penalties when residents have died or been seriously injured as the result of eloping from a long-term care facility.

Reducing the risk for restraint-related complications

Restraints are one method facilities sometimes use to manage wanderers. Generally speaking, restraints increase the risk of complications for all residents, and should be avoided, except as a last resort. Residents with certain conditions and diseases develop disuse syndrome when the musculoskeletal system is immobile. Disuse leads to complications of immobility, including

- weakness

- contractures

- atrophy

- increased risk of pneumonia and other lung infections

- blood clots

- pressure ulcers

- osteoporosis

- kidney stones

- urinary retention

- indigestion

- constipation and fecal impaction

- insomnia at night

- irritability, boredom, lethargy, depression, feelings of helplessness

Immobility can be caused by many internal and external factors, including complications of illness, surgery, lack of needed assistance with movement and ambulation, and use of restraints. Since the body works as a unit, complications of immobility will eventually affect all body systems, initiating a downward spiral of events in which one complication leads to another (and another and another). Anticipating, planning, and implementing interdisciplinary care to prevent complications of immobility is the *proactive solution* to the problem. The *reactive solution* is to wait until a resident experiences one or more complications, then trying to reverse them. The reactive method is much more common, and unfortunately it is also less effec-

tive, more difficult, expensive, frustrating, and time consuming.

Long-term care facility nurses must be acutely aware of the residents' risk factors for developing complications of immobility. Reduce the risks by planning and implementing preventive care. Several basic measures can be employed to preserve mobility in most residents:

- Exercising as many joints as possible through active, active assisted (assistive), and passive motion

- Avoidance of restraints

- Ambulation programs, such as "walk to dine," in which residents are assisted in walking from the dining room door to their tables, and sit in regular dining chairs with arms.

Sometimes our good intentions in keeping residents safe lead to further declines. For example, rather than strengthening the resident with exercise, we apply a restraint "to keep the resident safe" and "to prevent falls and injuries." Before applying restraints, you must consider whether a combination of restraint alternatives, assisted ambulation, and exercise would accomplish the same thing. If we strengthen the resident and maintain range of motion, would he or she be less likely to fall? *The resident who is not restrained is at risk only of falls. The risk of other injuries when using restraints is significantly higher than the risk of those same injuries when not using restraints.*

Staff with good intentions often apply restraints to protect the residents. All facilities should periodically review the care of at least one long-term resident who was admitted without restraints, but has subsequently been restrained. Work backward and track declines. You will find that many declines begin with application of restraints, and the deterioration became progressive. Consider this typical scenario:

A resident experiences several falls and is at risk of injury, so restraints are ordered and applied. Complications develop gradually. First, the resident becomes agitated or depressed. He or she loses bladder and bowel control. Next, he or she is hospitalized for urinary tract infection and dehydration. After returning to the facility, the resident becomes malnourished or experiences weight loss. He or she may be hospitalized several more times with dehydration (hypovolemia, hyponatremia, hypernatremia), and urinary tract infection. The resident is septic on one or more of these admissions. He or she will probably be hypothermic and in shock before the problem is identified and treatment initiated. Upon return from the hospital, the resident begins to develop contractures. There is a known, direct relationship between contractures and pressure ulcers. Pressure ulcers come next. The ulcers become infected, perhaps with a drug-resistant pathogen. By this time, the resident has deteriorated considerably and his or her prognosis is grim. His or her nutrition and hydration are probably not adequate to resist infection and promote healing. The use of psychotropic drugs worsens the problem, although this is not always readily apparent. When declines occur, we usually do not look past the short-term problems to see that application of restraints was the turning point. (Because of heavy turnover, staff may be unfamiliar with the resident's baseline status before the restraints were applied.)

If you perform one or more audits and identify a pattern of declines in restrained, dependent residents, take action immediately! Develop a plan to prevent the problem from recurring. If those residents are still under your care, develop a plan to gradually undo the damage. The following list can be used to complete the chart audit recommended above. It can also be used to assist in making decisions regarding whether to use restraints for the first time:

- Review the documentation on the medical record. The reader should be able to clearly determine the reason for physical restraint use from documentation, then track changes in restraint, medical, and physical condition, such as

- Safety of resident or others

- Impaired thought processes causing unsafe behavior

- Severe anxiety, depression, or other psychological condition

- Need for physical immobility, body positioning, or other rehabilitative or activity needs *that cannot be met in any other manner*

- Unsteady gait or unsafe ambulation, refusal (or inability) to call for assistance with ambulation; problems cannot be managed in another manner

- Consider convenience of staff if unable to determine another reason

- Resident discipline, punishment, or mistreatment

- Resistance to treatment, medication, or mechanical device

- Psychotropic drug use

- Emergency circumstances to eliminate an immediate or serious problem

- Recurrent eloping from the facility that cannot be managed in another manner

- Any decline in functional status related to loss of mobility or balance or muscle tone, increased agitation, reduced social contact, hearing/vision impairment, or communication deficit.

Determine whether

- The benefits of using restraints outweigh(ed) the risks.

- Staff can meet unmet needs or manage the behavior leading to restraint use in a different manner, thereby eliminating the need for restraints.

- Less restrictive alternatives were tried first, and were ineffective. No other viable alternatives exist.

- The environment was manipulated to eliminate the need for restraints, and the results of this manipulation were documented.

- The resident was toileted regularly. (Regular toileting eliminates ambulation attempts to use the bathroom, a common cause of injury in residents using restraints.)

- Staff have evaluated the effects of, and responses to, physical restraints, and documented the resident's response, including

Common singular event problems

– Physical side effects

– Psychosocial side effects

– Mental side effects

– Resident's level of functioning resulting from physical restraints, has improved, stayed the same or declined

– Resident's response to attempts to eliminate restraints

– The resident's plan of care, including alternate interventions, has been communicated to all direct care staff, and this is evident from signatures on the plan, flow sheets, or another component of the medical record or legal document.

Common side effects of restraints are:

Risks and Complications of Restraints	
Potential Physical Problems	**Potential Psychosocial Problems**
Decreased independence	Worsening of behavior problems
Pressure sores	Withdrawal, loss of social contact
Weakness	Depression
Decreased range of motion	Forgetfulness
Muscle wasting, atrophy	Fear
Contractures	Anger
Loss of ability to ambulate	Shame
Edema of ankles, lower legs, feet, fingers	Agitation
Decreased appetite, weight loss	Acute mental confusion or worsening of existing confusion
Dehydration	Combativeness
Distended abdomen	Restlessness
Urge to void frequently, dribbling, overflow	Sense of abandonment
Incontinence	Loss of self esteem
Urinary tract infection	Screaming, yelling, calling out
Constipation	
Fecal impaction	
Lethargy	
Shortness of breath	
Pneumonia	
Bruising, redness, cuts	
Falls	
Impaired circulation	
Blood clots	
Choking	
Strangulation	
Death	

Prerequisites to applying restraints were (are) met, including:

- Obtaining a physician's order

- Documented explanation given to resident or responsible party

- Documented reason why resident was not involved in explanation about physical restraint use

- Documented explanation regarding physical restraint side effects

- Documented choice for use of physical restraint by resident

- Documented acceptance or refusal of restraints by resident or responsible party

- Obtain written consent for use of restraints from resident or responsible party

- Document alternatives to restraints tried previously, and describe their effectiveness

Restraints do not reduce the need for supervision

Restraints do not eliminate the need for direct observation and supervision. In fact, the need for observation and supervision is increased if you follow the letter of the law. It takes more nursing time to care for a resident in restraints, than to care for a resident who is not restrained. When a resident is using restraints, staff must visually observe him or her every 15 to 30 minutes. The restraint must be released every two hours for at least 10 minutes. These things are often more time-consuming than supervising the resident. Nursing personnel are responsible for protecting the health, safety, and welfare of residents. This includes preventing complications of immobility and avoiding restraints whenever possible. Being

restraint-free is an attainable goal, but it takes a commitment from all staff. However, your initial goal should be to ensure that your facility is restraint appropriate. Begin with ensuring all restraints are appropriate for the residents and work from that point. Seeing the need for this commitment begins at the top and moves down. You have a number of great minds working with you. Each should be able to make a recommendation to avoid the use of restraints and maintain mobility. Try the following measures:

- If restraints must be used, consider them a temporary measure. Develop other alternatives.

- Make sure you know what alternatives are available. You may be surprised and pleased to learn of the many new, effective devices. Investigate online, in various catalogs, and with vendors to learn of new devices and items you are not familiar with. You may be delighted to see the scope and breadth of alternatives available.

- Network with your peers for best practices.

- Regularly assess the residents for complications. Determine whether other methods can be used to maintain safety. Gradually work on measures to reduce (and eliminate) restraints.

- Remember to periodically audit the records of residents who have been restrained for prolonged periods of time.

Restraint reduction activities

Note to reader: The information on restraints applies to the chronically ill or the healthy but mentally confused resident. The approaches listed may not be appropriate for an individual with delirium, acute medical illness, or an acute exacerbation of mental illness.

All long-term care facility nurses have had requests to use restraints and side rails on the residents from concerned family members. The most common reason is "to keep them safe." The loved one making the request is usually very sincere, believing the resident will fall without intervention. If the request is not immediately honored, it is common for the family member to make threats, such as, "I'll sue you if he falls. I'll own this whole facility." No long-term care facility has been successfully sued for failure to restrain a resident. Since the passage of OBRA 1987, lawsuits involving the inappropriate use of restraints have far outnumbered lawsuits involving unrestrained residents.[14] To successfully sue a facility for injuries to unrestrained residents, the plaintiff must demonstrate at least one of the following:[15]

- Failure to provide for a resident's safety as evidenced by a pattern of improperly assessing a resident's needs

- Failure to properly supervise or monitor the resident

- Failure to respond to a fall

- Failure to respond to an incident of eloping in a timely and professionally acceptable manner.

- Staff conduct endangered a resident

Family members commonly form opinions about the safety and protective features of restraints and side rails based on what they have seen in the acute care hospital. The nature of the care, patient acuity, patient complexity, manifestations of acute illness, and staffing patterns are vastly different from the long-term care setting. Since 10%–40% of all hospitalized elderly persons develop delirium, this is like comparing apples with lemons.[16] Reeducation is in order! Unfortunately, family members do not understand the significance of these differences when demanding restraints and side rails in the chronic care setting. Restraints may be appropriate, at least temporarily in many hospitalized

elderly patients. The family may have difficulty understanding why the long-term care facility cannot use side rails for the resident in the same way as in the hospital. Your job is to educate them in the realities of the chronic care setting.

Side rails are also more common in hospitals, where patients receive preoperative sedatives, and hypnotic drugs are more commonly used. Although hospitals also try to avoid restraints, side rail use is more common. Most hospital facilities use split rails, whereas most long-term care facilities use full length rails. Despite the safety of using split rails, they have been implicated in the death of some individuals. Because of this, all facilities must be attentive to the inherent dangers of using any type of bed rails, especially with air mattresses or mattress overlays, which are more malleable than a regular mattress and increase the risk of entrapment.

Try to remember that the family members who request restraints have their loved one's best interests at heart, and rightfully assume that side rails and restraints will always keep their loved one safe. They do not have your inside knowledge about the risks inherent with their use. This is a complex, sometimes emotional situation in which much family education is usually needed. One brief session may not be adequate. Repeated teaching, written handouts, and audiovisuals may be more effective. Staff and physician education is also necessary. If restraints or rails are used, you must get physician orders for them. Ask the resident or responsible party to sign a written consent advising of the benefits and risks of the device selected. Many long-term care facilities get routine orders for side rails "for turning and repositioning." Avoid these orders whenever possible. A comparison of the restraint documentation, MDS, and other information on the record will make it readily apparent that the resident is not able to reposition independently using the rails. The result is that surveyors will cite you for inadequate assessment and care planning, based on conflicting data on your medical record.

Avoid telling concerned family members, "We just can't restrain these people because of the law." Help them to understand the problem. Families requesting, demanding, and threatening personnel in an effort to cajole them into applying restraints has long been a difficult, sensitive issue in long-term care facilities. The interpretive guidelines for the use of restraints (F221/222) state, *"In the case of a resident who is incapable of making a decision, the legal surrogate or representative may exercise this right based on the same information that would have been provided to the resident. (See §483.10(a)(3) and (4).). However, the legal surrogate or representative cannot give permission to use restraints for the sake of discipline or staff convenience or when the restraint is not necessary to treat the resident's medical symptoms. That is, the facility may not use restraints in violation of the regulation solely based on a legal surrogate or representative's request or approval."*[17]

Restraints and side rails are medical treatments, not benign safety devices. Although one component of your teaching plan involves informing family members of the accrediting body standards and state and federal laws, this should not be the only approach. You must also include quality-of-life issues, and the magnitude of the various risks associated with restraint use. Solicit their input into the resident's care, and ask for suggestions for distractions and restraint alternatives. Restraint reduction and maintaining a restraint-free facility is a systematic process, in which family teaching is one step. Many other issues must be addressed when reducing resident, family, and staff dependence on side rails and restraints.

Medical symptoms and restraints

Medical symptom is defined as an indication or characteristic of a physical or psychological condition.

The resident's medical symptoms should not be viewed in isolation, but rather the symptoms should be viewed in the context of the resident's condition, circumstances, and environment. Objective findings derived from clinical evaluation and the resident's subjective symptoms should be considered to determine the presence of the medical symptom. The resident's subjective symptoms may not be used as the sole basis for using a restraint. Before a resident is restrained, the facility must determine the presence of a specific medical symptom that would require the use of restraints, and how the use of restraints would treat the medical symptom, protect the resident's safety, and assist the resident in attaining or maintaining his or her highest practicable level of physical and psychosocial well-being.

Medical symptoms that warrant the use of restraints must be documented in the resident's medical record, ongoing assessments, and care plans. While there must be a physician's order reflecting the presence of a medical symptom, CMS will hold the facility ultimately accountable for the appropriateness of that determination. The physician's order and a brief progress note are usually not sufficient to warrant the use of the restraint.

It is further expected, for those residents whose care plans indicate the need for restraints, that the facility engage in a systematic and gradual process toward reducing restraints (e.g., gradually increasing the time for ambulation and muscle-strengthening activities). This systematic process would also apply to recently admitted residents for whom restraints were used in the previous setting.

Other restraint-related considerations that cause injury

Other restraint-related considerations that have the potential for causing serious injury are

- restraint size

- proper restraint application, according to manufacturers' directions

Some restraints, such as vests and ponchos, are applied based on restraint size guidelines determined by the resident's weight. Many manufacturers have colored piping on the margins of the restraints to denote size, such as:

- yellow - small

- green - medium

- large - red

- extra large - navy

The manufacturer guidelines will provide a color code for restraint size. Also, each restraint should have an inner tag denoting the size. Always consider restraint size when selecting restraints. Applying a restraint that is too small or too large can be very dangerous. Facilities should have a selection of sizes available.

Staff must know how to apply restraints correctly to prevent injuries. For example, most tie restraints are applied by using a slip knot or quick-release knot. However, personnel commonly thread the straps through the armrests and tie the restraint in the middle of the chair back, where it can be reached and untied by the resident. If you look closely at the manufacturers' directions, you will see that for many tie-type restraints, the ties are threaded *between the seat and the bottom of the armrest, instead of through the armrests.* Applying the straps in this manner keeps the hips down so the resident cannot stand up. After the straps are threaded between the seat and the armrest, they are tied in slip knots to the kickspurs on opposite sides of the wheelchair.

Another safety hazard is applying a restraint when a resident is in bed. The straps are tied to the inner springs, where the resident cannot reach them, not the bed frame. A slip knot is used. The manufacturers' posters clearly show proper application of straps and ties. The restraint must be tied to a movable area so the resident's breathing is not restricted if the head of the bed is raised or lowered.

All manufacturers have an abundance of free teaching aids, videos, and posters to teach staff proper restraint selection and application. Upon request, most will send a representative to your facility to do an inservice.

Going restraint free

In reality, there is no panacea to restraint removal. Long-term care facilities face difficult problems and walk a fine line in keeping residents safe without violating their rights. Since there are many reasons for restraint use, the resident's individual situation must be assessed and care personalized. Despite admirable attempts to eliminate them, restraints are sometimes necessary. In general, however, the least amount of restraint necessary to keep the resident safe should be used. Many excellent restraint alternatives are available. Skil-Care Corporation has a wide variety of alternate devices and free training materials. This company can be contacted at 1-800-431-2972. The Posey Company also has a variety of restraint alternatives and other materials. They can be contacted at 1-800-44-POSEY (447-6739).

The Kendal Corporation has been a leader since the beginning of the restraint elimination movement. Their recommendations[18] for facility-wide restraint elimination are

Chapter thirteen

Introductory Phase

- Absolute support of the administration and governing body of the facility must occur.

- Gain their full commitment and establish a facility-wide policy.

- Designate a responsible, dedicated, supportive staff person ("Change Agent" or "Cheerleader") to oversee the process.

- Together with the Administrator, gain cooperation from Medical Director. (Change Agent)

- Introduce the topic to staff in all departments. (Change Agent)

- Inform families of policy change (Administrator/Change Agent)

- Facilitate Restraint Reduction Committee (Change Agent)

Implementation Phase (Restraint Reduction Committee)

- Customize formal education programs for each group interfacing with facility

- Examine present use of restraints on a case-by-case basis

- Development of individualized care plan

Evaluation Phase

- Reexamine staff perceptions regarding restraint elimination. (Administrator/Change Agent)

- Reexamine resident, family, and physician perceptions regarding restraint elimination (Administrator)

Team approach to care

A team approach is essential to making good side rail and restraint decisions. Select an interdisciplinary committee to address both facility and individual resident restraint issues. Include direct care staff, such as nursing assistants. These valued staff members know the residents better than managerial personnel, and their insights can be invaluable. The social worker and physical and occupational therapists are also assets to your restraint committee because of their insights into behavior management, seating systems, wheelchair fit, positioning, and use of adjunctive devices. The social worker can recommend behavioral approaches, and therapists can recommend postural supports, strengthening, or restorative nursing programs to increase independence and reduce the risk of falls. All team members must make a personal commitment to the elimination of restraints and side rails. The restraint team should determine whether facility policies are realistic and appropriate. They should routinely review incident reports for falls, as well as incidents involving the use of side rails and restraints, making recommendations as necessary. Initially, frequent meetings may be necessary. Infrequent meetings, such as the quarterly quality assurance meeting, are not usually adequate.

After the policies have been reviewed and revised, the education department must work with facility staff to ensure that all employees understand their responsibilities. Family education sessions and meetings are also essential. A key to the success of your program is teaching staff how to work with families who demand restraints and side rails. Physicians may also need education in this area. Families commonly turn to the physician when there is a difference of opinion with staff. The physician orders whatever they ask for, to placate the family, regardless of facility policies or resident needs. Because of this, work with the medical director to provide physician information and education.

Protocols

Many facilities effectively use protocols that describe situations in which restraints and bed rails can be used. Protocols should be approved by medical staff and nursing administration. Initiation of a protocol usually requires a physician order within a designated time frame. The elements of a restraint protocol may include

- rationale for restraint use

- criteria for application of restraints

- staff authorized to conduct restraint assessments and make decisions

- documentation requirements

- consideration of resident's rights

- frequency, extent, and nature of monitoring and observation to address the resident's needs

Most protocols include the following elements:

I. Description of protocol, and conditions in which the protocol is implemented.

II. Definition of restraint

III. Criteria for applying restraints, including resident's decision-making ability, surrogate decision making, and resident teaching activities.

IV. Description of resident removal from restraint. This includes releases according to facility policy and removing the device when it is no longer necessary.

V. Protocol policy for assessment, reassessment, and documentation.

Like everything else, the nursing process forms the basis for your assessment and care. An interdisciplinary team approach to assessment is invaluable. If a family member requests a restraint

- Each team member assesses the resident.

- The entire team meets with the family member and resident. Ask for their assistance and involvement in developing a safe, acceptable plan to meet the resident's needs.

- Explain facility policies, accrediting body standards, and applicable state and federal laws.

- Define the terminology used in the policies that family members may not be familiar with. Avoid assuming that they understand. Most policies state that restraints and side rails are used to treat "medical symptoms." They are not used for "staff convenience." Make sure that family members understand the definitions for these terms. For example, medical symptoms are indications or characteristics of a physical or mental problems. Compare this with *staff convenience*, which is any action taken by the facility to control or manage a resident's behavior with a lesser amount of effort and not in the resident's best interest. To be successful, the family must be on the same page with the staff regarding policies and procedures. To get there, begin with definitions.

- Explain that restraints have been viewed as safety devices for years, but current research has proven that restraints increase the risk of injury and reduce quality of life. The staff seeks more positive and therapeutically beneficial alternatives for keeping the residents safe. Some of the magazine television programs from the early 1990's describe restraint use from the family perspective, and show why restraints may increase the resident's risk. You may wish to check available videos from shows such as 20/20 and Dateline to see if these are currently available. Check with staff members to see if any videotaped these programs. Since the shows were produced for the general public, they do an excellent job of meeting the needs of concerned family members, and are produced at a level that may be more appropriate than showing a medical video. Audiovisuals are powerful teaching tools. Investigate this potentially valuable source of information.

- Define your objective in seeking alternatives to restraints. Explain that preventing all falls is impossible, and one primary goal is to reduce the magnitude and severity of injuries from falls.

- Make the resident or responsible family member a valued member of the team, and solicit their assistance with the decision-making process. Reinforce that you value their input, knowledge and expertise in caring for the resident. Negotiate with them, if necessary. If a family member insists that you double the dose of a medication, you would teach and explain why doing so is unsafe. Do the same with requests for restraints and side rails. Try to find a compromise if there is a conflict of opinion.

- Suggest that the recommended restraint/side rail approach will work best if the family member is involved and assists during the transition period.

- Develop a list of reasonable alternatives to restraints and side rails. Use team members' assessments, knowledge of the resident, and healthcare expertise to suggest those that are most likely to work in preventing falls and injuries. Actively solicit family suggestions and document their participation and response.

- Determine whether environmental adjustments are necessary.

- Emphasize the importance of quality of life. Explain that the facility cannot isolate the residents in a risk-free, protective sanctuary. Some risks must be assumed by both the resident and facility to ensure that the resident achieves and maintains the highest practicable quality of life. In fact, the resident has a legal right to take risks, if he or she chooses to do so.

- By this time, the team assessment has identified the resident's risk factors and approaches to reduce the risk as much as possible. Assure the family that you will work with them to reduce the risk of injury as much as possible, but tactfully explain there are no guarantees. Taking this approach will assist you in maintaining or improving the resident's quality of life, while reducing risks, and keeping the resident as safe as possible.

- Develop a clear plan of care with short time frames for reassessment and modification of the plan. A frequent, individualized schedule for reassessment and care plan modification is crucial when the program is initiated. This is particularly true in facilities that normally review their care plans quarterly. In the early stages of restraint reduction, a quarterly reassessment is risky, at best. Daily or weekly assessment is essential. The short time frame for reassessment and revision of the plan is much more realistic and greatly reduces the risk of injury to the resident.

- Communicate the plan with appropriate staff members, and refer to it regularly. Reinforce the importance of using the plan. One of the greatest drawbacks of developing a restraint-reduction plan is that staff do not read or follow the plan. This is a problem of enormous proportion that plagues the entire long-term care industry. We spend an inordinate amount of time writing plans that no one uses. Each facility must have a method for ensuring that staff follow the plan, or the risk of injury (and liability) is greatly increased. Depending on the circumstances, ensuring that staff read and follow the plans may need to be your first step, not the last. Stress that over the long-term, you will reduce the time staff spend caring for restraints. (This is not a typographical error; if staff follow the letter of the law for caring for residents in restraints, they spend more time caring for the restraint than for the resident). Additionally, you will reduce the risk of injury, improve quality of life, and increase resident and family satisfaction.

- Explain the facility philosophy on restraints to all new admissions. Provide a copy of the policy.

When your facility accepted and began caring for the resident, they did so with the knowledge that chronically ill, elderly, and confused residents sometimes fall. The staff is charged with, and the facility has accepted the obligation of, ensuring safety and protecting the residents as much as possible. Personnel have the duty to take every reasonable action to minimize falls and injuries. If an injury occurs, an unbiased legal reviewer must be able to determine that you took every reasonable action possible to prevent falls and injuries. (He or she will do this by reviewing the medical record.) Document your assessment and daily care with every reasonable action in mind. Documenting your reasonable actions after an injury occurs is too late. Likewise, late entries and blatant efforts at repairing the medical record create additional legal risks, including potential exposure to criminal penalties.

Documentation

When residents are restless or agitated and require restraints, documentation must support the need and use of alternatives. The frequency of documentation varies with facility policy. In general, restraints must be ordered by the physician. The order should state the

- type of restraint (vest, belt, etc.; make sure you do not mix up vests, ponchos, and similar devices)

- time it is to be applied (when up in chair, when in bed, at all times, etc.)

- reason for the restraint (avoid "safety"; list a concrete, resident-specific reason)

- release (such as every two hours, or according to facility policy)

Documentation that the resident was visually observed every 15 to 30 minutes, and the restraint released every two hours for 10 minutes is also necessary. Check with your state survey agency for side rail release. Because side rails fall under the definition of physical restraints, they must also be released every two hours. Develop a method for doing this. Check your state laws to determine whether this requirement applies to night time, when residents are asleep, and whether it applies to side rails. The easiest way to document the visual checks and releases is by use of a flow sheet that states the resident was visually observed every 15 (or 30, or according to facility policy) minutes this shift, and released every two hours for 10 minutes. This eliminates the need for multiple entries. One flow sheet entry covering the entire shift may be adequate. Check your facility policies and state requirements. Documentation must be present, but save time by consolidating it in one place, and using flow sheets as much as possible. **Example forms are on your CD-ROM.** Make sure documentation is honest and consistent. Avoid gaps.

Chapter thirteen

Side rails as restraints

The answer to the question, "Are side rails restraints?" is not a simple one. Most experienced long-term care nurses will admit that side rails are restraints most of the time. They are not necessarily benign safety or enabling devices. In some facilities, all side rail orders state "for turning and repositioning." A review of the therapy documentation and MDS's reveals that many of the residents are incapable of doing this. Obviously, orders of this nature increase legal exposure. If a resident is incapable of using the bed rails for repositioning, a solid care plan should be formulated with progressive steps for teaching the resident this skill. A therapy or restorative nursing assessment should validate the need for this teaching. Documentation should reflect evaluation of the resident's progress and modification of the plan when necessary. However, there are situations in which side rails are used for valid reasons, such as turning and positioning. If the resident requests rails for this purpose, the request should be honored, but documentation should support the need. In this situation, the rails are enablers; they are not considered restraints. Documentation should reflect the resident's choice. A resident's or family's request to raise the side rails does not absolve the facility of the responsibility for resident teaching, informed consent, and continuous use of the nursing process in assessing, planning, implementing, and evaluating the use of bed rails and the resident's reaction to them. However, there is a gray zone in between clear indication and clear contraindication, and this is the area in which many residents fall. Consider this example:

Mr. Huynh is a cognitively impaired 72-year-old resident with Parkinson's disease. He has four half rails on his bed. All of the side rails are raised when he is in bed. The resident does not want them raised. He uses the bathroom frequently. When he feels the urge to void, the need is urgent. Although he calls for help, he does not like to wait for staff to arrive to assist him. The Parkinson's disease has caused him to be unsteady on his feet. Although he uses a walker, staff feel he cannot safely ambulate without supervision. Facility staff explain that the side rails are raised for three separate purposes. These are

- facilitating independent bed mobility

- providing support during transfers

- keeping the resident in bed when he wants to climb out of bed to use the bathroom

In Mr. Huynh's situation, consider the rails restraints, and manage the resident accordingly. Although two of the three purposes listed here assist the resident to maintain his highest level of function, the third causes them to be a restraint.

The key to side rail use lies in proper assessment of the resident. Having a policy that states that rails will be raised in all bedfast residents, or something similar, is not in compliance with the law. Likewise, assumptions such as "all cognitively impaired residents need side rails" are incorrect. Studies have shown that in some cases, rails worsen agitation and isolation. Some residents perceive them as bars in a jail cell. When a resident climbs over raised side rails, he or she falls quite a distance before reaching the floor. The risk of fracture or other serious injury is much greater than falling from the mattress height. Additionally, the feet or legs may become tangled between the bars on the rail, worsening the injury. Documented instances of strangulation have occurred both with and without the use of other types of restraints, such as vests and belts. Another consideration is the risk of entrapment of the head and/or body between side rails and mattress. Some of these instances have resulted in death.

After an assessment, but before rails are raised, consider alternatives to keeping the resident safe, such as low beds with a frame height five to 7.5 inches from the floor, placing the mattress on the floor, or using a pressure-sensitive alarm system. The approaches listed here are for example only, and are often effective. However, they may not be satisfactory for some residents, in some situations. If alternative approaches are tried and deemed ineffective, explore others. Attempt to determine the cause of the resident's behavior for which you believe side rails are necessary. Behavior problems are often the result of unmet needs. If the cause of the behavior is identified and eliminated, raising the rails may not be necessary. The need to use the bathroom is a common cause of climbing over side rails. In many situations, the resident cannot communicate this need, or staff do not respond immediately to calls for assistance. Make sure that your care plan tracks the alternatives tried and approaches used for managing the resident's behavior. Make sure that all staff are aware of the plan, and use the approaches consistently.

Side rail evaluation and assessment

When considering the use of side rails, add three questions to your regular restraint evaluation, in order:

- *Can the resident identify the edge of the bed?*

    – If you are unsure about the resident's ability to identify the edge of the bed, ask your therapists for assistance. If the resident can identify the edge of the bed, he or she is not in grave danger of rolling over and falling out of bed. Consider alternatives, such as foam bolsters, a body pillow, or a low bed.

- *Why is the resident getting out of bed?*

    – The nursing assistant staff may know the answer to this question. Elderly persons

tend to eliminate more fluid when they are in bed at night with their legs elevated. Often, they are getting up to use the bathroom! Other reasons may be hunger, thirst, pain, inability to sleep, fright, or wanting to investigate a noise. The answer to this question will drive your care plan. These are unmet needs! Write (and implement) a plan to meet the resident's needs. If you understand and ignore the resident's motivation for getting out of bed, the continued use of side rails is meaningless, and most likely dangerous.

- *If you understand why the resident is trying to get out of bed, why are you keeping him or her in bed?*

    – Answering this question may provide the key that unlocks the door to finding effective, resident-specific restraint alternatives. Having data on the resident's balance, coordination, and mobility are ineffectual. These data are only meaningful when the resident gets up! Going back to questions one and two will help solve the problems and eliminate the need for side rails.

Preventing injury and entrapment in side rails

Long-term care facility residents are at high risk for injury and entrapment from use of bed rails. In 1995, the FDA issued a warning regarding hazards of entrapment in hospital beds. The FDA and several advocacy groups continue to actively address this issue. To reduce the risk of hospital bed entrapment and injury, facilities should always assess the resident's needs thoroughly before making the decision to use side rails. If side rails are considered safe, beneficial, and appropriate for the resident, follow the FDA recommendations for checking for potential sources of injury:

- Inspect bed frames, side rails, and mattresses regularly to identify areas of possible entrapment.

- Remember that gaps can be created by movement, compression of the mattress, and other factors such as the resident's weight or position.

- Check mattresses. Mattresses wear out much more quickly than beds. Because of this, many facilities have replaced mattresses numerous times. The mattresses may have dimensions different from those of the original equipment supplied or specified by the bed-frame manufacturer. Variations in side rail design and mattress thickness/density affect the potential for injury and entrapment.

- Check side rails. Make sure they are properly installed and fit correctly. Avoid bowing, and ensure the rails are the correct distance from the head and foot of the bed.

- Ensure that the resident's overall body size, height, and weight are appropriate for the bed's dimensions.

- Although the mattress, bed frame, and side rails appear safe, a resident's limbs can become caught in small side rail openings, causing injury. To reduce the risk, assess the resident, discuss options with other staff members, the resident and responsible party, then plan the resident's care accordingly. Many adjunctive devices are available to keep residents safe, such as bed bolsters, guards, and pads. Adjuncts and alternatives are available from the restraint manufacturers. Select the appropriate device, then install it securely and correctly to eliminate gaps between rails and mattress.

See your CD-ROM for the FDA guidelines on side rails.

Other bed-related liability considerations

Although most of the information in this book discusses the risk of legal exposure with resident injuries, using low beds is an area in which you must also consider injuries to your workers. This is another clear example of how fixing one problem creates another. Low beds are used to reduce the risk of injury if the resident falls from the bed. Some facilities place pads on the floor next to the bed to further reduce the risk of fall-related injuries. Overall, the beds are excellent for reducing resident injuries, but pose a risk to the workers. Nursing assistant staff must use good body mechanics to prevent back injuries when lifting, moving and caring for residents, and when making beds. They must also be careful to avoid bending at the waist when performing any procedure, especially moving the resident. A few manufacturers supply beds with high-low features, but many low beds are stationary, which greatly increases the risk of worker injury.

A floor mat reduces the risk of injury if a resident falls, but the mat creates a fall hazard for staff, who may be entering the room in the dark. Leaving a night light on, or turning the light on when entering reduces the risk. Teach staff to squat or kneel on the floor mat when caring for the resident, and to avoid bending at the waist. Use good body mechanics, a transfer belt, or a mechanical lift when assisting residents into and out of the beds. List resident-specific instructions on the plan of care. The procedure for making the bed is the same as it is for hospital beds. To make this task easier, advise staff to

- Mentally plan the procedure before beginning.

- Organize work well to reduce the total number of motions required to complete the task.

- Make sure to bring all needed items and equipment when entering the room.

- If a high-low bed is used, elevate the bed when caring for the resident or making the bed. (When purchasing beds, an electric high-low model is best. Staff tend to leave the manual beds in the low position because of difficulty raising and lowering them.)

- Place linen and needed items on a chair within close reach. Remember to avoid placing clean items on the floor.

- Bend from the legs, not the waist, and maintain a neutral posture; avoid twisting.

- Kneel, squat, or sit on the mat when making the bed, or providing resident care if this is easier.

- Remove the bed linen several pieces at a time. Avoid removing all the linen in one bundle. The weight of the linen and your posture increase the risk of back injury.

- Make one side of the bed at a time to reduce the number of movements, improve efficiency, and conserve energy.

- Use a fitted bottom sheet to reduce the number of movements necessary for making the bed.

- If a plastic mat is used on the floor to prevent injuries when the resident is in bed, fold it and move it out of the way when the resident is out of bed so that no one trips on it.

Choking

Resident choking is the cause of some singular-event lawsuits against long-term care facilities. All staff must be taught to perform the current obstructed airway procedures for responsive and unconscious residents. The American Heart Association guidelines changed in 2005. Make sure your employees are familiar with current standards. Generally speaking, you should relieve airway obstructions caused by foreign bodies and food. In almost every situation, this is a medical emergency, not an expected terminal event. Because of this, your DNR orders probably do not apply to this situation. If you have residents for whom choking is an expected terminal event, clarify appropriate action in advance and ask the physician to leave specific orders in the event it occurs. Otherwise, know and follow all emergency facility policies and procedures. A 2005 court decision upheld a CMS deficiency with civil monetary penalties for a facility who failed to clarify the DNR order (which was written on an unsigned transfer form) on admission. The resident had no advance directive. When the resident experienced a cardiac arrest, nurses spent 15 minutes phoning the physician to clarify what action to take. The court viewed the situation as substandard care planning in violation of federal regulations, and upheld the citation and monetary fines.[19] The principles applied are the same as those in which nurses fail to treat a choking resident.

Drowning

Sadly, drowning is a common cause of lawsuits against long-term care facilities. Drowning is the second leading cause of accidental death in young adults, but statistics are erratic for nursing facility residents. However, each year long-term care facility residents drown in bathtubs, whirlpool tubs, and similar bathing units. This commonly occurs when the resident is left unattended, or the safety belt and lift on the whirlpool seat are not in good working order. The only way to address this risk is to firmly enforce a policy of remaining in the tub room with the resident for the duration of the bath. Staff should never leave the resident unattended, even for a few seconds. Develop policies and procedures for bathing residents and inservice staff. Additional safeguards are to

- Check the whirlpool apparatus and seat belts monthly or more often.

- Post signs in the tub rooms, such as "Never leave a resident unattended."

- Specify the water level for bathing residents.

- Mount cabinets in the tub room and keep them well stocked with necessary items, such as washcloths, towels, bath blankets, and shampoo.

- Make sure all professional staff have current CPR cards.

- Keep oxygen, suction, and emergency equipment in good working order in an accessible location.

Teach personnel to use the normal basic life support procedures for drowning or near-drowning. At one time, several methods were recommended for removing water from the lungs before beginning rescue breathing and CPR. The routine use of abdominal thrusts or the Heimlich maneuver for drowning victims is not recommended. Attempts to remove water from the airway, throat, and lungs by any means other than suction (e.g., abdominal thrusts or the Heimlich maneuver) are unnecessary and potentially dangerous.[20]

Fire ants and other pests

In June 2004, a jury awarded $1.2 million to a Florida woman who was attacked by fire ants in her long-term care facility bed. Although the resident had cognitive impairment, she remembered the fire ant bites, which she described as very painful. A facility nurse initially documented that the resident was itching. He subsequently noted multiple red blotchy areas, which turned into "numerous pustules over her upper torso areas, arms, back and neck as a result of uncon-

trolled fire ants." When interviewed, the nurse told the newspaper reporter, "She ended up suffering longer than she should have because they didn't have enough staff." The facility was sold 11 days after the attack and no longer does business in Florida. Another Florida resident died at age 87, after being stung more than 1,600 times by fire ants in another Florida long-term care facility in 2000. The autopsy listed the stings, heart and lung disease, and kidney failure as contributing factors in the death of the resident. The facility was closed for a month after the attack. Another 83-year-old Florida resident was attacked and stung 50 times by fire ants in a Florida hospital in 2002.[21]

In October 2005, the jury awarded a resident of a Dallas, Texas facility $156,000 for injuries she received in a fire ant attack. This case was slightly different, because she also sued the pest control company, which denied responsibility for the problem. The jury believed differently, and stated the pest control company was indeed partially responsible, and that they had failed to comply with the terms of the contract, finding them negligent. The jury found that the long-term care facility's benefit-of-the-bargain damages were $6,000. Initially, the jury had tried to return a verdict that the breach-of-contract award was zero and the negligence award $150,000. However, the judge, over the pest control company's objection, instructed the jury that those findings were in conflict. In a note, the jury asked if the two findings must be the same, and the court, again over defense counsel's objection, answered yes. The jury finally awarded the resident $150,000 for breach of contract and $150,000 for negligence. There was no jury award for malice, which was alleged.[22]

A resident of a Galveston, Texas, facility was stung repeatedly while in her bed. Ambulance personnel found hundreds of ants inside her adult brief. Ants had been found in a room on the same wing several days earlier, and the plaintiff contended the facility was negligent for failing to ensure the ants were eliminated. The resident had severe emphysema and heart problems, and died under hospice care several weeks after the incident. A jury awarded $136,000 to the daughter, who appealed the ruling as an inadequate dollar amount, blamed partially on the fact that the judge would not allow a physician expert witness to testify in the probate court. The court of appeals upheld the original court decision for $136,000.[23]

Incidents of fire ants

South American fire ant attacks in long-term care facilities are increasing in the southern states. Many of the resident victims have died within one week of the attack. Initially, it was believed that the ants are cold intolerant and would not move north. However, they are hardy, resilient, and capable of change. The ants can reproduce in temperatures as low as 0° F.[24] Fire ants (*Solenopsis wagneri*; may also be called *S. invicta*, *S. richteri*, and *S. invecta x richteri*) are spreading quickly to the north and are expected to cover the entire contiguous United States within the next few years. The ants live and forage for food through a series of underground tunnels. A nest is actually a full network of tunnels and chambers occupying a vertical column 12 to 18 inches in diameter and approximately 36 inches deep. The queens burrow deep in the colony and are fairly well protected from baits and insecticides used at the surface. During the spring and fall, the ants clear the tunnels and expand their chambers, creating a mound of loose soil on the surface of the ground. The ants live in the above-ground area when the temperature is right for breeding, moving below ground (or indoors) when it is cool or rainy. They will also move indoors if the weather is extremely hot, very dry, or during heavy rain.

One of the greatest dangers posed by fire ants is that they invade electrical systems, damaging circuit breakers, relays, motors, and other electrical devices, and causing fires. No one seems to understand why electrical systems are attractive to the ants, but researchers at Texas Tech University are researching and addressing the problem. In the long-term care facility, the ants target spilled and uneaten food, and are attracted to chairs and surfaces with body oil buildup, soiled linen, IV tubes, and needles. If fire ants are noted in or around the facility, obtain professional exterminator services immediately. One Texas facility was fined $255,000 per day for 55 days for failing to eradicate fire ants after a resident was attacked.[25]

The ants reproduce rapidly, producing many hundreds of new queens each summer. Colonies containing multiple queens are the norm in Texas, making eradication difficult.[26] When the queens mature, they fly about, dropping into many areas to breed. Fire ants are very aggressive, and when a colony is established, they eliminate most other competing ants. The ants have no natural enemies in the United States. However, the problem has become so severe that in some areas, the U.S. Department of Agriculture has released phorid flies, tiny Brazilian insects, in an effort to eradicate the ants. The flies lay eggs on the ants and when the larvae hatch, they eat the ants. This method is believed superior to insecticide because the flies affect nothing other than fire ants.[27]

Fire ants are tiny—about one-eighth to one-quarter inch long. They move very quickly, and are able to crawl rapidly through tiny cracks in the facility foundation. They are also very defensive, and will sting most anyone they contact, stinging about 60% of the human population in affected areas annually.[28] The bites are very painful. A single ant sting is rare. When fire ants attack, many swarm the body and attack simultaneously. Initially the stings appear to be small, red welts. These progress to pustules the size of a pin's head within eight to 10 hours. Initially, they burn and hurt, but subsequently cause severe, maddening pruritus. The itching and burning may respond to diphenhydramine (Benadryl®) cream or a topical steroid product. Home remedies that have been reported to be effective are dabbing fresh bites with a straight household strength sodium hypochlorite solution (bleach) or pure cooking vanilla (not extract). About two percent of the population has a true allergy to fire ant stings, but deaths related to an allergy are less common than complications caused by the residents' underlying medical problems and overall fragile condition. The bites have the potential for causing anaphylactic shock in affected, sensitive individuals.

Fire ant control

Note to reader: Fire ant prevention and control is an ongoing area of research. In some areas of the United States, there are pesticide restrictions. Check current sources of information for standards related to extermination and control.

A professional exterminator is essential to good fire ant control. Make sure your contract specifies inspection and control for fire ants. This was an issue in the Galveston lawsuit, noted above. Begin by baiting and eliminating fire ants in outdoor nesting areas. An area 25 to 50 feet surrounding the building is a key area. However, baits may work slowly, taking up to three months depending on the chemicals applied. Other recommendations for outdoors include

- Facilities should check the grounds weekly for signs of fire ants, and maintain a log of the inspections.

- Maintain at least 20 inches of space between the building and outdoor plants, shrubs, and bushes.

- Make sure sprinkler heads are facing away from the facility; avoid soaking the foundation and walls.

- Grade the soil so water flows away from the building.

- Keep downspouts clean and make sure the water flows away from the facility.

- Have an exterminator regularly inspect and treat the perimeter of the facility for signs of infestation.

- Remove trash from the facility daily and keep dumpsters closed; avoid accumulation of boxes and trash next to the building.

- Maintenance personnel should monitor for and repair water leaks regularly.

Thorough cleaning indoors is essential. The precautions for fire ants are things that facilities do routinely when cleaning and satisfying the requirements of the regulatory bodies. No special precautions have been recommended. Move tables for cleaning to avoid food accumulation under the base plates. Keep beds and furnishings pulled out slightly from the walls, and keep linen off the floor. Clean mattresses and bed frames regularly and monitor for food accumulation. Food should be conscientiously removed from floors and resident beds after meals. Store food in sealed containers. Staff should monitor for open or spilled foods in night stands and drawers in residents' rooms. Nursing assistants should be instructed to monitor for signs of ants when positioning and moving the residents or changing the bed linen. Keep the outsides of intravenous fluid and catheter drainage bags dry.

If ants are noted on a resident, staff should apply gloves and gowns. Eliminate the ants by compressing them with a wet cloth, then wiping them away. Move the resident out of the bed, and do a complete body check, including all external orifices. Monitor for signs of hypotension and respiratory distress. Inform the physician and responsible party promptly. Complete an incident report and implement ongoing monitoring, or transfer the resident to the emergency department, depending on the severity of the attack, signs and symptoms, and resident response.

Facilities should maintain an ongoing log of pest sightings for the exterminators. However, in the event that fire ants are sighted, a special plan of action must be put into place. Require exterminator response within 24 hours, with daily inspections for the following week. Logging is fine, but immediate action is needed to prevent injury to the residents from these aggressive pests. If ants are spotted in a resident room, move the residents until an exterminator treats the area. Check all resident rooms in the facility for signs of infestation, paying close attention to rooms in the proximity of the sighting.

Until a method for eliminating fire ants is identified, they will continue to pose serious problems and risks for long-term care facilities. Vigilant monitoring and aggressive action if ants are noted provide the best line of defense. Although most fire ants are red in color, some are black. Other aggressive species may also be black. If an ant must be identified, store it in alcohol for the exterminator. Avoid making assumptions about the ants based on color.

Suicide

For some elderly individuals, death may seem like the only option to suffering from chronic disease, many losses, and ongoing physical or emotional pain. In some residents, any sudden loss increases the risk. Silent suicide is defined as "the intention, often masked, to kill oneself by nonviolent means through self-starvation or non compliance with essential med-

ical treatment."[29] The resident must be distinguished from terminally ill residents who are refusing intervention to avoid prolonging the act of dying. Behavior such as a sudden refusal to eat may be a sign of silent suicide in elderly residents. Relocation stress may be a contributing factor.

The polypharmacy problem

Polypharmacy is the use of multiple drugs simultaneously. This is a common occurrence in elderly, long-term care facility residents. Drugs provide many positive effects, including improved quality of life, alleviating symptoms, and curing some infections and diseases. Despite the benefits, polypharmacy is a great concern to those caring for the elderly in the United States. Consequences of polypharmacy may include

- Adverse drug reactions

- Drug-to-drug interactions

- Noncompliance with the drug regimen

- Decline of quality of life or functional ability

- Deterioration in mental status.

Some common drugs used for treating medical problems can cause symptoms and signs of depression. Of these, antihypertensives and sedatives are the most common. Polypharmacy is the most common cause of treatment-induced symptoms of depression. The environment in which medical conditions are treated is also a consideration, and can predispose the resident to depression because of the isolation, sensory deprivation, and forced dependency.[30]

Some residents will express their desire to die. Long-term care facility residents have committed suicide by hanging, hoarding medications and overdosing, and even using creative methods such as consuming large quantities of Epsom salts, which have been provided by a well-meaning family member for use as a laxative. A few have eloped and deliberately walked in front of moving vehicles. If a resident expresses a desire to die, promptly notify the social worker and attending physician. Request a mental health evaluation. Implement suicide precautions. Facilities have a duty to assess the resident and attempt to determine the degree of risk. When assessment suggests a need for concern over the possibility for suicide, the facility has a legal duty of reasonable care to try to prevent harm. Facility residents may lack full mental capacity, creating a special relationship with the resident, and imposing a duty on the facility to take appropriate steps to attempt to prevent voluntary acts of self-destruction.[31]

Additional information about suicide precautions is on your CD-ROM.

Injury at the hands of another resident

F224 states, "Each resident has the right to be free from mistreatment, neglect and misappropriation of property. This includes the facility's identification of residents whose personal histories render them at risk for abusing other residents, and development of intervention strategies to prevent occurrences, monitoring for changes that would trigger abusive behavior, and reassessment of the interventions on a regular basis."[32] Most facilities have policies, procedures, education, and other programs to prevent staff abuse of residents. Facilities sometimes fail to consider resident-to-resident abuse, which is a growing problem. Each year, the popular press reports long-term care facility resident murders that have occurred at the hands of another resident.

Census is the lifeblood of the facility. Occasionally, long-term care facilities pressured or anxious to fill beds have knowingly admitted criminals, including sex offenders. (A few special facilities in the United States are contracted with their respective State Department of Corrections to accept only criminals; these facilities are exempt from the present discussion.) The most notable inappropriate placement is that of a 23-year-old female resident at a Connecticut facility, who ignited her mattress with a cigarette lighter, starting a fire that engulfed part of the long-term care facility, killing 16 residents. Subsequently, the resident who started the fire was found not competent to stand trial for murder.

In 2000, a nurse in an Oklahoma long-term care facility discovered a resident who had been strangled. He could not be resuscitated. Police arrested a 34-year-old resident, described as having "the mental capacity of a 1-year-old," who had been a resident since the facility opened 13 years previously. The men were not roommates but saw each other daily. The murdered resident's mother contended that the day before her son's death, the perpetrator was seen dragging him through the center's hallways with a belt wrapped around the victim's legs. The belt was allegedly taken away, but given back the next day. This facility had previously been cited after a resident's death went undiscovered for six days. A housekeeper found the 48-year-old resident in her room. She was last seen alive six days previously. After the murder, the state of Oklahoma closed the facility, and the residents were moved elsewhere.[33]

In 2000, a 53-year-old resident of a Dallas, Texas long-term care facility was arrested on charges of first-degree murder and aggravated assault after the bludgeoning death of his 54-year-old paraplegic roommate. A nursing assistant was also injured, when she responded to a commotion in the residents' room. Upon her arrival, she was hit in the head with a cane, causing a head injury. In this same facility in 1997, a nursing assistant entered a room and discovered an HIV-positive male resident sexually assaulting a female resident with Alzheimer's and heart disease.[34]

In 2005, a Connecticut resident with a diagnosis of dementia was arrested for the murder of his roommate. Sometime during the night, the 88-year-old resident bludgeoned his 82-year-old roommate with a footboard from the bed. No one heard anything unusual. The roommates were described as "good friends who went everywhere together."[35]

Researchers estimate that only one in 14 incidents of elder abuse is reported to law enforcement or human service agencies. Abuse of older adults is one of the most under-recognized and under-reported social problems in the United States. It is far less likely to be reported than child abuse, because of the lack of public awareness. Nationally, it is estimated that more than 55% of elder abuse is due to self-neglect of individuals living in the community.[36]

Several reasons are given for the increased resident-to-resident violence in long-term care facilities:

- Young, strong, physically capable residents are being admitted to geriatric facilities; some of these residents are mentally ill.

- Facilities are caring for greater numbers of residents with Alzheimer's and other forms of dementia. These residents can be both aggressors and victims.

- Residents with dementia lose their inhibitions and may be more prone to aggressive behavior. They get agitated more easily and afraid. Some have delusions and hallucinations, believing others will harm them.

- Some residents wander and rummage through or take others' belongings, causing residents to

respond with violence.

- Residents with dementia may become agitated with change in facility, in caregiving personnel, with roommates, or changes in rooms, causing them to react violently.

- Some residents are delusional and believe others are stealing from them or plan to harm them.

- Many facilities have admitted felons, including those with a history of violence and sexual assault.

Residents with violent tendencies or a potential for violence increase the liability exposure of facilities and their personnel. The court system has imposed harsh penalties on facilities in ruling that they failed to provide a safe environment for the residents. In resident-to-resident abuse, lawsuits are common. The plaintiff usually alleges that the facility was aware of the perpetrating resident's potential for violence, but failed to act on it or properly address it, thereby failing to protect other residents from harm. The following suggestions are helpful in reducing your legal exposure related to residents who are aggressive:[37]

- Establish a clear philosophy of individualized care for the facility. Plan all interventions, interactions, and programming around this philosophy of care.

- Clearly identify the acuity level for which the facility can safely provide care.

- Set resident admission criteria and policies that enable staff to address behaviors.

- Whenever possible, evaluate the resident in his or her environment prior to admission. Ideally, a nurse and social worker will assess each resident. Consider the potential resident's anxiety level and orientation within a familiar setting.

(Agitation will probably worsen in a new setting). Request a history and physical for facility staff to review prior to admission. Question family members about aggressiveness, wandering, safety factors, etc.

- If a resident is on the border between two levels of care on admission, offer admission to the higher level. After he or she successfully makes the transition to his or her new surroundings, reevaluate the resident for a lower level of care.

- Be consistent, and accept only those individuals whose needs can be met by your staff.

- Establish a system for monitoring residents to ensure that residents qualify for the level of care the facility provides. Upon admission, formulate a plan to move the resident to a higher (or lower) level of care if needed. Clearly explain the admission criteria, monitoring system, and potential transfer plan to the resident and responsible party prior to admission.

- Educate the resident and responsible party about the resident's diagnoses and expectations when transitioning to a new environment. You may wish to caution the responsible party about the potential for delirium and relocation trauma.

- Educate staff in the care of residents with dementia. Include content on

  - What dementia is and how it affects function and behavior.

  - How to approach residents with dementia and use calming communication techniques (such as validation therapy, distraction, redirection, etc.).

  - How staff should modify their own behavior in response to the resident's behavior.

  - How to provide assistance with ADLs, such as sequencing tasks and breaking procedures down into smaller, more manageable steps.

  - Keeping the residents' environment as simple and structured as possible (avoid clutter, distractions, etc.).

  - Keeping residents' routines redundant and consistent.

  - Identifying and managing pain and other stressors.

  - Using techniques for managing behavior problems and avoiding triggers to difficult behavior.

  - Following a consistent care plan, taking each step in order if signs of aggression begin. Emphasize the importance of implementing the plan before the aggression is out of control.

- Assess each resident's ability and develop a plan of care to meet his or her needs. Negotiate and discuss the plan with the resident, responsible party, and staff. Regularly review the plan. Document changes in behavior or condition, and modify the plan as often as necessary.

- Assess the environment and modify it to eliminate conditions that are stressful to the resident, such as extremes in lighting (bright or dim), too much stimulation or lack of stimulation, loud noises, temperature extremes, etc.

- Ensure that nursing care and activities meet the needs and abilities of each resident. Provide a wide range of purposeful activities (such as providing towels to fold or socks to match, wrapping silverware, folding napkins, etc.).

- Inform the physician promptly if the resident experiences acute behavioral changes suggesting a medical problem (such as UTI or dehydration). Obtain orders for lab work (including urinalysis) to pinpoint the problem.

- Develop a system for monitoring and documenting difficult behaviors.

- Keep communication open with the responsible party, physicians, and interdisciplinary staff.

- Assign sufficient staff to meet the needs of residents. Make sure staff are knowledgeable about the residents' needs. Assign extra staff at problematic times, such as during the early evening when residents are sundowning.

- Thoroughly investigate any incident involving resident aggression or potential abuse allegations immediately. Report outcomes to the proper individuals.

The bulleted list above is modified with permission from Williams L. Liability Landscape: When residents attack residents. Nursing Homes/Long Term Care Management 2004;53(August):2.

Accidents outside of the facility

Lawsuits are filed every year as a result of transporting residents outside the facility in a bus or van which is either owned or leased by the facility. In most cases, facility personnel are accompanying the resident. The most common problems creating legal exposure when transporting residents are

- Personnel are not properly trained in transporting residents, fastening wheelchairs to the floor, or securing the residents in a vehicle. Residents fall from chairs during turns or sudden stops, usually sustaining multiple lower-extremity fractures.

- The wheelchair is not strapped securely to the floor, leaving slack in the straps. Wheelchairs tip to the side during turns, causing residents to hit their heads or fall out of the wheelchair.

- Personnel are careless when operating the van lift, resulting in fractures and other injuries to the feet, including amputation of toes and metatarsals.

- Wheelchairs are secured to the floor of the van, but residents are not secured in the wheelchair with a seatbelt or shoulder harness. When questioned post-injury, most of these personnel state they did not fasten the safety device because of prohibitions against using restraints and residents' rights in the facility. (Facility rules regarding prohibition of restraints clearly do not apply to moving vehicles, or states in which seat belt laws are mandatory. Jurors typically do not believe this excuse.)

Standard of care for transporting residents

Standard of care for transporting long-term care facility residents by bus or van

Each facility must have policies and procedures for transporting residents to appointments and activities. Personnel accompanying residents must be thoroughly trained in routine and emergency procedures. The standard of care for long-term care facility personnel transporting residents on a vehicle is the same, whether the vehicle belongs to the facility, a private company or party, or a governmental entity. Consider a random audit system in which a manager periodically rides in the van and reviews driver safety and other security issues. Consider incorporating the following into facility policies and procedures:

- Implement a drug testing policy and procedure

for employees responsible for resident transportation.

- Facility personnel accompanying residents should be properly trained or oriented regarding taking residents on outings away from the facility.

- The facility must ensure the vehicle or personnel are equipped with communications equipment, such as a cell phone or central dispatch radio.

- Complete annual driving record checks on personnel driving the vehicle. Keep the insurance carrier informed of driver changes. Follow the laws in your state regarding driver's license and the need for a chauffeur's license in some situations.

- Provide a defensive driving or other safety course for all designated drivers.

- Develop a checklist for routine preventive maintenance and safety checks when using a facility-owned van. List equipment that must remain in the vehicle at all times, such as a certain number of seat belts and/or shoulder harnesses, and a first aid kit. Inspect the vehicle daily, weekly, or monthly, depending on frequency of use. Maintain a log or file for all safety checks.

- Keep utility scissors or a web cutter in the van in case cutting restraining straps is necessary.

- One or more personnel from the long-term care nursing facility should accompany residents who are being transported by bus or van.

- Always park the vehicle on a flat area, outside the flow of traffic, where it is safe to load and unload residents.

- Under most circumstances, the driver should operate the wheelchair lift, with other personnel assisting residents as necessary. Monitor

movement of personnel to prevent injuries from the lift.

- After moving wheelchairs onto the lift, check the positions of the wheelchair wheels and the resident's feet to ensure the lift can be moved safely, without tipping or crushing injury to the feet.

- Ensure employees are familiar with all necessary procedures, such as loading and unloading the vehicle, securing wheelchairs to the floor, and securing residents to the wheelchairs.

- All residents, including those who are in wheelchairs, should be fastened into the appropriate safety restraint. This includes seat belts, shoulder straps, or a combination thereof. In general, seeing that residents are properly secured is the responsibility of facility personnel, and not the driver of a leased vehicle, such as a bus. Facility personnel are expected to know the residents' medical problems and needs, whereas the driver would not be familiar with them. If personnel do not know how to operate the particular restraining devices used on the vehicle, they should ask the driver for assistance. Since the use of seatbelts is required in the United States, the long-term care facility rules regarding the residents' right to refuse restraints does not apply in any moving vehicle. Residents must agree to use of seat belts and/or shoulder harnesses, or transportation will be refused. Most residents feel more secure with a safety belt, and refusals are seldom a problem.

- Wheelchairs must have the wheels properly secured to the floor with an appropriate locking system before the vehicle is moved. Several effective locking systems are available. The type selected depends on the vehicle. The wheels to the wheelchairs are secured by an individual who has been trained in the operation of the locking system. This may be the driver or facility personnel, depending on the vehicle or situation. However, facility staff are always responsible for securing residents in chairs. This is not the leased carrier's responsibility.

- After all residents have been seated on the vehicle, and before the vehicle is moved, a staff member should do a walk-through to ensure that they are properly secured in seat belts, shoulder harnesses, or other restraining devices. (This walk-through is similar to that done by flight attendants on an airplane).

- After the safety walk-through, the staff member is seated and fastens his or her seat belt. After this individual is seated and secured, he or she gives the command to the driver to move the vehicle. However, he or she should visually monitor the residents throughout the trip to ensure that their needs are met.

- In the event that one staff person is present, he or she should sit at the back of the vehicle, in a position to supervise the residents during the trip.

- In the event that two staff persons are present, one should sit at the front, and one at the back of the vehicle. Both should supervise residents during the trip. They should not sleep, read, or focus on other distractions.

- When the vehicle arrives at its destination, and the vehicle has completely stopped, all passengers may remove their seat belts/shoulder harnesses.

- Facility personnel must assist residents as needed to remove restraining devices and to safely exit the vehicle.

Managing an emergency when transporting long-term care facility residents by bus or van

If a medical emergency situation occurs while residents are being transported by bus or van, facility personnel should

- Request that the driver pull off the road and stop the vehicle as quickly as possible.

- Remove their seat belts or shoulder harnesses and go at once to the ill or injured resident.

- Determine the nature of the emergency by assessing the resident for airway, breathing, circulation, bleeding, fractures, or other illness or injury.

- Immediately provide emergency care for the illness or injury to the extent possible. Do not move the resident unless imminent danger is present. In the event of suspected fractures, immobilize the extremity. Apply pressure to bleeding areas with a clean cloth. Apply the principles of standard precautions and avoid direct contact with blood or body fluids.

- Instruct the driver to radio or call for help (i.e., 911 ambulance) through dispatch or by using a cellular telephone.

- Provide necessary information to ambulance personnel and assist ambulance personnel as necessary to remove the resident from the vehicle.

- After the ill or injured resident has been removed from the vehicle, do a walk-through to ensure that all other residents on the vehicle are properly secured in their seats. Reassure and calm residents as necessary.

- Return to their seat, fasten their seat belt, and instruct the driver to continue to the destination.

- Upon return to the facility, personnel should notify the physician and responsible party of the illness or injury, prepare and fax a transfer form and other medical information and documents to the emergency receiving agency, and complete an incident report. List all witnesses to the incident in the incident report. Document the incident in the resident's medical record.

Recommendations for day trips and transporting residents on a bus or leased carrier

- Staff members/group participants are required to carry cash or credit cards to purchase amenities and comfort items in the event of delays, emergencies or breakdowns.

- Smoking is prohibited on buses at all times.

- No alcoholic beverages are allowed on buses.

- Each person participating in the scheduled outing must return with the group to the destination (pickup location). No participant may leave the group to stay at any location other than the original pickup point.

- The bus driver is not permitted to accept gifts or tips. Please do not offer money, gifts, or gift certificates.

Resident and staff conduct on leased carriers

Bus drivers have specific procedures they must follow in the event of misconduct by persons using the bus:

- The bus driver will notify the leader or person responsible for the group of the problem. This individual must take the necessary steps to correct it.

- If the responsible person is unable to correct the problem, the bus driver will make preparations to leave the event and return to the facility or original pickup location.

- The bus driver will make a detailed written report of the problem upon return.

- Misconduct reports may result in the inability to use bus transportation for group activities in the future.

Passenger safety on leased carriers

The bus driver is responsible for checking the bus prior to the trip to ensure that all safety equipment is operational, including windshield wipers, turn signals, headlights and reflectors. Unsafe conditions will be corrected before beginning the trip.

- All passengers must be secured in seat belts or safety harnesses before the bus is moved. Wheelchairs and similar mobility devices must be secured to the floor with the appropriate restraining device. Facility personnel are responsible for securing seat belts and safety harnesses to residents.

- A list of all individuals on the trip must be drawn up and given to the bus driver upon arrival at the pickup facility. Each individual riding the bus must sign his or her own name to this record. In the event of a resident who is cognitively impaired, the facility must make arrangements for the responsible party to sign the form. *(NOTE: consider preparing a separate release form for families of cognitively impaired residents to sign in advance of the trip—some may not be able to be present at the time the bus arrives)*

- One staff member must remain on the bus at all times when residents are on the bus or leased carrier.

Leased carrier procedures at the pickup location, and each time the bus stops at a destination

- Ambulatory residents are placed on the bus first, including those using walkers, canes, crutches, and other adaptive equipment.

- Residents in wheelchairs are placed on the bus last.

- The bus driver or qualified transportation employee operates the wheelchair lift.

- Facility personnel must be in place to receive the wheelchairs inside the bus and move them to their designated location.

- The bus driver or qualified transportation employee must secure wheelchairs to the floor with the appropriate safety restraint.

- Facility personnel will ensure that all passengers are properly secured in their seats with seat belts or shoulder harnesses. The bus driver will instruct facility personnel in the operation of these devices, if necessary. However, he or she is not familiar with residents' medical conditions or problems, such as gastrostomy tubes and colostomies under clothing. Facility personnel are responsible for applying restraints to residents.

- After all residents are properly secured, facility personnel must conduct a walk-through to check all seat belts. After walking through the bus, personnel take their seat and secure their own belt. It is recommended that personnel sit in the back of the bus so they have visual control over residents during the trip. If more than one staff member is present, one may sit in back and the other in front.

- After all residents have been secured and facility personnel have walked through to check, the person in charge instructs the driver that he or she may move the bus.

- Upon reaching the destination, the bus driver will stop the bus. All passengers are expected to remain in their seats with belts fastened until the bus has completely stopped and parked, and the driver instructs the responsible employee that it is safe to move.

- Facility personnel will assist passengers to remove their seat belts and exit the bus. The bus will be off loaded in order of accessibility. If wheelchairs are in front, remove them first to prevent trip hazards for ambulatory residents. If space is not a consideration, unload in this order:

  – Ambulatory residents first

  – Residents with mobility devices such as canes, walkers, and crutches second

  – Residents in wheelchairs last

- The bus driver is responsible for releasing the belts or other devices restraining the wheelchair wheels to the floor of the bus. He or she will prepare to operate the wheelchair lift. Facility personnel are responsible for moving the resident to the door and positioning the wheelchair on the lift. The bus driver will raise and lower the lift.

Leased carrier emergency procedures

In the event of an emergency during a bus trip, the driver will stop and park the bus at the nearest safe location upon request. He or she will contact central dispatch, police, fire, or ambulance as appropriate. Follow the driver's instructions for remaining on the bus or exiting the bus, as appropriate to the emergency situation.

In the event of an injury or medical emergency, the driver will contact dispatch and EMS. An ambulance will be dispatched to the scene of the emergency and the ill or injured passenger will be removed from the bus. Facility personnel are expected to care for the ill or injured resident to the extent of their ability, until the ambulance arrives. The bus driver is not permitted to provide emergency care. The driver is not permitted to move the bus until ill or injured passengers have been removed.

After the ill or injured passenger is removed from the bus, facility personnel must conduct another walk-through to ensure that all passengers are securely fastened in their seat belts or shoulder harnesses. Follow the steps above to double check passenger safety before the bus is moved. After being advised that all passengers are safe, the driver will continue to the destination. Unload the bus according to established procedures at the destination.

Wandering risk for cognitively impaired residents on day trips

In January 2006, a 13-month-long search for a missing facility resident ended in the marshy woods in Tennessee. Dental records confirmed that remains found by hunters belonged to a facility resident who had disappeared from a day trip to a casino a little more than a year earlier. The ambulatory resident was confused after having experienced a series of TIAs or strokes. She had been on a day trip with a facility group and was videotaped leaving the casino. That was the last time she was seen alive. A private investigator, $50,000 reward, and signs on billboards on major highways produced no results. Early in the investigation, helicopters, dogs, and heat-seeking devices were used in an unsuccessful attempt to locate the resident. The body was found less than two miles from the casino.[38]

Because of the risk of harm or injury to cognitively impaired residents, the facility must ensure the resi-

dents have adequate supervision when on day trips away from the facility. For example, avoid taking a bus load of cognitively impaired residents unless you have sufficient staff to oversee them. Depending on the resident, you may need one-on-one or one-on-two supervision. Volunteers may fulfill this responsibility. You are not required to take a group of licensed or certified personnel away from the facility to monitor otherwise healthy residents. You may also wish to write a policy and procedure for doing periodic "head counts" during day trips. Formulate procedures for locating residents who wander off during trips in the community. Make sure that all activities personnel and other staff involved in day trips are familiar with these policies and procedures. For reduced legal exposure as well as enhanced resident safety, try to anticipate everything that could go wrong in advance, and take steps to reduce the risk and eliminate problems.

Other considerations for day trips

The facility should develop policies and procedures for medication administration and dealing with medical problems when the residents are out of the facility. In most states, a licensed nurse or certified medication aide must administer medications. Determine whether your activities personnel can administer medications during day trips. You may find that you must send a nurse or medication aide along.

Another consideration is residents with allergies to food items. Provide a list of allergies and special medical problems to the activity director or person responsible for the trip. You may also wish to list which residents have DNR orders. When determining the information to list, identify information you consider essential, such as food allergies. Then determine whether listing the desired information is a violation of the HIPAA rules. You may need to modify the listing, depending upon which personnel accompany the residents, as well as the circumstances of the trip.

References

1. This modified "Hippocratic Oath" was composed in 1893 by Mrs. Lystra E. Gretter and a Committee for the Farrand Training School for Nurses, Detroit, Michigan. It was called the Florence Nightingale Pledge as a token of esteem for the founder of modern nursing. Online. *www.nursingworld.org/about/pledge.htm.* Accessed 12/26/05.

2. Iyer P. (2003). Liability in the care of the elderly. *JOGNN*, 33, 124-131; 2004.

3. Legal Eagle Eye Newsletter for the Nursing Profession(5)11 Nov 97. Online. *www.nursinglaw.com/sexualassault1.htm.* Accessed 12/6/05.

4. United States District Court, Louisiana. (1996). Schenck vs. Living Centers-East, Inc., 917 F. Supp. 432 (E.D. La., 1996).

5. Predators in America's Nursing Homes. (2005). A Perfect Cause. Online. *www.aperfectcause.org/.* Accessed 12/27/05.

6. Morris EA. (1997). Medical code of silence threatens the lives of Alabamians. Montgomery Advertiser, July 13, 1997.

7. Lachs MS and Pillemer K. (1995). Current concepts: Abuse and neglect of elderly persons. 332 *NEJM.* 437 (1995).

8. Marks D T. (1996). Neglect in nursing homes. *Trial,* Feb 1996 v32 n2 p60(3).

9. 661 So. 2d 873 (Fla. Dist. Ct. App. Sept. 29, 1995).

10. Cannon vs. Rehabilitative Services, Inc., 544 N.W. 2d 790 (Minn. App., 1996).

11. Guide One Insurance. *Resident elopement facts.* Des Moines, IA. Briggs Corporation brochure.

12. Perlmutt D. (2006). Missing patient found, but dies: Woman, focus of 4-day search, was in nursing home storage room. Charlotte Observer. Online. *www.charlotte.com/mld/charlotte/13733659.htm.* Accessed 01/28/06.

13. Nursing home employee charged in missing woman case. *www.wsbtv.com/news/5859523/detail.html?rss=atl&psp=news.* Online. Accessed 01/05/06.

14. Schnelle JF. Total quality management and the medical director. *Clinics in Geriatric Medicine* 1995;11(3): 433-48.

15. Miles SH, Meyers R. Untying the elderly: 1989-1993 update. *Clinics in Geriatric Medicine* 1994;10(3): 513-25.

16. Delirium is a global disorder of attention and cognition. It is commonly caused by metabolic problems, dehydration, and medication reactions. It is present in 10% to 40% of elderly persons at the time of hospital admission; the incidence rises to 25% to 60% during the stay. (Inouye SK. (1998). Delirium in hospitalized older patients: recognition and risk factors. *J Geriatr Psychiatry Neurol.* 1998;11:118-125, 157-158.)

17. State Operations Manual. Interpretive Guidelines §483.13(a)

18. For a complete description of the Kendall Corporation program, see *www.ute.kendal.org/index6.htm,* or contact Untie the Elderly®, The Kendal Corporation P. O. Box 100, Kennett Square, PA 19348.

19. Omni Manor Nursing Home v. Thompson, 2005 WL 2508547 (6th Cir., October 11, 2005).

20. Rosen P, Stoto M, Harley J. The use of the Heimlich maneuver in near-drowning: Institute of Medicine report. *J Emerg Med.* 1995;13:397–405.

21. Patrick R. (2004). Woman awarded $1.2M in ant attack. *Herald-Tribune. www.heraldtribune.com.* Jun 4,2004.

22. Juliette Fowler Homes, Inc., d/b/a Pearl Nordan Care Center v. The Terminix International Limited Partnership, d/b/a Dallas Pest and Termite Services, Inc., No. 03-9060-F. Online. *www.verdictsearch.com.* Accessed 10/27/05.

23. Estate of Jose de Alminana v. Gulf Health Care Center District Court, Galveston County, Texas. 14-04-00715-CV.

24. Siddiqi Z. (2001). Spreading menace: Fire ants on the move. Nursing Homes, Sept. 2001.

25. Siddiqi Z. (2001). Spreading menace: Fire ants on the move. Nursing Homes, Sept. 2001.

26. Siddiqi Z. (2001). Spreading menace: Fire ants on the move. Nursing Homes, Sept. 2001.

27. United Press International. (2005). Fly latest weapon in war against fire ants. Online. *www.sciencedaily.com/*. Accessed 12/30/05.

28. Siddiqi Z. (2001). Spreading menace: Fire ants on the move. Nursing Homes, Sept. 2001.

29. Simon RI. (1989) Silent suicide in the elderly. Bulletin of the American Academy of Psychiatry & the Law, 17, (1):83-95.

30. Kane R L, Ouslander JG, & Abrass IB (Eds). (1999) Essentials of clinical geriatrics New York: McGraw-Hill.

31. Klein vs. BIA Hotel Corporation, 49 Cal. Rptr. 2d 60 (Cal. App., 1996).

32. State Operations Manual (Intent) §483.13(c), F224

33. Reynolds D. (2000). Man charged with murder as facility closes. Inclusion Daily Express. September 13, 2000. Online. *www.inclusiondaily.com/news/institutions/choctaw.htm.* Accessed 01/03/06.

34. Anderson K. (2000). Man, 54, killed at nursing home: Roommate in wheelchair held in beating death of paraplegic. *Dallas Morning News* July 24, 2000. Online. *www.nursinghomelawyer.com/nursing_home_law_firm/nursing_home_news/nursing_home_death.htm.* Accessed 1/03/06.

35. Christoffersen J. (2004). Nursing home killing shows wider problem. Phillyburbs.com. Online. *www.phillyburbs.com/pb-dyn/news/1-10062004-378108.html.* Accessed 1/03/06.

36. Iowa Department of Human Services. (2005). Dependent adult abuse: A guide for mandatory reporters. Online. *www.dhs.state.ia.us/dhs2005/dhs_homepage/docs/depend_adult_abuse.doc.* Accessed 01/03/06.

37. Modified from: Williams L. (2004). Liability landscape: When residents attack residents. Nursing Homes, August 2004, Vol. 53, No. 8

38. Staley O. (2006). Remains confirmed as those of woman missing since 2004. The Commercial Appeal. Online. *www.commercialappeal.com/mca/local_news/article/0,1426,MCA_437_4362048,00.html.* Accessed 01/04/06.

Infection-related complications

Infections

Infections are cited in many lawsuits as both a primary and secondary complication. Generally speaking, plaintiffs view infection as a result of prolonged neglect, in which inadequate precautions were used over a long period of time. Infections and complications commonly seen in lawsuits include

- infected pressure ulcers

- Gram-negative septicemia as a complication of infected pressure ulcers or surgical wounds

- Gram-negative septicemia; as a complication of ongoing urinary catheter use (usually cited as a long-term failure to monitor and provide proper catheter care)

- Gram-negative septicemia as a complication of urinary tract infection

- Gram-negative septicemia as a complication of other localized infection

- Aspiration pneumonia

- Gram-negative or -positive septicemia as a complication of pneumonia

- gangrene

- septic shock

- osteomyelitis related to Stage IV pressure ulcers

- overuse of antibiotics resulting in drug resistance

- drug resistant infections; most commonly MRSA

- failure to use the correct antibiotic based on a culture and sensitivity report

- failure to ensure an infection was eliminated (by rechecking culture and sensitivity testing) after a course of antibiotics is administered

Another common infection control problem that does not result in lawsuits, but is problematic nonetheless, is the presence of isolation signs on residents' doors. Sometimes interested family members see isolation signs, then call the state reporting hotline to note that, "infection is widespread and out of control in that facility." The presence and need for isolation signs should be addressed periodically (and in advance) in meetings, newsletters, family council, and educational programs. Be proactive by informing families that the isolation signs make conditions safer and contain potential pathogens to a single room. You may also want to clarify the fact that sometimes the isolation sign has been posted as a preventive measure only, such as when an infection is suspected, but you are waiting on the lab. This further reduces the risk to other residents, and the sign will be removed if the lab results are negative. In any event, teach staff, residents, and families about the importance of good hand washing and preventive infection control.

Infection control

§483.65 Infection Control—The facility must establish and maintain an infection control program designed to provide a safe, sanitary, and comfortable environment and to help prevent the development and transmission of disease and infection.

§483.65(a) Infection Control Program—The facility must establish an infection control program under which it

(1) Investigates, controls, and prevents infections in the facility;

(2) Decides what procedures, such as isolation, should be applied to an individual resident; and

(3) Maintains a record of incidents and corrective actions related to infections.

Intent §483.65(a)—The intent of this regulation is to assure that the facility has an infection control program which is effective for investigating, controlling, and preventing infections.

Interpretive Guidelines §483.65(a)—The facility's infection control program must have a system to monitor and investigate causes of infection (nosocomial and community-acquired) and manner of spread. A facility should, for example, maintain a separate record on infection that identifies each resident with an infection, states the date of infection, the causative agent, the origin or site of infection, and describes what cautionary measures were taken to prevent the spread of the infection within the facility. The system

must enable the facility to analyze clusters, changes in prevalent organisms, or increases in the rate of infection in a timely manner. Surveillance data should be routinely reviewed and recommendations made for the prevention and control of additional cases. The written infection control program should be periodically reviewed by the facility and revised as indicated.

Surveillance

Infection surveillance is the foundation of the infection control program in long-term care. The purpose of an infection surveillance program is to identify infections, plan control activities, and prevent outbreaks.[1] Effective surveillance consists of data collection, data analysis, data reporting, and decision making.[2] The need for infection control must be balanced with the residents' quality of life, and need for socialization and mobility.[3]

The facility must have an ongoing system for collection of information about infections in the facility. At the very least, conduct surveillance weekly and obtain data through communication with the staff and a review of lab reports and 24-hour logs, or other reporting tools. Pay particular attention to culture and sensitivity reports, treatment orders, and physician progress notes. Walking rounds and staff-communication clipboards at the nurses' station may assist in this effort. Collect surveillance data to calculate and analyze infection rates, looking for patterns, trends, and unusual occurrences. Surveillance data may also be used for planning infection control activities, staff education, and to detect outbreaks.[4] When reviewing infections, consider specific individual factors such as age, underlying diseases, treatments with antimicrobials, corticosteroids, or other immunosuppressive agents, irradiation, and breaks in the first line of defense. Mechanisms caused by operations, anesthesia, and indwelling catheters will also increase the risk for infection.

Infection control practices and isolation precautions are designed to prevent transmission of microorganisms by many different routes in healthcare facilities. Because agent and host factors are more difficult to control, interruption of transfer of microorganisms is directed primarily at transmission. Most recommendations for interrupting the spread of infection are based on this concept.[5] In long-term care, the use of standard precautions provides the foundation for the standard of care. It is important for the designated infection control practitioner to understand the difference between universal precautions, body substance isolation, and standard precautions. Many individual workers use a combination of these systems rather than using standard precautions exclusively. Standard precautions have been available for more than 10 years and provide the highest level of protection. Older systems and combinations of systems must be eliminated.

Documentation stating, "Universal precautions in use" is a red flag to a medical-legal reviewer, and often is used as proof that the facility did not provide care in keeping with the current standards.

Additional information on Infection control practices and Standard Precautions can be found on your CD-ROM

Example criteria for infections

- Criteria are guidelines or definitions used by the infection control nurse to determine the presence of infection for surveillance purposes.

- These criteria are not intended to be used as guidelines for medical diagnosis or treatment.

- Surveillance criteria are approved by the infection control committee.

- Criteria are used by the infection control nurse to differentiate infection from colonization (the presence of microbes in or on the resident but without tissue invasion or damage).

- Unless diagnosis by a physician is specifically designated as a criterion for a specific type of infection, a physician's written or verbal diagnosis does not, without supporting data, justify counting the condition as an infection.

- If infection appears at a new and different site in the same resident, it is counted as a new nosocomial infection.

- An infection will be considered nosocomial (facility-acquired) only if there is no evidence that the infection was present or incubating on admission or readmission (after hospitalization or community visit). Also, there must be no evidence that the infection began as the result of a procedure carried out in a hospital, physician's office, or other healthcare facility.

- Infections that are not nosocomial are referred to as community-acquired infections.

  – Community-acquired infections are included in surveillance, since they may alert personnel to the need for preventive measures. However, they are grouped separately from the nosocomial infections in the statistical summaries.

- See "Criteria for Infection" for definitions adopted by the facility for surveillance purposes.

Example criteria for infections

Example criteria for infection can be found in Figure 14-1, which appears on your CD-ROM. These criteria are a basic part of the infection surveillance program. They are used to identify infections in the absence of any other known reason for the signs and symptoms. Infections must meet these criteria to be counted in the surveillance statistics. These criteria are intended for surveillance purposes only and are not to be used as a basis for medical diagnosis or treatment.

Urinary tract infection

Urinary tract infection (UTI) is a symptomatic infection that can occur anywhere in the urinary tract. It is more common in women, but men may also experience UTI. The increased risk of infection in women is believed to be related to the female anatomy and short urethra, compared with males. The incidence of UTI increases with age for males.

Geriatric long-term care facility residents are at greater risk of infection than their peers who live in the community.[6] Inadequate fluid intake greatly increases the risk. In long-term care facilities, UTI is the

- Most common cause of infection.[7,8]

- Most prevalent source of bacteremia.

- Most common reason for hospital transfer.

- Most common condition for which antibiotics are given.[9]

Vaccines are being developed to prevent urinary tract infections. Additional studies are needed to determine effectiveness and long-term effects. Other potentially effective suggestions for preventing UTI are

- Encourage and help residents to drink sufficient fluids. All residents should meet the dietitian's minimum calculated requirement daily. Monitor and assess intake and output if fluid intake is inadequate.

- Ensure that nursing assistants and direct care personnel use standard precautions and aseptic technique for perineal care. Monitor and spot check their performance periodically.

- Bathe/wash the genital area daily from front to back. Shower instead of taking a tub bath.

- Cleanse the genital and urinary areas from front to back with soap and water after each bowel movement.

- Avoid tight-fitting pants.

- Wear cotton underwear (or underwear with a cotton liner in the crotch); change daily.

- Wear pantyhose with a cotton crotch; change daily.

- Avoid powder, bath oil, and feminine hygiene sprays. Keep all products containing perfumes, fragrances, or other potential allergens and irritants away from the genital area.

- If sanitary napkins are used, change after each voiding.

- Encourage and assist residents to urinate frequently.

An area of ongoing study is the usefulness of an estrogen vaginal cream, intravaginal estradiol suppositories (Vagi-Fem®), or estrogen-releasing vaginal ring (Estring®). Research suggests that estrogen prevents infection by increasing the number of lactobacilli (a microbe that resists infection by lowering the vaginal pH levels and preventing *E. coli* from adhering to cells). Consult the dietitian and physician about the use of cranberries (and/or blueberries). Cranberries and blueberries contain chemical substances called tannins, or proanthocyanidins. These substances prevent *E. coli* from adhering to cells in the urinary tract. Studies suggest that consumption of cranberry juice or cranberry tablets or capsules daily reduces the incidence of UTI.[10] (Capsules and tablets have varying amounts of tannin. Preparations made from spray-dried cranberries contain tannin, but those derived from extracts may not.) Other effective alternatives are cranberry sauce and dried cranberries. Cranberry juice cocktail is also effective. Fructose, which is present in all fruit juices, may also interfere with bacterial adhesion.

- There is no evidence that cranberry consumption will eliminate an established infection.

- Avoid cranberry products if the resident is taking anticoagulants.[11]

- Taking vitamin C daily makes urine more acidic. The acidity is inhospitable to bacteria, but there is no evidence this prevents UTIs.

Definitions

Bacteriuria is characterized by the presence of bacteria in the urine with no evidence of tissue invasion in the lower or upper urinary tract. *Simple bacteriuria* in the absence of UTI symptoms or obstruction is called *asymptomatic bacteriuria*. Asymptomatic bacteriuria does not require treatment unless the resident is about to undergo an invasive procedure in the genitourinary area. More than 50% of female residents with asymptomatic bacteriuria develop recurrent bacteriuria within four weeks of antibiotic treatment. Treating asymptomatic bacteriuria is not beneficial. Treatment increases the risk of developing antimicrobial-resistant organisms. There is little evidence to suggest that asymptomatic bacteriuria leads to other complications. However, residents known to have this condition should be regularly monitored for signs and symptoms of infection.[12] Residents with indwelling urinary catheters for more than 30 days are commonly colonized with more than 50,000 colony-forming units of bacteria per mL of urine.[13] A resident with asymptomatic colonization does not have an infection, but should be regularly monitored.

Urinary tract infection is bacteriuria accompanied by signs and symptoms.[14] Many nurses use the terms UTI and "symptomatic bacteriuria" interchangeably, but they are not the same condition. Typically, a labo-

ratory confirmation of >100,000 colony-forming units (CFU)/mL of one or more organisms is the standard for a positive urine culture. However, if the resident is symptomatic or highly significant pathogens are present, lower counts are diagnostic for infection, particularly in high-risk or debilitated residents. Factors affecting the colony count include the method of specimen collection, resident symptoms, overall hydration, frequency, presence of an obstruction, and recent or current antibiotic therapy.[15]

Three or more episodes of symptomatic bacteriuria within one year are defined as *recurrent UTIs*. Recurrent UTIs may be caused by either relapse or reinfection. A *relapse UTI* is bacteriuria within two weeks of completion of antibiotic therapy. A *reinfection UTI* is bacteriuria that develops in four or more weeks after a previous infection has been treated and eliminated. The causative agent may be the same or different. A *complicated UTI* is one in which the infection is not completely resolved (or recurs) after standard therapy.

Common causes of UTI

UTIs are most commonly caused by *Escherichia coli, Proteus* or *Klebsiella species*. In chronically ill residents, *Enterobactor* species, *Staphylococcus aureus*, coagulase-negative *Staphylococci, Enterococcus*, and other Gram-negative bacilli are common causative agents.[16,17] Catheter-associated UTI accounts for 40% of nosocomial infections.[18] When an indwelling catheter is present, polymicrobial flora are common, including various Gram-negative bacilli such as *Providentia stuartii, Pseudomonas aeruginosa,* and *Enterococci*.[19,20] Drug-resistant pathogens are a great concern in all healthcare settings. The increased incidence of vancomycin-resistant *Enterococcus* (VRE) is a significant problem. The Centers for Disease Control and Prevention have issued guidelines for the use of vancomycin to reduce the spread of resistant strains of

Enterococcus.[21] Because of the diversity of pathogens implicated in UTI in elderly persons, the facility must ensure that urine specimens are properly collected.

Complications of UTI are associated with increased morbidity and mortality.[22]

Any unresolved infection has the potential to cause sepsis, which may be serious or fatal in elderly persons. Early recognition and treatment of signs and symptoms of infection are the best prevention. UTIs are the most frequent cause of sepsis in elderly persons, so nurses must take monitoring seriously.[23,24]

Signs and symptoms

Unfortunately, identifying signs and symptoms of UTI is often difficult in residents with communication problems and those who are cognitively impaired. This increases the risk of both over- and under-treatment. Symptoms of a UTI may be mild or absent. They are usually atypical. The resident may not mount a febrile response.

In fact, the resident may become hypothermic or the temperature may be below normal.[25,26] Because elderly persons may not mount a febrile response, fever may be defined as any increase over the upper limits of the resident's usual or normal daily temperature range. If infection is suspected, use the most accurate method available for taking the temperature. The rectal method is preferred. Avoid the axillary method unless no other alternatives exist. If a tympanic thermometer is used, make sure the technique is meticulous to prevent inaccurate readings. Signs and symptoms of infection vary widely and the resident usually presents differently than a younger adult. Common, nonspecific symptoms of UTI are

- unexplained deterioration of physical function

- change in mental status

- new or worsening cognitive impairment, increasing confusion

- delirium

- agitation, restlessness

- lethargy

- anorexia

- decline in mobility

- falls

- nonspecific complaints of feeling ill

- new episode of incontinence, increased frequency of incontinence, and/or nocturia

- cough

- nausea, vomiting

- abdominal pain

- change in appearance, color, odor of urine that does not promptly respond to increased fluids

- body language or other behavior suggesting pain

These signs and symptoms suggest sepsis, regardless of whether the resident is febrile. Monitor the resident carefully and notify the physician promptly if you encounter the following:

- hypothermia

- hypotension

- tachycardia

- dyspnea, respiratory distress

Diagnosis

Because of the wide range of presenting symptoms, the misdiagnosis of UTI in the geriatric population ranges from approximately 20% to 40%.[27,28] Some physicians use the McGeer & MSHD definitions for LTC nosocomial infections to diagnose a symptomatic UTI:[29]

A resident without an indwelling catheter should meet three or more of these criteria:

- Fever (>38° C) or chills

- New or increased burning pain on urination

- New flank or suprapubic pain or tenderness

- Changes in character of urine, and worsening mental function

A resident with an indwelling catheter should meet two or more of these criteria:

- Fever (>38° C) or chills

- New flank or suprapubic pain or tenderness

- Changes in character of urine

- Worsening mental function

Nurses sometimes believe that malodorous or dark, concentrated urine are diagnostic of UTI. There are many plausible reasons for these problems in the absence of an infection. These symptoms are commonly related to inadequate fluid intake. Push fluids and observe the resident every shift for 24 hours. If the urine does not clear with increased fluids, consider a urinalysis. If the resident becomes symptomatic or his or her condition worsens, notify the physician promptly.

All long-term care facilities should develop, adopt, and adhere to an evidence-based policy for identifying and managing potential urinary tract problems. The medical director and quality assurance committee can develop and help enforce this policy to ensure that facility practices are consistent with current research. Related procedures must address issues such as

- Documentation to support a diagnosis of symptomatic UTI (this is necessary for Medicare billing)

- Accurate and precise monitoring of the resident's condition

- Accurate and precise documentation of signs, symptoms, and other findings

- Criteria for physician notifications by phone and fax

- Minimum information to report to the physician

- Prerequisites for requesting antibiotic orders

- Documentation to support ongoing monitoring and care of the resident with a UTI

Also consider asymptomatic residents with recurrent *E. coli* infection. Repeated instances of *E. coli* may also be an indication of improper collection technique. To rule this out, a catheterized specimen may be necessary. Using a tiny catheter with a closed system collection device, such as Medline's SpeciCath®, is more comfortable for the resident and poses the least risk of complications.

Reagent strip testing

Some facilities perform reagent strip (dipstick) tests for screening, or before sending a specimen to the lab for culture. This is a controversial practice. Some problems, such as pyuria, are readily identified by the leukocyte esterase dipstick test. The presence of pyuria or a positive leukocyte esterase test is *not adequate* confirmation of a UTI. However, the *absence of pyuria* or a *negative leukocyte esterase test* strongly suggests that a UTI is *not* present.[30] Unfortunately, there are many variables. One study concluded that reagent strip testing is *not sensitive enough* to identify UTI in all high-risk residents for whom missed diagnosis would have serious implications. Although reagent tests will identify bacteriuria, they will not detect Gram-positive organisms such as *Enterococcus*.[31] Because of this, dipstick testing should not be done routinely, and the need for laboratory urinalysis should be determined on an individual basis.

When performing reagent strip testing, always follow

manufacturer's directions for the product you are using. Perform the test as soon as possible after the sample is collected. Store the strips in a tightly sealed container to prevent accumulation of moisture, away from direct sunlight or heat sources. The test strips are stable at room temperature until the expiration date on the vial. Never touch the test pads on the reagent strip with your fingers.

Interpreting a urinalysis

Basic information to evaluate and consider when reviewing a urinalysis is:[32]

- **Specific gravity**—provides information about the concentration of urine. Usually elevated in dehydration, low in fluid overload.

  – Dilute and concentrated urine will affect dipstick test results.

  – A reagent strip is commonly used for this test in the facility. Abnormal urine color may alter the results. If the color is abnormal, consider using another method or sending the specimen to the lab for analysis.

  – Large amounts of glucose/protein, recent tests with contrast dye, and recent alcohol consumption can cause altered values.

- **pH**—For reliable results, the urine specimen must be fresh. (Urine is usually considered stable at room temperature for one hour or refrigerated for four hours.) Elevation with *Proteus* most commonly occurs with bacterial infection.

- **Nitrates**—Dietary and endogenous nitrates are excreted in urine. When an infection is present, some (but not all) bacteria will reduce them to nitrite. In a normal urine sample, nitrates are usually low. They are elevated if an infection is present, or if the sample has been adulterated

in some manner. If dipstick testing is done, best results are obtained by using the first specimen of the day. False negatives are possible with low colony-count infections.

- **Protein**—Values are commonly elevated in UTI, uncontrolled diabetes, hypertension, or primary kidney disease. Protein is commonly seen in urine in febrile response or in the presence of protein-containing substances such as white blood cells, bacteria, mucous. In UTI, values are usually trace to 30 mg/dL (1+). They can reach values greater than or equal to 100 mg/dL, but this is rare.

- **Urobilinogen**—Significant amounts suggest liver disease. However, a number of drugs interfere with the results, causing false positives.

- **Leukocyte esterase**—Infection is almost always indicated with the elevation of this bacterial infection-related enzyme. The resident will experience decreased sensitivity to this test with increased urinary glucose concentration, elevated urinary specific gravity, and presence of antimicrobial drugs in urine.

- **Casts**—Nonspecific hyaline casts will be present; other casts may indicate glomerulonephritis or inflammatory conditions of the kidneys.

- **Red blood cells (RBC)**—An elevation occurs in many different renal conditions. Values of less than 10 RBC per high-powered field are usually of limited concern in elderly persons.

- **White blood cell count (WBC)**—Values are commonly elevated in UTI. Values of greater than 10 WBC suggest infection.

- **Bacteria**—A bacterial count of more than 1+ suggests infection. Lesser amounts in the presence of WBCs (and/or a symptomatic resident) may also warrant treatment.

- **Epithelial cells**—These cells are found outside the urethra; this finding suggests specimen contamination.

- **Glucose**—Positive values suggest poorly controlled diabetes. Normal urine has no glucose.

The most important diagnostic values in identifying a possible UTI are

- Nitrates

- Leukocyte esterase

- White blood cells

- Bacteria

Reporting to the physician

Notifying the physician of laboratory values is the responsibility of the long-term care facility. Do not assume the laboratory will make physician notifications. Follow facility protocols for obtaining a urinalysis and contacting the physician with laboratory results and a status report of the resident's condition. If the resident is acutely ill or the urinalysis is markedly abnormal, prompt physician notification by telephone is a priority. Be prepared to give the physician an accurate and complete overview of the resident's condition in the past 24 hours, including vital signs. Faxing a copy of the laboratory report and allergy information is helpful, but you must make phone contact as well.

In a non-emergent situation, the facility may fax the laboratory report to the physician. However, the facility should have a system in place to ensure the report was received and that appropriate follow-up action is taken within a reasonable period of time. Document all lab results, physician notifications, and the physician response in the clinical record.

Nurses and physicians frequently order follow-up culture and sensitivity testing following antibiotic treatment. Facility nursing personnel should ensure that assessment and resident monitoring support the need for continuing antibiotics. Making an entry each shift that states "no adverse reaction to antibiotic" is not adequate or appropriate. Document your observations and focused assessment of the urinary system (and atypical symptoms, such as delirium, if present), the resident's overall status, and how the urinary tract infection affects his or her total well-being.

Indwelling urinary catheters

Centers for Disease Control and Prevention Guideline for Prevention of Catheter-Associated Urinary Tract Infections[33]

Indwelling urinary catheters have been implicated in many long-term care lawsuits, usually as a result of sepsis or other serious complications. Occasionally residents develop skin problems and other conditions necessitating catheter insertion, but this should be a last-resort skin treatment, not an early response to new breakdown. Many infections follow instrumentation of the urinary tract, mainly through urinary catheterization. In 1999, news reports indicated that many of the bacteria responsible for causing urinary tract infections have become drug resistant.

Although not all catheter-associated urinary tract infections can be prevented, it is believed that the incidence can be reduced by proper management of the indwelling catheter. The following recommendations were developed for the care of *patients with temporary indwelling catheters in the acute care hospital.*

The CDC has not published a separate guideline for management of catheters in the long-term care facility. In the absence of a separate guideline, surveyors often follow this guideline when determining whether proper catheter care was provided.

The CDC criteria for catheter-related infection can be found on your CD-ROM.

Septicemia, sepsis, and septic shock

Sepsis is a serious problem in the elderly. Unfortunately, it is seen with increasing frequency in long-term care facility residents with urinary tract infection and pressure ulcers. This condition is commonly implicated by the plaintiff in lawsuits against long-term care facilities. Widespread, systemic infection is a potential problem with any unresolved infection. Early identification, treatment, and management of signs and symptoms of infection are the best prevention. The terms sepsis, septicemia, and septic shock are sometimes used interchangeably by healthcare providers. However, these are not synonyms. The definitions are not interchangeable. Understanding that septic shock must be prevented is important, so begin with accurate terminology:

- *Sepsis* is a severe infection caused by the presence of toxins; it can occur anywhere in the body. Sepsis kills more than 200,000 people annually in the United States alone—more deaths than from lung and breast cancer combined. Muppets creator Jim Henson died from this condition. Sepsis is estimated to affect 18 million people worldwide each year and kill 1,400 people each day. In the United States alone, 750,000 people yearly develop sepsis, and about 30% of them die.[34]

- *Urosepsis* is a generalized sepsis caused by leakage of urine or toxic urine by-products into the bloodstream. This is a generalized infection that originates in the urinary tract.

- *Septicemia* is a systemic infection in the bloodstream. Bacteria multiply and release toxins into the bloodstream, which spreads the toxins throughout the system. This condition was formerly called "blood poisoning."

- *Septic shock* is the outcome of serious infection. It is caused by serious infections, usually those caused by Gram-negative bacteria. Like other forms of shock, we cannot predict exactly when it will occur. Also, like other types of shock, it reaches a point when it becomes irreversible. One goal of treatment for infection is to prevent septic shock. The onset of septic shock is heralded by hypothermia, low blood pressure, rapid pulse, inadequate tissue perfusion, hemodynamic changes, and compromised organ function. In the long-term care facility, these are sometimes the first definitive signs identified by nurses suggesting treatment is necessary. At this point, the infection is well advanced, and the prognosis may be poor.

Causes of septic shock

Septic shock occurs when the body attempts to destroy an invading pathogen. The causative agent is usually a Gram-negative bacteria (75% of the time), but Gram-positive organisms, *Rickettsia*, fungi, and viruses have been implicated as well. Sepsis typically starts as a bacterial infection that can originate from pneumonia, skin infections (cellulitis), and urinary infections. The infections often begin with bacteria inside the body that grow out of control or from invading external pathogens that enter the body through wounds, urinary catheters, or IV lines.[35] In about 20% of all cases, the source is never found.[36] The cell walls of the Gram-negative pathogens contain toxins that are liberated when the immune system attempts to destroy them. Other toxic substances are released in response, creating massive shock, organ failure, and death.

Signs and symptoms of septic shock

Septic shock usually occurs when the resident is being treated for a known infection. Signs and symptoms depend on how far advanced the condition is when it is identified. Fever, tachycardia, hyperventilation, and warm, dry, flushed skin are early signs. Remember that elderly persons do not mount a strong febrile response, so do not depend on normothermic temperature as a diagnostic sign. The resident may have shaking chills. *Hypothermia is common.* As the condition progresses, the resident becomes hypotensive and hypoxic, with rapid, shallow respirations, tachycardia, and cool, clammy skin. In this stage, the temperature drops. The pulse becomes weak and thready. Pulmonary edema occurs. You may auscultate crackles in the lungs. Urine output decreases. Oliguria will occur, and mental changes will be evident as a result of decreased oxygenation. Blood clotting abnormalities (disseminated intravascular coagulation, DIC) may develop. Alterations in liver function may cause jaundice. Hyperglycemia or hypoglycemia may develop, even in residents who are not diabetic. The body's compensatory mechanisms progressively fail, and death ensues.

Treatment

A resident with septicemia should be transferred to the hospital. Aggressive treatment, consisting of broad-spectrum intravenous antibiotic therapy, fluids, and oxygenation is required. In this situation, it is better to start treatment than to wait 72 hours for culture and sensitivity test results. (Verify that the correct antibiotic is being used after blood culture reports are returned.)

In the early stages of treatment, antibiotics may exacerbate symptoms as the bacteria are destroyed. Long-term care facilities are not equipped to treat this condition properly. IV vasopressors are often needed to support blood pressure and tissue perfusion. After the resident has been stabilized, he or she may be treated in a subacute unit, but the acute care hospital is best for the initial management. Several products

will effectively treat shock caused by Gram-negative bacteria. However, they are ineffective if the condition is caused by other pathogens. These products are called antiendotoxin monoclonal antibodies (MABs).

Other treatments, such as receptor antagonists and interleukins are being researched for efficacy. However, the elderly do not respond well to *any treatment* when the infection is well advanced. In the event treatment is effective, complete recovery takes a long time. The best option is prevention, including close monitoring of at-risk residents, and early intervention.

An excellent slide presentation describing sepsis, as well as other resources is available at *www.sepsis.com/.*

Methicillin-resistant *Staphylococcus Aureus*

Methicillin-resistant *Staphylococcus aureus* (MRSA) has become a prevalent nosocomial pathogen in the United States. In long-term care facilities, the most important reservoirs of MRSA are infected or colonized residents.

Although long-term care facility personnel can serve as reservoirs for MRSA and may harbor the organism for prolonged periods, they have been more commonly identified as a link for transmission between colonized or infected residents. The primary mode of transmission of MRSA is via the healthcare workers' hands, which are often contaminated by contact with

- colonized or infected residents
- colonized or infected body sites of the personnel themselves
- devices, items, or environmental surfaces contaminated with body fluids containing MRSA

Standard Precautions, as described in the "Guideline for Isolation Precautions in Hospitals" (*Infect Control*

Hosp Epidemiol 1996;17:53-80), should control the spread of MRSA in most instances.

Colonization Versus Infection

Colonization occurs when the staphylococcus (staph) bacteria are present on or in the body without causing illness. Approximately 25 to 30% of the population is colonized in the nose with staph bacteria at a given time. Infection occurs when the staph bacteria cause disease in the person. People also may be colonized or infected with MRSA, the staph bacteria that are resistant to many antibiotics.

Culturing personnel and managing carriers of MRSA

Unless the objective of the long-term care facility is to eradicate all MRSA carriage and treat all personnel who are MRSA carriers, whether or not they disseminate MRSA, routine cultures and screening are not recommended. It may be prudent to culture only personnel who are implicated in MRSA transmission based on epidemiologic data. MRSA-carrier personnel who are epidemiologically linked to transmission should be removed from direct resident care until treatment of the MRSA-carrier status is successful. If the long-term care facility elects to culture all personnel to identify MRSA carriers

- Surveillance cultures should be done frequently; and

- It is likely that personnel colonized by MRSA who are not linked to transmission and/or who may not be MRSA disseminators will be identified, subjected to treatment, and/or removed from resident contact unnecessarily.

Because of the high cost attendant to repeated surveillance cultures and the potential of repeated culturing resulting in serious consequences to healthcare work-

ers, long-term care facilities should weigh the advantages and the adverse effects of routinely culturing personnel before doing so.

Control of MRSA Outbreaks

When an outbreak of MRSA occurs, initiate an epidemiologic assessment to identify risk factors for MRSA transmission. To do this, clinical isolates of MRSA should be saved and submitted for strain typing. Colonized or infected residents should be identified as quickly as possible, appropriate barrier precautions instituted, and hand washing before and after all resident contacts strictly enforced.

Schedule the following inservices to review appropriate precautions for residents colonized or infected with multiresistant microorganisms:

- The importance of hand washing, including how and when to wash hands;

- Proper use of barrier precautions (standard precautions) in preventing contact transmission.

If additional help is needed by the long-term care facility, consultation with the local or state health department or CDC may be necessary.

This information was modified for long-term care from the Centers for Disease Control Fact Sheet on methicillin resistant *Staphylococcus aureus*.[37]

Drug-resistant pathogens

Drug-resistant microbes have become a serious problem. Understanding the mode of transmission is critical to prevent their spread. Use Table 14-1 to guide you. Apply the principles of standard precautions in all resident care.

Drug resistant pathogens

Table 14-1

Organism	Common location(s)	Mode of transmission	Prevention	Other information
Methicillin-resistant *Staphylococcus aureus* (MRSA)	• Nasal secretions • Skin • Produces toxins that facilitate invasion of body tissues and cause serious illness.	• Direct and indirect contact. • Hands most common • Contact with contaminated environmental surfaces	• Proper, frequent hand washing or use of alcohol-based hand cleaner • Standard precautions • Contact precautions (in addition to standard precautions) • Droplet precautions if MRSA in respiratory secretions • Gloves when entering the room • Change gloves if contact with infective material • Gown if close contact with the resident, linen, or environmental surfaces, or if soiling or splashing of clothing is likely • Some experts advocate wearing a mask if MRSA has been confirmed; CDC does not recommend this practice unless the resident is known to have a respiratory infection	• For known MRSA infection, consider using dedicated staff to care for the resident. • Vancomycin is the most effective treatment, but other drugs may be used.
Vancomycin-resistant *Enterococcus* (VRE)	• Common organism in the intestinal tract and female genital tract.	• Direct and indirect contact. • Hands most common • Contact with contaminated environmental surfaces	• Proper, frequent hand washing or use of alcohol-based hand cleaner • Standard precautions • Contact precautions (in addition to standard precautions) • Gloves when entering the room • Change gloves if contact with infective material • Gown if close contact with the resident, linen, or environmental surfaces, or if soiling or splashing of clothing is likely	• For known VRE infection, consider using dedicated staff to care for the resident. • <None>If infection occurs, treatment options are extremely limited.
Penicillin resistant *Streptococcus pneumoniae*	• Upper respiratory tract • Produces toxins that facilitate spread to other areas	• Droplets	• Proper, frequent hand washing or use of alcohol-based hand cleaner • Standard precautions • Droplet precautions (in addition to standard precautions) • Door to room may remain open if the resident is more than 3 feet from doorway • Mask upon entering the room, or when working within 3 feet of the resident (according to agency policy) • Limit transport of the resident to other areas. If transport essential, the resident should wear surgical mask when out of room • Notify the receiving area in advance, so they can make preparations for the resident's arrival	• During an outbreak, you may be required to screen residents and staff for nasal colonization of this organism. If colonized, treat with topical agents.

Necrotizing fasciitis

In 2005, 13 residents and staff members at a facility in Virginia were diagnosed with *Streptococcus A*. One resident's daughter chronicled her mother's problem for a newspaper reporter, describing how she became progressively ill. An emergency amputation was needed to save the resident's life. However, she became so unstable during surgery that the procedure had to be abandoned. The resident survived, but lost a leg, and experienced many surgeries, pain, and suffering. Several other residents experienced amputations, myocardial infarctions, and other complications. Some died. At least one of these residents filed a lawsuit requesting $1.5 million in damages.[38] The facility did not notify the families because they had been given an instruction sheet by the health department regarding how to manage the condition. The instruction sheet did not instruct them to make any notifications, and the facility believed the disease was controlled and isolated.[39]

A Gainesville, GA, long-term care facility had an outbreak of *Streptococcus A* in 2004. Several residents died.[40,41] Long-term care facilities in Colorado and Texas have also had outbreaks resulting in resident deaths in 2004 and 2005.[42] At least one resident of a Chicago-area facility contracted *Streptococcus A* as a result of infected pressure ulcers and died. The family sued.[43]

In 2006, a 44-year-old nursing assistant was seen by a physician for complaints related to a swollen thumb. She had sustained the injury at the long-term care facility where she worked, while cleaning wheelchairs. The pain was so intense that she feared she had dislocated it. The physician gave her pain medication and sent her home. Over the next three days, the swelling worsened, involving her entire hand and arm. In fact,

her husband noted that the "arm was twice as large as normal and looked like it would burst." Fluid leaked from her elbow and wrist, and she complained of excruciating pain. She returned to the emergency room three days after her initial visit. The physician diagnosed her with *Streptococcus A*. By the time she arrived, the infection had spread farther down the left side of her body. Doctors amputated her arm at the clavicle and removed all the muscle and tissue around her left breast, torso and thigh in a futile attempt to save her life. She died later that night.[44]

Etiology

Necrotizing fasciitis may also be called "flesh eating strep," or "man eating strep." The condition begins as an invasive skin infection caused by *Streptococcus*. The bacteria attack soft tissues, usually in response to very minor trauma. Occasionally it occurs after surgery, most often abdominal surgery. Occasionally, the signs and symptoms are mistaken for the flu, which delays treatment. Pain out of proportion to the injury is usually the first sign that the pathogen has invaded soft tissue. At this point, the condition spreads rapidly, and almost always becomes life-threatening. In the elderly, amputation is often necessary, and many individuals do not survive. The symptoms are varied, but often include the following:[45]

Early symptoms (usually within 24 hours):

- Usually a history of minor trauma with a skin injury, although there have been reported instances with no visible break in skin integrity

- Pain in the general area of the injury, but not necessarily at the site of the injury

- Pain is usually disproportionate to the injury; it may initially feel like a pulled muscle, but progressively worsens

- Flu-like symptoms, including vomiting, diarrhea, dehydration, general malaise, weakness, confusion, muscle pain, and fever

- Thirst; may become intense as resident begins to dehydrate

- Resident may complain of feeling worse than he or she has ever felt, but does not know why

- Increasing/progressive pain/tenderness

- Edema and redness; the affected area feels hot and very painful

- Condition worsens without any improvement of the above conditions

- Reduced urinary output

- Sunburn-type rash

Advanced symptoms (usually within 3–4 days):

- Edema and pain at the area of injury, progressively increases in size; may develop a purplish rash

- Large, dark blisters filled with blackish fluid

- Wound may have a necrotic appearance with a bluish, white, or dark, mottled, flaky image

- Large, dark boil-like blister(s) may or may not develop

- Signs and symptoms of shock progressing

Critical symptoms (usually within 4–5 days):

- Profound hypotension

- Unconsciousness

- Toxic shock

In addition to the tissue decay, the bacteria cause septic shock. This results in respiratory failure, heart failure, hypotension, and renal failure. Every body system will be affected rapidly. About 60,000 incidences are diagnosed annually in the United States, although statistics are elusive and may not be reported. The incidence may be much higher.

Streptococcus A bacteria are spread through direct contact with mucus, mucous membranes, and nonintact skin. (This type of contact is prevented when standard precautions are used.) The single, most important preventive measure is keeping the skin intact! Some people are carriers. A carrier may not be symptomatic, but most have a recent history of having strep throat. The bacteria may also be spread by coughing and sneezing or by coughing into the hand and then touching an object that someone else touches later.

At any time, 15% of people in the community are infected with *Strep A.* However, most of the time, the immune system staves off infection. Individuals with chronic illnesses, such as cancer, diabetes or kidney problems, residents with open wounds, and those who are immunocompromised are particularly susceptible to the development of necrotizing fasciitis. The injury that initiates a rapid, serious deterioration may be as tiny as a clip from the nail clippers, a splinter, or a paper cut.

Prevention

As you can see, the incidence of *Strep A* outbreaks have been increasing in long-term care facilities. This condition is prevented by conscientious use of standard precautions. However, staff must be aware of and alert to potential signs and symptoms of the infection, which are dissimilar to infections caused by other breaks in skin integrity. In this situation, maintaining a high suspicion index and providing early intervention are the best defense to endemic conditions and poor outcomes.

Legionella

Long-term care facilities in both the United States

and Canada had outbreaks of Legionnaires' disease in 2005. We have learned that there is a relationship between colonization of water systems with *Legionella pneumophila* and the development of Legionnaires' disease. Studies have shown that 12%–85% of hospital water systems have been colonized.[46,47] In two of three outbreaks in long-term care facilities, *Legionella* was isolated from the potable water.[48,49,50] In another outbreak, eating pureed food was considered a significant risk factor for *Legionella*, consistent with aspiration originating from a swallowing disorder.[51] In two additional studies of long-term care residents who were hospitalized with pneumonia, 6.5% of patients in a U.S. study,[52] and 1.4% of patients in a Canadian study[53] were found to have Legionnaires' disease.

Legionnaires' disease is contracted through breathing aerosolized water containing the *Legionella* bacteria. Exposure may occur in the shower, tub or whirlpool, or areas with spray nozzles. Cooling towers, evaporative condensers, fluid coolers, and domestic hot-water systems are water sources that frequently provide optimal conditions for growth of the *Legionella* bacteria. To prevent transmission of the pathogen in hot water systems, OSHA recommends

- Good work practice includes appropriate maintenance of water systems, as recommended by the OSHA Technical Manual: Legionnaires' Disease.

- Store hot water at 140° F. To avoid scalding problems, install appropriate, fail-safe scald protection equipment, such as preset thermostatic mixing valves.

- Inspect the hot-water system annually to ensure equipment is functioning properly.

For domestic cold-water systems, OSHA recommends

- Maintain cold-water lines below 68° F.

- Eliminating water tanks that hold water uncirculated for a prolonged period of time, or reducing storage time to a day or less.

- Cover the water tank and protect it from temperature extremes.

- Avoid cross-contamination of the domestic cold-water system with other systems.

- If the cold-water lines have significant contamination, hyperchlorination by a qualified professional can eradicate *Legionella*.

- Clean and disinfect cooling towers at least twice a year.

- Periodic application of biocides by a qualified professional to control bacterial growth.

- Visually inspect and periodically maintain the water system to prevent a buildup of scale, sediment, and bio-fouling, which support *Legionella* growth.

OSHA also recommends developing an employee awareness program to educate staff about the dangers of *Legionella*, inform employees of any outbreaks, educate about the disease, and provide early identification of the disease.

For additional information on *Legionella* and environmental infection control, see *Morbidity and Mortality Weekly Report*, June 6, 2003 / Vol. 52 / No. RR-10, Guidelines for Environmental Infection Control in Health-Care Facilities: Recommendations of CDC and the Healthcare Infection Control Practices Advisory Committee (HICPAC). Additional information about Legionella can be found in Chapter 9.

Pseudomembranous colitis

The colon is full of many bacteria in healthy people. Most of the resident bacteria are harmless. Some help with digestion. However, some normal flora are troublesome if they escape the colon and go to another area of the body, such as the bladder. They may also be troublesome if the balance of normal flora in the colon is upset and certain bacteria grow unabated or out of control. Taking antibiotics is a common method of upsetting the normal balance in the colon. Developing a brief bout of diarrhea from antibiotics is fairly common, but the situation resolves quickly on its own.

Pseudomembranous colitis is a serious condition in which diarrhea is caused by a bacterium called *Clostridium difficile (C. difficile)*. It is commonly called by its nickname, "C. Diff." Diarrheal illness develops in residents who have been on antibiotic therapy. The friendly bacteria die as a result of the antibiotic, and the harmful bacteria (C. diff.) flourish, reproducing rapidly without the friendly bacteria to hold them in check. In this situation, the antibiotic destroys the normal bowel flora, except *C. difficile*, which is a virulent pathogen. As the C. diff. breeds, it produces toxins that affect the intestinal lining, causing serious illness.

C. difficile is usually picked up on the hands, on bedpans, bedside commodes, toilets, sinks, countertops, bed rails, door knobs, and other surfaces that have been contaminated by stool (or by gloves that have been contaminated by stool). It spreads into the body (most commonly the mouth) by unwashed hands.

Signs and symptoms

Pseudomembranous colitis can be difficult to diagnose, developing several weeks or months after an antibiotic is completed. The resident will experience sudden, explosive, severe, foul-smelling, watery diarrhea. Unfortunately, the damage has already been done, and stopping the antibiotic will not stop the diarrhea. Stools may be so frequent and severe that the resident rapidly becomes dehydrated and develops a serious electrolyte imbalance. Other signs and symptoms are

- cramping and colicky pain in the lower abdomen; this may begin several days before the diarrhea starts

- fever

- mucus, pus or blood in the stool

- abdomen very tender to touch

- in severe cases, low blood pressure and signs of shock develop rapidly

Diagnosis and treatment

Pseudomembraneous colitis must be rapidly treated. Ignored, it has the potential to cause ruptured bowel and severe distention with retention of stool. The resident will become rapidly and profoundly dehydrated. If pseudomembranous colitis is suspected, the physician will order one or more stool cultures. If possible, the antibiotic causing the problem will be changed to another drug. Antimicrobials, such as Flagyl, may be used to restore the bacterial balance in the colon. Giving the resident yogurt and lactobacillus tablets may be useful in restoring the normal flora. (The tablets are an over-the-counter product that must be stored in the refrigerator.) Although this course of treatment usually eliminates the problem, it may recur, making a second course of therapy necessary. Place the resident in contact precautions until 72 hours after the appearance and frequency of stools returns to normal, or as ordered by the physician.

Prevention

In 2002, the CDC published the results of extensive

hand washing studies, as well as new recommendations for cleansing hands.[54] Each recommendation is categorized based on existing scientific data, theoretical rationale, applicability, and economic impact. The recommendations call for routine use of alcohol-based hand cleaners during resident care, with two notable exceptions:

- When hands are visibly dirty or contaminated with proteinaceous material or are visibly soiled with blood or other body fluids, wash hands with either a non-antimicrobial soap and water or an antimicrobial soap and water.

- *Note: If the resident has a condition caused by spores, such as* Clostridium difficile *or* Clostridium botulinum, *wash hands with soap and running water. Alcohol will not eliminate spores. The friction and running water will remove them from your hands during hand washing.* Because of this, use good hand washing (only) if *Clostridium difficile* infection is known or suspected. Some facilities have posted signs, such as a photo of alcohol hand cleaner with a circle and slash through it, indicating the product should not be used in certain rooms. Some facilities remove the alcohol hand cleaners from the room or affix the sign directly to the bottle. Others use signs that state something like, *"Hand Hygiene: Use Soap and Water Only."* The terminology alerts staff that the resident has *C. difficile* or another condition spread by spores without releasing diagnostic information.

Cimex lectularius (Bedbugs)

Many adults believe that bedbugs are imaginary creatures in a common nursery rhyme. In fact, *Cimex lectularius* (bedbugs) are hearty, resilient pests that have been with us for centuries. In 2005, widespread sightings of bedbugs were reported throughout the United States. The stealthy and fast-moving nocturnal creatures have been found in hospital maternity wards, private schools, long-term care facilities, five-star hotels, and physicians' offices. The pests have been found throughout the world, except Antarctica. Ideal conditions for most hatching, nymphal development, and adult activity all occur between 55° F and 59° F (13° C and 15° C), but they can survive in both hot and cold environments. A temperature of 70° F is ideal for bedbugs. Only adults survive in temperatures below 50° F.

Bedbugs have an anticoagulant in their saliva to prevent blood from clotting during a meal. This substance causes sensitivity in some people, causing irritation, itching, and inflammation. Other people can live with bed bugs and not be aware of them. Some people develop welt-like bite marks, similar to flea or mosquito bites. The bites commonly feel itchy and look like little red bumps. They may appear in lines, similar to the pattern of scabies in which the insects are following the blood vessels. The average life span is about 10 months, but they have been known to live as long as 18 months, and are capable of breeding at least three generations per year. Adults can survive for up to a year without blood, allowing infestations to persist unabated, even if the property is vacant.

The pests were essentially eradicated in the United States and other developed countries when DDT use was widespread, but have made a strong comeback as various industrial-strength pesticides have been eliminated or banned. Today's bedbugs are resistant to many over-the-counter insecticides, and setting off cockroach bombs may scatter them farther about.

Because they are active only at night, many people do

not discover them until there are hundreds or thousands of them in an area. They leave little excretion droppings on the sheets, and if the infestation is heavy or very serious, the bugs may give off a sickly sweet smell.

A bedbug is tiny. They are visible to the eye, flat in shape, and clear or white in appearance before feeding. After feeding they take on a reddish-brown hue. The insects will expand, shedding their exoskeletons (similar to a snake shedding its skin) as it grows. Bedbugs are primarily parasitic on humans, but will also live on bats, chickens, pigeons, other birds, laboratory animals, and some domestic pets. The insects have long been suspected of transmitting disease in humans and bats, but this has not been verified. They tend to cluster on dry, rough surfaces. They avoid wet surfaces. When not feeding, they usually remain in their nests or in tiny holes and cracks in rooms or furnishings. They avoid light if possible, but they will feed in daylight when hungry. You may occasionally see bedbugs, but more commonly staff will find tiny bloodstains on the linen from crushed bugs, or dark spots from the droppings.

Although bedbugs do not fly or hop, they run fast and multiply quickly. Bedbugs travel easily from one place to another, in luggage, through walls, and hidden in the seams of clothing. They may spread to cracks and crevices in mattresses, bed frames and box springs, behind headboards, inside nightstands, behind baseboards, window and door casings, pictures, and moldings. They have also been found hiding in couches, chairs, and other furnishings, loosened wallpaper, and cracks in plaster and floors. They can and do hide in clutter, such as piles of books, papers, boxes, and items near sleeping areas. When checking for bedbugs, shining a flashlight and aiming a hot hair dryer into the crevices will help force the insects out.

Cimex lectularius are all but impossible to eliminate without exterminator treatments. Even then, elimination is difficult, and eradicating the pests involves throwing out as many objects in the room as possible, then either freezing nonwashable items for 48 hours or exposing items to high temperatures. Thorough washing of all clothing and furnishing, and sealing cracks in the walls and floors also helps. The most difficult part of the eradication effort is finding and eliminating the eggs. The exterminator must return seven to 10 days after the initial treatment, and repeat the application to eliminate newly hatched bugs.

Control measures

Maintain a high degree of suspicion for bedbugs (and/or scabies) if staff or residents have rashes, or if the appearance of the bed linen has tiny blood stains. Inservice your staff about the potential problems related to these pests. Contact a professional exterminator immediately. Determine whether your community requires reporting infestations to the local health authority. Temporary control measures include

- Vacuuming all carpeting, furnishings, and cracks and crevices in walls and floors thoroughly. When finished, discard the vacuum cleaner bag in a sealed plastic bag.

- Using a pesticide known to eliminate the bugs. Some pesticide sprays can be applied to infested areas. Before spraying, remove all residents from the area. Make sure the person applying the product uses an appropriate respirator system. Close doors and windows as tightly as possible. Remove the mattress from the bed frame or box springs. Open dresser drawers and bedside stands to allow the pesticide fumes to penetrate the surfaces. Spread clothes and other items about.

- After applying a pesticide product, residents and staff should stay out of the area for at least four to eight hours, or according to product directions.

- After widespread room spraying, apply a light application of an approved pesticide to mattresses, stuffed chairs, clothes, etc., to kill surviving bugs. Check the mattress for cracks, which provide a potential hiding place for bugs and their eggs. If the mattress of an infested resident is cracked, discard it. Before using the mattress, wash and dry the surface to remove residual product, then apply fresh linen.

- Treat all cracks and crevices. Repeat the applications if you see signs of bugs again after two weeks.

At the time of this writing, no known long-term care facility lawsuits have implicated bedbugs. However, suits have been filed against five-star hotels, correctional institutions, and other facilities. Bedbug infestations have been found in hospitals and long-term care facilities. It is only a matter of time before this issue is added to the growing list of infection-control related problems noted in lawsuits. Maintain a high degree of suspicion and be vigilant for the appearance of these annoying pests.

Scabies

Outbreaks of scabies have been implicated in long-term care facility lawsuits. Scabies also have the potential for creating serious problems with surveyors, and are generally very difficult for long-term care facilities to identify and manage. They spread rapidly, and outbreaks are not uncommon in long-term care facilities. One administrator said, "It is no shame to get them; it is a big shame to keep them." Scabies is caused by the human itch mite, *Sarcoptes scabiei*, a parasite. The mite is microscopic, and cannot be seen with the eye, making diagnosis difficult. Residents are often treated for a variety of rashes and skin conditions over a prolonged period of time before an accurate diagnosis is made. In the early stages, signs of scabies are often mistaken for allergies, aging changes, and dryness of the skin. The condition is typically not diagnosed until it is extensive, with skin lesions and other symptoms. Many residents and employees are usually exposed before the condition is accurately identified.

The scabies mite

Infestation begins when a pregnant female mite is transferred to the skin of an uninfested person. Transfer is done by direct or indirect contact with an infected person or object, such as a cracked mattress. The parasites usually spread rapidly under crowded conditions where there is frequent skin-to-skin contact between people, such as in hospitals, child-care facilities, and long-term care facilities. The mites cannot be transmitted to or from pets. They cannot hop, jump, or fly, but they can run quickly. The mites wander about on the skin, then tunnel beneath the surface and lay eggs.

The life span of the female mite is approximately two months. During this period of time, the mite continues to wander about, laying two or three eggs a day in the burrows. The eggs incubate for about a month, then hatch, producing larvae. The larvae make their way to the area just beneath the skin surface, where they feed on the host's blood. The mites become sexually immature adults during the next month. Four days later, they molt, becoming sexually mature adults. The males will die within two days. However, they mate during this time, and the cycle perpetuates itself.

Many eggs are unknowingly removed from the skin during bathing and scratching. Mites leaving the skin will die within several hours to several days, depending on environmental conditions. Since the host is not symptomatic during this time, he or she can transmit mites to many others before proper diagnosis is made.

Scabies infestation

The severity of an infestation is determined by the

- total number of mites on the skin
- interval between infestation and treatment

The mites will continue to multiply until the host is finally diagnosed and properly treated. Scabies are hearty, and mites have become resistant to some scabicide products, so infestation may persist after treatment, or if proper treatment procedures are not followed. Untreated, the parasites continue to multiply, and signs and symptoms worsen. Residents with diabetes, mental retardation, renal failure, and immunosuppression may progress to heavy infestation within two or three months.

Norwegian scabies, or keratotic scabies, is a severe form of infestation. The skin develops thick crusts, each containing thousands of mites. The problem is commonly misdiagnosed. Persons with AIDS often develop Norwegian scabies. Some sources suggest that this type of scabies may be more infectious, because shorter contact times resulted in transmission of this mite. Prolonged contact is normally required for transmission of the scabies mite. The shorter contact times may be due to heavy concentrations of mites in the crusted lesions. In most long-term care facilities, outbreaks are usually typical scabies, with low mite loads, however.

Transmission

The scabies mite is transmitted by direct and indirect contact. Skin contact with an infected person, or contact with clothing and linen, have the potential for spreading the mite. In long-term care facilities, scabies is often introduced by workers, who may contract them from their children. Occasionally, newly admitted residents introduce the parasite. Family members and visitors may also transmit the mite to residents. Scabies is usually transmitted to staff by skin contact with residents. Infected staff continue to pass the mites to additional residents.

The scabies mite can survive for a short time on inanimate objects, but many factors affect survival. Moist surfaces seem to increase the life expectancy. A common problem in long-term care is that the mite crawls through cracks in the mattress covers to the foam below, which is often wet from repeated episodes of incontinence. This is a common source of repeated transmission until the mattresses are replaced. Using sprays to eliminate the mite are not recommended. The National Pediculosis Association recommends vacuuming. For infection control purposes, wipe the surface with disinfectant after vacuuming. Unfortunately, this will not eliminate mites that have migrated into the mattress. Replace cracked mattresses immediately. Check mattresses in rooms of residents known to be infested, and replace if cracked or torn. In heavy infestation, and with Norwegian scabies, other furnishings may also transfer the mite. Otherwise, furniture is not usually associated with the problem. Vacuum the surface to be safe.

Signs and symptoms

Residents who have previously contracted scabies may be symptomatic as early as 48 hours after exposure. Healthy residents who have never contracted scabies will be asymptomatic for up to four to six weeks from the time of infestation. Following the incubation period, the resident will complain of severe itching. He or she may scratch until the skin bleeds. The itching does not respond to topical moisturizers or antihistamines. The itching sensation often worsens when the resident is in bed.

Next, the resident develops rash-like areas on the skin. The most common locations are the webs of the fingers, inside the wrists, outside the elbows, in the underarm, waist, and nipple area. The rash may also be seen around the knees, lower buttocks, and the genital area in males. Norwegian scabies cause scaling of the skin on the hands and feet. Skin that has been exposed to moisture may be heavily involved. The skin may appear excoriated. As the rash progresses, it mimics many other skin conditions. Scratching may cause an infection, worsening the condition and contributing to misdiagnosis.

Diagnosis

Diagnosing scabies may be difficult in elderly persons with dry skin and conditions such as eczema or psoriasis. Scabies can imitate and may be misdiagnosed as many other skin conditions, such as insect bites, hives, eczema, folliculitis, contact or atopic dermatitis, impetigo, rosacea, psoriasis, lymphoma, and drug reactions. The first indication of scabies is often severe, maddening pruritus, accompanied by a rash. It may occur in multiple residents and staff concurrently. Be suspicious if many residents and employees develop a rash and itching in a short period of time.

To conclusively diagnose the condition, the mite must be present in a skin scraping. Scrapings must be collected by a properly trained person.

However, they are often negative, despite presence of the mites. Because of this, the absence of mites does

not guarantee that the individuals are free from infestation. Scrapings are almost always positive in Norwegian scabies, but this type is less common.

The burrow test may be useful in persons who are symptomatic but have negative skin scrapings. For this test, locate a burrow. If possible, select an area that is not excoriated or inflamed. Rub a black or green wide-tipped marker directly on the burrow. Immediately remove the ink using an alcohol sponge. In a well-lighted area, view the burrow under a magnifying glass. The ink that remains in the burrow will look like a threadlike line. This method of testing may, however, only be useful within a few days of onset of signs and symptoms. The test should be performed on at least one individual.

Another method of diagnosing scabies involves applying mineral oil to dry, scaly areas. Allow the oil to soak for a few minutes, then scrape the scaly skin surface gently with a scalpel. Apply the scrapings to a slide, then examine under the microscope.

If scabies is diagnosed, the infection control nurse should develop a list of every individual who has had direct contact with the affected person. If many persons are infested, start a separate contact list for each. Include roommates and employees who are no longer at the facility. Document

- employee or resident name

- room number

- date symptoms began

- results of diagnostic testing

- date of treatment/retreatment, and results

You should also

- Evaluate the infested person's activities for the

past four weeks, and identify others who have potentially been exposed.

- Identify staff who have cared for the resident. This may include hospital and ambulance personnel, hospice workers and volunteers. Determine whether these individuals are symptomatic.

- Notify the resident's family and visitors.

- Check all nursing units to determine whether individuals there are also symptomatic.

- Identify residents and staff needing treatment. Treat symptomatic persons first.

Infection control measures

- Isolate symptomatic residents in contact precautions for at least 12 hours after the first treatment. While the resident is in isolation, staff and visitors wear long-sleeved gowns and gloves when contacting the resident, and his or her bed, linen, and clothing. Make sure the cuffs of the gown are tightly covered with gloves. Change gloves after each skin contact, even if you will be performing additional tasks in the room. Workers may wear the same gown for an entire shift, then send it to the laundry. Use gloves only once, discarding them before leaving the room. Each time the gown and gloves are removed, wash hands and arms to the elbows.

- Apply the appropriate treatment (see below). Products containing Lindane are not recommended by the National Pediculosis Association,[55] and several activist and watchdog organizations.[56] Over time, the mites have developed resistance to Lindane. Also, this product has shown to be extremely neurotoxic to some persons, particularly in children and elderly individuals. Toxicity can occur with a single dose. Because of this, several states have banned Lindane treatment

products. Other products have found to be effective for eliminating the mites. In the past, bathing the resident prior to product application was recommended. This has proven controversial, as bathing enhances product absorption, increasing the risk of toxicity and side effects. Generally speaking, it is no longer recommended. Follow facility policies and physician orders.

- Apply the treatment product to all skin surfaces, from the hairline to the bottoms of the feet. Avoid the eyes, eyelids, and mucous membranes of the nose, mouth, and perineum. Clip the nails, then work the product under the nails with a cotton applicator or soft brush. Covering the entire body is important. If the resident washes his or her hands or eliminates while the product is on the skin, reapply it. Likewise, reapply the product if the resident perspires heavily. Repeat the application as often as necessary, or each time the skin becomes wet. The pediculicide should remain on the skin for 8–12 hours, or according to manufacturer's recommendations, then washed off. Give the resident a tub bath or shower. Wear gown and gloves during bathing.

After the pediculicide has been removed

- Discontinue contact precautions. Depending on the product used, a second treatment may be necessary. Wear gloves when applying this treatment. Further isolation is not necessary.

- Remove the resident's bed linen, including mattress pad, spreads and blankets. Bag all facility linen, such as washcloths and towels, and send to the laundry. Wash in very hot water.

- Vacuum the mattress, plastic pillow cover, bedside equipment, bedside chair and other furniture, and floor. Disinfect after vacuuming to remove microbes left by the surface of the vacuum.

- Check the mattress for cracks and tears and replace, if necessary.

- Apply clean bed linen.

- Disinfect community equipment such as blood pressure cuffs and gait belts.

- Discard creams, lotions, and ointments used by symptomatic residents.

- After treating the resident, collect all clothing worn over the previous week in sealed plastic bags, and transport to laundry. Instruct laundry personnel to avoid washing these clothes with other facility linen. Avoid handling or sorting them. Wash in hot water, and dry in a hot dryer.

- Bag nonwashable items, such as coats and shoes in plastic bags. Seal the bag for at least seven days. The scabies mite does not survive in very hot or cold temperature extremes, so placing the sealed bag outside in weather extremes is a consideration.

- If family does laundry, seal clothing in bags. Instruct family members to avoid handling them, and to wash them in hot water, and dry in a hot dryer. Dry-clean items should be sent to the cleaners, or sealed in a plastic bag for seven days. If dry cleaning is not possible, an alternative is to place them in a hot dryer for 30 minutes.

For residents with keratotic scabies

- Maintain contact precautions in a private room. Isolation continues until two or three consecutive negative skin scrapings have been obtained, according to infection control

committee guidelines. The first repeat scraping should be obtained when the lesions show visible improvement. Other procedures are the same as listed.

Treatment failures

Treatment failures almost always reflect inadequate application of the scabicide to appropriate body surfaces and not reinfestation from other residents or staff. Treatment failures occasionally result from resistance of mites to scabicides; failure for elderly, institutionalized persons may reflect immune deficiency.

Treatment of staff, visitors, and others

Mass prophylaxis will most probably not totally eliminate scabies, and the decision to use it should be based on the magnitude of scabies infestation in the facility. Follow-up examinations are recommended to assess overall effectiveness. Treat symptomatic contacts at the same time as residents.

The Centers for Disease Control and Prevention recommends restriction from resident care for personnel known to be infested until after they receive initial treatment, are medically evaluated, and determined to be free of infestation. These workers are advised to report for further evaluation if signs and symptoms do not subside. Consult the personal physician or healthcare provider prior to treating pregnant women or children.

Workers who have not had substantial contact with symptomatic residents do not need to be treated, but if insistent, should be supplied with enough product for a single treatment. Substantial contact means direct skin contact during transfers or bathing, or contact with bed linen. Family members and sexual partners of symptomatic employees should also be treated. Provide guidelines for washing clothing and bed linen, and vacuuming environmental surfaces. In outbreak situations in which transmission continues to occur, prophylactic treatment may be warranted for both residents and exposed personnel.

Treatment products

Follow physician orders and facility policies for resident and employee treatment. Avoid products containing Lindane.

Permethrin

- Treat all cases and contacts within the same 24–48-hour treatment period. Treat symptomatic cases first.

- Massage the product into the skin from the hairline to the soles of the feet. Include skin on the ears and neck. Avoid all mucous membranes.

- Reapply the product to any area that becomes moist or wet during the treatment period.

- Bathe and shampoo the resident after 8–12 hours, or as ordered.

- If a second application is ordered, it can be repeated immediately, or any time within the first seven days. Bathe and shampoo the resident 8–12 hours after the treatment is applied. Permethrin may be used repeatedly, if scabies is not eliminated following two applications. Follow physicians' orders.

Crotamiton (Eurax) 10%

Crotamiton is effective about 50% of the time. The risk of contact dermatitis is increased. Avoid using this product on open lesions or inflamed skin.

Ivermectin

Ivermectin has been used for scabies treatment, but is not marketed or recommended for this purpose. In one study, 15 of the 47 residents who had received ivermectin treatment for scabies died, compared with five of the age-matched and sex-matched cohort.[57]

Reassessment

If treatment is effective, pruritus should subside within the first three weeks after treatment. Triamcinolone and hydrocortisone may be prescribed for pruritus, but should not be applied when the scabicide is in place. The rash may persist for up to 30 days, but this does not suggest active infestation. No new burrows or rashes should appear 24–48 hours after effective treatment. If new lesions are identified, treatment failure is suggested, and the individual should be retreated.

Treatment failure

Treatment failures occur because of

- Immunosuppression

- Poor application technique

- Continued contact with infested individuals or environmental surfaces, such as mattresses with cracks, carpeting, and upholstered furniture.

- Use of topical products for pruritus when the treatment product is on the skin.

Reporting

Follow the reporting guidelines in your state for reporting scabies to the health department.

Prevention

The infection control committee should develop a preventive program for head lice and scabies. Suggested policies are to carefully assess the skin, hair, and nail beds of new admissions. Further evaluation is required if pruritus, lesions, or rash are present. Repeat the skin assessments periodically for all facility residents.

If scabies is suspected or confirmed, evaluate all residents and staff. Make sure employees are familiar with and can identify signs and symptoms suggesting scabies, and establish an immediate reporting mechanism. The infection control committee should designate a physician to order diagnostic tests and treatment of all residents and staff suspected of having scabies.

Guidelines for using transmission-based precautions for resident isolation can be found on your CD-ROM.

Infectious disease transmission risks associated with long-term care facilities

The draft guidelines make special note about the unique challenges faced by long-term care facilities:

The term "long-term care facility" (LTCF) applies to a diverse group of residential settings, ranging from institutions for the developmentally disabled to long-term care facilities for the elderly and pediatric chronic-care facilities. Long-term care facilities for the elderly predominate numerically and frequently represent the group. Approximately 1.8 million Americans reside in the nation's 16,500 long-term care facilities. HAI rates of 1.8 to 13.5 per 1,000 resident-care days have been reported, with estimates between three and seven per 1,000 resident-care days in the more rigorous studies.

LTCFs are different from other healthcare settings in that elderly residents at increased risk for infection are brought together in one setting and remain in the facility for extended periods of time; for most "residents," it is their home. An atmosphere of "community" is fostered, and residents share common eating and living areas and participate in various facility-sponsored activities. Able residents interact freely with each other. Controlling transmission in this setting is challenging. Residents who are colonized or infected with certain microorganisms may, in some cases, be restricted to their room environment. Such actions, if not fully justified, may be perceived as infringing on resident rights and quality of care.

Risk factors for infection abound in LTCF residents. Age-related declines in immunity may affect responses to immunizations for influenza and other infectious agents, or increase susceptibility to tuberculosis. Immobility, incontinence, dysphagia and age-related skin changes increase susceptibility to urinary, respiratory and cutaneous and soft tissue infections, while malnutrition impairs wound healing. Medications that affect level of consciousness, immune function, and gastric acid secretions, and normal flora heighten susceptibility to infection. Antibiotic therapy, invasive devices, and feeding tubes also contribute to infection risks in LTCF residents. Finally, total dependence on healthcare personnel for activities of daily living has been identified as an independent risk factor for colonization with MRSA and ESBL-producing *K. pneumoniae*. Several position papers have been published that provide guidance on various aspects of infection control and antimicrobial resistance in LTCFs.

Because residents of LTCFs are hospitalized frequently, they can serve as conduits for transmission of infectious agents between the healthcare facilities in which they receive care. Pediatric chronic care facilities also were the source of imported colonization with extended-spectrum cephalosporin-resistant Gram-negative bacilli in one PICU. Children from child care centers and pediatric rehabilitation units may also contribute to the reservoir of community-onset MRSA infections in pediatrics.[58]

Additional resources and information

The following Centers for Disease Control and Prevention guidelines and information can be found on your CD-ROM:

- **Using PPE, as well as the sequence for applying and removing PPE**

- **Summary of the 2002 handwashing recommendations**

References

1. Rusnak PG, Horning LA. Surveillance in the long-term care facility. In: Smith PW (Ed.). *Infection Control in Long-Term Care Facilities.* 2nd ed. Delmar Publishers, Inc.,: Albany, NY. 1994:117-130.

2. Smith PW, Rusnak PG. Infection prevention and control in the long-term-care facility. *American Journal of Infection Control* 1997;25(6):488-512.

3. Chinnes, L. Preventing infections in long-term care. Online. *www.infectioncontroltoday.com.* Accessed 11/17/03.

4. Chinnes, L. Preventing infections in long-term care. Online. *www.infectioncontroltoday.com.* Accessed 11/17/03.

5. Hospital Infection Control Practices Advisory Committee. (eds). (1997). *CDC Guideline for Isolation Precautions in Hospitals.* Baltimore. US Government Printing Office.

6. Smith P, Rusnak P. Infection prevention and control in the long-term-care facility. *Am J Infect Control* 1997;25:488-512.

7. Warren JW, Tenney JH, Hoopes JM, Muncie HL, Anthony WC. (1982). A prospective microbiologic study of bacteriuria in patients with chronic indwelling urethral catheters. *J Infect Dis* 1982;146:719-723.

8. Ouslander JG, Schnelle JF. Incontinence in the nursing home. *Ann Intern Med* 1995;122:438-449.

9. Emory University Center for Health in Aging Monograph. (2001). *Prevention and Management of Infections in Residents of Long-Term Care Facilities: An Agenda for Research.*

10. Lynch, D. (2004). Cranberry for prevention of urinary tract infections. *Am Fam Physician* 2004;70:2175-77.

11. Suvarna, R; Pirmohamed, M; Henderson, L. (2003). Possible interaction between warfarin and cranberry juice. *BMJ* 2003;327:1454 (20 December), doi:10.1136/bmj.327.7429.1454.

12. Beizer, J. (1996). Urinary tract infections in elderly long-term care residents. *Journal of the American Society of Consultant Pharmacists;* Supplement 5; 1996/Vol. 11.

13. Warren JW, Tenney JH, Hoopes JM, Muncie HL, Anthony WC. (1982). A prospective microbiologic study of bacteriuria in patients with chronic indwelling urethral catheters. *J Infect Dis* 1982;146:719-723.

14. Howes DS. Urinary tract infections. Tintinalli JE, Kelen GD, Stapczynski JS, eds. (1999). *Emergency Medicine, A Comprehensive Study Guide,* 5th Ed. New York, NY: McGraw-Hill; 1999.

15. Gleckman RA. (1992). Urinary tract infection. *Clin Geriatr Med* 1992;8:793-803.

16. Gleckman RA. (1992). Urinary tract infection. *Clin Geriatr Med* 1992, 8:793–803.

17. Emory University Center for Health in Aging Monograph. (2001). *Prevention and Management of Infections in Residents of Long-Term Care Facilities: An Agenda for Research.*

18. Gomolin, I; Kathpalia, R; Sangwan, A. (2002). UTI in long-term care and nursing home patients. *Current Treatment Options in Infectious Diseases* 2002, 4:7–13.

19. Grahn D, Norman DC, White ML, et al.: (1985). Validity of urinary catheter specimen for diagnosis of urinary tract infection in elderly. *Arch Int Med* 1985, 145:1858–1860.

20. Emory University Center for Health in Aging Monograph. (2001). *Prevention and Management of Infections in Residents of Long-Term Care Facilities: An Agenda for Research.*

21. Centers for Disease Control and Prevention. (1995). Recommendations for preventing the spread of vancomycin resistance. Recommendations of the Hospital Infection Control Practice Advisory Committee (HICPAC). *MMWR* 1995; 44(RR-12): 1-9.

22. Kunin C. (1997). *Urinary Tract Infections: Detection, Prevention, and Management,* 5th edition, Baltimore, MD: Williams & Wilkins, 1997, pp. 150-154.

23. Henkel, G. (2003). The ever-present UTI. *Caring for the Ages,* August 2003; Vol. 4, No. 8, p. 8-10.

24. Norman DC, Castle SC, Cantrell M. (1987). Infections in the nursing home. *J Am Geriatr Soc* 1987; 35: 796-805.

25. Gomolin, I; Kathpalia, R; Sangwan, A. (2002). UTI in long-term care and nursing home patients. *Current Treatment Options in Infectious Diseases* 2002, 4:7–13.

26. Orenstein R, Wong ES. (1999). Urinary tract infections in adults. *Am Fam Physician* 1999;59:1225-1234.

27. Nickel JC, Pidutti R. (1992). A rational approach to urinary tract infections in older patients. *Geriatrics* 1992;47:49-55.

28. Ackermann RJ, Monroe PW, (1996). Bacteremic urinary tract infection in older people. *JAGS* 1996;44:927-933.

29. Vance, J. (2002). Diagnosing & managing urinary tract infections: myths, mysteries, & realities. *Caring for the Ages,* October 2002, Vol. 3, No. 10, p. 18-21).

30. Levenson, S and Crecelius, C. (2003). Identifying and managing possible UTIs. *Caring for the Ages,* March 2003; Vol. 4 No. 3, p. 43-44.

31. Eidelman Y, Raveh D, Yinnon AM, et al. (2002). Reagent strip diagnosis of UTI in a high-risk population. *Am J Emerg Med* 2002;20:112-113.

32. Levenson, S and Crecelius, C. (2003). Identifying and managing possible UTIs. *Caring for the Ages,* March 2003; Vol. 4 No. 3, p. 43-44.

33. Wong, ES and Hooton, TM. (1981). Guideline for prevention of catheter-associated urinary tract infections. U.S. Department of Health & Human Services. Public Health Service. Online. *www.cdc.gov/ncidod/hip/guide/uritract.htm.* Accessed 6/13/04.

34. Tanner L. (2004). Docs aim to reduce blood infection deaths. Online. *http://cnn.netscape.cnn.com/ns/news/story.jsp?floc=FF-APO-PLS&idq=/ff/story/0001/20040213/2013373617.htm.* Accessed 01/06/06.

35. Tanner L. (2004). Docs aim to reduce blood infection deaths. Online. *http://cnn.netscape.cnn.com/ns/news/story.jsp?floc=FF-APO-PLS&idq=/ff/story/0001/20040213/2013373617.htm.* Accessed 01/06/06.

36. International Sepsis Forum (2002). *Promoting a better understanding of sepsis.* England and Wales. International Sepsis Forum.

37. CDC. (1999). MRSA - methicillin resistant staphylococcus aureus information for healthcare personnel. Online. *www.cdc.gov/ncidod/hip/ARESIST/mrsahcw.htm.* Accessed 7/16/04.

38. Nursing Home Law and Litigation Alert. (2005). Vol. 5, No. 6, Page 420. June 2005

39. McCaffery J. (2005). Anger breaks out after infections. *Roanoke Times.* Online. *www.roanoke.com/news/roanoke/20826.html.* Accessed 3/26/05.

40. Gilbert D. (2004). Necrotizing fasciitis. *Gainesville Times.* April 1, 2004.

41. Gilbert D. (2004). Nursing home: Infection no longer a threat. *Gainesville Times.*

42. Gunn J. (2004). Are Nevada's nursing homes safe?. *Nevada Observer.* Vol. 1, No. 6 Jan. 15, 2004. Online. *www.nevadaobserver.com/Archive/040115/Newsstory.htm.* Accessed 3/26/05.

43. Nursing home faces suit. (2005). *Chicago Tribune.* Online. *www.rednova.com/news/display/?id=219357&source=r_health.* Accessed 8/29/05.

44. Williams R. and Fuquay J. (2006). Flesh-eating bacteria kills Harnett County woman. Fayetteville (NC) Observer. Online. *www.fayettevillenc.com/article?id=228104.* Accessed 3/10/06.

45. National Necrotizing Fasciitis Foundation. Necrotizing fasciitis fact sheet. Online. *www.nnff.org/nnff_factsheet.htm.* Accessed 01/06/06.

46. Yu VL. (1998). Resolving the controversy on environmental cultures for Legionella. A modest proposal [editorial]. *Infect Control Hosp Epidemiol* 1998; 19:893–897.

47. Sabria M, Garcia-Nunez M, Pedro-Botet ML, et al. (2002). Presence and chromosomal subtyping of Legionella species in potable water systems in 20 hospitals of Catalonia, Spain. *Infect Control Hosp Epidemiol* 2002; 22:673–676.

48. Loeb M, Simor AE, Mandell L, et al. Two nursing home outbreaks of respiratory infections with Legionella sainthelensi. *J Am Geriatric Soc* 1999; 47:547–552.

49. Nechwatal R, Ehret W, Klatte OJ, et al. Nosocomial outbreak of legionellosis in a rehabilitation center. Demonstration of potable water as a source. *Infection* 1993; 21:235–240.

50. Maesaki S, Kohno S, Koga H, et al. An outbreak of Legionnaires' pneumonia in a nursing home. *Intern Med* 1992; 31:508–512.

51. Loeb M, Simor AE, Mandell L, et al. Two nursing home outbreaks of respiratory infections with Legionella sainthelensi. *J Am Geriatric Soc* 1999; 47:547–552.

52. Fang GD, Fine M, Orloff J, et al. New and emerging etiologies for community acquired pneumonia with implications for therapy: a prospective multicenter study of 359 cases. Medicine (Baltimore) 1990; 69:307–316.

53. Marrie TJ, Blanchard W. A comparison of nursing home-acquired pneumonia patients with community-acquired patients pneumonia and nursing home patients without pneumonia. *J Am Geriatric Soc* 1997; 45:50–55.

54. CDC. (2002). Guideline for hand hygiene in health-care settings. *MMWR* 2002; 51(No. RR-16).

55. Lyons, P. (1994). The most dangerous medicine: mothers have found that the cure can be worse than the complaint. June 1994. Ladies Home Journal. Online. *www.headlice.org/news/classics/lhjarticle.htm.* Accessed 7/24/04.

56. Public citizen criticizes fda for failing to ban topical lindane products used for treating scabies and lice. (2003). Online. *www.headlice.org/news/2003/pubcitizen.htm.* Accessed 7/24/04.

57. Barkwell, R and Shields, S. (1997). Deaths associated with ivermectin treatment of scabies. The Lancet v.349, 19apr97. Online. *www.headlice.org/news/1997/ivermectin-deaths.htm.* Accessed 7/24/04.

58. Draft CDC Guideline for Isolation Precautions: Preventing Transmission of Infectious Agents in Health-care Settings 2004. Online. *www.cdc.gov/ncidod/hip/isoguide.htm.* Accessed 8/1/04.

Progressive injuries related to nutrition and hydration

"This is a civil liability case in which it has become necessary for Plaintiffs to bring a lawsuit by reason of the profound neglect suffered by Jane Doe during her residency at ABC Care Center, which resulted in great physical and mental injuries, considerable consequential damages, and her untimely death. The serious bodily injuries and death made the basis of this lawsuit were proximately caused by the negligence and negligence per se of the named Defendants or their agents or employees acting in the course and scope of their employment."

Plaintiffs will show this Court that the Corporate Defendants, their employees, and agents violated these fundamental laws on a routine basis engaging in a pattern and practice of ongoing neglect. More specifically, Defendants' continuing course of repeated negligence included:

(a) Continuing failure to provide sufficient numbers of staff to meet said resident's fundamental care needs;

(b) Ongoing failure to properly monitor, observe and assess Jane Doe including ongoing assessments required by law;

(c) Repeated failure to hire and train appropriate personnel to monitor, supervise, and/or treat Jane Doe;

(d) Continuing retention of and assignment of unfit, unqualified and incompetent direct care staff;

(e) Ongoing failure to obtain and provide timely and appropriate medical treatment and nursing intervention to Jane Doe;

(f) Persistent failure to update and formulate health care plans in response to Ms. Doe's changes in condition and known medical problems, including those required by law;

(g) Repeated failure to notify the physician of significant conditions and changes in condition;

(h) Continuing failure to follow physician's orders;

(i) Ongoing failure to render proper treatment to Jane Doe for pressure sores;

(j) Continuing failure to accurately and timely assess and monitor Ms. Doe's skin condition;

(k) Repeated failure to turn Jane Doe every two (2) hours or as needed to prevent the formation and deterioration of decubitus ulcers;

(l) Ongoing failure to accurately and timely document Ms. Doe's pressure sores;

(m) Repeated failure to supervise and monitor the effects of Ms. Doe's wound treatments;

(n) Ongoing failure to follow up on initial skin assessments and provide treatment to Ms. Doe's pressure sores;

(o) Persistent failure to implement treatment orders despite knowledge that Ms. Doe was at high risk for delayed wound healing;

(p) Continuing failure to protect Ms. Doe from and prevent injury;

(q) Ongoing failure to assess and treat Jane Doe's pain by reason of the occurrence and advancing deterioration of Ms. Doe's pressure sores and other injures caused by Defendants;

(r) Repeated failure to provide adequate hygiene and provide minimal care to protect Jane Doe's dignity;

(s) Continuing failure to observe and comply with infection control precautions and protect Jane Doe from infection;

(t) Ongoing failure to provide ordered nutrition to Ms. Doe in violation of dietary and physician's orders;

(u) Repeated failure to adequately monitor Ms. Doe's hydration and ensure that she received sufficient amounts of fluid to meet minimum needs;

(v) Persistent failure to adequately monitor Ms. Doe's nutritional intake and ensure that she received sufficient nutrition to meet her minimum needs;

(w) Continuing failure to provide basis care planning for Ms. Doe's known medical problems;

(x) Ongoing failure to timely transfer Jane Doe to a facility that could properly treat decubitus ulceration;

(y) Repeated failure to establish and implement appropriate corporate budgeting policies which were consistent with the needs of residents including Ms. Doe that Defendants had accepted and promised to care for in accordance with the minimum standards prescribed by the Health and Safety Code and regulations promulgated under such statutes; and

(z) Continuing failure to establish and implement appropriate corporate safety, training, staffing, and fundamental nursing care policies to prevent harm to residents and avoid the known consequences of inadequate care."

(From a petition of an actual lawsuit alleging progressive failures and omissions of care.)

"Defendants knew or should have known from warnings, prior and concurrent victims such as (lists names of four other residents who have also filed suit), and their experience as nursing home operators that these acts or omissions, some of which occurred at ABC Care Center and some of which occurred at higher corporate levels, posed a serious threat to the safety and welfare of residents such as Jane Doe. Defendants' conduct was not occasional or fortuitous, but rather was the natural and predictable result of the decisions made at the higher levels of Defendants' corporate structure to maximize revenues and profits while at the same time reducing costs. Defendants' policies and financial decisions caused: a) ongoing dangerous levels of unqualified staff at the facility; b) patient population needs that continuously and grossly exceeded the capacity of the limited number of qualified care givers on duty; c) a total systems breakdown in the administration of basic care to all residents; and, d) widespread and ongoing neglect of multiple residents similarly situated to and including Jane Doe. Defendants then concealed these facts to deceive Ms. Doe and her loved ones. Overall, the systemic neglect which resulted in Ms. Doe's injuries and death was the product of Defendants' high-level corporate policy and the exercise of corporate control over said Defendants' nursing home.

Each and all of the aforementioned acts, both omission and commission as well as those yet to be discovered, constitute negligence and negligence per se and were a direct and proximate cause of the incident made the basis of this suit and Ms. Doe's resulting injuries, damages, and death."

(Continuation of petition from page one from an actual lawsuit alleging progressive failures and omissions of care. This lawsuit names the facility, corporate owners, administrator, director of nursing, and assistant director of nursing. It also alleges resident rights violations, gross negligence, malice, and violations of the penal code related to injuries of an elderly individual.)

Progressive injuries

Progressive injuries evolve gradually and a specific time of occurrence cannot always be identified. The nutritional problems in this chapter are considered progressive injuries. When they result in a lawsuit, the plaintiff will allege that the injury occurred as a result of pervasive, repeated, recurrent neglect by many staff members over a prolonged period of time. As a result, the resident suffered greatly and is entitled to punitive damages. The plaintiff will seek a negative ("No") answer to the question, "Without the neglect would the injury or death have occurred at this time?" The defense's objective will be to show the injury or death would have occurred despite the actions or omissions of the facility. The defense will assert that the nature of the elderly resident's complex medical problems, combined with his or her fragile state of health, age, and ongoing deterioration established, preordained, or caused the injury, making the negative outcome completely unavoidable.

American Nurses Association position statement on nutrition screening for the elderly[1]

Reprinted with permission from American Nurses Association, ANA position statement on nutrition screening for the elderly, www.nursingworld.org/readroom/position/social/scnutr.htm, ©1997 American Nurses Association, Silver Spring, MD.

Nutrition screening is the process of uncovering characteristics known to be associated with dietary or nutritional problems. Its purpose is to identify individuals who are at risk for nutritional problems or who have unrecognized malnutrition. Screening may be a basis for effective intervention.

Nutrition screening

In the past two decades, major efforts have been undertaken to alter nutrition practices and patterns of Americans with the goal of maintaining health and preventing illness and disease. As we begin the 21st century, major demographic shifts demand an emphasis on efforts to keep older people healthy, prevent illness, and to extend functional competence.

Nutrition takes on greater importance in the context of chronic illness. Some older persons are at increased risk because of multiple drug therapies, dental problems, economic hardship, and reduced social contacts. These problems arise from many varied environmental, social, and economic factors that are compounded by physiological changes of aging. A statement on nutrition screening is needed in order to:

- incorporate nutritional screening in the clinical care of older persons

- heighten awareness of the multiple risk factors having an impact upon nutritional status of older persons

The American Nurses Association (ANA) acknowledges the fact that some older persons are at risk for nutritional deficiencies. The ANA supports screening initiatives to identify nutritional risk and malnutrition. Incorporating nutrition screening in clinical care of older persons is critical to the prevention of disease and the promotion of health. Older persons must be informed consumers, and the American Nurses Association supports educational programs focusing on nutrition and the older adult. The ANA further supports linkages between other programs and initiatives directed toward improving nutritional status of older persons.

Research in the area of nutrition and the older adult should focus on food and drug interactions, iatrogenic causes of malnutrition, the role of nutrition in the aging process, and nutritional deficits existing in older persons in all settings. Studies have estimated that 10%–50% of the elderly in hospitals and nursing homes suffer from malnutrition. Because many nutrition patterns are established early in life, the American Nurses Association supports continued research in the area of nutrition with all age groups.

ANA recognizes that socioeconomic factors play a major role in the nutritional status of older persons. Maintaining and expanding community resources that contribute to the adequate nutritional status of older persons are essential. ANA supports nutrition sites, congregate meals, and home-delivered meals. The ANA strongly encourages recognition of the role of culture in nutrition.

Priorities and support

The American Nurses Association supports the prioritization of:

- routine nutrition screening and assessment of individuals on admission into the healthcare system

- a focus on the development of healthy nutritional patterns among the young and middle-aged community-based programs that address socioeconomic and cultural factors

Additionally, ANA supports

- nurses in their efforts to collaborate with other professionals in all settings to promote nutritional screening for older adults

- research in the area of nutrition and older persons

- educational programs focusing on nutrition for healthcare professionals and older consumers.

Rationale

Nutritional status is a "vital sign" of health. Maintaining adequate nutrition, thus avoiding the risks associated with nutritional deficiency, promotes a healthy American population. American healthcare practices have not incorporated routine nutrition screening and assessment. Nutrition screening is an essential step in the delivery of quality healthcare. Healthy People 2000: The National Health Promotion and Disease Prevention Objectives has an objective to improve nutritional status of all age groups in the next decade. Nursing's Agenda for Health Care Reform advocates for services specifically to assist population groups as well as health promotion and disease prevention strategies. Nutritional screening, assessment, interventions and research are necessary measure in achieving these objectives.

Weight loss and malnutrition

Weight loss and malnutrition are common problems in long-term care. Newly admitted residents often lose a few pounds within the first month. However, weight stabilizes soon afterward. Malnutrition, weight loss, and other weight-related complications may be unrecognized over time because staff do not compare the current weight with previous weights. This is a serious problem that is a common component of lawsuits, often in combination with pressure ulcers and other conditions that depend on nutrition to promote healing.

The plaintiff often alleges falsification of records, and produces flow sheets and other records showing inattention to weight monitoring, erratic and inconsistent weights, and substantial weight loss. In response, the facility may produce additional documentation that reveals a consistent food intake of 100% at every meal. Documentation supporting high caloric intake is often of questionable value in the face of substantial weight loss. Although the caloric requirements are largely determined by body size, activity, nutritional requirements, and disease process, in this situation the facility records often show caloric consumption of 3000 to 4000 calories a day. Despite the alleged high-calorie intake, weight loss persists. Juries are not stupid, and many question the veracity of these data when compared with the weight loss. The plaintiff may also produce flow sheets replete with documentation gaps, then allege, "The defendant nursing facility did not feed the resident 47 of 90 meals for this month." Other common problems the plaintiff will note are documentation that liquid nutritional products (Ensure®, Great Shakes®, etc.) were given and consumed by the resident three or four times a day.

If the resident is fed through a tube, the plaintiff usually alleges that the tube feeding intake and output records have been falsified if the ordered amounts of calories and fluids are adequate to support the resident's normal body weight and fluid balance. Sadly, malnutrition and dehydration are commonly seen in many tube feeders whose cases make it into the courtroom. These conditions almost always develop after the feeding tube was inserted. When this occurs, the defense will almost always allege that, despite the conscientious care provided, including tube feedings, supplements and adequate food intake, the resident experienced significant weight loss, therefore it must have been an underlying medical problem or a freak of nature. Next, the plaintiff will show the jury contradictions between the weights listed in various parts of the record. For example, the weight flow sheet reveals a weight of 150 pounds on March 1, but the MDS of that date lists the weight as 132. The plaintiff will also look for alteration of the resident's height in the record to learn whether the defendant deliberately falsified the height to reduce the average body weight range, thereby reducing the magnitude of the deficiency. Varied weighing techniques and different scales also present potential problems. Make sure residents are weighed on the same scale, using the same technique each time they are weighed. Pay attention to weight increases as well as declines. An incorrect weight gain of 15 pounds this week will become a weight loss next week. A loss of this magnitude may push your team into panic mode unnecessarily.

In 2004, a widely publicized study alleged that approximately 14,000 nursing home residents died of malnutrition and dehydration between 1999 and 2002, according to an investigation by the *Detroit News* which was based on federal records. A separate study by the Commonwealth Fund of Virginia noted that at least a third of the nation's long-term care facility residents "may suffer from malnutrition and dehydration." The Commonwealth Fund is a private foundation that supports research to promote improvements in healthcare.[2]

In 2000, the Health Care Financing Administration (HCFA; now CMS) spent an extraordinary amount of money to distribute materials for a comprehensive nutrition and hydration program to every nursing facility in the United States. Called "National Medicare Education Program: A Fact Pac for Nursing Home Administrators and Managers," the materials were geared toward direct caregivers, and included posters, bookmarks, and laminated pocket cards listing signs and symptoms to monitor and report, and describing methods of preventing dehydration and malnutrition in long-term care facilities. Materials were also provided to schools for nursing assistants and other long-term care personnel. Facilities could obtain unlimited copies of these materials, along with lesson plans and other instructional resources. It is evident that the government had identified malnutrition and dehydration as serious problems in facilities. Because the materials were widely distributed and free of charge, they continue to appear as exhibits in lawsuits. Most commonly, they are presented by the plaintiff, who alleges that the defendant nursing facility deliberately ignored the wealth of information and free resources provided by the government.

Responsibilities of licensed nurses

The nutrition and hydration information in this chapter are solidly within the scope of nursing practice, including identifying signs and symptoms of malnutrition and dehydration and recognizing abnormal laboratory values consistent with nutritional and hydrational abnormalities. Likewise, weighing residents at a specified frequency, pushing fluids, and monitoring intake and output are within the nursing purview. No physician's order is needed, although the physician must be kept apprised of changes in the residents' conditions.

Many nurses believe the sole responsibility for identifying and treating weight loss, malnutrition, dehydration, and related problems lies with the physician or dietitian. In court, they will testify they did not monitor intake and output because there was no physician order. (They try to omit details of their own omissions, such as failing to request a physician order, or failure to consider monitoring I & O as a part of the nursing process.) In any event, these are nursing responsibilities. As you can see, the nursing diagnoses listed in Table 15-1 are an essential part of nursing practice.

Table 15-1	*NANDA Nursing Diagnoses Related to Nutrition and Hydration*	
Pattern	**Taxonomy Code I**	**Taxonomy Code II**
Altered nutrition: more than body requirements	1.1.2.1	00001
Altered nutrition: less than body requirements	1.1.2.2	00002
Altered nutrition: risk for more than body requirements	1.1.2.3	00003
Risk for fluid volume imbalance	1.4.1.2	00025
Excess fluid volume	1.4.1.2.1	00026
Deficit fluid volume	1.4.1.2.2.1	00027
Risk for deficient fluid volume	1.4.1.2.2.2	00028
Adult failure to thrive	6.4.2.2	00101
Feeding self-care deficit	6.5.1	00102
Impaired swallowing	6.5.1.1	00103
Readiness for Enhanced Fluid Balance (new 2003)		00160
Readiness for Enhanced Knowledge (Specify) (new 2003)		00161
Readiness for Enhanced Nutrition (new 2003)		00163

From: North American Nursing Diagnoses Association (NANDA). Philadelphia PA.

Nursing diagnoses are required parts of the care plan, according to most state nurse practice acts and the American Nurses Association Standards of Clinical Nursing Practice.[3] Identification and use of the correct nursing diagnoses are an integral part of the nursing process. The NANDA board believes that for development of the nursing profession, nursing diagnoses must be viewed as an essential component of any professional nursing/client interaction. As your plan of care evolves, you will implement, plan, and evaluate the individualized approaches to care, which often include weight monitoring and recording (and evaluating) the residents' intake and output. This is an area in which medical and nursing diagnoses overlap, but the terminology is different. We are comparing apples to apples when we consider a diagnosis of dehydration versus a nursing diagnosis of deficit fluid volume. However, weight loss and dehydration are conditions that are both signs and diagnoses. They are usually a small part of a larger, more complex medical problem. Nursing identification and management are critical to successful treatment and positive outcomes.

The table on your CD-ROM entitled "Adult normal body weight over age 51" is a useful resource for determining normal weights and calorie intake for weight gain.

Signs and symptoms of malnutrition

Some residents develop malnutrition in the long-term care facility. Signs and symptoms of malnutrition are:

- weight loss

- dull, dry hair

- hair loss

- red, swollen lips; may have fissures at corners

- red, swollen gums

- dry mouth with fissures of mucous membranes/tongue

- red or purple, inflamed tongue, smooth in appearance

- pale color, dry skin, sunken cheeks

- fragile nails; may be spoon shaped

- diarrhea, anorexia

- weakness, muscle wasting, peripheral neuropathy

- slow wound healing, ecchymosis, dry, flaky skin; may have edema as a result of low protein

- listlessness

Effects of malnutrition

Effects of malnutrition are:

- loss of muscle mass

- personality and behavior changes

- weakness

- fatigue, progressing to complete exhaustion

- depression

- immunosuppression

- apathy and lack of initiative

- increased risk of pressure ulcers

- increased risk of falls

- abnormal laboratory values, particularly albumin, total protein, cholesterol, hemoglobin, and hematocrit; magnesium and potassium may also be abnormal

- death

Conditions in which weight loss may be unavoidable

In most residents, weight loss and malnutrition are avoidable conditions. Residents with some medical problems and conditions may lose weight. The determination about the unavoidability of weight loss must never be made on diagnosis alone. The determination is made based on an evaluation of the resident's response to the plan of care, and the modifications made to the plan to enhance success. Another consideration is a physician progress note describing unavoidability. However, the whole package must be reviewed in context rather than depending on individual factors. If you believe you are caring for an at-risk resident, you must make sure that ongoing documentation (over a period of months) adequately supports the reason for the weight loss. Whatever the cause, to be considered unavoidable, your documentation must reflect:

- accurate assessment (and reassessment, if indicated) of the resident's problem

- the problem is adequately care planned, based on analysis of assessment findings

- the care plan is actually implemented

- interventions have been evaluated repeatedly and periodically and modified according to the resident's responses to interventions

If the weight loss persists after doing these things, it may be unavoidable. Conditions in which weight loss may not be prevented are:

- refusal to eat

- terminal illness

- cancer

- chemotherapy or other cancer therapies

- alcohol and drug abuse

- end stage renal disease

- gastrointestinal disease

- diarrhea, nausea, and vomiting that are not responsive to treatment

- increased calorie needs related to medical diagnosis

- HIV disease, AIDS, and medical conditions known to cause wasting

Common risk factors for weight loss and malnutrition

Residents who are at risk for weight loss and malnutrition usually have one or more of these risk factors:

- Need help eating and drinking

- Eat less than half of meals and snacks

- Have mouth pain, dental problems, or missing teeth

- Have dentures that do not fit

- Have difficulty chewing or swallowing

- Cough or choke while eating

- Depression, crying spells, withdrawal from others

- Wander and pace

- Diabetes, chronic obstructive pulmonary disease, cancer, HIV, Parkinson's disease, Huntington's disease, and other chronic diseases

Assessment

Attention to the resident's meal consumption, accurate recording of percentage of meals consumed, and periodic monitoring of weight is an important responsibility. Residents with some problems and conditions, such as wandering, Parkinson's disease, and Huntington's disease, require more calories to offset their increased physical activity. If a resident begins losing weight, assess:

- Hydration—weight loss and dehydration often go hand in hand

- Weight loss over the past six months

- Type of diet

- Resident's ability to feed self

    – If resident feeds self, evaluate ability to see the food

    – Dental problems interfering with ability to eat

    – Shortness of breath interfering with ability to eat

    – Distractions, noise, or other environmental problems interfering with ability to eat

    – Swallowing problems

    – Wandering interfering with ability to eat

    – Improper positioning (leaning, table too far away, table too high) interfering with resident's ability to eat

    – Determine whether factors such as tremors interfere with the resident's ability to bring the food to the mouth

- Feeding assistance available and given

- Cognitive loss

- Wandering and other behavioral problems increasing the resident's caloric needs

- Medical diagnoses, such as Huntington's disease, infection or pressure ulcer, increasing the resident's caloric needs

- Depression

- Medications affecting appetite; drugs that suppress the appetite but may not be considered are:

    – Aldactone

    – Antacids

    – Anticonvulsants

    – Antipsychotics

    – Aspirin

    – B-adrenergic antagonists

    – Barbiturates

    – Benzodiazepines

    – Bumex

    – Capoten

    – Carbidopa

    – Clonidine

    – Digitoxin

    – Digoxin

    – Dyazide

    – Flagyl

    – H2 blockers

    – Haldol

    – Iron

    – Levodopa

    – nonsteroidal anti-inflammatory drugs (NSAIDs)

    – Prozac

    – Theophylline

Evaluate:

- Accuracy of recorded food intake.

- Accuracy of recorded supplement intake.

- Accuracy of recorded quantity of tube feeding and need for increased calories.

- Is resident receiving a $1/2$ or $3/4$ strength tube feeding formula? If so, he or she is receiving only half or three fourths of needed calories as well (estimate calories in tube feeding 1 ml = one calorie).

- Check skin for presence of new pressure ulcers.

Nursing interventions

Notify the physician if weight loss is 5% within past 30 days or 10% within past six months. Consider drawing chemistry profile and CBC every three months. Discuss the need for vitamin(s), appetite stimulant, supplement, and/or change in diet with the physician and dietitian. Beware of "double portion" food orders. Some surveyors interpret this as two of everything on the plate. An order for "large portions" may be more appropriate. Complete a significant change MDS if weight loss is 5% within past 30 days or 10% within past six months.

Other approaches:

- Notify the family or responsible party.

- Update the care plan to reflect new approaches to prevent further weight loss.

- Increase the frequency of weight monitoring. Place the resident on weekly weight monitoring. Record weekly weights on the treatment sheet or other location in which they can be readily tracked and will not be overlooked.

- Ask the food service supervisor to reevaluate resident dislikes and preferences.

- Review the dietary notes. Determine whether the dietitian's previous recommendations are on the care plan and are being followed.

- Request a dietitian consultation at his or her next regular visit. Implement new recommendations.

- Evaluate the accuracy of meal intake recording over the next seven days.

- Evaluate I & O over at least one week. Compare with dietitian's calculations of the resident's minimum daily fluid requirements. If inadequate, continue I & O monitoring.

- Determine whether resident will benefit from psychological consultation, nursing feeding retraining program, occupational therapy, or speech therapy.

- Invite family to visit at mealtime, bring special meals from home, if allowed.

- Evaluate the care plan approaches for effectiveness weekly.

Low serum cholesterol in the elderly

Cholesterol levels that are not elevated are often overlooked by long-term care facility staff. Unfortunately, low cholesterol is often an indicator of nutritional problems, including malnutrition. Sometimes, the resident receives a medication to reduce cholesterol, which further reduces the number. Low cholesterol is an indicator that must be monitored in the at-risk elderly population. Elevated blood cholesterol has been shown to be a cause of increased mortality in middle-aged adults. However, some studies have shown that higher cholesterol levels decrease mortality in some adults. Adults with certain medical problems, such as dialysis, may also benefit from higher cholesterol levels. The authors of one such study conclude that low total serum cholesterol levels are an independent predictor of short-term mortality rates in hospitalized elderly patients, regardless of the presence or absence of malnutrition, frailty, inflammation, and comorbidities.[4] Other studies have been unable to replicate these findings, so this is an area for current discussion and further research. Levels of serum cholesterol below 156mg/dl are significant in elderly persons.[5] A combination of low cholesterol and low albumin is a predictor of increased mortality.

Until more conclusive guidelines are available, discuss the significance of cholesterol levels below 170 mg/dl with the facility medical director and dietitian, and establish policies and protocols for action. If a resident experiences low cholesterol levels, notify the attending physician promptly. Refer the resident to the facility dietitian for further evaluation on his or her next regular visit.

Guidelines for weighing the residents

Facility policies and procedures should specify the frequency of resident weights. If the resident is at risk, make sure the frequency is specified on the care plan. Use a flow sheet to document weight. If a flow sheet is used, professionals can tell at a glance if the resident has experienced a weight loss. This is not possible if the professional must search the record to find the various weight readings. Make sure the documented weights are consistent. If the March 1 MDS shows a weight of 150 pounds, we would expect the weight elsewhere in the record for the first week of March to be in the same range.

Take each resident to a private weighing area or take the bed scale to the resident's room. Residents may be weighed in the privacy of the shower room immediately before being showered. Some facilities routinely weigh residents at shower time. Others assign restorative nursing assistants to weigh all residents, as their schedule permits. Inservice your staff on questionable values, double checking potentially inaccurate weights, and reporting guidelines. Other considerations are:

- Determine usual scale type used for resident.

- If necessary, refer to instructions for the scale.

- A restorative nursing assistant, CNA, or other worker should be available to assist with weighing of residents who are difficult to weigh.

- Residents who are extremely overweight, non-ambulatory, and difficult to weigh may be weighed on a bed scale for resident and staff safety.

- Weigh residents at the same time of day.

- Use the same scale each time.

- Always balance the scale before weighing the resident.

- The resident should wear one layer of clothing.

- Have the resident wear similar clothing each time he or she is weighed.

- Have the resident empty the bladder before being weighed.

- If the resident is wearing an incontinent brief, make sure it is dry before weighing.

- If the resident has an indwelling catheter, make sure the bag is empty before weighing.

- If the resident has a cast, has recently had a cast removed, or has new onset edema, consult the nurse about possible weight discrepancies.

- If you are taking a standing weight and height on a balance scale, have the resident remove the shoes and stand on a paper towel.

- If the bed scale is used, make sure the sling and the resident's extremities clear the bed.

- If you are responsible for documenting the weight on a weight list on the resident's chart, compare it with the previous month's weight. If there is a difference of 5 pounds or more (or according to facility policy), recheck the resident's weight. If, after rechecking the weight, there continues to be a difference, inform the nurse.

Dehydration

Dehydration is the loss of at least 1% of body weight as a result of fluid loss. Dehydration is a much greater problem than malnutrition in long-term care, and its symptoms are often atypical and easily mistaken for other illnesses or delirium.[6] Measure blood urea nitrogen (BUN) regularly for all residents. All licensed nurses in the long-term care facility must be taught to identify abnormal BUN values and their implications, and recognize the signs of possible dehydration so that intervention may be instituted swiftly.[7]

Sadly, dehydration is seen in many long-term care facility lawsuits as a primary or secondary issue. Careful evaluation of fluid intake and output is important, yet it is often overlooked, misunderstood, or considered a means of paper compliance. Water is an essential nutrient that is needed by every system of the body for proper function. Residents who are at high risk for dehydration must be identified. Whenever possible, determine the reason for decreased fluid intake.

Fluid is eliminated primarily through the kidneys. Other sources of fluid loss are perspiration, in the stool, and through respiration. Without perspiration, the normal daily turnover of water is approximately 4% of total body weight in adults. Intake and output should balance within 250 ml. Intracellular fluid is lost with aging, resulting in a decrease in total body fluid, and reducing the margin of safety in fluid balance. Decreased fluid intake or increased fluid loss can quickly lead to fluid imbalance.

Conservatively, the minimum acceptable fluid intake for the elderly should be no less than 1500 ml to 1800 ml per day. More is desirable in many residents. Less than 1500 ml is unacceptable for most residents.

"This is a civil liability case in which it has become necessary for Plaintiffs to bring a lawsuit by reason of the profound neglect suffered by John Doe during his residency at XYZ Care Center, which resulted in great physical and mental injuries, cosiderable consequential damages, and ultimately, his death. Such serious conditions included, but are not limited to:

    (a) a massive infected Stage IV pressure sore to right hip measuring 6 cm x 10 cm with exposed femoral head, osteomyelitis, and MRSA;

    (b) a necrotic Stage IV left buttock pressure sore measuring 9 cm x 8 cm x 1 cm with exposed ischium and MRSA;

    (c) a Stage IV left shin pressure sore measuring 10 cm x 4 cm x .02 cm with MRSA;

    (d) a Stage IV right ischial pressure sore measuring 7.0 cm x 5.0 cm x 0.5 cm with MRSA;

    (e) a Stage III left tibial pressure sore measuring 10.0 cm x 2.3 cm with MRSA;

    (f) severe and painful contractures of his elbows, wrists, fingers, hips, knees, and ankles;

    (g) repeated dehydration requiring hospitalization despite the presence of a feeding tube;

    (h) malnutrition and unplanned weight loss despite the presence of a feeding tube;

    (i) urosepsis with MRSA requiring hospitalization; and

    (j) death.

The serious bodily injuries and death made the basis of this lawsuit were proximately caused by the negligence and negligence per se of the named Defendants or their agents or employees acting in the course and scope of their employment."

(From a petition of an actual lawsuit alleging progressive failures and omissions of care.)

Reasons for inadequate fluid intake in the elderly

Unfortunately, normal aging changes increase the risk for fluid imbalance and dehydration. The elderly are less capable of maintaining fluid balance compared with younger persons. Also, many elderly persons (especially women) deliberately limit fluids to reduce the risk of accidental or frequent urination. Some residents may refuse all fluids after the evening meal to avoid having to get up at night to urinate. Other common reasons for inadequate fluid intake and abnormal loss of fluids include:

- Decreased content of body water

- Age-related changes in thirst sensation; decreased thirst response

- Renal changes

- Dysphagia

- Poor dietary intake (food is up to 80% fluid)

- Lack of available fluid

- Warm environmental temperature

- Physical or mental inability to consume fluids independently

- Depression, alteration in mood or cognitive status

- Delirium

- Gastrointestinal distress

- Apathy

- Bedrest, causing physiological changes and fluid loss

- Immobility

Contributing factors to inadequate hydration

- Fever

- Infection

- Dysphagia

- Nausea, vomiting, diarrhea

- Malabsorption

- Polyuria

- Increased metabolic rate/excessive activity

- Excessive perspiration

- Edema

- Wound drainage

- Medications that cause fluid loss

- High osmolar feedings

- Uncontrolled diabetes

- Shortness of breath/mouth breather/respirator

- Enemas/irrigation

- Inability to consume fluids or refuses fluids

High risk conditions

Residents at the greatest risk of dehydration have one or more of the following conditions:

- Female

- Bedridden

- Acute illness

- Age 85 or older

- Four or more medications

- Four or more chronic illnesses

Signs and symptoms of dehydration

- Sunken cheeks

- Sunken eyeballs

- Dry, brown tongue and mucous membranes

- Furrows or lines in tongue

- Dry, inelastic skin

- Poor skin turgor (check forehead or over the sternum in the elderly)

- Weight loss

- Hypotension, postural hypotension

- Increased pulse

- Elevated temperature

- Weakness, particularly in the upper body

- Mental confusion

- Concentrated urine

- Constipation and impaction

- Nausea and anorexia

- Increased time for veins to refill

- abnormal laboratory values (elevated hemoglobin/hematocrit, potassium, chloride, sodium, albumin, transferrin, BUN, urine specific gravity)

- greater than 3-pound weight loss within 7 days

- delusions, dizziness, delirium

- unsteady gait

- headache

- flushed appearance

Sadly, by the time signs and symptoms appear and are evident to staff, most residents are already quite dehydrated, making the need for aggressive interventions essential.

Minimum fluid needs to prevent dehydration

Total water in the body decreases with age. However, the various body systems depend on water to function normally. Daily requirements are approximately:

- Intestines 125 ml

- Breathing 335 ml

- Lungs 500 ml

- Skin 500 ml

- Kidneys 1375 ml

The older female's body is approximately 46% water, whereas the younger female's is 52% water. The difference between young adults and the elderly can vary as much as 10%. The elderly can rapidly develop fluid and electrolyte imbalances. Likewise, they can exist in a state of chronic dehydration. In many long-term care facilities, the registered dietitian calculates the amount of fluid that each resident should consume daily. The dietitian usually calculates fluid needs based on weight. The formula follows:

100 Ml/kg for the First 10 Kg (22 Pounds) of Body Weight

Add

50 Ml/kg for the next 10 Kg of Body Weight

Add

15 Ml/kg after the First 20 Kg (44 Pounds) of Body Weight

Another, less precise method is to estimate 1 ml of fluid for each calorie of dietary intake. Thus, if a resident receives an 1800 calorie diet, he or she requires 1800 ml of fluid in 24 hours.

Determination of fluid needs

Residents who have fluid imbalances or are at high risk for dehydration should be monitored by accurately documenting, calculating, and assessing I & O each shift. Take I & O monitoring seriously. Set realistic fluid intake goals for the resident, and inform nursing assistants of the goal for each shift in report. Most fluid is consumed on the day shift, with the least consumed on nights. Setting a goal will tell the nurse at a glance whether the resident has consumed sufficient fluid on his or her shift. If not, the nursing assistant should have (or make) time to encourage fluids before leaving for the day. When establishing goals for fluid intake, fluid is usually divided as follows:

- Day Shift $^1/_2$ (one half) of total 24 hour fluid goal

- Second Shift $^1/_3$ (one third) of total 24 hour fluid goal

- Third Shift $^1/_6$ (one sixth) of total 24 hour fluid goal

For residents with a fluid restriction, total fluid allowance for each shift can be distributed in the same quantity listed above. Modify the amounts listed as necessary to personalize fluid intake to the resident's individual needs. The dietitian must be involved with calculating fluid intake for residents on dialysis and fluid restriction, because some of the fluids consumed are part of the food preparation process, and some food items have naturally high water content. Thus, nursing should never attempt to make a determination alone.

Fluid intake includes all fluids consumed during the shift. This includes fluids provided on meal trays, and fluids given during medication pass. If activities serves beverages, this fluid is included as well. These sources of fluid may not be recorded, resulting in inaccurate I & O readings. Staff often record only fluids consumed on the nursing unit. Asking staff which fluids are recorded on the I & O record may prove interesting. You may discover that the various staff members have different interpretations of what constitutes fluid recorded on the I & O record. Make sure that all staff are on the same page regarding which fluids to record!

The weight tables on your CD-ROM can be used as a quick estimate of fluid needs based on weight. The daily intake and output are cumulated every 24 hours, usually on the night shift. Comparing the resident's daily intake to the tables below will help you determine whether the resident's fluid is adequate to meet his or her body requirements.

Estimated fluid needs by weight

The formula used to calculate fluid needs in these tables may not be as precise as the formula used by the dietitian. He or she is your resident expert. Although this is a good resource for times when the registered dietitian is unavailable, the dietitian is always your final authority on nutritional, caloric, and fluid needs. Take advantage of the vast expertise this important professional has to offer! **Weights listed in the Weight and Fluid needs table on your CD-ROM were determined as follows:**

Resident's Weight in Kilograms x 30 Ml = Minimum Estimated Fluids in 24 Hours

Formula to increase fluids

A similar formula is used to determine fluid needs if the resident requires extra fluids, has a physician's order, or the care plan states to push (force, encourage) extra fluids. When a resident needs additional fluids, use this formula:

Resident's Weight in Kilograms x 35 ml = Total Fluid Needed in 24 Hours

Effects of food on hydration

Healthy adults need approximately 2500 ml of water daily. Of this, approximately 1500 ml are consumed orally, 700 ml come from solid food, and 300 ml come from oxidation of foods during normal metabolism. Many foods contain water that can be used by the body. For example:

Food Item	Water Content
• Lettuce	(96%)
• Asparagus	(92%)
• Whole Milk	(87%)
• Orange	(86%)
• Potato	(80%)
• Cottage Cheese	(79%)
• Veal	(66%)
• Chicken	(63%)
• Beef	(47%)
• Cheddar Cheese	(37%)
• Bread	(36%)
• White Sugar	(0.05%)

Effects of medications

The body uses water as a diluent and vehicle for medications. Drug dosages are calculated based on body weight. *Medication toxicity is a real possibility that is seldom considered in residents who are dehydrated.* A decrease in total body water will increase the medication concentration per kilogram.[8] Residents who are dehydrated may also experience more medication-related side effects. Some medications such as diuretics, laxatives, and other further deplete the body of fluids and increase the risk of dehydration. Use large cups during medication pass. Encourage each resident to consume at least eight ounces of water with medications. Document fluid intake as a nursing measure, if appropriate.

Laboratory values suggesting dehydration

Nursing personnel must be able to identify laboratory values suggesting dehydration. **An approximation of the degree of dehydration is seen in the Signs and Symptoms of Dehydration Table on your CD-ROM.** Contact the physician and dietitian for these values:

- BUN over 22 mg/dl
- Elevated hematocrit (greater than three times the hemoglobin)
- Potassium below 3.5
- Chloride over 107
- Sodium over 147 suggests severe dehydration
- Elevated serum creatinine
- A creatinine greater than 1.5 suggests renal disease. If so, determine the BUN/Creatinine ratio. Divide the BUN by the creatinine. Values over 23 suggest dehydration.

Suggested nursing interventions

Add appropriate nursing interventions to the plan of care pending more specific dietitian recommendations:

- Provide extra fluids with meals, including juice, soup, ice cream and sherbet, gelatin, water on trays.
- Serve beverages at activities.
- All staff should encourage at least 60 ml of fluid of the resident's choice upon entering each resident's room.
- Encourage the resident to consume at least 180 ml with medications. Residents who limit water intake may accept sugar-free juices during medication pass.
- Offer Popsicles between meals.
- Pass juice or fluid cart at least twice a day.

- Record accurate I & O. Cumulate each shift. Evaluate daily compared with resident's minimum fluid requirements.

Residents in need of intake and output monitoring

Intake and output monitoring is a simple procedure that does not require a physician's order. Sadly, nurses often view it as a means of paper compliance and do not take this important intervention seriously. Write the need for intake and output monitoring, as well as any special approaches or resident preferences, on the care plan. If the resident is known to be at high risk of dehydration upon admission, during illness, or at any other time, begin a temporary care plan to address this risk. Do not wait until the quarterly care conference! Facility personnel should routinely monitor fluid balance (intake and output) for:

- all residents receiving tube feedings

- residents with catheters

- residents with urinary tract infection

- residents with physician orders for fluid restrictions or orders to force (encourage) fluids

- residents with specific physician orders for additional liquid (fluid)

- residents who are known to be dehydrated or who are at risk for dehydration

- residents with certain heart and kidney conditions that are at high risk for fluid imbalance

- residents receiving intravenous fluids or parenteral nutrition therapy

Other components of resident care include:

- Develop an individualized plan of care that takes into account the resident's medical condition, medications, physical problems, catheter, tube feeding, and individual aging changes in hearing, vision, and mobility. Consider the resident's degree of cognitive impairment and ability to consume fluids without help. Communicate the identified risk of fluid imbalance and plan of care to all members of the interdisciplinary team.

- Identify patterns of behavior, individual likes and dislikes leading to fluid imbalance. Develop a plan of care to address these issues to prevent complications.

- Determine what fluids the resident likes and will consume most readily, and attempt to provide these items.

- Promptly meet resident needs. Offer fluids of the resident's choice each time staff are in the room. Place a straw in the resident's mouth and encourage him or her to drink, if necessary. Anticipate needs in cognitively impaired residents who have difficulty communicating.

- Assess for clinical signs and symptoms of fluid imbalance and document the results of this assessment daily, or more often, as indicated. Act immediately to reverse abnormalities.

- Ask the registered dietitian to calculate the resident's daily fluid needs. Write this number on the plan of care and intake and output record.

- Routinely record fluid intake and output for residents in whom monitoring is indicated (see above). Total the intake and output records each shift. At the end of 24 hours, the third shift nurse is responsible for cumulating the daily total. He or she should compare these figures with the resident's minimum body needs. If deficient, pass the information on in report, assess for dehydration, and update the plan of care if indicated. All nursing personnel should take corrective action if fluid consumption or urinary output are inadequate. Additional corrective measures may involve changing the plan of care or obtaining specialized consultations. The occupational therapist and dietitian are experts in problems of this nature.

Intake and output monitoring procedure

Intake and output monitoring is much more than paper compliance for residents with catheters! The answer is that all fluids the resident consumes should be recorded. Follow these guidelines:

- Document all fluid consumed by the resident during each shift on an intake and output flow sheet or worksheet. This includes fluids consumed on the nursing unit, fluids consumed with medications, fluids consumed during meals, and fluids consumed during activities.

- Record all fluid excreted in metric measurements (cc or ml). For the most part, this is urinary elimination. However, emesis, wound drainage, and liquid stools may also be included in output recording. For incontinent residents, this may be recorded in number of incontinent episodes. For more accurate values, incontinent pads can be weighed to provide an estimate of urinary incontinence fluid output. A metric scale is needed, such as an infant scale. You should post the dry weight of the pads or briefs used by the facility. Any weight above the dry weight is fluid. Use this formula to convert it to milliliters:

    One gram weight =
    approximately 1 ml fluid

- At the end of each shift, the nursing assistant assigned to collect the I & O totals the fluid intake and urinary output. He or she reports

the totals to the licensed nurse, who records them in the medical record.

- If, at the end of the shift, the nurse determines that the fluid intake and output are inaccurate or inadequate, he or she should question the assistants and attempt to reconcile the record. He or she may also instruct the nursing assistant to administer fluids immediately. Report the low liquid intake to the next shift, who should increase fluid intake and monitor the resident closely.

- Promptly obtain laboratory tests ordered by the physician to assess for the resident's fluid balance, electrolytes, and metabolic status, including hydration. The registered nurse should review the resident's laboratory values relating to hydration. If abnormal, make phone contact with the physician. Ask the registered dietitian to review the laboratory values and make recommendations. Repeat the laboratory tests periodically after that to ensure that abnormalities have been corrected or the resident is making improvement.

- Develop and implement an individualized plan of care based on the assessment of risk factors and the resident's individual needs.

- If the intake and output/fluid balance goals are not being met, determine whether the care listed in the plan has been or is being provided. Take appropriate corrective action.

Understanding hyponatremia and hypernatremia in dehydration

Many elderly long-term care facility residents are found to be dehydrated with *hypovolemia*, or low circulating blood volume. Some are diagnosed with hyponatremia, and others are diagnosed with hypernatremia. These conditions correspond with the following nursing diagnoses:

- Risk for fluid volume imbalance

- Excess fluid volume

- Deficient fluid volume

- Risk for deficient fluid volume

Long-term care facility nurses must be able to identify these conditions on laboratory reports, and know how to prevent them from developing.

Hyponatremia

Hyponatremia occurs when the sodium level in the blood is low, or the resident is in fluid overload. Although there are other causes, hyponatremia commonly develops in elderly residents as a result of:

- excessive intake or excretion of dietary sodium or water

- some diseases

- severe, prolonged, or uncontrollable diarrhea

- consuming a low salt diet for prolonged periods

- excessive sweating

- taking diuretics in combination with a low salt diet; diuretics implicated in the development of hyponatremia include:

  – furosemide (Lasix)

  – bumetanide (Bumex)

  – thiazide diuretics

Diuretics increase the excretion of sodium into urine. This is often necessary to correct high blood pressure. Elimination of too much sodium results in hyponatremia. If the resident is on a low sodium diet, severe hyponatremia can develop. Hyponatremia can be corrected either by increasing dietary sodium or by

decreasing body water. When a resident has edema, maintain a degree of suspicion for hyponatremia. Occasionally, fluid retention is the result of inadequate sodium or protein intake.

Signs and symptoms

The resident may be asymptomatic until the sodium level is well below normal. An astute nursing assistant may report an increase in the resident's normal urinary output. Symptoms of moderate to severe hyponatremia include:

- apathy

- feeling tired

- weakness

- confusion

- disorientation

- headache

- muscle cramps

- nausea

These signs and symptoms develop as a result of water moving into brain cells, causing swelling and disrupting normal function. If the condition develops rapidly (which is unusual in the elderly), signs of neurological irritability, muscle spasms, and coma occur.

Diagnosis

Hyponatremia is diagnosed from an abnormal lab test, usually routine electrolyte levels or a biochemistry profile. Monitor residents taking diuretics regularly for abnormal labs suggesting development of hyponatremia. The normal concentration of sodium in the blood plasma is 135–145 mM. Hyponatremia occurs when sodium in the blood falls below 135 mM. Plasma sodium levels of 127 mM or less can be very dangerous and may cause seizures and coma.

Prevention

Being aware of the resident's risk factors and providing close monitoring are always the best preventive measures. Regularly monitor the resident's laboratory values. Other nursing measures are:

- monitoring intake and output; never hesitate to order I & O as a nursing measure

- carefully evaluating fluid intake and output every 24 hours and comparing with dietitian's recommended fluid needs

- monitoring weight (and edema, if applicable)

- monitoring vital signs

- monitoring level of consciousness

- encouraging foods and fluids high in sodium

Treatment

Assuming that the condition is not caused by an underlying disease, hyponatremia is usually treated successfully. Severe hyponatremia is usually treated by hospitalizing the resident for fluid therapy. A solution of 5% sodium chloride in water is infused. Moderate hyponatremia may be corrected by increasing dietary sodium/drinking less fluid (which is usually not a problematic issue in the elderly). **A table for quantifying edema is on the CD-ROM that accompanies this book.**

Hypernatremia

Hypernatremia is almost always an indication of excessive fluid depletion. It usually occurs with inadequate fluid intake and increased water loss. It commonly develops in elderly residents as a result of:

- some diseases and medical conditions

- physical or mental inability to consume sufficient fluids

- lack of thirst

- conditions that override the body's volume control mechanisms, usually excessive diuresis or diabetes insipidus

- fever

- vomiting

- diarrhea

- loss of excessive water through the kidneys

- residents receiving tube feedings with inadequate free water

When calculating total fluid intake, be careful with tube feeding formulas and liquid nutritional supplements. Approximately 85% of the formulas are water. The formula is approximately 15% solid, which cannot be counted toward meeting daily fluid requirements. Ask the dietitian for assistance making calculations, if necessary. In most instances, the 15% solid content is not deducted from the total fluid intake cumulation.

Signs and symptoms

Signs and symptoms of hypernatremia can be very subtle. Reduced urinary intake is common. Urine appears dark and concentrated. Reduced level of consciousness is common. The signs and symptoms are usually neurological, including delirium, irritability, restlessness, lethargy, muscular twitching, spasticity, seizures, and hyperreflexia. The neurological problems are caused by decreased water content in the brain cells, which leads to shrinkage. If the condition persists over time, it can cause cerebral hemorrhage. Hypernatremic residents are often found to have an infection.

Diagnosis

Diagnosis is made based on laboratory monitoring. A serum sodium concentration greater than or equal to 145 mmol/L suggests the resident is hypernatremic.

This is an emergent condition that requires prompt physician intervention.

Prevention

Being aware of the resident's risk factors and close monitoring are always the best preventives. Regularly monitor the resident's laboratory values. Other nursing measures are:

- monitoring intake and output; never hesitate to order I & O as a nursing measure

- carefully evaluating fluid intake and output every 24 hours and comparing with dietitian's recommended fluid calculations

- monitoring weight

- monitoring vital signs

- monitoring level of consciousness

- restricting medications, foods, and fluids high in sodium

- encouraging fluids according to dietitian's recommendation; fluid consumption should exceed 1500 ml daily for all residents unless otherwise ordered

Administer sufficient water to residents who are fed by tube. Obtain dietitian recommendations and physician orders for free water. Administer a minimum of 30 ml to 50 ml water before and after each medication delivered through the tube. Document (and regularly evaluate) I & O on all residents receiving tube feeding.

Treatment

Assuming that the condition is not caused by an underlying disease, hypernatremia can usually be corrected with IV fluids. Normal saline is the most appropriate therapy. Early identification and treatment are always best. This must be done gradually in

the acute care setting. Rapid fluid replacement increases the risk of cerebral edema.

Comparison of dehydration

The Comparison of Dehydration table on your CD-ROM provides an overview of the various types of dehydration.

Dysphagia

Dysphagia is difficulty swallowing food, fluids, or oral secretions. Approximately 53% to 74% of long-term care facility residents have dysphagia. Residents who are at high risk for developing dysphagia include those who:

- have a neuromuscular diseases (Parkinson's Disease, Huntington's Chorea, or Multiple Sclerosis)

- have had a stroke

- have cancer of the head, neck, or esophagus

- have had radiation treatment to the face or throat

- are on medications that decrease saliva production, impair cognition, or increase sedation

- have dementia

Most people swallow at least 600 times each day. For persons with dysphagia, swallowing can be an insurmountable problem. These residents are at great risk for weight loss, malnutrition, dehydration, choking, and aspiration.

Signs and symptoms

Signs and symptoms of dysphagia are:

- difficulty controlling liquids and secretions in the mouth

- having a wet or gurgly sounding voice

- taking a long time to begin a swallow

- needing to swallow 3–4 times for each bite of food

- having a feeling of fullness or tightness in the throat or chest

- having a sensation of food sticking in esophagus or sternal area

- coughing

- frequent throat clearing

- lack of a gag reflex

- weak cough before, during, or after a swallow

- pocketing food

- spitting food out

- refusing to eat

- recurrent upper respiratory infections

- persistent low-grade fever

- unintentional weight loss

If a resident experiences any of these signs or symptoms, consultation with a speech language pathologist is needed. He or she will perform diagnostic tests, such as a modified barium swallow. Dysphagia may be treated with a combination of swallowing exercises, practicing swallowing techniques, and altering the consistency of food and beverages.

Diet textures

Nursing and dietary personnel must work closely with the speech language pathologist and dietitian to ensure food acceptance. Adults may resist eating pureed food because it resembles baby food. Some residents will not accept foods in which the texture has been modified. The goal is to ensure that the food is the proper consistency to meet the resident's needs and reduce the risk for aspiration. The food

should look and taste as close to normal as possible, and food consistency should be altered as little as possible, in consideration of the resident's safety needs. Extra gravies or sauces may be added to some foods. Molds and special methods of preparation are used to enhance the appearance of pureed foods, making them more acceptable to the resident. If pureed foods are used, the dietitian and speech language pathologist will prescribe the consistency needed by the resident. Generally speaking, pureed diets should not be watery or runny. When properly prepared, pureed items should be the consistency of pudding and support a plastic spoon in the upright position.

Altered texture diets, such as mechanical soft and pureed diets, are ordered for residents with dysphagia. Foods and fluids should be served in an appetizing manner, and be easy to swallow and nutrient dense. The National Dysphagia Diet Task Force (NDDTF) is developing standardized definitions for food and fluid consistencies for dysphagia treatment. The NDDTF has defined four diet levels:

- **Level 1**—Dysphagia Pureed: Pureed, homogenous, cohesive, pudding-like.

- **Level 2**—Dysphagia Mechanically Altered: Cohesive, moist, semi-solid. Requires some chewing ability. Ground or minced meats with fork-mashable fruits and vegetables. Excludes most bread products, crackers, and other dry foods.

- **Level 3**—Dysphagia Advanced: Soft-solid. Requires more chewing ability. Easy-to-cut meats, fruits, vegetables. Excludes hard, crunchy fruits and vegetables, sticky foods, very dry foods.

- **Level 4**—Regular: Any solid textures.

Food thickeners

The speech language pathologist will work with the resident and nursing personnel to teach the individualized approaches for eating and drinking to prevent aspiration and ensure proper intake. Liquids are usually the most difficult to swallow. The speech professional may recommend using food thickeners to slow the movement of fluid through the esophagus. He or she will prescribe thickening liquids to nectar, honey, or pudding consistency. High quality commercial thickeners do not leave an aftertaste, do not continue to thicken after they set, and are fully digestible. Thickening agents that are gum based, such as guar gum or pectin, are not recommended, as they will bind fluid so it is unavailable for hydration.[9]

Thickeners are commercially available products that slow the movement of fluid through the esophagus. They are ordered to make swallowing easier and reduce the risk of aspiration. The consistency of the liquid depends on the amount of powder added. There is a great margin of error in mixing powdered thickeners, so follow the therapists' instructions exactly. When using powdered thickeners, add the thickener immediately before serving the product. You should:

- use the correct product

- use the correct amount, according to therapist instructions and physician orders

- follow manufacturers' directions

- stir the thickener well

- follow the speech therapist's instructions and plan of care for positioning and feeding

An area of controversy

Nursing personnel must be aware that the use of food thickeners has fallen out of favor in some circles over the past few years. This is another longstanding practice for which further research is needed. Prethickened liquids are more expensive than powder-thickened liquids, but are usually better accepted.

We know that powder thickeners do not alter the taste of liquids, but many residents complain that powder thickeners intensify the taste, making it seem stronger. Some professionals believe that thickened fluids:

- are unpalatable and frequently refused

- do not supply adequate water and contribute to dehydration

- fill the stomach and reduce appetite

- will worsen lung problems if aspirated

Assisting residents with swallowing problems with meals

Residents with dysphagia will require a special plan of care, properly trained personnel, and one-to-one assistance, prompting, or supervision at meals. General approaches for feeding the resident are:

- Make sure the resident is fully awake and alert before serving food or beverages.

- Position the resident as upright as possible.

- Position the head facing forward, with the neck flexed forward slightly. Avoid hyperextending the neck.

- Reduce distractions and limit conversation at meals. Focus the resident on eating.

- If the resident has had a stroke, direct the food to the unaffected side of the mouth.

- Prompt or feed the resident slowly, offering small bites.

- Remind the resident to chew and swallow the food well.

- Check the mouth to make sure the resident has swallowed the food.

The speech language pathologist may order other special positions and exercises, depending on the resident's needs. Other approaches may be necessary, such as reminding the resident to tuck the chin in when swallowing. This changes the position of the airway, further reducing the risk of aspiration. This technique is effective for some types of dysphagia, but increases the risk of aspiration in other types. As you can see, dysphagia care is highly individualized.

Aspiration and pneumonia

Aspiration, pneumonia, and sepsis related to pneumonia are common components of many lawsuits. This sometimes occurs in residents with tube feedings whose head is not elevated, as well as those who have pulled the tube, causing it to migrate or dislodge. However, it is also common with residents who take nutrients and fluids by mouth. Attention to maintaining good nutrition and hydration is essential to good health. Inadequate nutrition and dehydration negatively influence quality of life, decrease resistance to infection, and suppress the ability to heal or to have sufficient energy to take part in activities of daily living. Many residents have problems swallowing liquids without choking. This is diagnosed and evident with some residents, such as those who have had strokes, and those with Parkinson's disease, but in many residents the condition is undiagnosed. Thin liquid, such as water, is the most difficult consistency to swallow without choking. The next most threatening is thin liquid mixed with a solid, such as vegetable soup, or dry cereal with milk. Because of this problem, liquid nutritional supplements have limited usefulness in some residents.

Residents with Alzheimer's disease are at high risk of malnutrition and dehydration. However, staff are expected to support and maintain nutrition, using a variety of approaches to maintain intake. Because of the strong pleasure response and quality of life issues associated with eating and drinking, tube feeding is the least desirable method of providing nutrition and hydration, if it can be avoided. Any time a tube is inserted, your initial goal should be to restore the resident's ability to eat normally.

Residents with Alzheimer's do not forget how to eat and drink. Swallowing is an involuntary action. However, the residents may lose the ability to move the food to the back of the mouth until it is in a position where it can be swallowed. Because of this, nursing staff must learn procedures and techniques for feeding residents to stimulate swallowing. This is not complex or difficult. Many experts have suggested that lack of proper staff training on how to feed the residents is a major contributing factor to malnutrition and dehydration in long-term care facilities.[10,11] Some studies have shown that tube feeding is of minimal benefit, and markedly increases the risk of aspiration, regardless of the type of tube used.[12]

Tube feeding tips and guidelines

- Use good hand washing before handling tube feeding equipment or solutions. If wearing gloves to check residual, wash hands well before gloves are applied and after gloves are removed.

- Avoid using a Foley catheter in place of a gastrostomy tube. Stomach secretions erode the catheter balloon more rapidly. The catheter length increases the risk of dislodgement and accidental removal.

- Check the position of the nasogastric tube before each feeding by withdrawing residual stomach contents. Avoid placing the end of the tube in a glass of water to check for bubbling. Another method is to inject 5 ml to 10 ml of air into the tube while simultaneously ausculating the epigastrium with a stethoscope. This method is useful in small bore tubes through which aspiration of stomach contents is difficult or impossible.

- Before an intermittent feeding, instill 30 ml of water into the tube to ensure patency.

- Check the position of a gastrostomy tube by withdrawing residual stomach contents.

- Aspirate residual stomach contents before each feeding, or according to facility policy. If you aspirate more than 100 ml, hold the feeding (or start the feeding at a slower rate, according to physician orders). Return aspirated residual to the stomach to maintain electrolyte balance. Avoid this method if the resident has a small bore tube.

- Discard dented or damaged cans of formula.

- Wash the outside of the can before opening.

- Never pour new formula on top of formula that has been hanging.

- Refrigerate open cans of formula. Cover the can, and label the date and time opened. If the contents are not used within 24 hours, discard them.

- Formula should be room temperature for feeding. If a partial can of solution is refrigerated, warm to room temperature in hot water. Avoid heating the solution to temperatures above room temperature.

- Formula should not hang for more than 6 hours if the open system of feeding is used. Closed system containers should not hang for more than 24 hours, or according to manufacturers' recommendations.

- The head of the bed should always be elevated during tube feeding and for 60 minutes after that. The recommended level of elevation is 45 degrees.

- If the resident has a tracheostomy, avoid deflating the cuff for at least two hours after feeding.

- If the resident becomes nauseated, stop the feeding. Notify the physician. He or she may order diluted formula, a different formula, or an antiemetic/antinauseant medication.

- If the resident is diabetic, monitor finger stick blood sugar every 6 hours, or according to facility policy, for the first week of tube feeding. After that, follow facility policy and physician's orders. Monitor regularly for signs and symptoms of hyperglycemia/hypoglycemia.

- Half- and three-quarter-strength formulas are usually not calorically adequate for long-term use. These are used in the early stages of tube feeding, until the resident can tolerate full-strength formula. Contact the physician and request an order change as soon as it becomes evident that the resident can tolerate the formula.

- Most tube feedings are not nutritionally complete at amounts less than 1500 ml–2000 mL in 24 hours. Evaluate nutritional adequacy of the formula.

- Tube feeding should be given to maintain the resident's body weight. Compare the number of calories with the resident's BEE, as calculated by the dietitian.

- Total fluid intake should meet the resident's minimum daily fluid needs, as calculated by the dietitian.

- In addition to formula, the resident needs free water. Residents with fever, diminished renal concentrating ability, and high osmolality formulas need extra fluids.

- Record *and evaluate* intake and output for all residents receiving tube feedings.

- For residents receiving a continuous feeding by drip method, mark the administration set with a time tape. If the feeding falls behind schedule, make a new tape. Do not increase the rate.

- Periodically evaluate the resident's chemistry profile and CBC.

- Flush the administration set before each feeding is added.

- Flush the tube after each feeding.

- Flush the tube before and after *each* medication.

- Change the administration set every 24 hours.

- The mucous membranes tend to dry out. Lubricate the lips, mouth, and nostrils regularly. Keeping the mouth clean is important for dental health, as well as to increase the bacteria in the mouth. Assist the resident with regular tooth brushing, or assign nursing assistants this task.

- If the tube is plugged, flush with 30 to 40 ml of fluid. Use a 30 ml or larger syringe. (A smaller syringe causes too much pressure.) *Exert gentle pressure.* Flushing the tube every 10 minutes for an hour may be necessary. Use fresh solution each time.

- Follow facility policy for irrigating and flushing tubes. Facilities commonly use water or cola. Studies have shown that cranberry juice is less effective than the others for irrigation.[13] Despite the well-published results of these studies, many nurses continue to use cranberry juice.

- After inserting a nasogastric tube, the most accurate method of determining proper tube placement is by x-ray. However, this method is not always realistic in long-term care facilities. Placement can be accurately determined by checking pH. In addition to determining whether the tube is incorrectly placed in the lungs, the pH of the stomach contents will suggest whether the tube is placed in the stomach or small bowel. The litmus paper used should have a wide range, from 0 to 10 (or higher). Paper with a lower range is not recommended. Usually, aspirates from the stomach will have a pH of 4 or lower. Aspirates from the intestine have a pH of 6 or higher. Although the results are sometimes inconclusive, an x-ray is recommended to determine placement if the pH exceeds 6.

- A nasogastric tube is a temporary tube. When a nasogastric tube is inserted in a long-term care facility resident, your goal should always be to return the resident to oral feeding. Obtain dietary, speech and occupational therapy evaluations as soon as possible. The time factor for evaluations is critical. If the enteral feeding continues over time, the resident may lose the ability for feeding, and a gastrostomy tube will be inserted.

Troubleshooting complications of gastrostomy tubes

Troubleshooting tips are listed in the Troubleshooting Complications of Gastronomy Tubes table on your CD-ROM.

Complications associated with enteral tube insertion

Infection control

Tube feeding systems and formulas are potential sources of infection. Contamination of the dispensing system account for most infections. However, improper handling and storage of nutrient solutions and faulty administration technique are also potential sources of serious infection. Enteral feeding has been implicated in the transmission and development of pneumonia, bacterial infections, *Clostridium difficile* (C. diff.) diarrhea, and other diarrheal illnesses. The length of time an enteral formula hangs is a significant consideration in the development of infection. Formula manufacturers have recommendations for maximum hang time of solution. The total hang time is partially determined by the type of delivery system being used. Instructions may be found on the can or bottle, package insert, or the manufacturer's web site. Never exceed the manufacturer's maximum recommendations. Each facility should have policies and procedures for infection control of the enteral feeding systems. Because of the changing nature of common pathogens, infection control recommendations change frequently. Review infection control policies for enteral feeding annually or when new information and recommendations are available to ensure the facilities delivers care that meets or exceeds current standards.

Buried bumper syndrome

A serious complication associated with PEG tubes is buried bumper syndrome. This condition results from an ulceration at the tube exit site or the internal mucosal layer of the gastric wall. It most commonly occurs when the tube has internal and external retention bumpers to hold the tube in place. Traction and excessive tension between the internal and external bumpers promotes ulceration and migration of the

tube into the muscular layer of the stomach, with the potential for very serious complications. Tube stress is commonly caused by excessive traction at the time of tube insertion, maintenance of a very tight skin disk, or failure to pull back and rotate the disk daily. Other common causes are failure to loosen the external bumper after weight gain and placement of padding or excessive dressings under the external bumper. Unrecognized and untreated, this condition can lead to peritonitis, gastrointestinal bleeding, and death. Signs and symptoms include:

- Bleeding from the stoma
- Formula leakage
- Leakage of gastric secretions
- Sudden onset of intolerance to formula that the patient tolerated previously

Reduce the risk for this potentially serious problem by leaving the healed stoma open to air. Rotate the disk daily, and pay close attention to the tension between the external and internal bumpers. Leave a small amount of space between the bumper and skin level.

Tube migration and peritonitis

The prevalence of tube placement errors reported in the literature varies from 1.3% to 50% in adults. Some tubes are more difficult than others to place and maintain. A 53-year-old patient sued a hospital for a misplaced nasogastric tube, which perforated his esophagus. The problem was not immediately identified. Transpyloric tubes are difficult to place initially and correct positioning is also difficult to maintain. All types of small-bore tubes dislocate easily, frequently with no outward sign that the dislocation has occurred. After the perforation was diagnosed, the patient underwent 11 surgeries to repair the damage. Doctors had to recreate part of his esophagus with a section of his colon.

The patient was fed through a gastrostomy tube for a year. Although his ability to swallow was eventually restored, he continued to have trouble eating and digesting food, and his blood sugar fluctuates wildly, causing him to feel tired and dizzy much of the time. The patient had to quit his job and must take an expensive medication for the rest of his life. In 2006, a jury returned a verdict for the plaintiff, finding that the hospital nursing staff was negligent. Although the physician was named in the original lawsuit, the jury did not find against him. The plaintiff was awarded $10,000,000 for medical expenses, lost earning capacity, pain and suffering, disfigurement, physical impairment. His wife was awarded approximately $700,000 for loss of consortium.[14]

Peritonitis is a common complication associated with tube migration and misplacement. The risk is especially great when a Foley catheter is used in place of a regular gastrostomy tube. However, as you can see from the lawsuit above, peritonitis can also develop as a result of misplaced nasogastric tubes.

Pay close attention to technique during feeding tube insertion. Frequent monitoring of the resident after placement is essential to minimizing complications.[15] If a gastrostomy tube is used, inflate the internal balloon with normal saline after inserting the tube. Document the amount of solution instilled. Carefully secure the feeding tube to avoid dislodgement or internal migration. Mark the tube at the exit site from the body with tape or indelible ink. Many tubes have markings imprinted into the tubing. If these are not present, measure with a tape measure and document the external length of the tubing. After the enteral feeding tube has been secured and measured, obtain an X-ray to confirm tube location. Then start feedings slowly, and monitor the resident for signs of aspiration, vomiting, or tube intolerance.

Tube displacement can be prevented through a combination of measures. Facility policies should address the frequency at which nurses should measure and document the length of the external tube. In most cases, this is done daily or weekly, although monitoring may be done every shift for a specified period of time immediately after insertion. If a gastrostomy tube is being used, check to be sure the disk or attachment device holding the tube externally is secure.[16]

Check and document the volume of fluid in the internal balloon every 7 to 10 days. The manufacturer's literature will specify the total fluid volume of the balloon. Withdraw the fluid, note the volume, then reinflate the balloon. Compare the amount withdrawn with the amount initially injected into the balloon. If the volume is less than previously, refill to the manufacturer's recommended volume. Document the date and time the balloon was checked and the amount of fluid instilled.[17]

The potential for peritonitis is very high related to feeding tube migration. Take your responsibility for tube placement checks and monitoring for migration very seriously. Undetected peritonitis quickly leads to serious complications, including death in the frail elderly population.

Tube removal and reinsertion

Facilities must establish whether licensed nurses are permitted to reinsert gastrostomy tubes into an established surgical tract. In the old days, this was standard operating procedure, because the original insertion procedure involved making an incision into the abdominal skin, through which the gastrostomy tube was threaded. A Foley catheter was commonly used as a feeding tube. Because the pH of the urinary bladder is different from the stomach, the use of Foleys required frequent tube replacement, as acids eroded the feeding tube (catheter) and inflation balloon. Reinsertion procedures and practices began to change when the percutaneous endoscopic gastrostomy (PEG) procedure became widespread. This is because a PEG is threaded from the inside out, versus threading a gastrostomy from the outside in.

Another improvement was that manufacturers began to make shorter gastrostomy tubes, which posed less of a chance for migration. The newer tubes are also better able to withstand the assault of the digestive enzymes, acids, and normal stomach contents.

Gastrostomy tubes are sometimes forcefully removed by confused residents. Occasionally, tubes plug and must be changed. Balloons occasionally rupture. Some facilities continue to routinely change/reinsert gastrostomy tubes into an established surgical tract, including the PEG tract. It is most likely time to abandon this old, unsafe practice and leave changing the gastrostomy tube to the physician, although doing so may be inconvenient. Going a brief time without formula and water will not hurt the resident. Inability to administer the feeding is comparable to keeping the resident NPO before any other surgical procedure. Medication administration may be a problem when the tube is out, however.

Resident 1's PEG tube was inserted surgically with an endoscope through his mouth and esophagus into his stomach. A stab incision was then made through the wall of the abdomen into the stomach, creating a track through which the tube exited. He was started on PEG feedings that he tolerated well without complications. At the time of his discharge from the hospital, his lungs were clear. Resident 1 was discharged to the facility at 7:00 P.M. on January 21, 2000, with orders that included PEG feedings and aspiration precautions. Although in restraints at the time of his admission to the facility, nursing notes describe him as "calm," and the restraints were removed. According to a treatment note, the resident's family was visiting that evening, but when they left the room, at 10:30 P.M., he pulled the PEG tube out. Resident 1's treating physician had delegated to his physician's assistant (PA) the authority to issue orders to care for patients, and, on the night of January 21, 2000, she was on call. According to treatment notes, at 10:35 P.M., facility staff called her to report the PEG's removal, and she issued orders to replace it. In her testimony, the PA flatly denied ordering facility staff to reinsert the PEG tube at the facility, but claimed that she instructed the LVN on duty to send Resident 1 to the emergency room.

On April 5, 2000, an individual called the Texas Department of Human Services (State Agency) to complain that the facility had provided inappropriate care to one of its residents (Resident 1). According to the complainant, Resident 1 pulled out a recently-inserted feeding tube. Instead of transferring him to an acute care hospital for reinsertion of the tube, as his family requested, the facility's director of nursing (DON) performed the procedure, but, according to the complainant, she incorrectly reinserted the tube so that it did not go into his stomach. The resident became acutely ill, was hospitalized, and died shortly thereafter. Responding to the complaint, the State Agency conducted a complaint investigation survey on May 9, 2000, and determined that from

January 21 through 22, 2000, the facility was not in substantial compliance with the requirements set forth in 42 C.F.R. § 483.20(k)(3)(i), because services provided to Resident 1 did not meet professional standards of quality. CMS agreed, and, by letter dated May 31, 2000, advised Petitioner of its decision to impose a per-instance civil money penalty (CMP) of $10,000 based on this instance of noncompliance.

Both the LVN and DON challenge the PA's testimony. According to the DON, the LVN on duty called her home at 10:30 to say that Resident 1 had pulled out his PEG tube. She instructed the LVN to ask the PA to come into the facility to replace the tube. The DON further testified that the PA also called her at about 10:30 P.M. and they specifically discussed that the tube was new. Because the DON lived closer to the facility, she agreed to go in and replace it. The DON did not document the conversation.

Moreover, in a statement dated February 14, 2000, the DON described her 10:45 P.M. telephone conversation with the PA, but did not mention any discussion of the PEG tube. According to the DON's February 14 statement, she and the PA discussed whether to use wrist restraints. The surveyor notes reflect the surveyor's May 2, 2000, interview of the DON. According to the notes, the DON called the PA and they discussed restraining with hands and body wrap. Again, the DON did not mention any discussion of the tube. The PA flatly denied having a conversation about the PEG tube with the DON. When she was interviewed by the surveyor, she said that if she'd been told the tube was new, she would have insisted that Resident 1 be sent to the emergency room (ER). On the other hand, the LVN told the surveyor that she told the PA that she could not replace the tube because it was new and she did not replace new tubes, indicating that the PA knew or should have known that this was a newly inserted tube.

In any event, both parties agree, and the treatment records confirm, that at 11:00 P.M., the DON came into the facility and reinserted the PEG tube. The DON testified that she inserted the tube, expressed stomach contents, instilled 30 cc's of air and listened with her stethoscope over the stomach to hear air. She did not document that she checked for tube placement, but an 11:00 P.M. nursing note signed by the LVN states: "PEG tube #22 Fr. [with] 15 balloon insert per RN, DON [without] any difficulty. Gastric secretions noted - aw part flushed [with] 50 cc H2O -Resident tol (sic) procedure well." Subsequent notes signed by the LVN describe the resident as "constantly picking" at his abdomen. At 3:00 A.M. he again pulled out the PEG tube. The PA was again notified, and the nursing note states: "orders to replace peg tube or transfer to ER." Again, in her testimony, the PA denies having ordered tube replacement at the facility. A 3:25 A.M. entry signed by the LVN states: "unable to insert PEG tube at present time," suggesting that she attempted, but failed, to reinsert the tube. In her affidavit, the LVN does not mention or explain this entry, although, according to the survey report form, she told the surveyor that she unsuccessfully attempted to replace the tube after the DON told her that "a new G/T is the same as [an] old GT." However, the LVN affidavit includes no reference at all to her early morning telephone call to the DON.

The DON testified that she went home after reinserting the tube at 11:00 P.M., but that at 3:30 A.M., the LVN called her at home to say that the resident had again pulled out his tube. The DON returned to the facility, reinserted the tube, and, according to her testimony, she checked for gastric juices, instilled air, flushed with 50 cc's of water. Both she and the LVN auscultated. Again, she did not document. A 3:45 A.M. entry in the treatment record confirms that the DON inserted the PEG tube, and the tube was flushed, but says nothing about her (or the LVN) checking for appropriate placement. A 4:00 A.M. entry indicates that the resident tolerated feeding. At 5:00 A.M., the LVN's last entry describes the resident as resting quietly in bed, but "rubs" abdomen at "intervals - Denies pain." Entries made by different staff at 6:00 A.M. and 9:00 A.M. indicate that the LVN checked on PEG placement. The 6:00 note contains no detail, but the 9:00 note indicates that the LVN checked the PEG tube via aspiration of stomach contents and air auscultation, that the PEG was in place, and that she administered medications and fed him. However, when the LVN next checked on the resident, at 11:15 A.M., her note describes rapid respiration and bilateral lung congestion. She states that the PEG tube is in place, but does not explain the method by which she made that assessment. The facility called the PA, who instructed staff to send the resident to the emergency room.

The resident was picked up by ambulance at 11:40 A.M. According to the EMS (emergency medical services) report, the facility reported that Resident 1 rapidly developed difficulty breathing. He is described as in respiratory distress, skin pale, very diaphoretic, rales up and down, right and left lobes. When Resident 1 left the facility, he was in critical condition. He was admitted to the hospital at 12:10 P.M. on January 22, 2000, in respiratory distress, with aspiration pneumonia. The Emergency Room physician listed sepsis among his clinical impressions. The admitting physician also noted Resident 1's recent PEG tube placement and history of aspiration, "which could obviously have occurred with this episode."

Soon thereafter, the hospital noted problems with Resident 1's PEG tube, which was placed on wall suction at 3:30 P.M. the afternoon of January 22. Treatment records from then through January 23, 2000, indicate that PEG tube suction was draining "thick cloudy material," later described as "thick purulent type material," with "large amounts of mucous," which continued to drain from the PEG tube throughout the day and into the next day. By evening, the staff withheld his Depakote because of the large amount of output from the PEG tube. It appears that the Depakote was the only medication he received at the hospital by tube. Most of his medications were administered subcutaneously or through an IV. Throughout his time at the hospital, he was given a total of four doses of Depakote, but did not receive tube feedings.

An abdominal x-ray taken January 24 showed "leakage into the free peritoneal cavity from the PEG tube." The radiologist opined the free peritoneal air was explained by recent placement of a PEG tube. On the morning of January 24, Resident 1's family signed permission for an exploratory laparotomy, which was performed and confirmed that he had "peritonitis due to intraperitoneal tube feedings."

Resident 1 died on January 29, 2000. His final diagnoses included pneumonia, acute respiratory failure, pulmonary embolism and infarct, anoxic brain damage, gastrostomy complication, peritonitis, (8) rib fracture, disorder of the peritoneum, Alzheimer's disease, dementia, and fracture of the clavicle.

(From: IN THE CASE OF IHS at Theron Grainger - v - Centers for Medicare & Medicaid Services. June 20, 2002. Docket No.C-00-606, Decision No. CR922.)

Lawsuits associated with gastrostomy tubes

Surprisingly, gastrostomy tubes are implicated as a factor in many lawsuits. Failure to feed or hydrate the resident was noted above, and the example above is not an isolated problem. Aspiration and inhalation of formula are also problematic. A surprising number of legal actions occur as a result of gastrostomy tube migration as a result of using (longer) Foley catheters in place of gastrostomy tubes, and improper insertion and placement check procedures.

The case history here is from the State of Texas,[18] but situations similar to this have occurred and are applicable in every state. The very real plausibility for gastrostomy tube migration exists, with the potential for aspiration, peritonitis, and resident death. When developing policies and procedures for gastrostomy tube replacement, begin by learning your state nursing board position on the procedure. In this situation, the State of Texas *does permit* nurses to reinsert gastrostomy tubes into an established tract. However, the operative term here is "established." The resident in this situation had a fresh tract. The Texas Board of Nurse Examiners notes:

> *"The Board approved curriculum for both vocational nurses and registered nurses does not provide graduates with sufficient instruction to ascertain that a nurse has the necessary knowledge, skills and ability to reinsert and determine correct placement of a permanently placed feeding tube (such as a gastrostomy or jejunostomy tubes). The Board does allow LVNs and RNs to expand their practice beyond the basic educational preparation through post-licensure continuing education and training for certain tasks and procedures. One of the main considerations in determining whether or not a nurse should consider reinsertion of a gastrostomy, jejunostomy or similar feeding tube is how long the original tube was in place before becoming dislodged. Though sources vary, most give a range of 8–12 weeks for maturation/healing of the fistulous tract and stoma formation. The method of initial insertion (surgical, endoscopy, or radiographic guidance) may impact the length of healing. Orders should be obtained from the patient's physician regarding reinsertion guidelines. It is the opinion of the Board that LVNs and RNs should not engage in the reinsertion of a permanently placed feeding tube through an established tract until the LVN or RN successfully completes a competency validation course congruent with prevailing nursing practice standards. Training should provide instruction on the nursing knowledge and skills applicable to tube replacement and verification of correct and incorrect placement. The BNE does not define nor set qualifications for competency validation courses."* [19]

Establishing facility policies and procedures

If your facility policies and procedures permit nurses to change tubes in established gastrostomy tracts, consider adding the following to your required protocols:

- Pay close attention to insertion technique and monitoring of the resident after placement. [20]

- Prohibit the use of Foley catheters. Use a tube that has been manufactured for use in a gastrostomy. Made of silicone and polyurethane, gastrostomy tubes are very durable and less likely to be damaged by gastric secretions than latex tubes (such as an indwelling catheter).[21]

- Carefully secure the feeding tube to prevent dislodgement or internal migration. After initial placement, mark the tube with tape or indelible ink. Most long-term tubes have markings imprinted into the tubing. Document external length of tubing.[22]

- Prevent tube displacement by using the external marks on the tube, noting the length of the tube where it exits from the body. If the tube has no permanent marks, measure from the level of the exit site to the external end. Document this length. A nurse on each subsequent shift should measure and verify the external length. The nurse should also check to be sure the disk, suture, or attachment device holding the tube externally is secure.[23]

- Confirm proper tube placement by x-ray before initiating feeding. Start feedings slowly.[24]

- Assess the residual tube fluid for presence of GI secretions (gastric juice or bile) to determine that the tube is within the GI tract. If you are unable to aspirate fluid from the tube and suspect it has migrated, confirm placement by x-ray before feeding. A number of tube anchoring devices are available to help secure the tube.[25]

- If the resident has a gastrostomy tube with a balloon, check the fluid volume in the balloon every seven to 10 days. Withdraw fluid, document the volume and compare with the amount previously instilled, and return liquid to reinflate the balloon. Consult the manufacturer's literature to determine what the balloon volume should be and make sure the fluid volume is the same amount as originally instilled. If the volume is less, visually assess for a leak and refill to the manufacturer's recommended volume. [26]

Gastrostomy tube plugging

Gastrostomy tube plugging is a common reason for changing the tube. Your objective should be to eliminate risks for tube plugging to reduce the frequency of tube changes. Begin by reviewing the medication regimen. Make sure that liquid medications are used as much as possible. If pills must be given, inservice nurses on proper administration techniques, and follow up with direct observation at the bedside. In practice, medications are often not given correctly when the resident has a gastrostomy tube. The two most important considerations are:

- Crush each pill to a fine powder in a separate cup. Dilute the pill by mixing with warm water before administering through a feeding tube. Administer each pill separately.

- Administer 30 to 60 mL water *before* and *after* each medication.

Many anecdotal methods are used to unplug feeding tubes. Facilities commonly irrigate the tube with cola, cranberry juice, or distilled water. Some report using enzymatic contact lens cleaners. A combination of Viokase and one sodium bicarbonate tablet is also reportedly effective. Warm water is most often recommended.[27]

Never leave the management of gastrostomy tubes to chance or nursing judgment. Consider all potential risks and complications associated with tube feeding practices, and address them through the quality assurance committee and educational programs. Check the current literature to ensure your facility protocols and practice meet the applicable standards of care!

References

1. American Nurses Association. (1997). Position statement nutrition screening for the elderly. Washington, D.C. American Nurses Publishing.

2. November 29, 2004. Study: Nursing home residents dying of hunger, thirst. *Consumer Reports*. Online. *www.consumeraffairs.com/news04/nursing_home_neglect.html.* Accessed 01/11/06.

3. American Nurses Association (eds). (1998). *Standards of Clinical Nursing Practice 2nd Edition.* Washington, D.C. American Nurses Publishing.

4. Onder G, et al. Serum cholesterol levels and in-hospital mortality in the elderly. *Am J Med* September 2003;115: 265-71.

5. Grant MD; Piotrowski ZH; Miles TP. Declining cholesterol and mortality in a sample of older nursing home residents. *J Am Geriatr Soc*, 44:31-6.1996.

6. Chidester JC and Spangler AA. (1997). Fluid intake in the institutionalized elderly. *Journal of the American Dietetic Association* 97:23-28. 1997.

7. Campbell-Taylor I. *Malnutrition and dehydration in the elderly*. Online. *www.seniorhealthcare.org/.* Accessed 9/26/03.

8. Priddle, M. Nature's Ale . . . Water and hydration. *PHARMAwise* newsletter. Online. *www.classiccare.on.ca.* Accessed 09/10/03.

9. Kendall KA; Leonard RJ; McKenzie SW. (2001). Accommodation to changes in bolus viscosity in normal deglutition: a videofluoroscopic study. Ann Otol Rhinol Laryngol 2001 Nov; 110(11): 1059-65

10. Porter C; Schell ES; Kayser-Jones J; Paul SM. (1999). Dynamics of nutrition care among nursing home residents who are eating poorly. *J Am Diet Assoc*: 1444-6. 1999.

11. Kayser-Jones J; Schell E. (1997). The mealtime experience of a cognitively impaired elder: ineffective and effective strategies. *J Gerontol Nurs*;23:33-9. 1997.

12. Mitchell SL, Kiely DK, Lipsitz LA. (1998). Does artificial enteral nutrition prolong the survival of institutionalized elders with chewing and swallowing problems? J Gerontol A Biol Sci Med Sci 1998 May;53(3):M207-13.

13. Methany N, Eisenberg P, McSweeney M. (1998). Effect of feeding tube properties and three irrigants on clogging rates. *Nurs Res.* 1988;37(3):165-169.

14. After surgery, man's esophagus punctured by nasal tube. (2006). *Verdict Search*. Online. *www.verdict-search.com/jv3_news/newsletter/nat/053106/1.jsp.*

15. American Gastroenterological Association. (1994). American Gastroenterological Association Medical Position Statement: Guidelines for the Use of Enteral Nutrition 1994.

16. Bowers, S. (2000). All about tubes: Your guide to enteral feeding devices. *Nursing* 2000, December. Springnet Publications.

17. Guenter, P. (2001). Mechanical complications in long-term feeding tubes. *Nursing Spectrum*. Online. *http://nsweb.nursingspectrum.com/ce/ce201.htm.* Accessed 9/3/01.

18. IN THE CASE OF IHS at Theron Grainger - v - Centers for Medicare & Medicaid Services. June 20, 2002. Docket No.C-00-606, Decision No. CR922.

19. Texas Board of Nurse Examiners. (2005). 15.24 Nurses engaging in reinsertion of permanently placed feeding tubes. *www.bne.state.tx.us/position.htm.* Accessed 01/06/06.

20. American Gastroenterological Association. (1994). American Gastroenterological Association Medical Position Statement: Guidelines for the Use of Enteral Nutrition 1994.

21. Bowers, S. (2000). All about tubes: Your guide to enteral feeding devices. *Nursing* 2000, December. Springnet Publications.

22. Bowers, S. (2000). All about tubes: Your guide to enteral feeding devices. *Nursing* 2000, December. Springnet Publications.

23. Guenter, P. (2001). Mechanical complications in long-term feeding tubes. *Nursing Spectrum.* Online *http://nsweb.nursingspectrum.com/ce/ce201.htm.* Accessed 9/3/01.

24. Bowers, S. (2000). All about tubes: Your guide to enteral feeding devices. *Nursing* 2000, December. Springnet Publications.

25. Guenter, P. (2001). Mechanical complications in long-term feeding tubes. *Nursing Spectrum.* Online *http://nsweb.nursingspectrum.com/ce/ce201.htm.* Accessed 9/3/01.

26. Bowers, S. (2000). All about tubes: Your guide to enteral feeding devices. *Nursing* 2000, December. Springnet Publications.

27. Methany N, Eisenberg P, McSweeney M. (1998). Effect of feeding tube properties and three irrigants on clogging rates. *Nurs Res.* 1988;37(3):165-169.

Injuries precipitated by progressive failures and omissions of care

This is a civil liability case in which it has become necessary for Plaintiffs to bring a lawsuit by reason of the profound neglect suffered by Mary Doe during her residency at MNOP Health Services, which resulted in great physical and mental injuries, considerable consequential damages, and ultimately, her death. The serious bodily injuries and death made the basis of this lawsuit were proximately caused by the negligence and negligence per se of the named Defendants or their agents or employees acting in the course and scope of their employment. These acts or omissions were the acts or omissions of Defendants themselves, and not simply the acts or omissions of Defendants' lower level employees. Additionally, or in the alternative, the conduct complained of was:

(a) authorized by Defendants;

(b) the conduct of employees Defendants employed in a managerial capacity who were acting in the scope of that capacity;

(c) the conduct of unfit employees Defendants recklessly employed; or

(d) ratified by an employee or manager of Defendants.

Additionally, or in the alternative, the conduct complained of was a vice-principal of Defendants or was conduct that breached non-delegable duties of Defendants.

(From a petition of an actual lawsuit alleging progressive failures and omissions of care.)

Restorative nursing care and the OBRA '87 legislation

Rehabilitation (rehab) and restorative nursing care (restorative) is given to assist residents to attain and maintain the highest level of physical, mental, and psychosocial function possible in light of each resident's individual, unique situation. Rehab and restorative care are based on a belief in the dignity and worth of each resident. The residents' individual abilities, strengths, and needs are considered. To understand restorative nursing, you must first understand the purpose and philosophy of the OBRA '87 legislation. In fact, reading the MDS manual from cover to cover should give you an idea of the commitment the government has made to holistic, restorative care.

Holistic care

The medical model of care emphasizes diagnosing and treating the residents' illness or medical condition. To some extent, nurses in many long-term care facilities practice under this model, because this is the way they were educated, and may be the only way they know. OBRA '87 was designed to eliminate the medical model, replacing it with holistic care. Rehabilitation and restoration are important parts of holistic care. These services improve self-esteem and quality of life. To use the holistic model, nurses must look at the entire person. If one body system becomes weak, the other systems will initially compensate for it. Over time, one weak system will adversely affect other systems and cause declines throughout the body. Likewise, one unmet psychosocial need can, over time, affect the entire person.

When caring for residents holistically, view each resident as a whole person, a complex being with many strengths and needs, both physical and mental. Recognize and identify unmet needs (either psychosocial or physical) that affect the resident. Avoid viewing residents as medical conditions (e.g., "the hip fracture in 208")! Each is a unique individual, a member of a family and a community. Their families love them. They were children once. They have a past. They have contributed to society. No two residents are exactly alike. When providing holistic care, the nurse sees the uniqueness and value of each resident. Look for the value and stress the importance of seeing the whole person to the nursing assistant staff. This is what OBRA '87 is all about.

Declines

An important part of OBRA '87 addresses declines in condition. The ANA standards note, "Gerontological nursing practice involves assessing the health and functional status of aging adults, planning and providing appropriate nursing and other health care services, and evaluating the effectiveness of such care. Emphasis is placed on maximizing functional ability in activities of daily living (ADLs); promoting, maintaining, and restoring health; preventing and minimizing disabilities of acute and chronic illness; and maintaining life in dignity and comfort until death."[1]

Declines may be large or small. When using the medical model of care, nurses accept declines as unavoidable. Under the medical model, declines are a normal part of the aging process and the effects of chronic

illness. Under OBRA, declines are not permitted in any area of the resident's life, unless they are medically unavoidable. Although a decline may be truly unavoidable, the facility remains responsible for taking measures to slow and delay deterioration. If a progressive decline develops, the facility should take steps to minimize the effect of the decline on overall function as much as possible. Documentation must support unavoidability and show the facility tried to prevent or slow the decline. This is usually tracked by reviewing the care plans.

Risk factors are conditions that have the potential to cause the resident's health to worsen, or suggest a problem may develop. Identifying risk factors is a key nursing responsibility. Risk factors are identified through a combination of common sense, various assessments, physical findings, and medical diagnoses. The presence of one or more risk factors does not equal inevitability of any condition. Once the risk of developing complications is known, nursing care is given to reduce the risk, thus preventing the complication or mitigating its effects. Planning preventive care is an important nursing function that is essential for positive outcomes to be achieved.

Some declines are obvious immediately, such as skin tears and injuries. However, these are reversible. Of great concern are the many subtle, progressive problems such as contractures and incontinence that develop gradually, over a period of time. Many long-term care facility residents have declined gradually over a period of years. Because of turnover, and the expectation that aging residents will decline over time, staff members may not realize the significance of the deterioration. Ask long-term staff how residents were several years ago. Compare their former conditions with the residents' conditions today in major activities of daily living. You will probably notice many declines, particularly in the area of bowel and bladder control. This is a particular problem in long-term care facilities, where many staff become desensitized to residents' incontinence. It is estimated that 50% of all long-term care residents have urinary incontinence. Surprisingly, one study revealed that 22% of female residents and 56% of males who were continent on admission had become incontinent at the end of a year in the facility. The reasons for the deterioration were identified as deterioration in mobility, cognitive decline, and normal adjustment to the facility environment. Once a pattern of incontinence begins, reversing it is difficult.[2]

Because of staffing and other problems and priorities, residents may not be taken to the bathroom regularly. Nurses routinely document that residents are toileted every two hours, but many admit this is because toileting is the care that is *supposed to be given,* not the care that was *actually* done. Some residents display behavior problems when they need to use the toilet, but staff may not recognize and connect the problem with the discomfort of needing to use the bathroom. Thus, residents lose control over bowel and bladder after admission to the long-term care facility. Another facet of this problem is caused by lack of familiarity with assessment-based management and the many different, effective approaches to use for managing incontinence.

OBRA requires facilities to use all of their resources to assist residents to attain and maintain the highest level of function possible in their unique, individual situation. Resources can be internal or external, from within or outside of the facility. As you can see, OBRA requirements are almost identical to the definition of rehabilitation and restoration.

The plan of care

Thoughtfully developing, maintaining, and using the care plan is a key to making restorative nursing care work. This may be a surprisingly difficult notion, because many long-term care nurses provide care without ever looking at the care plan. Nursing assistants must be familiar with the residents' goals and approaches. For restorative nursing to succeed, all care must be in keeping with the restorative goals and approaches. Using this method of care provides continuity, because all staff must be moving in the same direction. Some residents progress quickly when proper restorative care is given. Others make slow, steady progress. Another group will remain stable and not decline. The key here is that all the residents benefit, and many make progress! This is what the OBRA legislation really wants! Many facilities have a position called "Restorative Nursing Assistant." This is admirable. However, delivering proper restorative care and meeting the intent of the OBRA legislation takes a team! One nursing assistant cannot be expected to meet each resident's restorative nursing needs each day. The scope of the need is simply too great. Additional keys to successful restorative nursing are

- consistency

- all staff understanding and implementing the restorative philosophy

- continuity of care, based on an accurate, individualized care plan used by staff daily

- good communication

Range of motion

§483.25(e) Range of motion.
Based on the comprehensive assessment of a resident, the facility must ensure that §483.25(e)(1) A resident who enters the facility without a limited range of motion does not experience reduction in range of motion unless the resident's clinical condition demonstrates that a

reduction in range of motion is unavoidable; and §483.25(e)(2) A resident with a limited range of motion receives appropriate treatment and services to increase range of motion and/or to prevent further decrease in range of motion.

Contractures

Contractures are a shortening and deformity of muscles or connective tissue around joints from lack of use. This shortening prevents extension and normal range of joint movement. Range of motion is the normal movement that muscles go through during activities of daily living. Passive range of motion maintains muscle flexibility, but does not improve strength. A contracture develops when the muscle fibers become unable to flex. Each muscle has an antagonist that works in the opposite direction. If the muscle group is not moved for a period of time or if proper body alignment is not maintained, the stronger muscles will predominate, causing contracture deformities.[3] Risk factors for contractures include nerve or muscle disease, including stroke, head injury, and neuromuscular diseases.

"This is a civil liability case in which it has become necessary for Plaintiffs to bring a lawsuit by reason of the profound neglect suffered by John Doe during his residency at ABC Care Center, which resulted in great physical and mental injuries, considerable consequential damages, and ultimately, his death. Such serious damages included, but are not limited to: severe and painful contractures of his elbows, wrists, fingers, hips, knees, and ankles."

(From a petition of an actual lawsuit alleging progressive failures and omissions of care.)

Most residents are weaker than they were when they were living independently in the community. Con-

tractures place already-weakened muscles in a position of mechanical disadvantage. As the contracture progresses, movement is limited, and the joint becomes fixed, making the contracture permanent. Residents with neurological problems and existing contractures are at high risk for developing additional contractures. Contractures also present as an additional risk factor for pressure ulcer development. The muscle rigidity and tightening promote capillary occlusion in the bony prominences. One source has estimated that 60% of all wounds involve some sort of unattended contracture.[4] In any event, contractures are serious complications of immobility, making voluntary movement painful, difficult, or impossible, and complicating the nursing care delivered by unlicensed staff. Contractures make ADL care, dressing, grooming, moving, and positioning the resident much more difficult and painful.

Assessment of joint range of motion is an important part of restorative nursing. You must have some type of baseline knowledge of the resident's joint motion to show you have maintained or improved function. Residents can begin to develop contractures in as little as four days. Most nurses do not recognize a contracture until it is Stage III, at 45 degrees. Reversing a contracture at this point takes months, but can take years. Most contractures can be reversed if detected before the joint is immobilized completely.

Contractures are often painful, feeling much like cramps that athletes get from overexertion. An athlete with a muscle cramp can stretch and work it out. A resident with this type of pain cannot, so he or she is forced to endure the pain in silence. Women who wear high heels all day often complain of pain when they remove the shoes and place their feet on the floor. This is because the muscles have contracted and are being stretched out again. This discomfort is comparable to the pain from a foot drop contracture, but the resident is unable to flex and extend the muscle repeatedly, which is necessary to relieve the pain. Women who remove high heels do this effortlessly when they begin to walk. Many malpractice suits against long-term care facilities involve residents with both contractures and pressure ulcers. However, the presence of contractures is a serious deterioration for which the facility can be sued, despite the presence of other problems. This makes the case for prevention clear.

Measuring joint mobility

Assess joint range of motion on initial (admission) assessment and quarterly after that. For accuracy, a therapist should measure joint mobility with a goniometer. Some nursing forms have pictures that show degrees of joint mobility. These are used for screening by comparing the resident's degree of joint mobility to the picture. If the angle is abnormal, the resident is referred to therapy for follow-up and possible intervention. If the resident is at risk, a restorative nursing program is developed to prevent or reverse the contractures. Restorative care of the resident involves using pillows, props, and supportive devices, maintaining good body alignment, and providing range of motion exercises two to three times daily.

Preventive care

Risk factor identification and contracture prevention are major nursing responsibilities. Nursing interventions to prevent contractures include

- encouraging and helping residents to be as active as possible

- repositioning every two hours or more often

- providing active and passive range of motion exercises

- using pillows, props, and adaptive positioning devices to keep the extremities properly positioned in extension

- using splints, cones, and other orthotics to maintain joint position and function

- recognizing risk factors and signs of impending contracture and consulting with therapists and other professionals to develop a viable plan of care

Avoid homemade devices such as rolled washcloths to prevent hand contractures. The texture of the washcloth promotes squeezing, worsening the contracture. Consult an occupational therapist for alternatives or use commercial handroll devices.

Incontinence, inadequate personal care

> Plaintiff, in this case, seeks punitive damages in an amount commensurate with: (a) the nature of the wrongs committed by Defendants; (b) the inhumane character of Defendants' course of conduct; (c) the degree of culpability of the wrongdoers herein; (d) the helpless and dependent nature of the victims in this case; and (e) the severity, frequency, and degree to which the conduct described hereinabove offends the public sense of justice. Defendants' conduct alleged hereinabove justifies an award of exemplary damages in an amount sufficient to deter Defendants from engaging in the conduct referenced herein in the future.
>
> *(From a petition of an actual lawsuit alleging progressive failures and omissions of care.)*

Problems with urinary elimination overlap slightly in Chapters 9, 14, and 16. Several distinct issues are seen in lawsuits:

- The facility was not properly cleaned and was known to have pervasive, permeating urine odors.

- Failure to keep the resident clean and failure to provide bathing, personal hygiene, and incontinent care are common factors. (These issues may be related to a primary physical problem, such as pressure ulcers.)

- Mental anguish and loss of self-esteem related to failure to manage incontinence, failure to provide incontinent care, and failure to maintain the resident's personal hygiene. (This is associated with the self-esteem and quality of life issues relating to being soiled with excretions and having an odor.)

- Recurrent urinary tract infections (The plaintiff may also allege mismanagement of an infection, such as when the facility administers a drug to which the causative organism is resistant.)

- Failure to support dignity and quality of life related to failure to provide a proper retraining or management program.

- Urosepsis and related complications resulting from failure to identify and properly address signs and symptoms of infection or mismanagement of an infection.

Urosepsis

When urosepsis is a component of the lawsuit, the attorneys will also investigate

- the resident's overall condition prior to illness (chronic medical conditions, immunocompromised state)

- whether the facility provided sufficient fluids to maintain and support hydration in the presence of UTI; if the resident is dehydrated, his or her condition is more fragile, and he or she is susceptible to renal failure from insufficient fluid

- whether the facility accurately documented, monitored, and assessed the meaning of intake and output values; in some states, documenting I&O is a component of Medicaid reimburse-

ment for UTI management. Nurses record the numbers as a means of paper compliance, but fail to analyze their meaning associated with the infection and overall renal function

- the resident's overall nutritional status; whether there is an associated weight loss

- whether the facility provided alternative methods of nutrition (if needed)

- whether a dietary consult was requested in presence of weight loss or dehydration

- appropriate and timely recognition of illness/signs and symptoms of infection

- whether nurses recognized the significance of hypothermia, if present

- appropriate and timely notification of physician and responsible party

- appropriate and timely laboratory diagnostic testing obtained and results timely reported to the physician

- appropriate and timely interventions/cultures/ antibiotic treatment sensitive to specific organisms

- monitoring and documenting the resident's response to antibiotics (improvement vs. need for different therapy)

- validation of proper personal hygiene, perineal care, incontinent care, or Foley catheter care (if present)

- urology consult requested and obtained, if recurrent episodes of infection

- other infection control measures employed, such as contact precautions (if indicated)

- assessment of kidney function, CBC, blood and urine culture

- presence of other concurrent infections (pressure ulcers, respiratory infections, etc.)

- administration of medications that make the resident more prone to infections (i.e., steroids, recurrent antibiotics for treatment of asymptomatic UTIs); if so, whether special monitoring was done and identified on the care plan

- timely notification of the physician for changes in condition, such as fever, hypothermia, urine with sediment, foul-smelling urine, increased WBC

- evidence of septic shock (diminished mental status, confusion, labile blood pressure, decreased output, organ failure, hypothermia)

- evidence the facility monitored for signs of infection during and after treatment for urinary infection; evidence the facility rechecked the urinalysis 72 hours post-antibiotic to ensure the pathogen was eliminated

Facility cleanliness

Facilities are expected to keep the environment clean and the residents clean. There is not much more to say on the subject. A pervasive odor of urine or stool in the facility suggests that cleanliness is not adequate, and provides a negative impression to all who enter the facility. The problem must be corrected by eliminating odors at the source, rather than covering them up. Pervasive odors may be multifactorial, such as

- soiled personal clothing in open containers in residents' closets

- open trash cans and linen hampers

- cracks in mattresses through which urine has leaked and collected

- unclean residents

- residents wearing soiled clothing

- urine has seeped under floor tiles in bathrooms and other areas

- residents voiding in plants and other inappropriate areas

- check the residents' shoes; athletic shoes and leather shoes tend to retain urine odors

All contributing factors must be identified and eliminated to eradicate a pervasive odor problem permanently.

Other considerations

Industry-wide, application of incontinence management programs has been suboptimal.[5] Nurses are often aware that more resources are needed to address incontinence problems adequately. When questioned, staff listed the following reasons as barriers, causing them to be unable to provide more effective incontinence management programs:

- lack of available time and staff resources

- lack of authority to change existing staff (or facility) practices

- lack of administrative support

- lack of physician support

- lack of support from other staff

- increased cost of an effective incontinence management program; one study revealed the cost was $9.09 per patient day; of this 50% of the cost was labor[6]

One study revealed that continence could be improved through a combination of incontinence management and exercise, without increasing facility costs.[7] In considering the listed reasons for not providing improved incontinence care, improved resident self-esteem and quality of life are the primary reasons for initiating a program.

Chapter sixteen

The incontinence problem

Urinary incontinence is a major problem in long-term care facilities. Incontinence is a decline, according to the OBRA '87 definitions. Incontinence is a medical problem that is typically beyond the resident's control. Incontinence is not a normal consequence of aging, and can frequently be cured or improved. Many treatable problems contribute to incontinence. Some residents have several coexisting problems. To manage the incontinence successfully, all must be identified and treated.

Many facilities use medical aids when caring for residents with incontinence. Staff sometimes call the medical aids used for managing incontinence *"diapers."* This term is demeaning. Instead use *"adult brief,"* *"garment protector,"* or *"clothing protector,"* or call the product by the brand name. Avoid actions or words that affect the resident's self-esteem.

The problem of incontinence in long-term care facilities is often related to failure of staff, although we are not willing to admit it. Over time, staff become insensitive to incontinence. Remember that the sensation of needing to use the toilet is *one of the last to be lost* in cognitively impaired residents. The problem is often one of communication. The residents cannot express the need to use the bathroom. Some scream, pull at clothing, disrobe, or display other behavior problems. These stop when the resident eliminates, but the staff may not realize it. If the resident is taken to the bathroom and seated on the toilet, he or she usually knows what to do.

Australian researchers have divided bladder control into three categories. Some facilities in the United States are successfully using these terms in their care plans.

- *Independent continence* is ability to maintain continence without assistance from others

- *Dependent continence* applies to residents who are kept dry by staff because of physical or mental impairments

- *Social continence* applies to residents who are continent because of regular toileting by staff or those who depend on incontinent pads to contain urine.

Incontinence management versus active bladder retraining

Many nurses believe that toileting residents every two hours is the best means of keeping them dry, when in fact this is a dated method of management. Some believe toileting every two hours constitutes a formal retraining program. Likewise, this is an old wives' tale. Despite the prevalence of incontinence in long-term care, there is a dearth of efficacious, accurate information for nurses with which to address the programs. Avoid making assumptions about your staff's knowledge about incontinence management and retraining. Ask questions and see if their knowledge is accurate and current! Effective urinary management is assessment-based and individualized to the resident. *Incontinence management is a "catch" program that keeps residents dry. It is assessment-based, but it does not involve retraining or relearning. It involves toileting the resident at times in which he or she is most likely to eliminate.* Many residents will not be able to participate in active bowel and bladder retraining programs, but most will benefit from a regular, assessment-based toileting schedule.

Retraining is an active program that involves teaching the resident to identify sensations and relearn how to control the bladder. The key term here is relearning. Retraining is used only for residents with a potential to relearn. The relearning process involves learning how to resist the urge to void and become used to emptying the bladder at progressively increasing intervals. This is also an assessment-based program that is done according to an individualized resident schedule. This method of management does not involve toileting every two hours. The toileting schedule may be erratic, depending on the resident's need. Residents who have been recently admitted to the facility after an acute illness are often good candidates for active retraining. Most of these individuals have been living at home, and have only recently lost bladder control. Beginning treatment early optimizes results.

Overview of individualized bladder-management programs

If a resident is admitted with bowel and bladder control, the long-term care facility is expected to maintain this continence. If the resident is incontinent upon admission, the facility must assist him or her to attain and maintain the highest level of well-being possible. Typically, this means the facility can reduce the total number of incontinent episodes, with a proper plan of care and use of the nursing process. Bladder management is one of the most important restorative nursing programs that facilities carry out. As you can see, the old school of toileting residents every two hours is not effective. Developing an individual program based on the resident's needs is the key to success. Begin with an assessment. This involves taking an elimination history, evaluating the resident's incontinence pattern, and developing an individual toileting schedule. Using the nursing process, develop a plan based on the assessment results. Implement the plan for several days to a week, then reevaluate. You will probably find that modification and adjustment of the plan are necessary. Modify and implement the plan again. Continue evaluating and modifying until maximum success is achieved.

Initiating a facility continence management program

Individualized management programs work! Be enthusiastic, and make your enthusiasm contagious. Develop a reward system for your staff, such as a pizza party for successfully implementing this program. If staff are serious about this process, almost all residents show an improvement, regardless of the type of plan used. Sometimes paying close attention to the residents' elimination needs is all that is necessary to initiate improvement. Use caution, however. Developing individualized management and retraining programs creates a lot of work and requires exacting performance from your staff. The programs will increase their recordkeeping responsibilities. Do not be tempted to place an entire wing of residents on a management plan simultaneously, or you are setting the scene for failure. Begin with a few residents, or one from each section, depending on staffing. Teach your staff their responsibilities, make your expectations clear, and above all, *listen to their ideas.* They probably know the residents well. Start with residents with the greatest chance of success. As they complete the assessment and care plan modification period, begin assessing another resident. Do this, one resident at a time, until all residents have been assessed.

Management and retraining plans

There are two basic types of bladder management programs. For success, teach your staff how to differentiate between the two types. Eliminate "q2h" toileting from facility vocabulary and practices. The *incontinence management program* is used for residents who have no potential for retraining, but will eliminate successfully on the toilet (or bedpan, urinal, commode) if assisted by staff. *Bladder retraining* is an active program in which the resident learns to regain control of bladder function.

Begin with an assessment. Evaluate the history and other factors listed in the Assessment for Bowel &

Bladder Management, (on your forms CD-ROM) or use your facility forms. Simultaneously, instruct staff to check the resident hourly and record whether he or she is wet or dry. Document findings on the Assessment for Bowel and Bladder Management Programs, or use your facility forms. When you begin the program, clearly advise them not to offer to toilet the resident. During the initial assessment, their responsibility is to do nothing other than observing the resident, and cleaning incontinent episodes as they occur. However, if the resident asks to be taken to the bathroom, staff should honor the request.

During the assessment period, a pattern of fairly regular incontinent episodes usually emerges. The pattern may also provide clues regarding the type of incontinence. Advise staff that accurate completion of this analysis and good record keeping are very important. This is much more than paper compliance, because you depend on them to gather accurate data you will use to develop the plan of care. The toileting schedule is developed largely from the information and data they document, so checking hourly and recording the results accurately is critical. An erratic pattern of checks, gaps in data, inaccurate or poor record keeping will doom the plan to failure from the outset. For seven to 14 days, staff check the resident hourly and record their findings. Fourteen days is an arbitrary time frame. Sometimes a pattern will emerge in less time.

After the assessment period, gather all of the assessment data. Take it to a quiet area and study it. If you have questions, ask the staff. Do not worry if the pattern is erratic, such as voiding every three hours when in bed, but voiding every four hours when up. This is normal! If no pattern emerges, try to find out why. This is seldom due to cognitive impairment. Residents with no distinct pattern often have a urinary infection, neurogenic bladder, or another medical

problem. Prostatic enlargement is a common problem in male residents. Treat correctable problems, if possible, and make necessary environmental modifications. For example, if the assessment uncovers signs and symptoms of a urinary tract infection, do not attempt a management program until the infection is treated and eliminated. Reassess the incontinence pattern again before proceeding. You may wish to review the RAP guidelines to give you an idea of methods for management at this juncture.

Developing the plan

Develop the bladder management plan based upon the resident's

- previous habits

- routines

- recorded times of incontinent episodes

- patterns or preferences that emerge during the assessment period

Write a toileting schedule listing specific times to toilet the resident. Base the schedule on the resident's needs. A needs-based, individualized assessment may list erratic, or irregular toileting times. Some people can wait for five hours before urinating. Others urinate more often. The individualized schedule may reflect this type of pattern. Develop the schedule accordingly. For example, if the resident was incontinent at 9:00 a.m. four out of seven days, schedule toileting for 8:30 a.m. or 8:45 a.m. If the resident had a bowel movement five out of seven days immediately after lunch, schedule toileting 15 to 30 minutes before the approximate elimination time. An example of individualized, 24-hour assessment-based toileting times is

- 6:15 a.m., 9:00 a.m., 12:45 p.m., 2:15 p.m., 5:30 p.m., 9:30 p.m., 11:30 p.m., 2:30 a.m., 4:30 a.m.

Instruct nursing assistants about the toileting program, and describe how to implement it for the resident. Write a simple, clear plan of care. Punctuality, consistency, flexibility, a positive attitude, being available at toileting times, and accurate record keeping promote success. Motivate the staff. Believe that the program will succeed. Maintain your motivation and theirs. Instruct staff to toilet the resident at the designated times, recording each successful elimination and episode of incontinence. Again, emphasize the importance of staff availability at toileting times, and importance of accurate record keeping. Describe how nursing assistants should approach the resident. Teach them to avoid scolding the resident for failures, and sincerely compliment the resident for success.

Next, begin the program, reassessing the resident every three to seven days, or as often as necessary. Adjust the times as needed. The revision time schedule will vary, depending on how successful the resident is. Be patient and flexible. It may take several months for the resident to reach the highest level of independence. Continue adjusting the schedule until success is achieved. Be empathetic and supportive. Encourage the residents and staff. A coordinated team effort will help maintain the resident's dignity and self-esteem. Nursing assistants, too, will benefit if you sincerely compliment them on a job well done. Although the early stages of a toileting program are more work for staff, over the long-term, their jobs will be much easier. Your facility will remain in compliance with the OBRA '87 requirements, odors will be reduced, supply budgets decrease (glove and brief budgets can be used for other needed items), and your residents and staff will feel better about themselves.

Some facilities do not practice management or retraining during the night, but many believe that a 24-hour program is best for the residents. In these facilities, retraining continues at night, but the interval for toileting is increased to longer intervals when residents are asleep.

Importance of fluids

Encourage fluids during bladder management and retraining programs. Offer residents fluids they like and are most likely to accept. Restricting fluids to reduce voiding does not help the resident. Some facilities schedule and adjust fluid intake, but do not withhold fluids. Fluids are also given at scheduled times, allowing the bladder to fill. Initially, the goal is to wait for about two hours. The goal is progressively increased to every three to four hours. Scheduling toileting times and fluid times may be too labor intensive and too rigid/restrictive for some residents and facilities. Follow your facility policies and keep the residents' best interests in mind.

Recording the residents' intake and output is important. List this approach on the plan of care. Evaluate the intake and output daily during bladder management and retraining. This is more than recording numbers. Total the number each shift and cumulate the totals each 24 hours. Compare them with the dietitian's calculation of minimum daily fluid requirements. Write this number on the care plan. Ensure that daily fluid intake is adequate, based on the dietitian's calculation of the resident's fluid needs. Some facilities reduce fluids during the late evening and nighttime hours for residents on bladder management programs. This is a facility decision. The important consideration is that the resident meets his or her minimum body requirements each day.

Residents with catheters

Have you ever wondered why your residents are admitted to the hospital without a catheter, then return to you with a catheter in place? No good reason was identified in a comprehensive study of 1,586 hospital-ized senior citizens ages 70 and older at two Ohio hospi-tals.[8] In this study, 24% of the patients were catheterized unnecessarily. Of patients 85 or older, the rate of un-necessary catheterization was 32 percent. Patients with five or more risk factors had a 50% risk of being catheterized unnecessarily. Researchers noted that the risk of medically inappropriate catheterization was high-er among women, patients with disability or dementia, and patients admitted with a geriatric condition such as confusion or frequent falls. None of the 378 catheter-ized senior patients studied had a medical condition indicating a need for a catheter. The study's principle investigator, Seth Landefeld, MD noted that, "the people who are most likely to suffer the adverse effects of a urinary tract infection are exactly the peo-ple who seem to be getting unnecessary catheteriza-tions." This study identified nine specific risk factors for unnecessary catheterization:

1. female gender

2. chronic illness

3. cognitive impairment

4. incontinence

5. inability to carry out common activities of daily living

6. a physician's order for bed rest

7–9. three geriatric conditions–confusion, falls, and failure to thrive at home

The study did not examine the question of why un-necessary catheters are being placed. Dr. Landefeld stated, "Other studies have found that most doctors don't know whether their patient has a catheter in place or not," Landefeld notes. "It's something that happens frequently for reasons that have not been fully teased out. We need very obvious approaches that will

get people to think three times before placing the catheter—and once it's in, to think how quickly they can get it out." This is an area for which current research with medical and nursing guidelines is badly needed. Until that time, long-term care facilities should follow CMS guidelines and eliminate urinary catheters whenever possible. An abundance of medical and nurs-ing evidence exists to suggest that long-term catheter use is detrimental to the residents. In fact, catheter-related sepsis is seen in many lawsuits. One study was completed to learn whether the use of urinary catheters in long-term care facility residents affected morbidity and mortality. The researchers conducted a one-year prospective study among 1,540 residents in a stratified random sample of facilities. Resident mortality was assessed at one year in relation to the presence or absence of a catheter at entry to the study, acquisition of a catheter, and the proportion of long-term care facility days spent catheterized during the study year. At entry, 10.5% of residents had catheters. With few exceptions, these residents remained catheterized dur-ing most of the study year. An additional 10% were catheterized during the year. The following factors were found to have an independent relationship with increased mortality:

- urinary catheter

- age

- mental status

- activities of daily living

- cancer

- cardiac disease

- diabetes

- skin condition

During the study year, there was a progressive increase in mortality with duration of catheterization. Residents who were catheterized for 76% or more of their days in the long-term care facility were three times more likely to die within a year. The number of hospitalizations, duration of hospitalization, and use of antimicrobial drugs were all three times greater among catheterized residents.[9]

Urosepsis is a common problem in long-term care lawsuits. The Centers for Disease Control and Prevention (CDC) have published guidelines for prevention of catheter-associated urinary tract infections in hospitalized patients (Chapter 14). No such definitive guidelines exist for long-term care facilities, and the hospital recommendations generally are applicable and used to identify the standards of care for catheterized residents in long-term care facilities.[10]

One longstanding practice that needs medical clarification and nursing research is the prevalent practice of changing catheters monthly in the long-term care facility. The CDC guidelines state, "Indwelling catheters should not be changed at arbitrary fixed intervals." One source notes, "Although residents with newly placed catheters have quantitatively less bacteriuria, *routine catheter changes may not alter the course of bacteriuria or culture results and are not advocated.* Catheter-related bacteriuria is ever changing and not amenable to prophylactic antibiotics."[11] Consider the frequency of routine catheter changes in your quality assurance committee and develop an evidence-based plan.

Eliminating the catheter

Some long-term care facilities place residents on bladder management or retraining programs to remove an indwelling catheter. Several schools of thought are employed to manage these programs. One school removes the catheter and begins an assessment. This is the preferred method of retraining. Some facilities clamp and unclamp the catheter regularly. Theoretically,

this enables the resident to get used to the sensation of urine in the bladder. The catheter is opened to drain urine every two hours, then is immediately reclamped. The interval for draining the catheter is progressively increased until the resident is comfortable holding urine for three to four hours. The catheter is removed and a plan developed to keep the resident dry.

Evaluation

Successful bladder management or retraining does not happen overnight. However, a successful program is rewarding for both the residents and staff. As you can see, many individuals and departments are needed for successful bladder management and retraining. Your desire and commitment to assisting residents with bladder management will benefit many residents and the facility.

Resident cleanliness

When resident incontinence, hygiene, and cleanliness are components of a lawsuit, your flow sheets may become an important part of the discovery and trial. Flow sheet documentation is a perpetual problem in long-term care, so a proactive approach to this documentation is essential.

Interpretive Guidelines §483.75(l)(1)

A complete clinical record contains an accurate and functional representation of the actual experience of the individual in the facility. It must contain enough information to show that the facility knows the status of the individual, has adequate plans of care, and provides sufficient evidence of the effects of the care provided. Documentation should provide a picture of the resident's progress, including response to treatment, change in condition, and changes in treatment.

Nursing assistants usually work from an assignment sheet and some type of bath schedule. They document ADL care on a flow sheet. Because flow sheet documentation is problematic, licensed nurses are often required to document the ADL procedures. If this is the policy of your facility, ask yourself the purpose of this documentation. Are nurses documenting care *that has actually been given* or are they documenting care because they know *it is supposed to be done*? In most facilities, the ADL care is given by nursing assistants. The nurses have no way of verifying that every documentable procedure was done as ordered or required. If this is the case, you are probably on shaky legal ground. At the very least, make sure this documentation meets the spirit and intent of the requirements in your state. Signing or countersigning the nursing assistants' documentation generally means the nurse has verified that all required resident care has been provided. Facility policies must address the meaning of countersigned documentation; i.e., whether by documenting on a flow sheet the licensed nurse is verifying the care was provided, or simply that the nursing assistant had the authority and competence to perform the procedure.[12] Some facilities have solved the flow sheet problem by installing touch-screen computer terminals in convenient areas in which nursing assistants can document procedures and ADL care immediately after completing them.

Care that is not documented creates a legal inference that the care was not given. All nurses are familiar with the old maxim, "If it is not documented, it was not done." However, in practice, documentation may be omitted because resident care is the priority. This subsequently places the nurses in a precarious position of having to prove the care was given in the face of absent documentation. When this occurs, nurses usually use a "charting by exception" (CBE) excuse. The nurses will insist they had provided the required care and argue they only charted when significant changes occurred in the resident's condition. Charting by exception is a formal documentation system. It is not a haphazard excuse for failing to document. A legal nurse consultant can

readily determine whether the facility truly did have a formal CBE system. Most facilities do not. It should also be noted that juries have formerly found facilities using CBE to be negligent and higher courts have upheld the jury's decision on appeal.[13] Medicare intermediaries and third-party payers have denied claims when CBE was used. Objective, clear, and precise documentation is only one source of information. In a lawsuit situation, facility employees will also be questioned. Although they can probably attest to the fact that Mrs. Geary had a shower Saturday, remembering each and every shower over a prolonged period of time is impossible. Cases work their way through the courts slowly. It is inconceivable to think a staff member will accurately remember that the resident had a shower on any given day three years ago (or more).

Nothing remains to be said on the ADL issue. This is another area in which the facility may be judged by the public for things they use their five senses to identify. To prevent allegations of improper personal care, each facility must emphasize the need for facility cleanliness and resident hygiene. Residents with unusual odor problems may respond to administration of one of the chlorophyll preparations on the market. A body of research exists supporting the efficacy of chlorophyll for odor nullifications, but the product has never gained widespread acceptance, despite the relatively low incidence of side effects. Chlorophyll is not a substitute for cleanliness, but is a good adjunct to use when the resident has an offensive odor that does not respond to normal hygienic measures. Remember to evaluate the documentation system you are using to ensure it is accurate, thorough, concise, and supports the high-quality care the facility provides.

The nursing assistant care plan on your CD-ROM may be a useful adjunct for solving documentation problems.

Emotional distress

In the heat of battle, the plaintiff in a lawsuit will often ask for punitive damages because of injuries sustained at the hands of the defendant facility. The plaintiff commonly alleges that the nature of his or her injuries caused emotional torment, which developed as a result of inhumane conditions and negligent care of a persistent and longstanding nature.

> "This action is maintained by Plaintiff Jean Doe in her individual capacity, and by and through her next friend and power of attorney agent, Frances Doe, for all damages which Jean Doe may be justly entitled to because of the wrongful conduct made the basis of this suit, including but not limited to damages for the past and future: (a) pain; (b) suffering; (c) torment; (d) destruction of dignity; (e) disfigurement; (f) mental anguish; and (g) reasonable medical expenses caused to Jean Doe by reason of Defendants' wrongful conduct detailed hereinabove. Plaintiff seeks punitive damages in an amount commensurate with: a) the nature of the wrongs committed by Defendants; b) the inhumane character of Defendants' course of conduct; c) the degree of culpability of the wrongdoers herein; d) the helpless and dependent nature of the victim in this case; and e) the severity, frequency, and degree to which the conduct described hereinabove offends the public sense of justice. Defendants' conduct alleged hereinabove justifies an award of exemplary damages in an amount sufficient to deter Defendants from engaging in this conduct in the future."
>
> *(From a petition of an actual lawsuit alleging progressive failures and omissions of care.)*

The platinum rule

All nurses are familiar with the Golden Rule, which states, "*Do unto others as you would have them do unto you.*" An alternative to the *Golden Rule* is the *Platinum Rule: "Treat others the way they want to be treated."*[14] This may be one of the best kept secrets of guest relations, because applying the platinum rule inevitably has a positive impact on resident and guest attitudes and satisfaction. The Platinum Rule is more individual than the Golden Rule, so it fits well into the OBRA requirements. It shifts the focus from treating everyone alike to providing highly individualized care. Find out what the residents want, and give it to them, as much as possible, in keeping with their plans of care. The goal of the Platinum Rule is personal chemistry and productive relationships. To apply the rule, there is no need to change your personality or roll over and submit to others. You must simply understand what drives people and recognize your options for dealing with them.[15] The Platinum Rule divides behavioral preferences into four basic styles:

- Director

- Socializer

- Relater

- Thinker

The good part is that everyone possesses some qualities from each style, although everyone has a single dominant style. If you are honest with yourself, you can probably think of instances in which personal comfort and convenience potentially interfered with the resident care you delivered. By placing the residents' interests ahead of your own, you are fulfilling the ethical and legal obligations of your practice, protecting resident safety, enhancing resident comfort and satisfaction with care, and reducing your personal risk of legal exposure.

The Platinum Rule is a powerful life skills tool that will serve you well at work, as well as all your personal relationships, including your friends, family, spouse, and children. Improved relationships create infinite possibilities. The author compares it with the words of John Lennon's song, "Imagine." One of the verses could be, "Imagine there's no conflict, it's easy if you try." This is a potential inservice and philosophical area that has the potential for paying great dividends for your facility. It is well worth your consideration.

Emotional distress is another area in which little more can be said. Applying the Golden Rule and Platinum Rule is always helpful. Objective supportive documentation related to resident quality-of-life issues and psychosocial support usually helps mitigate potential claims for emotional distress or mental anguish.

Aggregate of issues

"Aggregate of care" is a consideration when determining whether a resident's stay will be covered under the Medicare payment program. Aggregate of care is also a component of a formal pain management program. When using concept mapping for care plans, the resident's history is mapped on a storyboard template that describes the current care episode (total care for the resident). Each care episode is an aggregate of care event (periods of active care, or resident response) based on the nursing process. Aggregate of care interventions are specific resident interventions. If you are familiar with this method of care planning, you will understand how an aggregate of issues applies to lawsuits.

When the plaintiff makes aggregate of care allegations, he or she is suggesting the facility has provided an overall pattern of poor care in all life activities. This is a serious charge to make, consisting of a storyboard chronicling the staff's misdeeds and implying the facility did nothing right! Like the other issues in this chap-

ter, your best defense is a strong offense. Become intimately familiar with your state nurse practice act and the state and federal rules for long-term care and follow them! If things seem to be broken in your facility, think outside of the box and find a way to fix them. This is achievable, and operating a compliant facility is definitely an attainable goal!

Pain management and legal exposure

Two well-published long-term care facility civil cases were related to inadequate pain assessment and management. In the first of these, a resident was admitted to a North Carolina facility with prostate cancer that had metastasized to the left femur and spine. The resident had an order for oral morphine elixir every three to four hours, but this was not given. A facility nurse determined on her own that the resident was addicted to morphine, so the facility substituted a tranquilizer for the pain medications, gave Darvocet infrequently, or withheld pain medication all together.[16]

In 2001, a California jury returned a $1.5 million dollar verdict for the undertreatment of pain at the end of life. This was a particularly sad case, because the resident's pain was ignored by so many individuals during his treatment in the hospital and a long-term care facility. Nursing personnel, a nurse practitioner, and several physicians failed to assess/manage the resident's pain. Nursing assessments routinely placed the resident's pain between seven and 10 on a 10-point scale, yet no analgesics were given. The resident suffered greatly over a prolonged period of time. The resident finally decided to die at home. At the time of discharge, nurses assessed his pain as 10. The physician provided a prescription for oral Vicodin, but refused to prescribe higher levels of opioids. (At trial, the physician defended his actions, because the resident had previously experienced breathing problems after being given Demerol during a procedure. The physician, who had virtually no pain management training, said he feared respiratory depression if strong pain medications were administered.) (The American Geriatric Society guidelines for pain management firmly state that Demerol should not be given to elderly persons.) In frustration, the family found another doctor, who prescribed morphine, which brought immediate relief. The resident died comfortably at home several days later. In addition to being found negligent at the jury trial, the attending physician was found reckless and was disciplined by the medical board for not relieving the pain of a dying, elderly man.[17]

The pain problem

As a group, elderly individuals are frequently under-medicated. This is ironic, because most have at least one painful, chronic condition that is known to cause pain. The pain problem is complicated by existing delirium, dementia, and cognitive impairment in some residents. The well-published results of one study revealed that 71% of residents in long-term care facilities said they experience pain.[18] Most were unhappy with the quality of nursing pain management.

Nurses should consider pain the fifth vital sign, and assess all residents regularly. Quarterly assessments are fine for screening, but infrequent assessment increases the facility's legal exposure and reduces quality of life. In an informal study, nurses administered acetaminophen three times a day to 10 residents with difficult behavior, who were also receiving psychotropic medication. This study showed a 63% reduction in behavioral symptoms over the course of a month. 75% of the psychotropic drugs were discontinued.[19]

In a 1998 study, researchers found that 47% of the alert residents had a routine pain medication order. Only 25% of the cognitively impaired residents had analgesic orders. Additionally, cognitively impaired residents were given less pain medication compared with those who were alert.[20] When residents with recent postoperative hip fractures were studied, 12 cognitively impaired persons received less opioid analgesia than did alert individuals during the first 48 hours postoperatively. After the initial 48-hour postoperative period, persons with cognitive impairment received significantly less acetaminophen than the alert persons in the study.[21]

In another study, 14 cancer patients over age 85 were less likely to receive narcotic analgesics than patients 65 to 74 years of age. Of those who experienced daily pain, 26% received no analgesia. Cognitively impaired persons received significantly less pain medication, either PRN or routine, compared with patients who were alert.[22] Another study found that 60% of the residents in one long-term care facility, with at least one painful diagnosis, had received no pain medication during the previous month.[23]

Some residents believe that pain is part of normal aging. Evaluating cognitively impaired residents may be especially difficult. Pain decreases quality of life, and can have a devastating effect on the resident's ability to achieve the highest level of function. Monitoring for pain, and developing, and implementing a pain-relieving plan of care, is essential. The undertreatment of pain has the potential for numerous harmful effects. The maxim "no pain, no gain" has proven dangerously wrong. Research has shown that unrelieved pain can inhibit the immune system and enhances tumor growth. Pain increases oxygen demands, causing respiratory dysfunction, and decreases gastrointestinal (GI) motility. It increases confusion. Severe acute pain is a major risk factor for chronic neuropathic pain.[24]

Pain is a major preventable public health issue that slows recovery, and increases healthcare costs.[25] Pain is never normal. It is always sign of something wrong. Unrelieved pain is a serious problem, with many significant physical and psychological consequences. It interferes with the resident's optimal level of function and self care. It contributes to immobility, increasing the risk of pneumonia, skin breakdown, contractures, behavior problems, depression, and many other complications. The most common nursing diagnoses for residents with pain are

- Activity intolerance (related to decreased muscle tone and strength from inactivity)

- Disturbed sleep pattern and sleep deprivation (related to pain and anxicty)

- Ineffective coping (related to persistent pain)

- Risk for disuse syndrome

- Impaired physical mobility

- Acute pain

- Chronic pain (although persistent pain is the preferred terminology, the nursing diagnosis has not been updated)

Types of pain

There are four basic types of pain:

- *Acute pain*—Occurs suddenly and without warning, but usually dissipates over time. This type of pain commonly occurs because of an injury or surgical procedure.

- *Persistent pain* (this is a newer term that replaces "chronic" pain)—This type of pain persists for more than six months. It may be constant or intermittent. It is often caused by chronic disease, residual from an old injury, or multiple medical problems. Unrelieved, it decreases quality of life, causes hopelessness, and may cause anxiety, depression, and a feeling of helplessness.

- *Phantom pain*—Develops as a result of an amputation. The pain is real and not imaginary. 95% of amputees who participated in a Johns Hopkins study experienced amputation related pain during the previous four weeks.[26]

- *Radiating pain*—This pain moves from the site of origin to another area of the body.

Identifying residents in pain and those at risk for pain

All residents have the right to appropriate pain assessment and management. Upon admission, nurses must identify residents who are having pain, as well as those who are at risk for pain. They must monitor residents after invasive procedures and identify and treat residents who are having pain. Use common sense. For example, pressure ulcers are painful conditions. The standard of care for pressure ulcer pain was identified by government guidelines many years ago. This standard has not changed:

"The goal of pain management in the pressure ulcer patient is to eliminate the cause of the pain, to provide analgesia, or both. Assess all patients for pain related to the pressure ulcer or its treatment. Caregivers should not assume that, because a patient cannot express or respond to pain, it does not exist. Manage pain by eliminating or controlling the source of pain. Because pain may be evoked or may be especially acute during dressing changes and debridement, the caregiver should try to prevent such discomfort or take steps to prevent it. Provide analgesia as needed and appropriate."[27]

Pain assessment

If pain is present, determine the location, duration, character, and frequency. Other considerations for pain assessment are

- pain quality

- pain intensity

- radiation, if any

- variation or patterns of pain

- aggravating and alleviating factors

- pain management history, if any

- present pain-management regimen, if any, and its effectiveness

- effect of pain upon activities of daily living, sleep, appetite, relationships, emotions, concentration, etc.

- physical assessment and direct observation/ examination of the site of the pain

- side effects of analgesic medications, if applicable

- response to analgesia and other forms of treatment, if applicable

As part of your assessment, monitor for and document

- behavior changes

- facial expressions

- body language

- verbal indications of pain (such as moaning)

Document your pain assessment in a manner that promotes regular reassessment and good communication. A flow sheet may be used for this purpose. Pain assessment should be simple and frequent. Asking residents to complete a pain questionnaire may be helpful. When assessing residents with delirium or cognitive impairment, look for body language or facial expressions suggesting pain. Question nursing assistants and family caregivers about nonverbal indicators, such as changes in mood or behavior suggesting pain. Monitoring nonverbal behavior is useful in delirium and cognitively

impaired adults, but these signs and symptoms apply to all residents having pain. Always suspect pain if the resident's behavior changes. In residents with mental illness, be aware that mental and behavioral problems cannot be adequately addressed until pain is controlled. Your observation, assessment, and reporting skills are particularly important with these residents.

Using a pain-assessment scale

Since pain is subjective, consistent pain assessment is a concern. Using a pain-assessment scale prevents subjective opinions, provides consistency for the resident and the nurse, provides consistency between nurses, and gives the residents a means of describing the pain accurately. Your facility should have a variety of tools available to meet the needs of a diverse group of residents. Having one scale is inadequate. Many nurses ask residents to rate their pain from one to 10, with one being least pain and 10 being intolerable pain. Some residents cannot do this accurately. Number scales can be especially problematic with cognitively impaired residents. Some residents respond best to word scales, whereas others find that pictures or number scales help them describe their pain intensity accurately. A pain rating scale is a communication tool. You must have more than one scale available. Allow the resident to select the scale that helps him or her *best express* and describe the pain.

Pain assessment scales and other tools can be used to assess residents of all ages and cultures. Test each resident to identify the scale that is most effective in helping the resident describe his or her pain. Select a tool that is appropriate for the resident, and is easy to use and document. If possible, teach the resident about the pain scale when he or she is not having pain. After the resident understands the pain scale, agree with him or her on a pain control goal, and develop a plan of care to achieve this goal. Keeping a pain assessment flow sheet may also be helpful. Document the pain-assessment tool used, the resident's score, analgesics administered, side effects, and the resident's response to the medication.

Studies have shown that some cognitively impaired residents can report pain reliably by using a pain intensity scale.[28] Pain scales with pictures of faces are often effective for cognitively impaired residents, and those with delirium who do not understand other pain scales. Residents with aphasia and those who have limited English skills also do well using picture scales. Elderly residents relate well to word scales, the 0-10 scale, and the Wong-Baker FACES pain scale. Although the FACES pain scale has faces of children, most adults do not find it offensive or demeaning, although some nurses disagree with the use of this particular tool in elderly residents. Many facilities use the Wong-Baker FACES scale successfully with cognitively impaired adults, as well as those with delirium. Facilities may consider adopting a nonverbal pain scale for assessing residents who are severely impaired, such as the one developed by Karen Feldt, PhD, RN.[29] The most important consideration is whether the tool helps the resident accurately communicate important information. Remember, the resident should be permitted to select the pain scale. He or she will not select a scale that is demeaning. Some residents do best with a vertical number scale, rather than a horizontal one. As you can see, use of a pain scale can be highly individualized!

When assessing pain by using a pain scale, consider the resident's hearing and vision. Scales with large print can be indispensable. Enlarging the scales on the copy machine may be helpful. Make sure the resident can hear you, and allow adequate time for him or her to process your questions and respond. Residents with cognitive impairment and delirium may surprise you. Avoid assuming that the resident cannot understand.

Experiment with several different pain scales. Be patient and do not give up quickly. Many can describe their pain accurately.

Nursing responsibilities for managing pain

Nursing responsibilities for managing pain include

- determining the nature of the pain and its impact on the resident

- identifying factors affecting the resident's perception and expression of pain

- determining when to administer analgesics

- deciding which analgesic to administer, if more than one is ordered

- determining the dose of analgesic medication to administer, if a range is prescribed

- evaluating the effectiveness of the analgesic

- assessing for and managing side effects of the medication

- determining why the analgesic was ineffective, if applicable

- determining the need to change the dose, timing, or medication and reporting this information to the physician

- using nursing interventions to promote comfort and relieve pain

- making sure the plan of care describes pain assessment and management

- documenting pain assessment and intervention noted herein to reflect use of the nursing process[30]

When you meet residents, inform them that you will provide attentive analgesic care. Advise residents that pain management is an important part of their care and that you will respond promptly to complaints of pain. Assess and document the intensity of pain at regular intervals, depending on severity. Quickly and attentively assess and manage each new report of pain. Consider administering routine analgesics to residents with chronic pain. The resident will be more comfortable, and you will avoid the peaks and valleys associated with PRN drug use.

Barriers to effective pain management

Sadly, numerous barriers to effective pain management exist in the average long-term care facility. For a pain management program to be effective, long-term care nursing personnel must understand barriers to effective pain management, and be particularly sensitive to resident needs and nonverbal signs of pain. This is especially true when caring for residents with cognitive impairment/impaired communication. Analyze the cause of behavior problems and address them! One small study revealed residents were less withdrawn and had fewer behavior problems after they were given acetaminophen. Although the residents' overall level of agitation did not improve, their isolation, activity, and social skills showed positive changes after taking three daily doses of acetaminophen daily for four weeks.[31] This is another area in which additional medical and nursing research is badly needed.

For some residents, behavior problems are the only means of communicating pain. If the pain is relieved, the behavior stops. For example, some residents cry for no apparent reason, and staff assume they are upset or depressed. You may be surprised to find that some residents with regular crying or other behavior problems improve dramatically after they are given pain medication! Many residents with cognitive impairment cannot express pain verbally, while others aren't taken

seriously if they do. Some residents with dementia will clearly verbalize their complaints of pain, or will admit to having pain if asked directly. Always give the resident the benefit of the doubt. *Unrelieved pain can cause (or worsen) confusion and other complications!* You may be surprised to find the mental status improves when pain is controlled. Assess the resident's pain systematically and regularly, including those who are cognitively impaired.

Fear of addiction

Fear of drug addiction is another major barrier to pain management. This fear may also be present in residents, family members, physicians, and nursing personnel. *Narcophobia* is the irrational fear of prescribing, administering, or using narcotic analgesics *(opioid drugs)* to treat pain. Physicians and nurses alike experience narcophobia. The term *opioid analgesics* is synonymous with *narcotic analgesics. Opiophobia* is sometimes used synonymously with narcophobia. Drugs in this category include morphine, codeine, fentanyl, and opium derivatives. Narcophobia is most prevalent when caring for residents with chronic pain. Sadly, many nurses believe that residents who use narcotic (opioid) analgesics for chronic pain are addicted to the drugs. Avoid assuming that residents with chronic pain are chemically dependent or addicted. By withholding drugs, many nurses believe they are preventing addiction. You will not do the residents a favor by withholding analgesic medications. *This is a myth with no basis in fact.* In fact, a study done in the early 1990s showed erroneous definitions and misinformation about addiction and pain management, including information in many popular nursing school textbooks![32] One study showed the following facts:

- 40% of cancer patients have undertreated pain. One in four elderly cancer patients in long-term care facilities receives no treatment at all for daily pain.

- Oregon's medical board disciplined a doctor for treating a dying cancer patient's pain with acetaminophen when a stronger medication was needed. The patient died in pain.

- 9% of all Americans suffer chronic pain. Experts say four of every 10 people with moderate to severe pain do not get adequate relief.[33]

Inadequately treated cancer pain was cited in several long-term care facility lawsuits. Interestingly, the pain was not listed as a consequence of the injury but as the injury itself.[34] Pain medications improve the quality of life in residents with chronic pain. Individuals with chronic pain become physically dependent on the drugs and go through mild withdrawal if the drugs are abruptly discontinued. However, this is not the sole indication of addiction. *In fact, less than 1% of all chronic pain patients become addicted to narcotic analgesics.*[35] Many nurses believe the percentage is much higher, particularly if the person has used narcotic analgesics for six months or more.[36]

Addiction is an all-consuming, drug-seeking behavior. Another condition, called *pseudoaddiction* is often mistaken for addiction. Most nurses have seen "clock watchers." In this condition, pain is partially relieved, but relief is inadequate or breakthrough pain begins immediately when the blood level of the analgesic drug drops. The resident fears pain, and worries that he or she will not receive the medication. The resident will watch the clock and request pain medication as soon as it is due. Clock-watching behavior stops when pain is adequately controlled.

Drug tolerance

Tolerance is a phenomenon that may occur after receiving the same analgesic drug regularly over a long period of time. Increasing the dose or changing the drug will relieve the pain. This is *not* a sign of addiction. Tolerance and dependence are common side effects of the analgesic regimen. *Pain-relieving drugs should never be withheld from residents in chronic pain out of fear of causing addiction.* If tolerance develops, contact the physician. The dose can usually be in-creased as much as 25% to 50% to improve control.[37,38] In fact there is no upper dosage limit to many narcotic analgesic drugs. However, you must be careful when providing drugs containing non-prescription items such as aspirin and acetaminophen because of the potential for toxicity and complications. Drug dosages should be increased gradually.

Age-related barriers

Some staff believe that *no complaint of pain means no pain.* In fact, lack of complaints of pain is a common excuse used by defense attorneys and nurse defendants in lawsuits when no pain assessments were done. Nursing personnel fail to assess for or identify pain because the resident does not complain. The current generation of residents may be culturally conditioned to suffer in silence. One of the greatest barriers to adequate pain management is staff who have been taught (and believe) the myth that pain sensitivity and perception decrease with age. In the absence of disease, aging does not alter pain sensitivity and threshold. Avoid making assumptions about whether the resident is having pain. Always ask. Asking is not offensive. The pain may have no visible effect on the resident. Vital signs may be normal. Avoid assuming that residents who are smiling, laughing, or sleeping are not having pain. *The resident's self report of pain is the most accurate indicator of the existence and intensity of pain, and should be accepted and respected.*[39] *If residents complain of pain, believe them!*

Cultural barriers

Always consider culture and age when assessing pain.

Culture affects the resident's beliefs and outward responses to pain. Residents from some cultures believe that displaying outward signs of pain signifies weakness, so they are very stoic. In other cultures, residents will be very dramatic or cry loudly when having pain. Religious beliefs may also affect the resident's perspective about pain. Sadly, some believe it is a punishment from their higher power, so will not complain or volunteer that they are having pain. However, if asked directly, they will often admit to having pain.

Semantics

Learn to adjust your terminology and use a variety of synonyms during your pain assessment. Select terms that the resident is likely to respond to. If a resident denies pain, try other terms such as soreness, discomfort, burning, heaviness, tightness, aching, and others. If he or she admits to having another type of discomfort, further assess the resident and use a pain scale to identify the intensity of the pain accurately.

Cognitive impairment

If the resident clearly does not understand your questions about pain, evaluate body language. Look for restlessness, or irregular or erratic respirations, such as intermittent breath holding, dilated pupils, and sweating. The resident may clearly favor one extremity, or show signs of irritability, withdrawal, fatigue, or anorexia. Often, the resident will act opposite of normal. For example, a resident who is normally very noisy becomes quiet and withdrawn. A resident with disjointed communication will accurately describe his or her pain. The quiet, nonverbal resident becomes agitated and combative. The friendly and outgoing resident cries easily and withdraws. The resident who is normally physically active, who moans and rocks, becomes still and quiet. Always suspect pain if the resident's behavior changes, then use pain assessment tools and physical assessment to confirm your suspicions. If,

after assessing the resident, you are still not sure, administering a mild analgesic will not hurt the resident. If his or her behavior reverts to normal, this further confirms your beliefs.

Side effects

Misinformation, misunderstanding, fear, and denial are also barriers to effective pain relief. Residents may deny pain because they fear it means worsening of disease. Some believe that taking narcotic analgesics is wrong, even for medical treatment. Some fear sedation and other side effects. Most side effects become less severe over time. Sedation is often managed by reducing the dose, but increasing the frequency of administration. Sedation usually subsides spontaneously in three to four days. However, *constipation is a major side effect of opioid drugs that never goes away.* Monitor the resident's bowel movements carefully to prevent fecal impaction and bowel obstruction. If your residents are on an opioid regimen, make sure bowel management is carefully addressed on the care plan, and make sure nurses monitor his or her elimination closely.

Fear of causing respiratory depression

Nurses fear causing respiratory depression in residents taking narcotic analgesics. The risk of this complication is highest when opioids with long half-lives are used. The greatest offenders are drugs such as methadone and Demerol, which are not recommended in this age group. Elderly persons are more sensitive to sedation and respiratory depression, most probably as a result of altered distribution and excretion of the drugs. This is especially true in opioid-naive patients. Avoid long-acting drugs for this reason. Start low and go slow, titrating upward as needed and as tolerated. This enables the resident to adjust to the increased dosage gradually, and respirations will not be significantly affected. Subacute overdose is more common than respiratory depression in the elderly. In this condition, sedation builds gradually, followed by a slowing of the respiratory rate and ventilatory failure. *The degree of sedation is a better indication of complications than counting the respiratory rate.*[40] Clients of all ages should be frequently monitored when beginning an analgesic regimen. The elderly are not distinct in this regard. Regularly review the medications, effectiveness, use patterns, and side effects.

Continuity of care

Breakdown in the continuity of care is another barrier to effective pain management. Many individuals care for each resident. Residents may be reluctant to discuss their pain with unfamiliar staff. They may become frustrated when many people ask the same questions about their pain. Excellent verbal and written communication help promote continuity of care. Be sensitive and compassionate to each resident's needs.

Effective pain management

Uncontrolled pain profoundly affects the residents' health and functional status. Provide analgesic medication promptly when a resident complains, before pain becomes severe and out of control. Anticipate and prevent pain by administering routine analgesics, whenever possible. Avoid passing judgment about residents receiving narcotic analgesics. Opioids are the treatment of choice for acute pain and chronic pain.

The quality of pain control is notably influenced by the education, expertise, experience, and attitude of the team of healthcare providers caring for the resident. Normal aging changes affect how the body metabolizes and eliminates drugs. Since water is a diluent for many medications, this is a particular concern for residents whose fluid intake is inadequate, or those known to be dehydrated. Manufacturers do not provide dosing guidelines specific to elderly individuals. Optimum dosing and side effects are difficult to predict from one resident

to the next. Beginning with a low dose and titrating upward gradually is usually the best approach.

WHO analgesic ladder

The WHO analgesic ladder (see Figure 16-1 on next page) is an excellent tool for selecting and administering analgesic medications. Although it was originally developed as a guide to managing cancer pain, the ladder was subsequently endorsed by the American Pain Society and United States Agency for Health Care Policy and Research (AHCPR). The steps in the ladder represent pain intensity. If several drugs are ordered, begin analgesic therapy at the bottom of the ladder. Before moving up, try substituting drugs within a category. Use the easiest modalities and simplest dosing schedule first. For mild to moderate pain, use aspirin, acetaminophen, or NSAIDs. If the pain persists or increases, move up a step. Opioids combined with other drugs such as acetaminophen, are the logical next step if the nonopioid drug relieves some, but not all, of the pain. If pain increases in intensity or persists, move to step three, increasing the dose or potency of the drug.

The ladder is designed so that it builds upon previously used drugs before introducing new ones. Combining smaller effective doses of several drugs may be safer than higher doses of a single medication in the elderly. The WHO scale also advocates administering "adjuvants." Adjuvant drugs are ordered to enhance the efficacy of analgesics, treat symptoms that exacerbate pain, or provide an independent analgesic effect. Examples are drugs to calm fear and anxiety, or drugs such as gabapentin for neuropathic pain. For persistent pain, administer short-acting analgesics "by the clock," or every 3–6 hours, rather than PRN. This three step approach of administering the right drug in the right dose at the right time is inexpensive and 80%–90% effective. Surgical intervention may be considered later if drugs are not wholly effective.

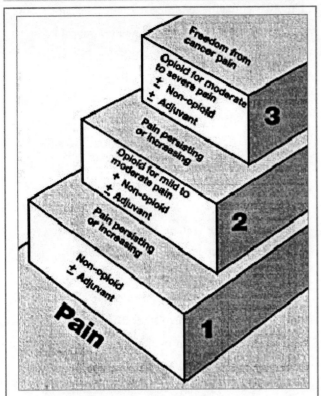

The WHO three-step analgesic ladder

Reproduced by permission of WHO, from: Cancer pain relief, 2nd ed. Geneva, World Health Organization, 1996

American Geriatric Society Guidelines

An excellent resource is the "Management of Persistent Pain in Older Persons" guideline published (revised) by The American Geriatrics Society (AGS) in May 2002.[41] The guideline provides advice on the management of persistent pain in elderly persons with limited social and financial resources. Four broad pain categories and generalized approaches for treating each are described in the guideline. Residents with persistent pain may respond best to around-the-clock (ATC) dosing, rather than waiting to medicate until the pain is out of control. Short-acting analgesics may be given for breakthrough pain, or before activities known to exacerbate pain. Residents with some types of pain respond well to non-traditional treatments

and combinations, such as antiarrythmics, antidepressants, and anticonvulsants. The physician will order drugs that have the greatest chance of pain relief with the fewest side effects.

Acetaminophen is the first choice for treating mild to moderate pain. Most elderly residents tolerate acetaminophen well, and this drug may be a better choice than NSAIDs. The maximum dosage of acetaminophen (from all sources) should not exceed four grams a day. For chronic use, three grams or less daily is best. Elderly residents, those with liver and renal disorders, and individuals who consume alcoholic beverages, should take much less, or not use the drug at all. Evaluate the resident's total drug regimen to ensure he or she does not receive other drugs containing acetaminophen. Make a notation on the medication administration record (MAR) and care plan warning staff not to exceed the daily dosage limits.

The risks and benefits of NSAID therapy should be carefully weighed against other available treatments. The resident may progress to nonsteroidal anti-inflammatory drugs (NSAIDS), unless this category is contraindicated due to underlying medical conditions. In the anti-inflammatory category, the COX-2 inhibitors are preferred to the non-selective NSAIDS for long-term use. Caution the resident about potential for and monitor for gastrointestinal bleeding. Administer the drug with food to reduce this risk. Encourage fluids and consider monitoring intake and output. When administering NSAIDS, monitor the resident for gastric and renal toxicity, and other unusual drug reactions including cognitive impairment, constipation, and headaches. Using "platelet sparing" NSAIDs should be considered to lessen the risk of gastrointestinal bleeding.[42]

According to the AGS, elderly adults with severe pain

can safely take opioid analgesics. Monitor the resident for side effects, including gait disturbance, falls, pruritus, nausea, sedation, and impaired concentration. Anticipate and prevent constipation with good fluid intake, ambulation, an exercise regimen, regular toileting, and drugs such as senna. Anticipate mild sedation and impaired cognitive function when the drug is initiated, and take fall precautions. Remember that the resident will probably experience a higher peak and longer duration of pain relief. [43]

Narcotic analgesics

Narcotic analgesics are being increasingly accepted for managing chronic pain. Those that are commonly prescribed for persons who are elderly include hydromorphone, hydrocodone, codeine, and oxycodone. Transdermal fentanyl is ordered for some residents who may be unwilling or unable to take drugs by other routes of administration. However, the drug may accumulate in the elderly over time, resulting in a longer terminal half-life. Since the drug is absorbed through the subcutaneous tissue, titration may take days to weeks. The physician may order the first patch applied when the last dose of a long-acting oral analgesic, such as morphine, is administered. Rescue medications may be needed to relieve pain until the patch takes effect. After prolonged administration, it may take up to 15 hours for the drug to be removed from body stores.

When titrating an opioid dosage, you must consider both the analgesic effects and side effects. Cognitive impairment is the most common, but other side effects of concern are urinary retention (particularly in residents with prostatic hypertrophy), constipation and intestinal obstruction, respiratory depression, or exacerbation of Parkinson's disease. Avoid using phenothiazines or antihistamines to manage nausea, if possible, because elderly people are very sensitive to anticholin-

ergic side effects including delirium, bladder and bowel dysfunction, and movement disorders.

The AGS guideline reinforces current research that the incidence of addiction is very low in residents taking opioids for painful medical conditions. Tolerance to opioids is slow to develop when the pain causing disease is stable. If an increased dosage is required, the resident should be evaluated for new or worsening disease.

Three "opioids of concern" are generally contraindicated in elderly individuals. *Propoxyphene* is much more toxic than aspirin and acetaminophen, and is no more effective. *Tramadol* is about as effective and safe as codeine or hydrocodone, but has the additional risk of inducing seizures. Using methadone is risky in elderly persons. Methadone is difficult to titrate because of the long and variable half life. Other drugs that have been known to cause delirium in elderly and terminally ill persons are levorphanol, morphine sulfate, and meperidine.[44] Pentocazine may cause agitation and delirium.

The key to using opioids successfully is in individualizing the dose. Begin with 25% to 50% less drug than you would use with a younger person, then increase upward. Evaluate the resident's response, then gradually increase the dosage for control. As-needed (PRN) medication is appropriate only for intermittent pain. Use ATC dosing for residents with constant pain.

For some residents, nonsteroidal anti-inflammatory (NSAID) analgesics will adequately control pain. For others, opioid medications will be necessary. Always individualize the schedule for analgesic medication to the resident. Teach residents about their pain and encourage them to take an active part in its assessment and control. Give residents information about various interventions and provide support in using them. Some residents will take scheduled medications around the clock, whereas others will be effectively managed using PRN dosing. Pain levels fluctuate throughout the day, and with activity. Residents taking long-acting analgesics may require a periodic rescue dose to manage breakthrough pain. For residents who cannot tolerate oral analgesics, rectal or parenteral doses may be given. After medicating the resident, determine and document the degree of relief and side effects, if any.

American Medical Directors' Association

The American Medical Directors' Association (AMDA) is the professional association of medical directors and physicians practicing in the long-term care continuum, dedicated to excellence by providing education, advocacy, information, and professional development. This group provides direction to long-term care facilities, and have advocated pain assessment and management. The AMDA first published guidelines for managing chronic pain in nursing facilities in 1999. The guidelines have been updated several times since then. The AMDA pain guidelines are in keeping with those of the APS and AGS. They further recommend

- Performing a comprehensive medical assessment to identify and diagnose the cause(s) of pain, including mouth inspection, diagnostic testing, and specialty consultation as appropriate.

- Teaching residents and families to report pain; educating staff to ask about pain and to listen.

- Using non steroidal anti inflammatories, including selective COX-2 inhibitors, only in short courses.

- Avoiding the use of placebos, which have no place in pain management.

- Documenting responses to the management plan systematically, using the facility's standard pain

ratings recorded -n standard formats at regular intervals.

- Monitoring pain management program effectiveness.

- Checking the accuracy of MDS Section J2 on pain symptoms for each resident.

- Adopting an interdisciplinary care plan that sets goals, delegates responsibilities to team members, and incorporates pharmacologic and non-pharmacologic strategies. The plan should be explained to and accepted by the resident or responsible party.

- Using the least-invasive route of administration first.[45]

Nurses and other healthcare professionals must unlearn the myths and other misinformation regarding pain assessment and management. Pain management is both a survey issue and a nursing ethics issue, and nurses must update their practice in this area.

Nursing comfort measures

Always provide nursing comfort measures in conjunction with analgesics and physician-ordered strategies. List comfort measures on the care plan and teach nursing assistants to use them when appropriate. Depending on the situation, providing information about alternative methods of pain relief, such as relaxation techniques, aromatherapy, music therapy, guided imagery, meditation, deep breathing, heat, cold, and massage. Instruct nursing assistants to schedule their care around the resident's analgesic medications, as much as possible.

Resident teaching

Teaching is integral to effective resident care. All licensed nurses are responsible for resident teaching, offering knowledge and skills residents need to meet their continuing health needs. Resident teaching should always be included on the plan of care, when appropriate. Teach residents that pain management is part of their treatment. As part of your teaching, help them to understand the importance of effective pain management. Be open and flexible. When assessing and planning for resident teaching, consider the resident's and family's values and beliefs, culture, literacy, educational level, language, emotional barriers to pain relief, physical and cognitive function and limitations, and financial implications of care. Provide teaching on the resident's level. Describe the implications of pain, and effective pain management techniques. If necessary, dispel myths about narcotic analgesics and teach residents the difference between addiction, physical dependence, and tolerance to pain-relieving medications. Teach residents about the low risk of addiction to opioid narcotic analgesics for pain relief.

Performance monitoring and improvement

Performance monitoring and improvement are important in healthcare facilities. You will also collect information related to pain assessment, and the effectiveness of pain management as part of your facility's quality assessment and assurance program. Data collected will be used to revise policies, procedures, guidelines, forms, and educational classes with the goal of improving the pain-management program.

Assess residents' pain relief to ensure that your nursing care is effective, and modify the plan PRN. Ask residents about their current pain intensity, the worst pain intensity in the past 24 hours, and the degree of relief obtained from pain management interventions. You may also wish

to question residents about their satisfaction with pain relief and staff members' responsiveness to their complaints of pain. Discharge planning and teaching should include information about pain management, according to the resident's condition. Include guidelines for when to contact the healthcare provider for further assistance, if needed.

Improving proficiency in pain assessment and management

Many excellent resources are available to assist you in becoming more proficient in pain management. Even if you are knowledgeable about pain assessment and management, consider reviewing current references. Pain management techniques are always changing as new drugs become available and research uncovers effective treatment information. Develop and expand your communication skills. Become familiar with various pain scales and how to use and interpret each.

Helping alleviate pain and suffering is an integral part of nursing care. Understanding and adopting a commitment to pain relief will enable you to provide optimal comfort and quality of life for your residents! Relieving pain has always been an important nursing responsibility. Becoming familiar with and following accepted guidelines will enable you to relieve older residents' pain and provide the highest quality of care possible.

Various pain assessment scales can be found on your CD-ROM. You may also wish to review the article "Addiction versus Pseudoaddiction," also on your CD-ROM.

References

1. American Nurses Association (eds.). Scope and Standards of Gerontological Nursing Practice. (1995). Washington, D.C. American Nurses Publishing.

2. Palmer MH. (2002). Urinary incontinence in nursing homes. J Wound Ostomy Continence Nurs. 2002; 29: 4-5.

3. DeLaune, Sue C. and Ladner, Patricia K. (2002). Fundamentals of Nursing: Standards and Practice, second edition. New York, Albany. Delmar Publishers.

4. Anderson, Peter. Contracture Care Management: An Emerging Healthcare Field. (1998). Medtrade News.

5. Berkowitz DR, Young GJ, Hickey EC, et al. (2001). Clinical practice guidelines in the nursing home. AM J Med Qual. 2001;16:189-195.

6. Frantz RA, Xakellis GC(Jr), Harvey PC, Lewis AR. (2003). Implementing an incontinence management protocol in long-term care. Clinical outcomes and costs. J Gerontol Nurs. 2003;29:46-53.

7. Schnelle JF, Kapur K, Alessi C, et al. (2002). Does an exercise and incontinence intervention save healthcare costs in a nursing home population? J Am Geriatr Soc. 2003;51:161-168.

8. Older Patients being given urinary catheters for no reason. (2006). Senior Journal. May 22, 2006. Online. *http://www.seniorjournal.com/NEWS/Alerts/6/05/22/OlderPatientsBeing.htm.*

9. Kunin CM., Douthitt S., Dancing J., Anderson J., & Moeschberger M. (1992). The association between the use of urinary catheters and morbidity and mortality among elderly patients in nursing homes. American Journal of Epidemiology. 135(3):291-301, 1992 Feb 1.

10. Wong ES, Hooten TM. (1981). Guideline for prevention of catheter-associated urinary tract infections. Infect Control 1981;2:125-130.

11. Nicolle LE, Mayhew WJ, Bryan L. Prospective randomized comparison of therapy and no therapy for asymptomatic bacteriuria in institutionalized elderly women. Am J Med 1987;83:27-33.

12. Tscheschlog, B. et al (eds). (1995). Mastering Documentation. Pennsylvania, Springhouse. Springhouse Corporation.

13. Lama v. Borras, 16 F.3d 473 (1st Cir. 1994).

14. Alessandra T. The Platinum Rule. Online. *www.platinumrule.com/aboutpr.asp.* Accessed 08/15/05.

15. Alessandra T. The Platinum Rule. Online. *www.platinumrule.com/aboutpr.asp.* Accessed 08/15/05.

16. Estate of Henry James v. Hillhaven Corp., Super. Ct. Div. 89CVS64, Hertford County, NC (Nov. 20, 1990).

17. Bergman v. Eden Medical Center, Cal. Super. Ct., No. H205732-1, June 13, 2001.

18. Long-Term Care Survey Monitor. December 2000. Online. *www.hin.com/.* Accessed 01/16/03.

19. Douzjian M, Wilson C, Shultz M, et al. A program to use pain control medication to reduce psychotropic drug use in residents with difficult behavior. Annals of Long-Term Care 1998;6(5): 174-179.

20. Kaasalainen S, Middleton J, Knezacek S, Hartley T, Stewart N, Ife C, Robinson L. Pain and cognitive status in the institutionalized elderly. *J Gerontol Nurs* 1998;24:24-31.

21. Feldt K, Ryden M, Miles S. Treatment of pain in cognitively impaired compared with cognitively intact older adults with hip-fracture. J Am Geriatr Soc 1998;46:1079-1085.

22. Bernabei R, Gambassi G, Lapane K, Landi F, Gatsonis C, Dunlop R, Lipsitz L, Steel K, Mor V. Management of pain in elderly patients with cancer. JAMA 1998;279:1877-1882.

23. Feldt K, Warne M, Ryden M. Examining pain in aggressive cognitively impaired older adults. J Gerontol Nurs 1998;24:14-22.

24. Pasero, C., Paice, J.A., & McCaffery, M. (1999). Basic mechanisms underlying the causes and effects of pain. Pain: clinical manual (2nd ed., pp. 15-34). St. Louis: Mosby, Inc.

25. JCAHO Press Release. (1999). Online. *www.jcaho.org/news/nb207.html*. Accessed 12/1/00.

26. Roniger LR. (2006). Study finds chronic pain a fact of life for amputees. Biomechanics. Online. *www.biomech.com/showArticle.jhtml? articleID= 175804025*. Accessed 1/12/06.

27. U.S. Department of Health and Human Services (Eds). (1994). Pressure Ulcer Treatment. Rockville, MD. Agency for Health Care Policy and Research.

28. Ferrell, B. (1996). An overview of aging and pain. In B.A. Ferrell & B.R. Ferrell (Eds.) Pain in the elderly, a report of the task force on pain in the elderly of the international association for the study of pain. Seattle. IASP Press, pp. 1-10.

29. Feldt, K. (2000). The checklist of non-verbal pain indicators. Pain Management Nursing. 2000; 1:13-21.

30. Adapted from Redmond, K. (1998). Barriers to effective management of pain. International Journal of Palliative Nursing, 4.6. Online *http://www.markallengroup.com/*. Accessed 1/16/00.

31. Pain masked by dementia may be eased with tylenol. (2005). Caregiver's Home Companion. November 2005. Online. *http://www.caregivershome.com/news/article.cfm?UID=765=VGFyZ2V0VVJM*. Accessed 11/29/05.

32. Ferrell, B. R., McCaffery, M., RN, & Rhiner, M. (1992). Pain and addiction: An urgent need for change in nursing education. Journal of Pain and Symptom Management, 7, 117-124.

33. American Broadcasting Company (ABC News). (2000, December 25). Easing the pain: hospitals told to treat patient's pain. Online at *http://abcnews.go.com/*. Accessed 7/01/04.

34. Tucker KL. A new risk emerges: Provider accountability for inadequate treatment of pain. Annals of LTC. 2001; 9:52-56. (Estate of Henry James v. Hillhaven Corp., 1990 and Bergman v. Eden Medical Center, 2001.)

35. Drayer, R., Henderson, J., & Reidenberg, M. (1999). Barriers to better pain control in hospitalized residents. *Journal of Pain and Symptom Management*, 17.6, June, 434-440.

36. McCaffery, M., & Ferrell, B.R. (1999). Opioids and pain management. Nursing 99, 29 March, 48-52.

37. Rhiner, M. (1999). Managing breakthrough pain: A new approach. *American Journal of Nursing*, 99.3, S3-14.

38. McCaffery, M., & Ferrell, B.R. (1999). Opioids and pain management. Nursing 99, 29 March, 48-52.

39. Agency for Health Care Policy and Research. (1992). Clinical practice guideline: Acute pain management: Operative or medical procedures and trauma. Rockville, MD. U.S. Department of Health and Human Services.

40. Agency for Health Care Policy and Research. (AHCPR). Management of cancer pain, AHCPR publication No. 94-0592. Rockville, MD. 1994, U.S. Department of Health and Human Services.

41. AGS Panel on Persistent Pain in Older Persons. (2002). Management of persistent pain in older persons. *J Am Geriatr Soc.* 50 (S6), 205-224. Copies of the AGS guideline can be purchased from: Elvy Ickowicz, MPH, Manager, Education and Special Projects, American Geriatrics Society, 350 Fifth Avenue, Suite 801, New York, NY 10118. Email: *EIckowicz@americangeriarics.org*.

42. Roth SH et al. (1989). Merits and liabilities of NSAID therapy. Rheum Dis Clin North Am 1989. 15(3): 479-98.

43. Kaiko RF. Age and morphine analgesia in cancer patients with post-operative pain. Clin Pharmacol Ther 1980;28(6):823-6.

44. Bruera E, Macmillan K, Hanson J, MacDonald RN. (1989). The cognitive effects of the administration of narcotic analgesics in patients with cancer pain. Pain 1989. 39(1): 13-6.

45. Excerpted from AMDA's Clinical Practice Guideline: Chronic Pain Management in the Long-Term Care Setting. ©1999 American Medical Directors Association.

Rights of the resident

Defendants knew or should have known from warnings, prior and concurrent victims such as (four other residents named), and their experience as nursing home operators that these acts or omissions, some of which occurred at FGH Care Center and some of which occurred at higher corporate levels, posed a serious threat to the safety and welfare of residents such as Eliza Doe. Defendants' conduct was not occasional or fortuitous, but rather was the natural and predictable result of the decisions made at the higher levels of Defendants' corporate structure to maximize revenues and profits while at the same time reducing costs. Defendants' policies and financial decisions caused: a) ongoing dangerous levels of unqualified staff at the facility; b) patient population needs that continuously and grossly exceeded the capacity of the limited number of qualified care givers on duty; c) a total systems breakdown in the administration of basic care to all residents; and, d) widespread and ongoing neglect of multiple residents similarly situated to and including Eliza Doe. Defendants then concealed these facts to deceive Eliza Doe and her loved ones. Overall, the systemic neglect that resulted in Eliza Doe's injuries and death was the product of Defendants' high-level corporate policy and the exercise of corporate control over said Defendants' nursing home.

In causing injury to Eliza Doe, Defendants flagrantly violated the following resident rights:

- the right to be free from abuse and exploitation;
- the right to safe, decent, and clean conditions;
- the right to reside and receive services in the facility with reasonable accommodation of individual needs;
- the right to a dignified existence; and
- the right to all care necessary for Eliza Doe to have the highest level of health.

(From a petition of an actual lawsuit alleging progressive failures and omissions of care.)

Resident rights

Maintaining residents' rights is one of the most important, and sometimes the most perplexing, aspects of managing a facility. **The rights listed under "Resident rights" on your CD-ROM** are a sample of many which vary from state to state and can be more encompassing but never be less than required in the federal statute. Residents are given a written copy of their rights upon admission. It is important that the written rights are in accordance with federal and state requirements, and all staff are taught to recognize those rights and ensure they are never violated.

Some of the biggest problems associated with resident rights lie in the staff's desire to do what is in the residents' best interest. Balancing a resident's needs with their rights is a complex and skillful art that must be learned. To sacrifice one for the other is a sure path to eventual litigation. It is also important to avoid the temptation to "threaten to begin discharge proceedings" everytime a resident is non-compliant. Such proceedings, although sometimes valid, should never be a "tool" used to coerce residents to "abide by the rules."

Other challenges arise when one resident's rights conflict with the rights of another resident. One resident's right to be free from restraints can easily conflict with another resident's right to privacy. It is never acceptable to violate one resident's rights to protect another. Hey, who said the job was easy?

Lawsuits alleging residents' rights violations usually focus on the right to be free from abuse and neglect. These issues have been covered in other chapters and will not be repeated here. The "rights" discussed here are those than have been problematic and/or confusing for nursing personnel. The other rights listed in the Residents' Bill of Rights (such as trust fund balances and private communications) are seldom, if ever, an issue in a lawsuit. However, facility personnel are responsible for knowing and adhering to the bill of rights. The issue of refusals of care directly or indirectly is a component of some lawsuits, such as when the resident refuses to reposition and develops a pressure ulcer. The resident's refusal may or may not absolve the facility of responsibility for the problem, depending on how the situation is handled. What is certain is that facilities cannot accept refusals at face value and stop providing care. The reason for the refusal should be investigated and alternate methods of managing the problem attempted.

§483.10 Resident Rights—The resident has a right to a dignified existence, self-determination, and communication with and access to persons and services inside and outside the facility. A facility must protect and promote the rights of each resident. §483.10(a) Exercise of Rights—§483.10(a)(1) The resident has the right to exercise his or her rights as a resident of the facility and as a citizen or resident of the United States. §483.10(a)(2) The resident has the right to be free of interference, coercion, discrimination, and reprisal from the facility in exercising his or her rights. §483.10(a)(3)—In the case of a resident adjudged incompetent under the laws of a State by a court of competent jurisdiction, the rights of the resident are exercised by the person appointed under State law to act on the resident's behalf. §483.10(a)(4)—In the case of a resident who has not been adjudged incompetent by the State court, any legal-surrogate designated in accordance with State law may exercise the resident's rights to the extent provided by State law.

Consent[1]

Residents have the legal right to make medical and health care decisions based on an explanation and understanding of the potential benefits and risks of treatment. The process of understanding the benefits and risks is called *informed consent*. The resident must give voluntary consent for most procedures. *Decision-making capacity*, or *competency*, means the resident understands the options and their implications, and can explain them, if asked. He or she can provide a rational reason for selecting an available option over the others. Performing a procedure without consent is called *battery*. This is a form of assault. Upon admission to a long-term care facility, the resident or responsible party signs a consent form that covers anticipated, routine, daily care. For more invasive risks and procedures, the patient may be required to sign an additional consent form that lists procedural risks and alternatives. Facility policies specify who is required to explain the procedure to the resident. Commonly this is the physician or other primary care provider. To give informed consent

- The primary care provider or designee must provide information about the procedure, the benefits and risks, and probability or likelihood that the benefits and risks may occur. He or she is not expected to provide every detail of the procedure.

- The person who explains the procedure should do so using language and terminology that the resident can understand.

- The resident must understand the information.

- The resident must understand the options, if any.

- The person who explains the procedure must answer questions.

- The resident must have the mental capacity or ability to make the decision based on the information provided and his or her medical condition. (Residents may have the capacity and ability to make some decisions, but not others.)

He or she must be able to understand the consequences of each option. He or she must be able to evaluate the risks, benefits, and costs of each and relate them to his or her personal values and priorities. Residents are legally permitted to make good or bad decisions.

- The resident must grant consent, and not be coerced to do so.

For full, informed consent, the resident should be given information about

- the medical condition that makes the procedure necessary

- the purpose and benefits of the proposed procedure

- an overview of how the procedure is performed, including potential complications

- alternative treatments and options, if any, as well as their potential benefits and risks

- the potential consequences of not consenting to or accepting the procedure

The written consent form should be signed and dated both by the primary care provider and resident or responsible party. In most facilities, invasive procedure consent is time-limited, such as for a 48-hour period. The resident should be given a copy of the signed form. In an emergency in which the resident is unable to give consent, a doctrine called implied consent may be used. This means that under normal circumstances the resident would consent to procedures that are done in emergencies to prevent serious, irreversible harm. Treatment is initiated and proceeds until consent can be obtained.

Admission documentation

At the time of facility admission, the resident or responsible party usually signs a consent authorizing routine facility care. Extraordinary and operative procedures are not usually covered by this type of consent. However, review your admission agreements to learn what they say. Consult the facility legal counsel if modification is needed.

The facility should also consider and make provisions for admissions in the evening and on weekends. Although this is not preferable, hospital discharge planners are often pressured to move patients out as soon as possible. Long-term care facilities are pressured to increase census. The result is that some residents are admitted after normal business hours. There have been occasions when discharge planners have neglected to notify family members of the resident's whereabouts. This may be a non-issue as far as admission agreements are concerned, if the resident is alert and can sign his or her own paperwork. It poses a potentially big problem if the resident is cognitively impaired and a family member must sign consent for treatment. Residents are being discharged much sicker than in years past. Having a resident death within 24 hours of admission is not unusual. Make sure your admission agreement and consent for facility treatment are in order!

Potential legal problems with admission paperwork

Each state has long-term care and business-practice statutes that define and describe actions constituting unfair and/or deceptive business practices. These are usually illegal practices that are not permitted. The Nursing Home Reform Act clearly states that long-term care facilities may not require a third party to guarantee payment to the facility as a condition of admission, expedited admission or continued stay. This applies to residents with Medicaid, Medicare, private pay, and any other payment source.

The California Court of Appeal has published its opinion that asking a family member or other person to sign as a guarantor of payment on a resident's long-term care facility admission documents is a deceptive (and therefore illegal) business practice. To require a relative or family member to guarantee payment, the facility must honestly advise the person signing the documents of his or her rights with respect to signing versus not signing the paperwork. However, this person must be informed that a cosigner is not required as a condition of admission. Another person can legally agree to co-signing the admission documents as a financially-responsible party for the resident. His or her co-signature is valid and binding if the cosigner was properly notified that their refusal to co-sign will not affect the resident's admission status. A person who co-signs admission paperwork voluntarily (such as a financially responsible party) is also entitled to advance written notice of discharge.[2] (Also see Chapter 3 for information regarding co-signing admissions documentation that includes mediation or arbitration agreements.)

Residents with cognitive impairment

Consent can be a thorny issue in long-term care, where many residents are cognitively impaired, and have no one designated to make healthcare decisions on their behalf. All residents have the legal and moral right to make bad decisions, including those that may cause serious injury and death. However, in a refusal situation the facility has certain responsibilities to the resident, including the responsibility for clearly explaining the consequences of the refusal. If the resident refuses a procedure, do not assume he or she is refusing all care. The healthcare provider should always offer explanations and other options if the resident refuses the recommended care. He or she should not be treated differently because of the refusal.

State laws vary on how incompetence should be handled. Each facility should anticipate consent problems in residents with cognitive impairment and designate an individual, such as the social worker to initiate guardianship or other proceedings, or obtain a durable power of attorney (healthcare proxy) designation to ensure procedural consent can be obtained, if necessary. If the resident has no known relatives, the facility must petition the court to designate a guardian. In most states, the spouse or an adult child makes decisions on the resident's behalf. Decisions made by surrogate decision makers are legally binding. Nursing assistants are particularly concerned when the resident refuses bathing or other ADL care. The assistant believes he or she should honor the refusal, yet the nurse invariably instructs the assistant to proceed with the activity. This is because the consents and contracts signed by the resident or responsible party at the time of admission cover the provision of ADL care. Obviously, there are better ways of handling this and soliciting the resident's cooperation, but in this situation, there is little likelihood of having battery charges filed.

Competency is the legal term denoting an individual has the cognitive ability to make and be held accountable for his or her decisions. Each state has a legal process by which an individual can be declared incompetent. Medical information is required to support the need for this declaration. The courts respect our individual freedoms (including the ability to make bad decisions), and the decision to declare someone incompetent is not taken lightly. A resident is never assumed to be permanently incompetent if he or she is temporarily unable to make decisions due to mental or physical illness. Technically, a person can only be declared incompetent by a court of law. A durable power of attorney for healthcare takes effect only if the resident is unable to make independent decisions. Because of this, staff should approach competent residents for permissions first, before turning to family members.

Myths and facts

A popular misconception is that the designated healthcare proxy can override the resident's healthcare decisions. This is not true if the resident is alert. He or she retains full decision-making ability, and conceivably may disagree with the durable power of attorney for healthcare. The healthcare proxy is not authorized to override the alert resident's decisions. The proxy's decision-making authority takes effect only if the resident becomes unable to make decisions. Even then, the proxy should make decisions based upon the resident's stated wishes, if known. However, it is conceivable that he or she would overturn the resident's decisions in certain situations, such as the healthy resident who requests a full code in the event of cardiac arrest. If the resident developed untreatable brain cancer and became confused, it is understandable that the healthcare proxy would request to change the full code to a DNR order.

Sometimes an alert resident becomes temporarily unavailable to make decisions, such as when he or she develops delirium because of anesthesia from a surgical procedure. During this time, the proxy would make healthcare decisions. When the delirium is resolved, the full decision-making authority reverts to the resident.

If a resident's family has financial power of attorney, he or she can write checks, pay bills, and make financial decisions. However, this type of power of attorney applies only to financial matters. The resident retains full decision-making authority for healthcare, or another person is designated to make healthcare decisions. Occasionally, a family member has full power of attorney, but this is not common. A full power of attorney enables a person to make all decisions, including medical and financial. This is similar to a guardianship situation with a minor child. The only way to find out is to ask for the guardianship or power of attorney papers and read them carefully. However, be reasonable. Documents of this nature are not normally carried in one's pocket or purse, and may be in a safe deposit box. Allow a reasonable time for the individual to produce them.

The nurse promotes, advocates for, and strives to protect the health, safety, and rights of the patient.[3]

Gay and lesbian partners

Be sensitive and compassionate to the problems experienced by residents with gay and lesbian partners. As a nurse, care for these residents without passing moral judgment. Consider the following true stories:

Rob and Steve were 20+-year partners upon which the movie, *Brokeback Mountain* is loosely based. They lived in a southwestern state, working as ranchers and cowboys. They built a home on an acreage that Steve bought before their partnership and lived and farmed there for many years. When Steve's parents were terminally ill, Rob and Steve moved them into their home and cared for them for three years until their deaths. Rob was a full partner in their care.

Rob and Steve thought they had their own affairs in order. They completed durable power of attorney for healthcare forms and living wills. To be on the safe side, they purchased a do-it-yourself will kit. Each filled out a will form, naming the other partner as the full beneficiary. Steve developed cancer and died. The do-it-yourself will did not meet the legal requirements in their state and was deemed invalid. The house, farm, and all Steve's possessions were given to distant cousins by the court. The cousins did not approve of

Steve's lifestyle. Steve barely knew them and had not seen them in years. However, they were blood relatives, and Rob had neither the benefit of blood, marriage, or a civil union. Rob lost both his partner and his home. The problem with the do-it-yourself will was that state law required that a will be signed in front of several impartial witnesses. Although the will was signed in front of a notary public, no other impartial witness was present. A single witness (the notary public) was not adequate to meet state requirements, so the will was considered invalid.

Ray (age 37) and Micah (age 29) were partners of eleven years. Ray was HIV-positive. Micah was HIV-negative. Over time, Ray developed full-blown AIDS. He also had longstanding hepatitis C, but his liver enzymes were reasonably low and stable. He was hospitalized with pneumonia, given Versed, Vancomycin, and put on a ventilator to relieve his congestion and allow him to rest and heal. He reacted to the Vancomycin, which caused liver failure. Ray had never designated Micah as his durable power of attorney for healthcare, although he had made his intentions verbally clear. He (wrongly) believed that Micah could make healthcare decisions on his behalf. He was superstitious and was afraid that making out a will was a bad omen. He was not ready to die. Prior to this hospitalization, he had been living at home in the community with Micah and was relatively healthy.

Since Ray had no healthcare proxy, his sister (age 47) was authorized to consent to his medical care as his closest living relative. She panicked when she learned of the liver failure and requested that the ventilator be removed. After the endotracheal tube was removed, Ray did not die. However, he was lethargic and somewhat confused. This was most probably due to residual Versed that was not clearing the damaged liver. This further distressed the sister, who said he did not want to "live like this as a vegetable in a nursing home." She was convinced that he was brain damaged. No one explained the drug clearance issues to her. She withdrew all but comfort care, and Ray died four days later. Micah was convinced that Ray was not confused, and although lethargic, he responded appropriately when awake. Sadly, he was devastated and powerless to do anything about the situation.

The problems experienced by gay and lesbian life partners are particularly heart-wrenching, because they are not afforded the legal protections of married couples. Monitor their advance directives closely and regularly to ensure they are current and reflective of their wishes.

Staying in touch

The facility must record and periodically update the address and phone number of the resident's legal representative or interested family member.[4]

Another concern is to make sure you have current contact information for each resident's surrogate decision maker. This is particularly problematic when family contact is infrequent or out of state. Review emergency contact information at each care conference. If the facility has had no direct contact with the surrogate decision maker since the last care conference, assign someone to check the phone number and make sure it continues to be valid. If not, send a letter to the responsible party requesting they contact the facility by a designated date. You may also consider printing pre-addressed postcards to hand out on admission or when an advance directive is signed. The back of the card can be completed with new address and phone numbers and dropped in the mail to notify the facility of a change of contact information. Your policies and procedures should address the steps the facility will take if a responsible party moves and does not provide forwarding information or a message

number. This inexpensive method is surprisingly effective, and places the responsibility for notifying the facility of changes squarely in the hands of the responsible party. If the family cannot be located to make a medical decision for a resident, the facility will have a record of steps or actions taken to maintain communication, thus reducing legal exposure.

Refusals of treatment

Residents who have the capacity to make healthcare decisions who withhold consent to treatment may not be treated against their wishes. The facility may not transfer or discharge a resident for refusing treatment unless the criteria for transfer or discharge are met. Refusal of treatment may constitute grounds for transfer if the facility is unable to meet the resident's needs or protect the health and safety of others. The best option is to fully and completely explain the consequences of the refusal in a manner the resident understands, offer alternatives, and see if you can reach a compromise.

Many facilities stop trying to provide proper care when a resident refuses treatment. This is not usually a wise decision. Refusal of turning and other basic care affecting the resident's well-being does not provide a license to withhold care. Although the resident refuses treatment, she has the right to change her mind at any time. Avoid closing the door to the potential change of heart. For example, a resident refuses to reposition off her back. The nurse informs her she will get a "pressure ulcer." No further explanation is given, and there is no indication the resident understands pressure ulcers, such as what they are, how they develop, how much they hurt, and the complications they cause. The resident's refusal persists. The nurse documents the refusal, and passes the information on in report. No one else addresses the issue with the resident. They assume nothing can be done for the resident and stop trying. (Some workers may also label the resident uncooperative.) Sometimes, they note the refusal on the care plan. Predictably, the resident develops serious, deep, infected Stage IV ulcers on her hips and torso. *The resident's refusal of treatment does not absolve a facility from the responsibility for providing care that enables her to attain or maintain the highest practicable physical, mental and psychosocial well-being in the context of making the refusal.*

Addressing refusals

To the extent possible, the facility must use the nursing process to address the resident's refusal. They must use all data available on the medical record and elsewhere to ensure that the plan of care is all inclusive and accurately reflects the resident's needs. Involve nursing assistants and activities staff and others who are close to the resident and have first-hand knowledge of the resident when reviewing options for managing refusals. These workers often have good insights into why the resident is refusing care and how to devise a better approach to the problem.

When planning care, view the resident holistically and anticipate other problems that may result from the refusal or decline. If it becomes evident that the plan is not working, they must reassess the resident and revise the plan. The frequency at which this is done will vary with the resident's needs, but in this situation a quarterly review is not adequate to prevent negative outcomes. The facility is expected to formally assess the reasons for the resident's refusal. Next, they must educate the resident and clarify the potential risks and outcomes. Try to compromise and find a way to satisfy the legal requirements while honoring resident preferences and accommodating needs. In this situation, the development and worsening of a

pressure ulcer is potentially quite painful. The resident is probably not aware that the consequences of her refusal may cause severe, unremitting pain, as well as the need for treatments that also have the potential to be even more painful. The facility should seek and offer alternatives to turning, such as providing a turn holder and other adaptive devices to make turning easier and providing support when she is repositioned. They should assure the resident they will do their best to make her comfortable after she has been repositioned. Make sure the physician and responsible party are informed of refusals in a timely manner.

The refusal problem becomes thornier if the resident has depression, mental health needs, or a mental health diagnosis. To manage the refusal and prevent injury to the resident, involving the social worker and/or mental health professionals may be necessary. These professionals may develop and implement a behavior-management care plan that is initiated in stepwise order on each refusal. Although the resident is refusing a single service, the facility should not give up, because doing so in this situation virtually guarantees a negative outcome. The facility must continue addressing the problem issue while providing all other services needed by the resident.

An exception to the refusal rules occurs if a resident's unanticipated violent or aggressive behavior places the resident, staff, or other residents in imminent danger. In this situation, the use of restraints is considered a measure of last resort to protect the safety of the resident or others and must not extend beyond the immediate episode.

The long-term care regulations support and affirm the resident's right to participate in care planning and to refuse treatment. However, the regulations do not affirm or create the right for a resident, legal surrogate, or representative to demand that the facility use specific medical interventions or treatment that the facility deems inappropriate. (For example, some facilities refuse to honor requests to withhold food, fluid, or tube feeding on moral, ethical, and religious grounds. If your facility has similar policies, inform all residents or prospective residents prior to admission.) The facility is ultimately accountable for the resident's care and safety, including clinical decisions. Document all refusals in the medical record. List interventions to minimize complications on the care plan. The point here is, a refusal of certain care does not necessarily absolve the facility of responsibility for the problem. Reevaluate the resident and modify the plan. The care plan must reflect the facility's ongoing efforts to find alternative means of addressing the refusal. Implement interventions to treat the resident for depression or other mental health problems, when indicated.

Involuntary discharge

When the facility accepts a resident for admission, it cannot arbitrarily decide to discharge the resident unless there is a medical need (see below), the facility is closing, or the resident cannot pay the bill and does not qualify for Medicaid or Medicare payment. A resident cannot be discharged for nonpayment if he or she has submitted information to a third-party payor and is waiting for their decision regarding whether the bill will be paid.

A 76-year-old long-term care facility resident had a history of 55 documented behavior problems on his medical record. The resident was diagnosed with Parkinson's disease and vascular dementia. One day, he wrapped the call signal cord around the nursing assistant's neck and tried to choke her. This was the final straw for the facility, who sent the resident to

the emergency department. They immediately notified the resident's son by phone and mailed him the required letter for involuntary discharge.

The resident spoke English as a second language, and hospital personnel were unable to assess his mental state thoroughly. They felt he was not a danger to others and notified the facility they were sending him back. The facility refused to accept the resident. The hospital admitted him to the mental health unit for 72 hours. Again, they believed he was no danger to others and attempted to return him to the long-term care facility, who continued to refuse to accept the resident. He was sent to another long-term care facility.

The resident's son filed an appeal with the state health department, but subsequently withdrew it because the resident did not want to return to the first facility. However, the health department issued a citation for wrongfully discharging the resident. Although the facility appealed, the California Court of Appeal upheld the citation.

The Court of Appeal ruled that prior notice requirements for involuntary discharge are "strictly mandatory." The federal requirement that applies to following state bed hold regulations are also mandatory. The rationale is that the bed must be held pending successful outcomes of treatment in the other facility (in this case, the hospital.) Since the facility had documentation of 55 previous episodes of acting out behavior, they may have been justified in sending him to a mental health center or more secure setting for treatment. However, sending him to the ER and refusing to take him back was not justified. The justices noted that the prior notice and bed hold requirements apply even in an emergency. In an emergent situation, the facility must give the resident and/or responsible party as much prior notice as practical in the situation.[5]

In a similar case, a facility transferred a resident with schizophrenia to a psychiatric hospital for treatment. They planned for and facilitated the transfer for a week prior to moving the resident. However, the resident was not notified until immediately before the transfer took place. His nearest relative, a sister, was not notified until three days later. Since no advance notification was given, the resident and family had no opportunity to refuse. The time limit for contesting the facility's actions administratively or in court does not begin until proper written notice is given pursuant to the law.[6]

Make sure your reasons for transferring or discharging a resident cannot be perceived as discriminatory. A resident was admitted to a long-term care facility with amyotrophic lateral sclerosis (ALS), a progressively degenerative condition. His wife was also admitted, and they shared a room. Upon admission, the resident signed a one-year contract with the facility. The resident used a wheelchair for mobility. The facility's policy was that residents must transfer from the wheelchair to a regular dining chair for meals. All wheelchairs were removed from the room. Initially, the resident with ALS transferred into a dining chair at mealtime. However, as his neurologic deterioration progressed, transfers became difficult and unsafe.

For a brief time, the resident was permitted to sit in his wheelchair for meals, but was assigned to a table by himself. His wife was assigned to another table. He was subsequently informed that his one-year contract with the facility would not be renewed because he refused to transfer from his wheelchair to a regular chair at mealtimes. After the couple was given notice of discharge, they stopped going to the dining room entirely, and took all their meals in their room, where they could eat together. At the end of the year, family members moved the resident and his wife to another facility.

The resident filed a disability discrimination lawsuit. The court ruling was in favor of the plaintiff. The long-term care facility denied discrimination and appealed the ruling. The Colorado Court of Appeals ruled that the state's fair housing law requires reasonable accommodation to the needs of disabled individuals to allow them equal opportunity for access to the use and enjoyment of a residential care setting. The court noted this law is almost identical to the U.S. Fair Housing Act.[7]

The involuntary transfer and discharge issue has been addressed by the courts in many states. Although the facility may have compelling reasons for discharging the resident, they must adhere to the letter of the law. If in doubt, the facility should check with legal counsel before acting. Make sure to give the proper written notice to the resident, responsible party, state agency or ombudsman and others. The resident has the right to assistance in making alternative arrangements, social work counseling and a written plan of action. Even then, the resident can request that the court to oversee the process to ensure that his or her rights are being honored. If not, the court can invalidate the entire process.[8]

Notification of transfer or discharge

The facility must promptly notify the resident and, if known, the resident's legal representative or interested family member when there is:[9]

- A decision to transfer or discharge the resident from the facility

The resident's attending physician must also be notified on plans to transfer or discharge the resident from the facility.

Give the resident as much notice as possible prior to a transfer within the facility (or to the hospital or other care setting) or complete discharge from institutional care. In most usual situations, the facility must give the resident a 30-day notice of its intention to transfer or discharge the resident. A family member must also be notified. The resident may voluntarily choose to waive the formal notice period and transfer or discharge immediately. If this is the case, you may wish to have the resident sign a waiver of the 30-day requirement. Document the details and circumstances.

In some situations, a 30-day notice of transfer or discharge is not realistic. In these situations, notice of intent to transfer or discharge the resident must be made as soon as possible, but may be less than 30 days:

- The safety or health of the other individuals in the facility would be endangered

- An immediate transfer or discharge is required by the resident's urgent medical needs

- The facility cannot meet the resident's needs due to a significant change in condition

    - If a potential transfer is due to a significant change in condition that is not an emergency, the facility must reassess the resident and determine if a new or revised plan of care would enable the facility to meet the resident's needs.

- The resident's health has improved markedly, safely allowing a more immediate transfer or discharge

- A resident has resided in the facility for less than 30 days

Refusal of treatment is not grounds for transfer or discharge, unless the facility is unable to meet the needs of the resident or protect the health and safety of others.

The facility must document the details of all transfers and discharges. However, if you are transferring or discharging the resident with fewer than 30 days notice, the attending physician must also document the reasons for transfer if the facility cannot meet the resident's needs, or the resident's health has improved to the point that facility care is no longer necessary. If the health and safety of other residents are jeopardized, any physician may provide documentation.

The written notice of transfer or discharge must include

- The reason for transfer or discharge.

- The effective date of transfer or discharge.

- The location to which the resident is transferred or discharged.

- A statement that the resident has the right to appeal the action to the state.

- The contact information of the State long-term care ombudsman. For residents with developmental disabilities, the contact information for the agency responsible for the protection and advocacy of these residents. For residents who are mentally ill, the contact information for the agency responsible for the protection and advocacy of mentally ill individuals.

The facility must promptly notify the resident and, if known, the resident's legal representative or interested family member when there is:[10]

- A change in room or roommate assignment

Give the resident as much notice as possible if a roommate is moving into or out of his or her room. A full 30-day notice is not required in this situation.

Preparing the resident for transfer or discharge

The facility must prepare the resident for transfer or discharge whenever possible. Document your efforts to make the transition as seamless as possible. Examples of methods for preparing the resident for transfer or discharge are

- informing the resident where he or she will be going

- arranging safe transportation

- involve the resident and family, to the extent possible, in selecting the new residence

- conducting trial visits, if possible

- allowing the resident to voice his or her concerns

- providing referrals to community resources, as appropriate

- ensuring the family or another responsible person transfers valued possessions

- informing staff in the new facility of the resident's routines and daily needs

- facilitating the discharge or transfer smoothly with the least disruption possible to the resident

Refusal of transfers within the facility

A resident has the right to refuse a transfer to another room within the facility, if the purpose of the transfer is to relocate[11]

- A resident of a SNF, from the distinct part of the institution that is a SNF to a part of the institution that is not a SNF, or

- A resident of a NF, from the distinct part of the institution that is a NF to a distinct part of the institution that is a SNF.

A resident's exercise of the right to refuse transfer does not affect the individual's eligibility or entitlement to Medicare or Medicaid benefits. This rule applies only to transfers and discharges *initiated by the facility*, and is a source of great confusion. It does not apply to residents who request a transfer from one unit to the other. *It applies to moving the resident into and out of the unit that is Medicare approved.* Some facilities attempt to force the transfer by asking the resident to sign a paper agreeing to such a move when he or she is no longer entitled to Medicare benefits. Consult your facility legal counsel before using an admission agreement of this nature. It may not hold water when challenged by the resident. If the resident wishes to remain in a Medicare bed after his benefits are exhausted or he is no longer eligible for Medicare, he may pay the entire bill privately. If he is a Medicaid recipient, Medicaid will pay the bill. If neither option is acceptable to the resident, the facility must give a 30-day notice of involuntary discharge.

Note that these provisions do not apply to residents moving from one room to another *within the Medicare unit*. For example, there is only one negative-pressure private room on the Medicare unit. All the other rooms are semi-private rooms. An alert, tube-fed resident (Resident A) who is eligible for Medicare upon admission requests a private room and is admitted to the only private room on the unit. Several weeks later, you find you must admit a resident (Resident B) with active tuberculosis. Resident A will be reassigned to a semi-private room within the Medicare unit. He or she cannot refuse to move from the only negative-pressure isolation room to another room on the same unit. Resident B will be admitted to the private room.

In some situations, this provision may also apply to residents returning to the facility after hospitalization.

For example, Resident C formerly resided in the non-Medicare section of the facility. She fell and broke her hip and had joint replacement surgery. She qualifies for Medicare benefits after returning from the hospital. If the resident wishes to return to her former room, she may forfeit the Medicare and return to her original room. If she was formerly a Medicaid recipient, Medicaid will resume responsibility for paying for the care. If she was formerly a private-pay resident, she reassumes responsibility for payment. *Do not issue a Medicare denial letter*. You recognize the resident qualifies for Medicare-covered services. The resident is refusing to use the Medicare benefit by returning to his or her former room. You are not denying benefits.

Notifications[12]

A facility must immediately inform the resident, consult with the resident's physician, and if known, notify the resident's legal representative or an interested family member when there is

(A) An accident involving the resident that results in injury and has the potential for requiring physician intervention;

(B) A significant change in the resident's physical, mental, or psychosocial status (i.e., a deterioration in health, mental, or psychosocial status in either life-threatening conditions or clinical complications);

(C) A need to alter treatment significantly (i.e., a need to discontinue an existing form of treatment due to adverse consequences, or to initiate a new form of treatment)

The facility must also promptly notify the resident and, if known, the resident's legal representative or interested family member when there is:

(A) A change in room or roommate assignment; or

(B) A change in resident rights under federal or state law or regulations

For additional change-of-condition information, review the communication guidelines in Chapter 10.

Bed hold policy and readmission

Before a facility transfers a resident to a hospital or allows a resident to go on therapeutic leave, the nursing facility must provide written information to the resident and a family member or legal representative that specifies

- the nursing facility's bed hold policies apply to all residents

- the duration of the bed hold policy, during which the resident is permitted to return and resume residence in the nursing facility

- the nursing facility's policies regarding bed-hold periods

The facility is required to furnish the resident with two bed hold notices. The first notice may be given well in advance, or as soon as transfer seems imminent. The second notice, which also specifies the duration of the bed hold policy, must be issued at the time of transfer. In an emergency, this means the family or responsible party are given written notice within 24 hours of the transfer, or a copy of the notice is sent with other papers accompanying the resident to the hospital.

If the resident exceeds the bed hold days, he or she may pay the bed hold privately. If the resident elects not to pay privately, the bed may be released for admission. However, the resident must be permitted to return to the first available bed if the resident

- Requires the services provided by the facility

- Is eligible for Medicaid nursing facility services

If the rules for bed holds written here contradict your state law, follow your state laws, or seek clarification from legal counsel.

Therapeutic leave

A physician's order is needed if residents wish to go on therapeutic leave. Therapeutic leave, such as a home visit or trip to the mall, can be a confusing subject for the facility. Facilities participating in the Medicaid program must give the resident and responsible party a copy of the bed hold policies before the resident leaves the facility. If the resident is on Medicaid, follow your state's guidelines for bed hold. They may stipulate a maximum number of overnight leaves per year. Bed hold for days of absence in excess of the state's bed hold limit are considered noncovered services. However, the resident is free to use his or her own income to pay for the bed hold. If the resident does not wish to pay privately, he or she must be permitted to return to the first available bed. Residents who are not on Medicaid may be requested to pay privately for all days of bed hold.

There is no bed hold for Medicare. However, this does not mean the resident cannot leave the facility for an outing, if doing so is safe considering the resident's condition. Some facilities believe residents under the Medicare payment program cannot leave the facility because of the lack of bed hold. Some also fear a denial of Medicare benefits because the resident does not receive his or her daily skilled service when out of the facility. Because of the need for daily skilled service, use discretion in allowing residents to go out on pass. Make sure the physician orders specify it is a "therapeutic" pass. Consider getting a new order for each pass instead of a routine, standing pass order

that is renewed each month. Document the reason for the pass, such as "to attend granddaughter's graduation," or "participate in a family gathering for Christmas." For overnight passes, trial home visits are certainly permissible, and are often recommended. Taking the resident home overnight will give the resident and family caregivers an opportunity to see if the resident's needs can be managed at home. If you are delivering the daily skilled service before or after the resident returns, there is no need to ask the resident to pay privately if he or she is out of the facility for an occasional night. However, if the resident is going on frequent or extended leaves, the facility should reevaluate the resident to ensure daily skilled services are still necessary.

Using interpreters

Non-English speaking residents have the right to having communications translated into their native language. The facility is required to furnish interpreters in certain situations, according to federal law:

F156

Guidelines: §483.10(b)(1)

"In a language that the resident understands" is defined as communication of information concerning rights and responsibilities that is clear and understandable to each resident, to the extent possible considering impediments which may be created by the resident's health and mental status. If the resident's knowledge of English or the predominant language of the facility is inadequate for comprehension, a means to communicate the information concerning rights and responsibilities in a language familiar to the resident must be available and implemented. For foreign languages commonly encountered in the facility locale, the facility should have written translations of its statements of rights and responsibilities, *and should make the services of an interpreter available.* In the case of less commonly encountered foreign languages, however, a representative of the resident may sign that he or she has explained the statement of rights to the resident prior to his/her acknowledgement of receipt. For hearing-impaired residents who communicate by signing, *the facility is expected to provide an interpreter.* Large-print texts of the facility's statement of resident rights and responsibilities should also be available.

Suggestions for working with interpreters

State laws may be more stringent than federal laws regarding requirements for furnishing an interpreter for residents. There are times, however, when using an interpreter will be essential, such as in obtaining consent for a procedure.

The guidelines for using interpreters in the healthcare facility are listed on your CD-ROM.

Resident work

Resident work and volunteer programs have been a source of confusion for some facilities. Many residents have "resident volunteer" programs through the activities department in which residents pass mail, meet and greet new residents, wrap silverware, set tables, and other tasks. Programs of this type are beneficial to many residents, and fulfill a need to contribute to the good of the community. The activities program is responsible for ensuring proper documentation and care planning.

The nursing department is only peripherally involved in the resident volunteer program. Since nursing is responsible for monthly physician order recaps, make sure you have an order that states, "May participate in therapeutic resident volunteer program per plan of care," or similar wording according to facility policy. If residents are doing tasks such as setting tables and wrapping silverware, make sure you teach them proper medical methods of handwashing, when to rewash the hands, or when and how to use an alcohol hand cleaner. Document this teaching.

Some facilities shy away from resident work programs entirely for fear of wage and hour law violations. Residents may choose to participate in a volunteer program. They may also choose not to participate. Few facilities pay residents for these services, which would be absorbed by regular personnel if they were not done by residents. However, the facility may choose to pay the residents the prevailing wage for the work they do. There is no requirement to have a "work for pay" type program. However, if residents are doing more substantial work, such as answering the phone on weekends, assisting with meal preparation, etc., more extensive preparation and education will be required. Since the nature of these jobs is more substantial than tasks such as wrapping silverware, the facility should consider paying the resident. A rule of thumb to use may be whether the facility will need to hire a person to do the job if the residents will not do it. If so, consider paying the resident as you would pay a new hire. If you would not hire someone to do the job, then you may wish to consider placing it under the auspices of the resident volunteer program.

Resident advocacy

Residents entering the facility are dependent on staff to provide care they formerly did themselves. Although they have medical challenges, they do not give up any rights of citizenship. Because of concerns about the legal and civil rights of facility residents, state and federal laws were carefully constructed to ensure the residents' rights are fully protected. If a resident cannot exercise his or her rights independently, staff must assist.

Violations of residents' rights subject the facility to administrative penalties and potential for legal exposure. Lawsuits alleging resident rights violations may be brought individually or in combination with other charges related to quality of care. In addition to the state administrative sanctions, a jury verdict in favor of the plaintiff commonly authorizes payment of

additional damages to the resident. Respecting the residents' rights is the law. However, the law is in keeping with the ANA standards, requiring nurses to advocate for the residents. Supporting, upholding, and advocating for the residents' rights are important ethical responsibilities that constitute a core part of nursing practice. You will also find that quality of care and quality of life are enhanced in an environment in which the residents' legal rights are acknowledged and respected.

References

1. The process described here applies to adult residents. Minor children may have decision-making ability, but are not legally empowered to make health care decisions independent of their parent or guardian.

2. Podolsky vs. First Healthcare Corporation, 58 Cal. Rptr. 2d 89 (Cal. App., 1996).

3. American Nurses Association (eds.). *Code for Nurses.* (1985). Washington, D.C. American Nurses Publishing.

4. State Operations Manual. §483.10(b)(11)(iii)

5. Kindred Nursing Centers West, LLC v. Calif. Health & Human Services Agency, 2005 WL 1460714 (Cal. App., June 22, 2005).

6. Anderson vs. Cabinet for Human Resources, 917 S.W. 2d 581 (Ky. App., 1996).

7. Weinstein vs. Cherry Oaks Retirement Community, 917 P. 2d 336 (Colo. App., 1996).

8. Robbins vs. Iowa Dept. of Inspections, 567 N.W. 2d 653 (Iowa, 1997).

9. State Operations Manual. §483.10

10. State Operations Manual. §483.10

11. State Operations Manual. §483.10

12. State Operations Manual. §483.10

Medication monitoring

Medication-related lawsuits

Entire books are devoted to medication safety. This chapter describes medication-related problems that commonly result in resident injury and long-term care litigation. Most residents receive one or more medications daily. One well-published study revealed that the average resident takes 5.85 medications daily.[1] The over- or under-use of medications can result in serious injury or death. Drug-related injuries in a long-term care facility lawsuit usually result from

- inappropriate prescribing

- failure of facility staff to follow physicians' orders

- failure to properly monitor the resident before and after administering medications; certain drugs such as warfarin account for the majority of medication-related lawsuits

- administering medications to the resident despite the presence of adverse symptoms that require prompt physician notification

- over- or under-medicating the resident

- administering medications to the wrong resident

One study revealed that as many as one in 10 long-term

care facility residents sustains a medication-related injury each month, a figure considered conservative by the lead researcher. When the data were applied to the nation's total facility population, the *Boston Globe* reported that 1.9 million drug related problems endanger long-term care facility residents annually, including more than 86,000 fatal or life threatening problems. The most common were confusion, oversedation, hallucinations, or bleeding. Drugs causing the most problems were warfarin and antipsychotics. The researchers in this study concluded that 42% of all the adverse drug events could have been averted, and 61% of the serious, life threatening and fatal adverse events were also avoidable.[2]

See your CD-ROM for a list of the "Six rights" of medication administration, medication errors, and causes of medication errors.

Action to take if an error has been made

- Recognize and admit that an error has been made. Covering up errors is never harmless. Failure to report errors is a violation of the standard of professional care owed to the residents.

- Assess the resident's condition and/or reactions to the medication.

- Report medication errors immediately, according to facility policy.

- Report the error to your immediate supervisor.

- Notify the physician. Give vital signs and a description of the event, and adverse reaction, if any.

- Follow the physicians' orders.

- Document physician notification and response.

- Notify responsible party.

- Document responsible party notification and response.

- Reassess the resident's condition; stay with him or her if untoward reaction or imminent danger.

- Consult the pharmacist, if needed.

- Complete an incident report.

- Document the event in the nurses' notes.

- Continue to assess and monitor the resident until he or she is stabilized.

- After the error is resolved, participate in a root-cause analysis. An investigation that focuses only on the actions or omissions of individuals is probably flawed and insufficient. In most cases, this is a learning process. Work with others to review systems and processes. Assist in development of processes and procedures that improve performance and reduce the chance of error.

Reducing the risk of medication errors

To reduce medication-related safety problems, caregivers should also

- Limit distractions to the person who is passing medications.

- Instruct nursing personnel to report suspected medication errors and omissions.

- Make sure the facility medication policies and procedures and a comprehensive drug reference book are accessible at the nursing station.

- Accurately follow the facility policies and procedures, physicians' orders and pharmacists' recommendations for medication administration. Contact the ordering physician if you have a question, problem, or concern. Use the pharmacist as a resource.

- Identify risk factors for safe medication administration, including a decrease in the ability to chew and swallow food or fluids, neurological and muscular deficits, oral health status, tube feeding, side effects of medications, or improper positioning. Consider risk factors when administering medication, and meet the resident's individual needs.

- Develop and implement a plan of care based on the resident's individual risk factors and unique needs. The plan should describe situations in which the drug is administered, when it should be withheld, laboratory monitoring, special precautions, and normal and abnormal observations to make. Modify the plan as often as necessary, depending on resident response.

- Some residents receive medications such as insulin or warfarin based on certain laboratory values. Monitor the results of laboratory or point-of-care testing closely. Know the implications of abnormal laboratory values. Inform the physician of complications, problems, or abnormalities. If you fax abnormal laboratory values to the physician's office, always follow up with a phone call. Document the fax and phone contact.

- Document administration of the medication on the medication administration record immediately after giving the scheduled dose. Never document medications in advance. Never document medications when the resident is in the hospital. Write a narrative description of special circumstances, complications, or problems encountered during medication administration. If the resident refuses medications, circle your initials in the administration box, and write a narrative note describing the circumstances of the refusal. Make sure all PRN doses are accurately documented.

- Assess the resident and notify the physician of missed doses, side effects, drug interactions, abnormal laboratory tests, problems, or complications related to administration of medications.

- Flag the MAR and care plan if special medication-related monitoring is indicated.

Atypical antipsychotics

A new category of medication-related problems has become problematic in recent years. This category involves failing to observe serious, unintended consequences related to administration of atypical antipsychotic drugs. Drugs in the atypical antipsychotic category have been found to cause an unusually high incidence of diabetes, stroke, endocrine abnormalities, cardiac problems and movement disorders. Drug manufacturers have admitted to misleading the FDA, physicians, and consumers about the side effects associated with these drugs. However, despite the risks, drugs in this category are routinely used. Atypical antipsychotics have been found to cause diabetes, even if the resident had no history of diabetes. A number of residents have died as a result of hyperglycemia, which was undetected until the resident was unresponsive and near death.

The atypical antipsychotic category of drugs is used to treat a variety of mental illnesses, including schizophrenia, bipolar disorder, dementia, psychotic depression, autism and developmental disorders. They are commonly administered to long-term care facility residents. In February 2004, the American Diabetes Association, American Psychiatric Association, American Association of Clinical Endocrinologists and the North American Association for the Study of Obesity joined forces in a published statement recommending judicious use of the following drugs:

- Zyprexa

- Risperdal

- Seroquel

- Abilify

- Clozaril

- Geodon

For some residents, the benefits of using the drug in this category may outweigh the risks. Physicians should screen residents before initiating atypical antipsychotic therapy, then reassess them again soon afterward, noting such things as a history of obesity and diabetes, and monitoring the resident's weight, blood pressure and cholesterol levels. The pharmacist should monitor the medical record for signs of untoward effects during the monthly drug regimen review. Monitoring must persist for the duration of therapy.

The FDA recommends testing residents taking antipsychotic drugs for signs of diabetes, especially if they have other risk factors such as obesity or a family history of the disease. However, residents with no family history of diabetes have developed elevated blood sugar and diabetic coma, so all residents receiving this category of drugs must be carefully monitored.

Diabetic ketoacidosis is an especially critical complication of atypical antipsychotic therapy. Take this issue seriously. Address blood-sugar monitoring through the quality assurance committee by developing broad, facility policies or through individual physician orders. Nursing personnel should monitor the resident's blood sugar regularly and maintain a high index of suspicion if the resident develops signs and symptoms of elevated blood sugar, including recurrent infection, weight loss, nausea, vomiting, rapid breathing and dehydration.

For residents with preexisting diabetes, monitor the blood sugar closely while he or she is taking the drug. Note the risks and additional monitoring on the resident's plan of care and medication administration record (MAR), and discuss concerns with the physician and pharmacist. Notify the physician promptly if signs, symptoms, or complications develop.

Case study

Case history excerpted from an expert report in a lawsuit in which Seroquel was implicated in the hyperglycemia diagnosis. Note the subtle but progressive signs and symptoms of new onset diabetes.

Sheila Doe was admitted to the JKL Village Health Care Center on May 26, 2003. The resident's family was highly involved in her care. Mrs. Doe was diagnosed with congestive heart failure (CHF), gastroesophageal reflux disease (GERD), osteoarthritis, Parkinson's disease, and dementia. Subsequent diagnoses of cellulitis, encephalopathy, atrial fibrillation, urinary tract infection, Alzheimer's disease, and right buttocks ulcer were added to the record later.

Mrs. Doe was mentally confused, and needed total care from staff for her activities of daily living. She became verbally abusive with behavior problems during the summer of 2003. No one considered her underlying painful condition (osteoarthritis), for which she took a mild anti-inflammatory drug each day. No one assessed her for pain or did a trial of increasing her pain medicine, which could have easily been done from the regimen ordered by the physician. No one considered that the change in her behavior was caused by physical illness, pain, urinary infection, or dehydration. Her left knee had been swollen, but no one monitored this condition or assessed whether knee pain was causing the change in behavior. The notes indicate she was combative with care, and did not voice complaints of pain. However, this resident had dementia and could not be expected to clearly articulate the presence or cause of pain.

No behavior management care plan was implemented. In July 2003, Mrs. Doe was found to have a urinary tract infection. The causative agent originates in the colon, suggesting the infection was caused by cross contamination. The resident was also quite dehydrated. She was sent to the emergency department for fluid replacement, then returned to the facility. No plan of care was initiated to ensure her hydration was sufficient, and no special monitoring was implemented. Laboratory work drawn on August 7, 2003 reveals values consistent with mild dehydration. In fact, most of the labs drawn while she was in this facility suggest the resident was maintained in a chronic state of (mild) dehydration. No one questioned the abnormal hydration values, and the problem was not addressed or explored with the physician. The problem was not noted on the care plan. The physician noted the need for additional fluids and ordered increased fluids in July 2002 and August 2003, but there is no evidence facility personnel followed these orders. Nursing personnel did not request a dietitian review of the laboratory values or evaluation of the resident's hydration.

When the physician ordered "complete" metabolic profiles (CMP), the facility ordered "basic" metabolic profiles (BMP) from the lab. This test provides less information. The physician was not informed of the omissions or failure to follow his orders. The facility failed to give the treating physician sufficient information to make accurate clinical decisions for the resident's care. They failed to inform the responsible party of their errors and omissions. This resident most probably needed routine (periodic) laboratory monitoring because of her diagnoses, risk factors, medication regimen, recurring infections, and other abnormalities. The facility failed to consult the physician, medical director, pharmacist, or dietitian about the need for routine laboratory monitoring.

A urinalysis of September 8, 2003 revealed an infection, for which the resident was treated. This urinalysis also revealed the presence of ketones, but no one explored the reason for this abnormality. On October 27, 2003, the resident became unresponsive, and was sent to EFG Hospital for treatment. She was diagnosed with urosepsis, and admitted. She was dehydrated on admission, and had a pressure ulcer that the JKL facility was not aware of. (In fact, they documented a routine skin check showing her skin was clear *during the time* she was in the hospital.) Mrs. Doe was treated, rehydrated, and returned to the nursing facility on October 30, 2003.

Upon readmission, Dr. Jones ordered a blood pressure check daily prior to a combination diuretic/antihypertensive medication administration. The physician order instructed nurses to withhold the drug if the systolic blood pressure was less than 120. Facility personnel documented the blood pressure daily, but repeatedly administered the drug despite values lower than 120, which exposed the resident to unnecessary risk of complications. They never once informed the physician, nor did they generate a medication error report. The drug was necessary to treat Mrs. Doe's underlying medical problems, but it further increased her risk of dehydration. Again no provisions were made to ensure her fluid intake or monitor her hydration status. Laboratory work done three days after her return to the facility, on November 2, 2003 again reveals mild dehydration. (Values were normal

---

upon hospital discharge.) Upon readmission, Dr. Jones also renewed the resident's previous medication orders, including the Vioxx, which was given daily for pain. The admitting nurse made an error, and the Vioxx was not ordered. No one identified the error, and the resident was not given routine pain medications for five full months, when the physician visited and changed the orders for routine pain medications. After the new drug was given, the resident's behavior was repeatedly described as "quiet." Mrs. Doe began a slow, steady weight gain upon admission to the facility. The admission Medicaid reporting form done on February 7, 2004 shows her weight to be 132 pounds, which is about her maximum weight in the facility. After this, she began a slow, steady decline. She weighed 111 in June 2005, then regained some weight to 122 in August 2005. No one explored the reason(s) for the weight loss. She experienced recurrent, very abnormal vaginal discharges suggesting infection, but the cause was not identified, and the condition was not treated. She experienced intermittent urinary tract infections. Management of the laboratory values and urinary infections is a grave concern to this writer.

The urinalysis of October 29, 2004 also showed the presence of ketone bodies, but the abnormality was once again not explored. There is no indication the facility notified the physician of abnormal culture reports promptly when they received them. The physician has signed off the urine culture reports, but they are not dated and there is no indication when he saw the reports. This is a concern because on several occasions, the drug ordered and administered to treat the infection was not the ideal/optimal drug to eradicate the infection. No nursing contact was made to inform the physician of the problem with drug sensitivities. The physician requested repeat urinalyses on several occasions, but these were not done.

Mrs. Doe continued to deteriorate. The record reveals she developed a contracture of one hand, which was splinted for a period of time until the facility lost the splint. There is no evidence it was ever found. In 2005, the resident began developing pressure ulcers. The most serious of these were ulcers on both her heels, which the facility notes were healed as of August 12, 2005. Mrs. Doe was given treatment for thrush, a fungal infection of the mouth in August 2005.

On August 24, 2005, Sheila Doe was found to be unresponsive, and was sent to the hospital. She arrived critically ill, and in generally deplorable condition. She had two large, deep pressure ulcers. One of these was the heel ulcer that the facility records noted was healed two weeks previously. No treatment was being done for this ulcer, because it was allegedly healed. This ulcer was necrotic. She was profoundly dehydrated with visible signs and symptoms, including dry lips and poor skin turgor. She had a fecal impaction, a serious condition. She had a urinary infection and sepsis. The physician describes her as unclean with fingernails that were "unkempt." She had multiple

Case study (cont.)

contractures. She was severely hyperglycemic and unresponsive, with a panic level blood sugar of 892. She was diagnosed with Hyperglycemic Hyperosmolar Nonketotic Syndrome (HHNK). She was admitted to the intensive care unit (ICU) in very serious condition. Gradual insulin doses were given to bring the blood sugar down, and the resident became responsive enough to drink some juice. Sadly, she did not respond well to treatment overall. A gastrostomy feeding tube was inserted, but she could not tolerate it. Hospice services were requested, and comfort care provided. She expired on September 12, 2005.

Normal blood sugar is approximately 70 to 110. Mrs. Doe had a hemoglobin (HbA1c) sugar value of 9.3. (Good diabetic control is 6.5; nondiabetic value is approximately 4 to 6). This test reflects the resident's blood sugar over the past two to three months, revealing that Mrs. Doe had been experiencing uncontrolled high blood sugars for a prolonged period of time. (The hemoglobin (HbA1c) sugar values reflect average blood sugars from approximately 240 to 275 during the previous three months; this is substantially above normal and represents uncontrolled diabetes). The presence of ketones in the urine suggests the diabetes was present as early as 2002. Her HDL cholesterol was 62 on hospital admission in October 2002 and 48 on hospital admission in August 2002.

Values over 35 warrant further testing for diabetes, in combination with Mrs. Doe's other risk factors, signs and symptoms. Had the facility obtained the comprehensive/complete metabolic profiles that were ordered, this value would have been available. The resident had experienced worsening mental status, pressure ulcers, numerous urinary infections, vaginal infections, and thrush during her residency in the facility. Had the JKL Village Health Care Center been attentive to the resident's total condition and reported their findings to the physician, screening and testing would have been done to identify the diabetes so that it could be properly controlled. Had they ordered more complete lab profiles when the physician requested them, additional information would have been available to cause the physician to test for diabetes.

Hyperosmolar Hyperglycemic Nonketotic Coma (HHNK) is a life threatening emergency with high mortality that frequently occurs in older persons with type II diabetes or in undiagnosed diabetes. HHNK occurs slowly and almost exclusively in elderly patients who are not getting enough fluids.[3] HHNK usually develops after a period of symptomatic hyperglycemia in which fluid intake is inadequate to prevent extreme dehydration from the hyperglycemia induced osmotic diuresis. The precipitating factor may be a coexisting acute infection or some other circumstance.[4] Although there are many possible precipitating causes, the final common pathway is usually decreased access to water.[5] The progression from poor glucose control to overt HHNK

Case study (cont.)

requires profound hyperglycemia for a significant period of time (two days to two weeks), which allows an extreme state of hyperosmolality and dehydration to develop. An acute illness is a common precursor of HHNK. The most common infectious causes involve the urinary and respiratory tracts. Some medications can contribute to the onset of uncontrolled hyperglycemia and precipitate HHNK.[6]

The JKL Village Health Care Center failed to prevent dehydration in Sheila Doe. They failed to provide sufficient fluids. One entry notes they offered her fluids when they entered the room on that day, but nowhere does it state her acceptance and consumption of fluids. Nowhere does it show a pattern of fluid consumption. There are no focused assessments for signs and symptoms of dehydration. They failed to monitor the resident for dehydration, and failed to implement a plan of care to prevent recurrence after the resident was treated at the hospital for dehydration in July 2003 and October 2003. Monitoring of the resident's hydration status is overall inadequate. They failed to follow physician orders to increase fluids. They failed to monitor her fluid intake and output. Without a means of monitoring, it is impossible to determine whether fluid consumption was adequate, or if it had been successfully increased. This is a nursing process failure, in that they did not evaluate the resident's response to their purported interventions.

The dietitian calculated the resident's fluid needs based on weight on admission to the facility. At that time, she required a minimum of 1539 cc each day. As her weight increased, so did her fluid needs. When her weight was 134, she needed at least 1809 cc each day. No hydration plan was put in place despite the resident's confused mental status, diuretic use, dependency on staff for the provision of fluids, and known high risk of dehydration. No one considered the dietitian's calculations, or the resident's minimum bodily requirements or incorporated them into the plan of care. No one consulted the dietitian on means of improving her hydration or prevent dehydration following her two hospitalizations for dehydration. No one monitored the fluid intake of this cognitively impaired resident, who could not verbalize thirst, nor could she drink independently. If fluids were not provided directly, she could not consume them. The facility failed to obtain comprehensive metabolic profiles, when these were ordered by the physician. They failed to analyze her laboratory values to determine if her hydration was sufficient. They failed to develop and implement a preventive plan of care. They failed to assess the resident for physical signs of dehydration, including dry mucous membranes, poor skin turgor, concentrated urine, sunken eyeballs, and worsening confusion.

Documentation does not reflect the use of the nursing process. The facility and its personnel failed to ensure the records contained sufficient information with which to evaluate the resident and develop or maintain a proper care plan, making it impossible for nursing personnel to provide proper care.

Case study (cont.)

They ignored data that were available, such as the dietitian's calculation of minimum daily fluid needs. They documented on her record during times when she was in the hospital. There are omissions in care during times when the resident was symptomatic for acute illness, including but not limited to August 14 to August 24, 2005. They failed to conduct focused assessments and monitor her vital signs. Nurses' notes are uninformative. There is no bowel monitoring record, and no assessment of the resident's bowel evacuation. There is no monitoring of the resident's fluid intake, despite having physician orders to increase fluid. There is no documentation of range of motion exercises and application of orthotics for contracture prevention. The resident's hand contracture had worsened markedly, and her fingernails would dig into the palm of her hand if not supported by a handroll. Laboratory tests were not obtained as ordered by the physician. Laboratory reports were not reviewed by nursing personnel as a means of evaluating the resident's hydration. Pain assessment and management were not adequate. Nursing personnel failed to collect and analyze pertinent information using the nursing process.

The polypharmacy problem

Polypharmacy is the use of multiple drugs simultaneously. This is a common occurrence in elderly, long-term care facility residents, and contributes to some problems seen in lawsuits. Drugs provide many positive effects, including improved quality of life, alleviating symptoms, and curing some infections and diseases. Despite the benefits, polypharmacy is a great concern to those caring for the elderly in the United States. Consequences of polypharmacy may include

- Adverse drug reactions

- Drug-to-drug interactions

- Noncompliance with the drug regimen

- Decline of quality of life or functional ability

- Deterioration in mental status

The American Nurses Association has issued a position statement entitled *Polypharmacy and the Older Adult.* This statement is online at the ANA Web site, *www.nursingworld.org.*

Warfarin therapy

Many residents in the long-term care facility receive oral anticoagulant therapy. Nursing personnel must have a healthy respect for drugs in this category, and be familiar with complications and side effects for anticoagulants.

Warfarin is the most commonly used anticoagulant in long-term care, so the generic drug name is used here. However, keep in mind that most of the information and protocols listed here apply to other anticoagulants as well.

Case Study

Case history from a lawsuit against an assisted-living facility involving warfarin administration; the following is excerpted from a state supreme court opinion.

Opinion

Plaintiffs/appellees, Darlyn Jill Stone, individually, and as representative of the estate of Donald G. Hill, and Richard J. Hill, individually, sued defendant/appellant, OPQ Retirement & Healthcare d/b/a OPQ Retirement Center, Ltd. for negligence in its care of Donald G. Hill. A jury returned a verdict awarding $999,999.99 to Hill's estate, but found that his children sustained no damages. The trial court entered judgment against OPQ and in favor of Hill's estate in the amount of $999,999.99, plus prejudgment interest of $169,191.71. We reverse and remand.

Background

Hill was a resident of OPQ, an assisted living facility, since 1995. Before his admission to OPQ, Hill had a multitude of health problems, including three prior strokes, diabetes, atrial fibrillation, and hypertension. He was in a wheel chair because of paralysis in his right arm and leg. Because of the atrial fibrillation, Hill was at risk for blood clots. His doctor, Dr. Love, prescribed Coumadin, a blood thinner medication, to reduce the risk of another stroke. Coumadin is an anticoagulant that helps prevent clots from forming and leading to strokes. A test known as Protime monitors the level of Coumadin. A low Coumadin level indicates a risk of stroke; a high level indicates a risk of bleeding problems.

In early July 1998, Hill developed a urinary tract infection. Dr. Love prescribed the antibiotic Bactrim, which did not cure the infection. On July 27, 1998, Hill continued to have problems with bowel incontinence. Dr. Love changed the antibiotic prescription to Cipro, which had the side effect of thinning blood. Dr. Love was aware that Cipro had an enhancement effect on the Coumadin to thin Hill'sblood even further. On July 27, Dr. Love ordered a Protime test to be run by Thursday, July 30.

The procedures for ordering lab work were as follows: Hill (or whoever took him to the doctor) would bring the doctor's order to OPQ. OPQ would then write that order into a lab book supplied by BCD Laboratories. As a courtesy to residents, so that they would not have to go to the lab, OPQ made arrangements for BCD to come to OPQ and take blood and urine samples from the residents. BCD would come to OPQ, review the order in the lab book, obtain the specimens needed to run the ordered tests, and fax a copy of the lab result to OPQ.

Case Study (cont.)

Prior to this lawsuit being filed, BCD's lab book disappeared. BCD admitted that one of its former employees took the lab book. It is unknown why Hill's Protime test, which Dr. Love ordered to be run on July 30, was not run until July 31. BCD performed Hill's Protime test on Friday, July 31, at 5:00 a.m.

A normal blood clotting time is 13–15 seconds. Hill's Protime test indicated that his time was 36.4 seconds, which is abnormal. Hill's results were faxed to OPQ on Friday, July 31, at 11:58 p.m., two minutes before midnight. The room where OPQ kept the fax machine was closed at 5 p.m. on Friday for the remainder of the weekend. OPQ contends that BCD should have faxed the lab result to Hill's physician because OPQ did not, and was not required to, have individuals on staff who were trained to interpret lab results.

After the weekend, on Monday, August 3, an OPQ medication aide, Edith Smith, saw Hill's abnormal lab report. She faxed the results to Dr. Love at 8:29 a.m. that morning. Upon receipt of the abnormal result, Dr. Love instructed OPQ to stop administering the Coumadin to Hill and inject vitamin K, which is designed to thicken the blood. Dr. Love did not request that OPQ bring Hill to the hospital. He expected that Hill's Protime result would return to normal within one or two days.

Pursuant to Dr. Love's orders, Hill did not receive any more Coumadin and instead received the vitamin K injection. Ms. Long, the director of assisted living at OPQ, testified that Hill was fine on August 3. He did not appear to be bleeding, dizzy, confused, or disoriented.

In the early morning of Tuesday, August 4, Hill was found on the floor. He was incontinent of urine and bowel. Later that morning, Hill began to experience difficulty breathing. OPQ called Hill's son and Dr. Love, who ordered him transferred to the hospital. The emergency room assessed Hill's condition as non urgent. The emergency room records indicate that Hill denied being in any pain. At the time of his admission, Hill's blood pressure was adequate. At 3:30 p.m., he was given a blood transfusion. That evening on Tuesday, August 4, at approximately 7:55 p.m., Hill died.

The cause of death listed on Hill's death certificate was CVA or cerebrovascular accident or stroke. Dr. Love agreed with the cause of death, opining that Hill did not begin bleeding until the morning of Tuesday, August 4. Dr. Hall, one of Hill's experts, disagreed, and instead opined that Hill bled to death. Dr. Hall testified that Hill had an overdose of Coumadin from July 31 to August 4, which resulted in Hill bleeding internally for a few days before his admission to the hospital.

Case Study (cont.)

Procedural History

Hill's children, individually and as representatives of Hill's estate, sued OPQ and BCD for negligence. OPQ filed a cross action against BCD for contribution. The allegations of negligence were that OPQ did not have lab work performed in a timely fashion, did not forward an abnormal test result to Hill's physician, and violated multiple provisions of the State Administrative Code pertaining to assisted living facilities. OPQ's claim against BCD for contribution was based on an agreement and BCD's course of performance to forward lab results directly to the residents' physicians.

Before the introduction of any evidence, plaintiffs announced that they had settled with BCD and dropped all claims against BCD. The trial court proceeded with plaintiffs' claims against OPQ, and OPQ continued to maintain its cross action against BCD. The jury returned a verdict awarding $999,999.99 to Hill's estate and no damages to Hill's children. The jury allocated 100% of the fault against OPQ and none against BCD. The trial court entered judgment against OPQ and in favor of Hill's estate in the amount of $999,999.99, plus prejudgment interest of $169,191.71. The court denied recovery to Hill's children in their individual capacities and denied OPQ's claim for contribution from BCD.

The dose of warfarin is individualized and resident-specific. The individualization is based on the specific indication for use and response to warfarin as indicated by the international normalized ratio (INR) testing.[7] Monitoring by experienced professionals reduces the risk of excessive (or inadequate) anticoagulation with the associated risks of bleeding (or thrombosis).[8]

The prothrombin time test (PT) and international normalized ratio (INR) are used to monitor the effectiveness of oral anticoagulation therapy. In addition to faxing the laboratory reports to the physician, facility nurses should review the reports closely to ensure that a crisis is not impending. If test values are abnormal, promptly follow up with a phone call to the physician. Follow physician orders and facility policies for frequency of laboratory tests. In early stages of therapy, very frequent tests may be ordered. After the

dosage is stabilized, the tests may be ordered weekly or monthly. Confirm that there are adequate safeguards in your system to ensure that the test is drawn regularly, and as ordered. *Anticoagulant therapy must always be noted on the care plan.* The plan should describe individualized approaches to prevent injury, specific bleeding precautions to take, and observations to make of signs and symptoms suggesting abnormal values and overdose.

Also carefully evaluate the resident's risk of falls and fractures and consider a care plan notation. Several studies have shown a relationship between warfarin and increased risk for osteoporosis-related bone fractures. This is an area in which further research is needed. In the interim, carefully monitor the bone health of residents taking warfarin and address the risk of osteoporosis, falls, and fractures.[9]

Factors affecting warfarin therapy

Many factors, alone or in combination, may affect the resident's response to anticoagulant therapy. Common factors causing an unpredictable response include

- change in diet

- change in environment

- overall physical condition

- many medications (also herbals)

The following factors, alone or in combination, may increase the PT response:

- cancer

- malnutrition, poor nutritional state

- acetaminophen

- NSAIDs, Aspirin

The following drug, alone or in combination, may decrease the PT response:

- trazodone

This list is not exhaustive. Warfarin interacts with many other drugs and herbals. See the package insert or a drug manual such as the *Physicians' Desk Reference* for a comprehensive listing. Since the drug is so sensitive to the effects of other drugs, as well as some herbs and botanicals, consider monitoring the resident's coagulation values any time a new medication is added. Since the residents may be exposed to any combination of these factors, the net effect on PT response may be very unpredictable. Consider more-frequent monitoring.

Other important considerations

In 2003, British researchers conducted limited testing, which prompted regulatory authorities to issue a warning to patients taking warfarin not to drink cranberry juice. The combination has been associated with unstable INR values, and excessive bleeding. One man reportedly died from this combination. Until the interaction has been more thoroughly studied, authorities recommend that persons taking warfarin avoid cranberry juice.[10]

The American Medical Directors Association and American Society of Consultant Pharmacists have published a list of the most common negative drug interactions in long-term care.[11] These drug combinations have the potential to produce harmful effects. The list includes

- Warfarin—NSAIDs

- Warfarin—Sulfa drugs

- Warfarin—Macrolides

- Warfarin—Quinolones

- Warfarin—Phenytoin

Warfarin necrosis

The major complication of anticoagulant therapy is bleeding. Less frequently, problems with skin necrosis may occur after initiation of therapy, particularly if the drug is administered in high doses. Become familiar with "warfarin necrosis." It may be identified because it looks like a necrotic pressure ulcer. However, the necrotic areas appear in non-pressure areas with no bony prominences, such as the abdomen, breast, or top of the thigh. Necrotic ulcers may also develop on the extremities, trunk, and penis (in males). This condition is more common in women than in men. In warfarin necrosis, skin lesions typically develop between the third and eighth day of therapy, although they may appear later. Avoid mistaking the lesions for pressure ulcers. They develop quickly (over a period of hours) from an initial central erythematous lesion.

Skin necrosis is usually associated with an underlying protein C deficiency. Although not a common complication, warfarin necrosis must be identified and reported to the physician promptly. No single treatment for the lesions exists, but the physician will probably order laboratory tests and may need to alter the anticoagulant medication or adjust the dosage. The physician will need to differentiate the lesions from other conditions, such as vasculitis and purple toes syndrome. Warfarin necrosis can be treated and most small lesions will heal by themselves, if an early diagnosis is made. However, failure to identify the condition quickly may result in the need for skin grafting and other surgical interventions including plastic surgery, mastectomy, and amputation. Undiagnosed, the condition may lead to death.

Other complications of warfarin

Always consider the possibility of hemorrhage when assessing a resident on anticoagulant therapy, even if signs and symptoms do not suggest an obvious problem. Bleeding that occurs when the PT is within the therapeutic dosage range warrants physician intervention and diagnostic investigation. The risk of bleeding is increased in those who are more than 65 years old, have a history of a stroke or gastrointestinal bleeding, or serious comorbid conditions such as renal insufficiency or anemia.[12] Early signs of warfarin overdosage that warrant monitoring and a call to the physician include

- suspected internal bleeding or overt abnormal bleeding

- blood in stool

- hematuria

- increase in menstrual flow

- new bruising

- persistent oozing from superficial injuries

- new or worsening confusion

Signs suggesting an emergency, warranting ongoing monitoring and an immediate call to the physician include

- excessive bruising

- unusually large amount of menstrual bleeding

- spontaneous bleeding

- hemorrhage from any tissue or organ

Signs and symptoms of hemorrhage vary depending on the location and extent of bleeding. These also warrant continuous monitoring and an immediate call to the physician. If he or she is not immediately available, send the resident to the emergency department via 911 ambulance if the resident experiences sudden onset of any of the following complications of internal hemorrhage:

- paralysis

- severe headache

- pain in chest, abdomen, or joints

- dyspnea, shortness of breath

- difficulty swallowing

- unexplained shock

Laboratory monitoring for anticoagulant therapy

Residents who are on anticoagulant therapy should have certain laboratory values monitored regularly. The frequency is determined by facility policies and individual physician orders. Recommendations for routine laboratory monitoring are

- CBC on initiation of therapy and every three months to monitor for anemia and blood loss.

- Prothrombin time (protime), INR daily until the dosage is stabilized, then weekly for two to three weeks after the dosage has been adjusted satisfactorily. After this, draw monthly levels. Draw stat levels any time complications are suspected.

- Stools for occult blood times three on initiation of therapy, then once every six months or according to facility protocol. (Some facilities monitor stools every three months.)

Warfarin has a very narrow therapeutic window and highly variable pharmacokinetics, both between individuals and within an individual over time.[13] Take the need for conscientious nursing and laboratory monitoring seriously. You will also find that surveyors often review residents receiving drugs such as warfarin that have a narrow therapeutic window.

Interpreting the prothrombin time test

The prothrombin time (protime, PT) test is done on blood plasma to detect the activity of prothrombin, or clotting factor II, which is part of the coagulation factor assay. Prothrombin time is most commonly used to monitor oral anticoagulant therapy. The normal control value is 11–15 seconds. For good control, *the resident's protime is normally maintained between 1.5 and two the normal control.*

Many drugs have the potential for causing false increases and decreases in the results of this test. A number of exogenous and endogenous factors have the potential to alter the resident's response. Review the prescribing information for a complete list. Monitor the resident closely for early warning signs of overdose, including blood in stools or urine, nosebleed, petechiae, persistent oozing from superficial injuries, and bleeding from ulcers or other lesions. Notify the physician immediately if these signs and symptoms are present. The facility must ensure that the INR

value is promptly communicated to the attending physician. The attending physician's follow-up orders and nursing response must be properly documented. The paper trail should be evident to all who review the resident's medical record.[14]

Vitamin K is administered if the protime is more than 40 seconds, or if bleeding occurs. Unfortunately, it may take several days to be effective. Subcutaneous Vitamin K is less effective than oral, and should not be used if possible.[15] Alternately, 0.5 mg of Vitamin K intravenously reliably reduces markedly prolonged INR values into the therapeutic range within 24 hours.[16] However, if early warning signs are ignored, the condition may progress very quickly, and may not be reversible in late stages. Facilities do not normally maintain a stock of Vitamin K. Consider adding this drug to your emergency box if warfarin is being administered to the residents.

Suboptimal laboratory monitoring can occur if the period between the prothrombin time testings is more than four weeks or if dosage change in response to a PT test result outside the therapeutic range is inappropriately great.[17] Keep track of coagulation tests. *If the lab has not notified you of the results within eight hours, contact them by phone.* Make sure the INR value is promptly relayed to the physician. If the value is abnormal, do not depend on fax notification. Call the physician and document his or her follow-up orders and nursing response carefully. Make sure the paper trail is available to and maintained by all who review and handle the resident's medical record.[18] Documentation should list the resident's signs and symptoms, laboratory values, nursing action, physician response. Some facilities use an anticoagulant flow sheet to provide an audit trail. The flow sheet contains data such as

- Warfarin dosage

- PT/INR results

- Physician notification (date, time)

- Physician response/dosage adjustment

- Date, time changes (new physician orders)
  were initiated

Nurses should initial or sign flow-sheet entries. Make sure the flow sheet is available when calling the physician so you can answer questions about previous results, dosages, and patterns. Another technique for documenting laboratory values is by using a stamp or printed label in the nursing notes, on which nurses write the information noted above. In any event, all communications with the laboratory, physician, pharmacist, or dietitian about the anticoagulant regimen must be clearly documented. If the facility uses agency or pool personnel, make sure they are familiar with the anticoagulant policies and procedures, including documentation.

The INR test

The International Normalized Ratio (INR) is a mathematical correction used to standardize the results of the prothrombin time. It was developed in response to concerns about wide variations in thromboplastin sensitivities.

By reporting prothrombin times as INRs, results can be interpreted with reasonable accuracy. Values are standardized from one laboratory to the next. This is important if the resident has the test drawn in more than one location, such as the hospital, physician office, and by the facility laboratory.

The INR is the prothrombin time ratio between the mean normal control sample raised to the power of ISI and the resident's sample. The denominator must be correct when the PT ratio is calculated. The laboratory should calculate this value for you. The recommended therapeutic range for anticoagulation with warfarin is listed in Figure 18-1 below.

See your CD-ROM for more information on bisphosphonates.

Figure 18-1	*Recommended Therapeutic Range for Anticoagulation with Coumadin® (Wafarin Sodium)*

Desirable Range	Medical Condition
INR 2.0-3.0	atrial fibrillation
	bioprosthetic heart valves
	pulmonary embolism
	venous thrombosis
INR 2.5-3.5	mechanical heart valves
	postmyocardial infarction

Acetaminophen toxicity

Acetaminophen is the most widely used pharmaceutical analgesic and antipyretic agent in the United States and the world. Acetaminophen may be administered plain or in combination with other drugs, and is an active ingredient in more than 200 prescription and over-the-counter products. As such, acetaminophen is one of the most common pharmaceuticals associated with both intentional and accidental poisoning.[19] Many healthcare providers view acetaminophen as a harmless, nonprescription drug. Slipping a resident a few tablets without an order is not unheard of. Most long-term care facility residents have orders for "as needed" acetaminophen for pain or fever, and some residents take it four times daily for chronic pain. Acetaminophen is routinely added to the standing order listing for pain or fever in facilities who use standing orders.

Unintentional acetaminophen overdose is the most common cause of acute liver failure in the United States, research from UT Southwestern Medical Center at Dallas shows. Most of the overdoses in the UT study were unintentional. Acetaminophen-induced liver failure is the second most common cause of hepatic failure necessitating liver transplant in the United States.[20] Patients are literally healthy one day, and need a liver transplant the next. In addition to liver failure, chronic analgesic use can also lead to a condition called analgesic nephropathy. In this condition, the analgesic drugs damage the kidneys over time. The offending agents here are usually acetaminophen and NSAIDs. Acetaminophen is commonly ordered for residents for mild pain and fever, but the resident may also have orders for other analgesics, such as Darvocet N 100, Lortab, Lorcet, Talacen, Vicodin, Midrin, and Percocet or their generic equivalents. These drugs contain 325 mg to 750 mg of acetaminophen per tablet.

Many over-the-counter cold preparations also contain acetaminophen.

Acetaminophen is absorbed quickly after ingestion. A single dose of 10 to 15 grams is considered toxic, although liver damage has been reported in adults with daily dosages as low as six grams. Elderly persons and those with preexisting liver disease may experience toxicity at lower doses, particularly those who consume alcohol regularly. Various sources report that doses exceeding four grams a day over a period of three months can cause potential hepatotoxicity. Doses of five to eight grams per day over two to three weeks have also been implicated in liver failure.

The maximum daily dosage of acetaminophen should not exceed four grams (4000 mg.). This means that as few as six tablets per day, over a period of several months, could lead to liver failure. Lower dosages are ordered for residents who are frail, small in stature, those who take acetaminophen daily for chronic pain, in residents with preexisting hepatic or renal disease, and individuals who drink alcohol occasionally. For example, when treating persistent arthritic pain in an 85-year-old woman weighing 110 pounds, most physicians would not exceed a dosage of 650 mg four times a day. Alcohol, anti-seizure medications (phenytoin, phenobarbital, primidone, valproic acid, and carbamazepine), and isoniazid may increase the risk of acetaminophen liver toxicity since all these drugs are potentially toxic to the liver. Acetaminophen may also potentiate the action of anticoagulants. Some physicians advise chronic alcoholics and individuals with heavy alcohol consumption to avoid the drug entirely.

Acetaminophen toxicity is often asymptomatic. The resident may have anorexia and mild nausea that progresses to vomiting. However, these signs are seldom associated with acetaminophen ingestion. Several days

later, the resident develops right upper quadrant tenderness, jaundice, and other signs of liver involvement.
By this time, damage may be extensive. Acetylcysteine
(Mucomyst, NAC) is the antidote for acetaminophen
overdose, and is most effective if given up to eight
hours after ingestion occurs, although it can and
should be administered anytime. Acetylcysteine may
be given orally or by IV. Use of emetics is not usually
recommended, although activated charcoal may be
used for recent overdosage. The resident should be
hospitalized if toxicity is suspected.

Before giving acetaminophen to any resident, review
his or her medical and medication history. *Nurses
must know how much acetaminophen is in each dose of
acetaminophen and combination medications.* Check
the drug profile to see if the resident routinely takes
other drugs containing this ingredient. If so, make a
notation on the MAR to warn others not to exceed
the daily allowable maximums. If the resident has
orders for multiple medications containing acetaminophen, ask the pharmacist to review the medication
regimen and make recommendations. If you discover
that a resident is ingesting more than four grams of
acetaminophen a day, notify the physician promptly.
Document your communication.

Remember, nurses are resident advocates. Never withhold analgesics to prevent toxicity. Pain is a treatable
medical problem, and relieving pain and making residents comfortable are important nursing responsibilities. Many excellent analgesics are available that
contain low-dose acetaminophen, or no acetaminophen. A healthy dose of education is necessary for
both residents and nursing personnel to avoid inadvertent overdose. Keep communication open with the
pharmacist and physician. Your attentiveness to the
use of a seemingly innocuous medication will prevent
potentially serious consequences for your residents.

Guidelines for antibiotic use

In recent years, much has been written about drug-
resistant pathogens. Over-prescribing of antibiotics is
a major cause of the problem. Drug resistance and
overuse of antibiotics has also been a major factor in a
number of lawsuits. Well-published studies have verified that antibiotics are often overprescribed in long-
term care facilities, leading to drug resistance.[21,22,23,24]
Geriatric residents are at greater risk of infection compared with younger persons because of nutritional
and hydration deficiencies, decreased immune function, comorbid or chronic diseases, and decreased
mobility. Facility residents are also at greater risk of
infection than their peers who live in the community.[25]
No official guidelines are available for antibiotic use
in long-term care facilities.

Bacteria, fungi, and viruses can become resistant to
drugs. Bacteria cause most of the drug-resistant problems in hospitals. Once a particular type of bacteria has
developed drug resistance, it can pass on this resistance
to other types of bacteria. The more often a drug is
used, the more likely bacteria are to develop resistance
to it. Consequently, and to combat the problem of
drug-resistant bacteria, the Centers for Disease Control
and Prevention (CDC) have developed recommendations to help ensure that antibiotic drugs are prescribed
only when appropriate. Nursing personnel should

- Ensure residents maintain sufficient nutrition
  and hydration.

- Maintain resident skin integrity; the skin is the
  largest organ in the body and provides a barrier
  against infection.

- Consistently emphasize the importance of
  handwashing. Have alcohol preparations readily
  available.

- Rapidly identify signs and symptoms of infection.

- Thoroughly assess the resident's signs, symptoms, and vital signs and provide the physician with an accurate report.

- Continue to monitor the resident's vital signs and focused assessment of symptoms until the infection is resolved.

- Obtain culture and sensitivity testing to verify the need for and appropriateness of antibiotic prescribing; report results to the attending physician as soon as they are available. If the report is faxed, always follow up with a phone call. Document physician response and orders.

- If an infection is identified, the physician will order antibiotics. Verify the ordered antibiotic against the sensitivity report to ensure the offending organism is not resistant to the drug.

- Avoid using antibiotics for viral infections.

- If a significant pathogen is identified, use the least amount of isolation needed to contain the pathogen. For example, a resident with MRSA may be placed in contact precautions. Always consider the roommate, if any. Move one resident if his or her roommate has any high risk condition or opening into the body, such as pressure ulcer, gastrostomy, tracheostomy, or catheter. Avoid overkill in selecting isolation precautions. Paper dishes and meltaway laundry bags are unnecessary if standard precautions are properly applied. Routine practices in the laundry and dish room will eliminate the pathogen with no special measures. The resident need not be confined to his or her room if the pathogen can be contained, such as in a dressing, incontinent brief, or urinary catheter.

- Avoid broad-spectrum antibiotics whenever possible; use antibiotics that are specific to the organism being treated.

- Make sure antibiotics are administered as ordered. If they are ordered four times a day, give them every six hours instead of on a four-hour daytime schedule, such as 8-12-4-8. Some facilities have each nurse sign for antibiotics administered on a narcotic sign-out sheet to ensure each dose is given. In any event, avoid skips in antibiotic administration; finish the entire prescription. Treat for the shortest duration possible.

- In some circumstances, such as wound and urinary infections, the physician may order a repeat culture and sensitivity test after the antibiotics are finished. Obtain this test five to seven days after the last antibiotic is given, unless otherwise ordered.

- The infection control nurse should review all culture and sensitivity laboratory reports at least weekly.

- Maintain a separate database for each pathogen identified by the laboratory culture and sensitivity testing. Include the resident's *a)* name, *b)* age, *c)* sex, *d)* date of transfer into facility, *e)* name of transferring facility, *f)* site(s) cultured, *g)* date(s) of culture(s), *h)* specific pathogen identified and the antibiotic resistance, *i)* antibiotic(s) prescribed and duration of therapy within two (2) weeks prior to a positive culture, *j)* presence of invasive devices (e.g., indwelling urinary catheters, vascular access lines, tracheostomy), *k)* room assignment(s), *l)* name of roommate(s), *m)* infection risk assessment (e.g., aspiration, chronic bronchitis, nonintact skin sites and bowel and bladder incontinence).

- Determine by chart review or physical assessment if the site cultured was infected or colonized and enter information into database.

- Analyze the databases prior to each infection control or quality assurance committee meeting to determine common relational factors such as the microorganism(s) cultured, antibiotic resistance patterns, relationship of new cases and old cases (e.g., room placement, activity times, etc.), transferring facility, sites of positive culture(s) such as urine, etc.

- Report the findings to the infection control committee, and implement their recommendations.

- Evaluate the recommendations implemented for impact on the number of identified infections over a defined period of time.

- Antibiotics, both oral and parenteral, should only be used to treat residents with suspect or documented clinical infections, not colonization. The infection control committee should monitor all antibiotics administered, the indications for which the antibiotic was ordered and the outcome of the resident receiving antibiotic therapy. Criteria for utilizing specific antibiotics should be developed and all physicians informed of the criteria. Anti-biotics such as vancomycin and second- and third-generation cephalosporins should not be used when the clinical effectiveness of another class of antibiotics has been described in the literature.

- Reserve the use of vancomycin only in specific situations in which other drugs are not available to eradicate the pathogen. Remember that vancomycin is ototoxic and nephrotoxic, and may cause liver damage in elderly persons.

Guidelines for nursing monitoring and documentation of antibiotics

Nursing personnel are responsible for regular, ongoing, monitoring of residents who have experienced an acute illness, infection, incident, or other event. Any change in condition, even if minor, falls into this category. Monitor the resident for as long as necessary to ensure that the illness is resolved, and the resident's condition is stabilized. Conduct focused assessments of the systems involved with the infection. Monitor vital signs. If abnormal observations are noted, take the appropriate nursing action and provide the necessary intervention. Notify the physician of abnormal observations as soon as practicable. Nursing personnel should

- Update the care plan to reflect the change in condition and monitoring required. Note any special preventive care, such as turning the resident to prevent skin breakdown.

- When residents are taking antibiotics for an infection, the narrative nurses' notes for each shift note repeatedly, "No side effects noted to antibiotics." This is a good observation, but it should never be your *only* observation. *The purpose of ongoing monitoring is to make observations of the condition for which the resident is receiving antibiotics.*

- Monitor the resident on all shifts until 24 hours after the acute event is completely resolved. Monitoring can continue for days or weeks, depending on the nature of the precipitating occurrence.

- Document the results of follow-up monitoring, observations, nursing interventions, and the resident's response in the nurses notes.

- Monitor vital signs every four to eight hours. Repeat vital signs and schedule more frequently if one or more of the values is abnormal, or the resident's condition warrants.

- Make sure fluid intake is sufficient to dilute the drugs and reduce fever; consider monitoring intake and output.

- Report results of the follow-up monitoring to the oncoming nurse in the change-of-shift report.

- Promptly notify the physician (and responsible party) if abnormalities are noted or the resident experiences further change in condition. Document your notifications.

- Conduct a focused assessment on the affected system every four to eight hours, depending on the severity of the resident's condition. For example, if the resident is taking antibiotics for a respiratory infection, assess lung sounds. Document positive and negative findings. For example, "Lungs clear, color pink, no shortness of breath, no cough." Examples of focused assessments are

  - Auscultation of lung sounds. Assess the nature of sounds and adequacy of chest expansion, rate, rhythm, depth of respirations, and use of accessory respiratory muscles.

  - Color of the resident's skin, lips, and fingernail beds.

  - Change in mental status or level of consciousness.

  - Increased restlessness.

  - Shortness of breath, or other difficulty breathing.

- In the presence or absence of signs and symptoms related to a suspected urinary tract infection, nurses would describe the color, odor, clarity, sediment, intake and output, and other factors related to the urine. They must identify positive and negative observations, such as frequency, burning, and pain.

- Document your assessment findings at least once per shift, or as often as necessary.

Drugs that are potentially inappropriate in the elderly

The federal long-term care regulations contain a list of potentially inappropriate drugs that were partially adapted from a paper entitled "Explicit Criteria for Determining Inappropriate Medication Use by the Elderly" by Mark H. Beers, MD This paper was published in the *Archives of Internal Medicine*, Vol. 157, July 28, 1997. The paper lists numerous drugs and diagnosis/drug combinations judged to place a person over the age of 65 at greater risk of adverse drug outcomes. The judgments in this paper were derived through an extensive review of the literature by a panel of experts.

The survey guidelines incorporate only *some of the drugs on the 1997 Beers' listing.* The list is regularly updated and researched. Many additional drugs are listed as having the potential for serious complications in elderly persons. Some drugs have been removed from the 1997 listing. A more comprehensive listing of drugs with potential for complications is provided here. Please note that cardiovascular medications; antibiotics/anti infectives; and diuretics account for more than 50 percent of all adverse reactions experienced by elderly persons.

See your CD-ROM for a listing of inappropriate drug and drug categories for use in the elderly.

The M3 project—top ten list

The Multidisciplinary Medication Management Project is an interdisciplinary professional group who developed and promoted a list of ten drug interactions that are problematic in long-term care settings. Each of these drug interactions involves medications that are commonly used in long-term care, and has the potential to cause significant harm if not managed appropriately. Medications chosen for the "Top Ten" list were based on their frequency of use in older adults in the long-term care setting, and on the potential for adverse consequences if used together.[26] The drugs and drug interactions on the "Top Ten" list are:

- **Warfarin—NSAIDs***—Aleve, Anaprox, Anaprox DS, Ansaid, Arthrotec, Cataflam, Clinoril, Daypro, diclofenac, diclofenac/misto-prostrol, diflunisal, Dolobid, etodolac, Feldene, flurbiprofen, ibuprofen, Indocin, Indocin SR, indomethacin, ketoprofen, ketorolac, Lodine, Lodine XL, mefenamic acid, meloxican, Mobic, Motrin, nabumetone, Naprelan, Naprosyn, naproxen, Orudis, Oruvail, oxaprozin, piroxi-cam, Ponsel, Relafen, sulindac, Tolectin, Tolectin DS, tolmetin, Toradol, Voltaren, Voltaren XR

- **Warfarin—Sulfa drugs**—Bactrim DS, Bactrim SS, Cotrim DS, Cotrim SS, erythromycin/sulfisoxazole, Gantanol, Gantrisin, Pediazole, Septra DS, Sulfatrim, sulfamethizole, sul-famethoxazole, sulfisoxazole, Thiosulfil Forte, trimethoprim/sulfamethoxazole

- **Warfarin—Macrolides**—azithromycin, Biaxin, clarithromycin, Dynabac, dirithromycin, E Mycin, erythromycin base, EES, erythromycin ethyl succinate, Ery Tab, Eryc, EryPed, Ery-throcin, erythromycin stearate, Ilosone, eryth-romycin estolate, Pediazole, erythromycin/sulfisoxazole, Tao, troleandomycin, Zithromax

- **Warfarin—Quinolones***—alatrofloxacin, Avelox, Cipro, ciprofloxacin, enoxacin, Floxin, gatifloxacin, Levaquin, levofloxacin, lomefloxacin, Maxaquin, moxifloxacin, Noroxin, norfloxacin, ofloxacin, Penetrex, sparfloxacin, Tequin, trovafloxacin, Trovan, Trovan IV, Zagam

- **Warfarin—Phenytoin**

  - Phenytoin - Dilantin, phenytoin

- **ACE inhibitors—Potassium supplements**

  - Ace Inhibitors—Accupril, Aceon, Altace, benazepril, Capoten, captopril, enalapril, fosinopril, lisinopril, Lotensin, Mavik, moexipril, Monopril, perindopril, Prinivil, quinapril, ramipril, trandolapril, Univasc, Vasotec, Zestril

  - Potassium Supplements—K+ Care ET, Kaon, K dur, Klor Con, K Phos, Micro K, potassium acetate, potassium acid phos-phate, potassium bicarbonate, potassium chloride, potassium citrate, potassium glu-conate, Urocit K

- **ACE inhibitors—Spironolactone**

  - ACE inhibitors—Accupril, Aceon, Altace, benazepril, Capoten, captopril, enalapril, fosinopril, lisinopril, Lotensin, Mavik, moexipril, Monopril, perindopril, Prinivil, quinapril, ramipril, trandolapril, Univasc, Vasotec, Zestril

  - Spironolactone—Aldactone, spironolactone

- **Digoxin—Amiodarone**

  - Digoxin—digoxin, Lanoxin

  - Amiodarone—amiodarone, Cordarone

- **Digoxin—Verapamil**

  - Digoxin—digoxin, Lanoxin

– Verapamil—Calan, Calan SR, Covera HS, Isoptin, Isoptin SR, verapamil, Verelan

- **Theophylline—Quinolones****

  – Theophylline—aminophylline, Choledyl SA, oxtriphylline, Phyllocontin, Slo Bid, Slo Phyllin, Slo Phyllin 125, Theo 24, Theo Dur, Theolair, theophylline, Uniphyl, Uniphyl CR

  – Quinolones—alatrofloxacin, Avelox, Cipro, ciprofloxacin, enoxacin, Floxin, gatifloxacin, Levaquin, levofloxacin, lomefloxacin, Maxaquin, moxifloxacin, Noroxin, norfloxacin, ofloxacin, Penetrex, sparfloxacin, Tequin, trovafloxacin, Trovan, Trovan IV, Zagam

  * NSAID class does not include COX-2 inhibitors

  ** Quinolones that interact include ciprofloxacin, enoxacin, norfloxacin, and ofloxacin

Suggested medication monitoring

Certain medications require special monitoring. Note special medication monitoring on the MAR and/or care plan. In absence of a facility policy or physicians order, the guidelines listed on your CD-ROM are suggested for monitoring certain drug categories.

See your CD-ROM for a sample list of policies and procedures for laboratory testing and medication monitoring.

Recommended medication-oriented laboratory tests for long-term drug therapy

Each facility should develop policies and procedures for laboratory testing and medication monitoring. The list on the accompanying CD-ROM may be useful in developing such a list. However, this is a

general guideline only. Seek the advice of the medical director when establishing the frequency for routine monitoring. Residents using specific drugs may need more frequent monitoring, especially in the early stages of drug therapy.

Drug-induced safety problems

The resident's drug regimen is often overlooked when assessing resident safety, particularly if the resident experiences falls and injuries. Personnel seem to favor assessment of environmental and behavioral factors, and may inadvertently overlook the effect of medications on the resident's cognitive status. A drug (or a specific drug combination) may also affect the resident's balance, causing weakness, dizziness, or other untoward signs and symptoms that make the resident less stable. Hip fractures affect older adults.

In the United States, one of every three adults over age 65 falls each year. Falls are the leading cause of injury-related deaths in the elderly. Of all fall deaths, at least 60% involve individuals who are over age 73. Of all fractures from falls, hip fractures cause the greatest number of deaths and lead to the most severe health problems. Women sustain 75% to 80% of all hip fractures. However, fall-related deaths are higher in men than women and differ by race. Caucasian males have the highest death rate, followed by Caucasian females. African American males have the third-highest death rate, followed by African American females.[27]

Medications can cause mental changes in all age groups, but drug-induced mental problems are most common in the elderly. Drugs can cause either delirium or dementia. Both conditions are associated with increased morbidity and mortality, so they are worthy of consideration and assessment. Residents with some conditions, such as Parkinson's disease, appear to have an increased risk of drug-induced cognitive decline.

The mnemonic, *"ACUTE CHANGE IN MS"* is useful for remembering the drug categories with the potential for causing cognitive decline in the elderly:

The Acute change in MS can be found on the accompanying CD-ROM.

Although we know that certain drugs and drug categories are likely to cause cognitive changes, polypharmacy is also an important consideration. The American Nurses Association (ANA) supports the safe and effective use of drug therapy for older adults resulting from collaborative efforts of those who prescribe, those who administer, and the older adults taking the drugs. In any event, they advise that a judicious approach to medication administration should be used with elderly individuals.[28] Most elderly persons have multiple chronic diseases and varying ability to metabolize and excrete drugs. Dehydration and inadequate fluid intake contribute to the problem. A combination of all these factors increases the likelihood of drug-induced delirium or dementia. An additional consideration is improper or inaccurate drug administration.

Delirium

Delirium has sudden onset and the course may fluctuate. Signs and symptoms of drug-induced delirium are change in cognition, disorganized thinking, altered attention span, changes in psychomotor activity, and abnormal sleep-wake cycles. The resident may experience hallucinations. Agitation is common, but delirium may also cause lethargy. If the resident experiences changes in level of consciousness, head injury and other neurologic causes should be ruled out.

Drug-induced delirium usually develops shortly after a new drug has been administered. Sometimes the delirium is related to drug dosage, but it may occur because of polypharmacy or for unknown reasons that are unrelated to dose. Fortunately, dosage-related delirium is short lived if detected early. When the drug wears off, the resident usually returns to baseline mental status. When a new drug seems to be causing delirium, consider interactions with other drugs and food. Apply aggressive safety precautions if you suspect drug-induced delirium. Many residents fall and fracture hips when they experience delirium. This situation often triggers a progressive, downward spiral of events from which the resident does not recover.

Because the residents' safety risk and mortality increase if delirium develops, identifying drug-induced delirium is essential. Estimates are that 22% to 39% of all cases of delirium are attributable to medications.[29] In fact, one study showed that medication administration was the most common cause of delirium in hospitalized adults.[30] Avoid assuming the signs and symptoms are caused by preexisting or worsening dementia. If the mental status changes, assess the problem, obtain laboratory tests, and consult the physician and pharmacist. Avoid making assumptions without first doing some detective work.

Classes of drugs most commonly associated with mental changes are benzodiazepines, anticholinergics, and antihypertensives. However, drugs in any category can cause mental changes, so predicting which drugs will cause delirium and dementia is difficult. The drugs listed below have been known to cause cognitive changes in elderly persons, but the effects are highly variable. Be suspicious if a resident develops mental changes following administration of any medication. Fortunately, drug-induced delirium is reversible. Stopping the drug or reducing the dose should solve the problem, but occasionally a prolonged period elapses before the resident returns to baseline.

Delirium may also occur when one or more drugs are

withdrawn. This problem usually occurs when the resident has used the same drug for a prolonged period of time. Confusion increases proportionate to a decreasing blood level of the drug. Suspect medication if the resident experiences confusion when a medication is discontinued.

Dementia

Dementia is a chronic form of cognitive impairment that includes impaired thinking, memory, safety judgment, and ability to learn. It interferes with daily function, emotional control, and problem-solving ability. Residents with dementia have deficits in their ability to process new information.

Substance use, abuse, and withdrawal can all cause varying signs of dementia. Substances include toxic chemicals and other sources of exposure, drugs of abuse, and medications. The relative odds of drug-induced dementia increase proportionately as the number of drugs ingested increases.[31] In one study, medication side effects accounted for 5% of reversible dementias in the over-60 population, but estimates range as high as 12% to 15%. Substance intoxication occurs when a resident develops maladaptive behavioral changes associated with recent exposure to a substance, including medications. The changes commonly include belligerence, cognitive impairment, impaired judgment, and emotional lability. This is another area where attention to the resident's underlying hydration and fluid consumption is critical.

To complicate matters further, delirium and dementia may coexist in the elderly. If a resident with dementia experiences a worsening mental status, medication-related delirium should be ruled out. If cognition improves when a potentially offending medication is withdrawn, the drug was the probable cause. If drug-induced delirium is not reversed, it may evolve into dementia.

Resident safety

It seems that part of the "judicious approach" to medication administration would be accomplished by evaluating the medication regimen as part of the routine safety and risk assessment in elderly adults. Evaluate each prescription, over-the-counter, and natural product individually and collectively. This requires a team approach, and may take some time. Employ a collaborative, interdisciplinary approach and recognize the increased risk that both polypharmacy and administration of certain medications pose to elderly adults. Incorporating a medication evaluation into your safety/risk/fall assessment will benefit many residents by reducing the risk of accidents and injuries caused by medication-induced cognitive impairment.

Medications that may cause cognitive impairment/delirium in the elderly

Type/Category of medication and generic name

- Alcohol

- Anesthetic agents: ketamine, all drugs in this class have the potential

- Antianginal: nifedipine

- Antianxiety agents

- Antiarrhythmic agents: disopyramide, quinidine, tocainide, lidocaine, procainamide, propanolol

- Antibiotics: cephalexin, cephalothin, metronidazole, ciprofloxacin, ofloxacin, imipenemcilastatin, trimethoprim-sulfamethoxazole, penicillin

- Anticholinergic agents: benztropine, homatropine, scopolamine, trihexyphenidyl

- Anticonvulsants: phenytoin, valproic acid, carbamazepine

- Antidepressants: amitryptyline, imipramine, desipramine, fluoxetine

- Antiemetics: promethazine, hydroxyzine, metoclopramide, prochlorperazine

- Antifungals: amphotericin B, ketoconazole

- Antihistamines/decongestants: phenyl-propanolamine, diphenhydramine, chlorpheniramine brompheniramine, pseudoephedrine

- Antihypertensive agents: captopril, clonadine, propranolol, metoprolol, diltiazem, atenolol, verapamil, methyldopa, prazosin, nifedipine, nitroprusside sodium

- Antimanic agents: lithium

- Antiulcer: cimetidine, metoclopramide, ranitidine

- Antineoplastic agents: chlorambucil, cytosine arabinoside, interleukin 2

- Anti-Parkinsonian agents: levodopa, pergolide, bromocryptine

- Antipsychotics

- Antiviral: acyclovir

- Benzodiazepines

- Bronchodilators: theophylline

- Cardiotonic agents: digoxin

- Corticosteroids: hydrocortisone, prednisone, any others have potential

- H2 receptor antagonists: cimetidine, ranitidine

- Immunosuppressive agents: cyclosporine, interferon

- Muscle relaxants: baclofen, cyclobenzaprine, methocarbamol

- Narcotic analgesics: codeine, hydrocodone, oxycodone, meperidine, propoxyphene, morphine

- Nonsteroidal anti inflammatory agents: aspirin, ibuprofen, indomethacin, naproxen, sulindac

- Radiocontrast agents: metrizamide, iothalamate, iohexol

- Sedatives: alprazolam, diazepam, lorazepam, phenobarbital, butabarbital, chloral hydrate

- Thyroid preparations: metronidazole

Note: These medications are listed as examples only. New medications appear regularly. Many compounds contain one or more other active ingredients. Changes in mental status may also be attributable to interaction between a new drug and the resident's existing medication regimen.

Drug diversion

Sadly, drug diversion occasionally occurs in long-term care. A 2001 study revealed substance abuse ranging from 2% to 18% among nurses.[32] A 1999 study reveal-ed misuse of prescription drugs was 6.9%.[33] The ANA had previously estimated the incidence of chemical de-pendency among nurses at 6% to 8%.[34] One Ohio law enforcement source states he arrests approximately one health care professional every six days. Some are not caught. Of those health professionals arrested in recent years, 70% were nurses.[35] The statistics suggest that there are more nurses diverting drugs than actually reported.

Working under the influence of any mind-altering substance places the residents at great risk and the facility is exposed to potentially serious liability. Experts on substance abuse in healthcare professionals note that a serious danger to residents exists when coworkers suspect drug abuse in a coworker, but ignore the problem and fail to act on their suspicions. Drugs are usually diverted for personal use. Occasionally, they are given to friends or sold to others, but this type of diversion is unusual. Most use drugs at work. The methods of substitution of the drug with another liquid or "split shots" are two methods where there is no waste discrepancy, making diversion very difficult to detect. When substituting injectable medicines, the perpetrator often replaces the active ingredient with water because it has a tendency to burn during injection, whereas normal saline does not. This gives the resident the false impression that he or she is receiving an active medication.

Some drug abusers will also substitute oral medications, such as acetaminophen with codeine with plain acetaminophen, or ibuprofen with hydrocodone for aspirin, because it is difficult to differentiate one generic tablet from another, and these drugs are very similar in appearance. Making the switch is easy to do if medications are supplied in bottles. Unit-dose drugs and bubble packs make diversion easier to detect, but do not prevent it.

Drug abusers can be very creative, using common items such as a glue stick and razor blade to tamper with packaging. Theft of narcotic analgesics, such as fentanyl, hydrocodone, codeine, and morphine has become increasingly common. Although few long-term care facilities maintain a floor stock of these drugs, they are ordered if prescribed for individual residents. The more frequently a drug is used for legitimate purposes, the less likely that diversion of the drug will be detected. The potential for diversion is one reason that facilities should discontinue and eliminate PRN medications that are not used for prolonged periods of time, such as 90 days. Review the controlled-drug sign-out sheets regularly even if there is no reason to suspect drug diversion. Ask the pharmacist to review the schedule drugs and documentation during his or her monthly visit.

Chemical dependency in nursing is a state of psycho-logical and/or physical addiction to a chemical substance or substances.[36] Substance use (whether the drugs are illegally or legally obtained), usually leads to the inability to practice according to established nursing standards. Most substance abusers exhibit several signs and symptoms. Seldom does a nurse have only one indicator of drug abuse. A combination of the signs and symptoms listed here warrants further investigation:

- The nurse tends to give more medication than others. Often holds the narcotic keys and counts narcotics more than others.

- Does not return the narcotic key when borrowed.

- The nurse frequently volunteers to pass medications to residents not in his or her assignment.

- The nurse seems to administer more PRN drugs than others. Other nurses note that they do not normally give these residents controlled substances for pain and sleep. (Although this is not a sign of guilt, it warrants further investigation.)

- The nurse may have higher rates of drug loss, waste or breakage than others.

- The nurse wastes drugs without a witness, then asks another nurse to sign for the wasted drug, often giving a plausible excuse.

- The nurse may be seen going to the bathroom soon after dispensing medications.

- The nurse takes long or frequent breaks, or simply cannot be located at various times.

- PRN medication usage seems to increase from usual patterns.

- Residents complain of inadequate pain relief, or not receiving his or her medications.

- The nurse documents giving controlled drugs to residents on the day of discharge, usually documenting after discharge or transfer.

- The nurse is frequently very tired (without apparent reason) or may be seen sleeping in his or her car.

- The nurse is frequently late for work.

- The nurse has dilated pupils, slurred speech, or other signs of impairment.

- The nurse volunteers for overtime, but calls off on scheduled shifts.

- The nurse complains of chaotic home life, many problems with spouse, children, finances, etc.

- Medications show signs of tampering such as torn packets, missing vial tops, puncture holes, and uneven fluid levels.

- The nurse may request reassignment to a higher-acuity unit, such as the Medicare unit, in which more pain medications are administered.

- If injecting at work, the nurse may have blood spots on clothes, but always has a rational explanation.

Other warning signs may depend on how well you know the employee. Changes in behavior that suggest drug abuse include

- Disregards standards of care and practice.

- Uses poor judgment.

- Disorganized, has difficulty setting priorities.

- Work pace inconsistent.

- Unreasonable excuses for poor performance or errors, often blames others.

- Experiences mood swings or changes; these often occur rapidly. May be accompanied by a change in energy level.

- Isolates self from other workers.

- Increasing anxiety or paranoia.

- Becomes overly emotional, belligerent, or cries.

- An overall change in attitude; not attributable to anything.

- Rapid mood swings or changes in energy levels.

- Gives implausible excuses for behavior if challenged.

- Job performance becomes inconsistent.

- Increasing rate of errors. These can be medication, documentation, or other types of errors.

- Forgetting where common items are kept, or forgetting how to use a common piece of equipment.

- Deterioration in handwriting or illegible handwriting.

- Regularly makes errors and omissions in documentation.

- Increasing absences or tardiness; often gives vague or implausible excuses.

- Feigns confusion about the work schedule.

- Appears on the unit on days off for no plausible reason.

- Requesting to work second or third shift.

- Shows trends in absences, such as during or after holiday weekends, the day after a scheduled day off, after periods of documented high medication use for residents, etc. The nurse manager may also notice trends in exchanging days off, in days worked, or overtime use.

- Deterioration in appearance.

- Wearing long-sleeved lab coats or sweaters when it is not appropriate.

- Does just enough work to get by.

- Frequent use of breath mints or gum. (This is common when alcohol is abused, but methamphetamine and some other drugs cause a condition called "meth mouth," which causes gingivitis and halitosis.)

- Depression.

- Defensiveness; overreacts to criticism.

Specific signs of drug diversion may also be evident on the nursing unit. These include

- Discrepancies on the narcotic count record.

- Unwitnessed or excessive waste of controlled drugs.

- Increased quantity of drugs being ordered for the unit.

- Schedule drugs being delivered for which residents do not have a specific physician order; this is usually blamed on pharmacy error.

- The nurse may write telephone orders for control drugs for several residents. Usually he or she will select a physician (such as the medical director) who has many residents in the facility, theorizing that the physician will not read each and every telephone order when signing.

- Tampering evident with drugs, unit-dose packages taped, abnormalities with vials or containers (such as a full vial with no cap and needle holes in rubber stopper.)

- Discrepancies between physician orders and controlled-drug records.

- Discrepancies between nursing notes, medication records, and controlled-drug records.

- Inconsistencies with individual resident PRN doses required from shift to shift.

- Changing back to the administration of IM or IV analgesic medication when the resident had progressed to oral pain medication.

- Defensiveness by a nurse when questioned about medications administered, phoned or faxed to the pharmacy, or medications picked up, delivered or stocked.

- Other nurses' signatures falsified on controlled drug records.

- One nurse is signing for most of the controlled drugs used on the unit.

Physical signs and symptoms of drug use that may disappear with drug use and are usually evident in the later stages of addiction:

- GI upset

- Slurred or difficult speech

- Increasing (or increased) anxiety

- Feels chronically hungover

- Abdominal cramps, rigidity

- Diarrhea

- Tremors, shakiness

- Difficulty focusing, inattentiveness

- Alcohol on breath

- Diaphoresis

- Sniffling, sneezing

- Clumsiness

- Face flushed

- Watery eyes

- Frequent, nonspecific complaints of not feeling well

See your CD-ROM for a list of commonly abused prescription medications.

In many states, nurses are mandatory reporters, if they suspect their colleagues are diverting drugs, or are working under the influence of drugs and alcohol. Years ago, boards of nursing revoked licenses for drug and alcohol abuse. Most boards now recognize addiction as a treatable illness. Although the board is responsible for protecting the public, most have recovery processes and referrals available. Completing a program of this nature will enable a nurse to keep his or her license, although it may be suspended or otherwise restricted during treatment.

If nurses become aware of or suspect medication diversion, they are obligated to report their suspicions to the Director of Nursing (DON) or nurse manager. If drug diversion is suspected, the DON must investigate the situation promptly by interviewing other nurses, checking floor stock and medication carts, and keeping meticulous notes of his or her findings. The DON should intervene quickly, by confronting the nurse with the facts gathered during the investigation. If necessary, suspend the nurse with or without pay pending the results of the investigation. The DON should include the following steps in his or her investigation:

1. Review unit records. Look for variances in scheduled drug administration, and deviations from known facility policies and procedures. Check trends on wastage and breakage.

2. Check the narcotic records for failure to properly sign out controlled drugs.

3. Check documentation for drug wasting and disposal, such as when a pill has been dropped on the floor. Have nurses obtained cosignatures when required?

4. If concerns or inconsistencies are identified on controlled drug sign-out sheets during the unit review, check individual resident records. If the sign-out sheets are inconsistent, you will usually find inconsistencies in the individual resident records. Check for medication administration patterns, pain relief notations, and accuracy and appropriateness of the nursing documentation.

5. Review nursing notes, medication administration records, PRN records, and other records pertaining to medication administration. Look for erratic handwriting, or signs the nurse was falling asleep while writing (stray pen marks, writing up or downhill, writing less legibly than usual).

6. If a nurse is suspected of diversion or impairment, review his or her personnel file. Look for trends such as frequent job changes. Also check the personnel file, log book, or quality assurance records for excessive incident reports that suggest problems such as inattention, impaired judgment or lack of control caused by substance abuse. Review annual performance evaluations to determine if there is a decline in job performance or a trend in disciplinary actions.

7. Review the employee's attendance records. Look for a pattern in sick-day use. Determine whether there is a trend in absences, such as after a weekend off, during or after holiday weekends. Compare the absences with the unit medication records and determine if there is a relationship between absences and documentation of high medication use for residents.

8. Objectively document all findings of your investigation. The employee may initiate or threaten a lawsuit. Objective documentation may defuse threats, and may be used to defend yourself or the facility if the employee follows through with legal action, although this is unlikely if allegations are proven and the investigation has been confidential.

9. Maintain confidentiality of all documentation. Keep the records in a file that is separate from the personnel file.

10. If you find objective evidence of diversion, such as containers of alcohol, syringes, or watered medications, check with legal counsel or law enforcement before discarding this potentially valuable evidence.

Intervention must be rapid to protect resident safety. As soon as the investigation is complete and the nurse manager is adequately prepared, he or she must notify the nurse that the facility is requiring a professional evaluation, including drug screening. Certain methods of diversion may be hard to detect. Facilities must anticipate this type of problem, and have approved policies and procedures for the nurse manager to follow. Do not wait until you are involved with an active drug investigation to formulate policies! Each facility should also be familiar with their state board of nursing guidelines and reporting mechanisms. Facilities should have procedures for reporting, tracking, and investigation of discrepancies in place.

Managers should be proactive and periodically review their narcotic control system in general. Consider periodic monitoring of narcotic administration by unit, by shift, and by person. This will help identify suspicious patterns. Random drug testing also promotes abstinence, but avoid singling any employee out for frequent testing. Follow facility policies and board of nursing guidelines exactly and do not deviate from them.

Another concern is that drug diversion is a crime. If the nurse is terminated and the police are called, the nurse may be charged with theft, forgery, or both. In addition to problems maintaining the nursing license, the employee has criminal charges as well. Obviously, the best approach is for nurses to avoid using alcohol and drugs altogether, but sadly, this may not be a realistic position. Let your conscience guide you. Discuss your concerns and suspicions with the administrator or your supervisor. Remind him or her of the mandatory reporting provisions. If the supervisor terminates the nurse in question, but fails to report him or her, there are possible legal consequences if the nurse goes to another facility and injures a resident because of the same problem. The best position here is a proactive one, although it is an uncomfortable position to be in.

Solid, research-based policies and procedures promote positive outcomes for the facility and the nurse, particularly if he or she seeks treatment. Although resident safety is your primary concern, the rehabilitation process for the nurse is an important aspect. A supportive environment is essential for reentry of the rehabilitated nurse at work. However, the possibility of relapse is always a possibility, and a system of safeguards and monitoring should be in place. One expert suggests that rehabilitation is usually more successful when it is tied to a person's employment and license.[37] An overall facility policy requiring random testing helps encourage abstinence.

Employers must also be aware of the Americans with Disabilities Act of 1990 (ADA), which prohibits discrimination against individuals with qualifying disabilities. Substance abuse is considered a qualifying disability in nurses if it is self reported. Nurses are not protected, however, if they subsequently abuse drugs at work, which potentially endangers residents. Under the ADA requirements, employers must keep records of substance abuse confidential, in a separate locked file cabinet with limited access.

Fentanyl diversion

Fentanyl deserves a mention because the route of absorption is subcutaneous and diversion of fentanyl (Duragesic®) patches has become increasingly prevalent in long-term care facilities over the past decade. Recipes for making fentanyl are available on the Internet, and labs are occasionally discovered by drug task forces. A common street name for fentanyl is "China White." Of the 100 different types of active fentanyl that potentially could be synthesized, only 10 derivatives have appeared on the black market.[38]

The analgesic effect of fentanyl is 100 to 300 times the potency of morphine.[39] Fentanyl transdermal patches have become common in long-term care, and this method of administering the drug has proven excellent for relieving acute and chronic pain. Patches are useful for residents with hypersensitivity to morphine, those who are unreliable, or who cannot take oral medications. Although patches are usually changed every 72 hours, analgesia may exceed this period in elderly individuals. Advantages are ease of compliance and infrequent dosing.

A pocket on the back of the patch contains fentanyl in a gel with ethanol and hydroxyethyl cellulose. This reservoir is separated from the skin by a nonporous ethylene vinyl acetate membrane. The design deters diversion, but abuse can and does occur. Patches diverted for abuse are usually opened and the fentanyl extracted.

The greatest opportunity for abuse of transdermal fentanyl probably occurs in the long-term care setting.[40]

Patches are retrieved from the trash. They may be stolen from unit stock or removed from the skin of residents.[41] Used patches may contain as much as 60% of the drug.[42] New patches are stolen, then used patches applied to residents' skin in their place. Another method of diverting the drug is to move a used patch to a new location on the resident's body, making it appear that the patch was rotated. Patches have also been removed and not replaced.[43] The media have reported many incidences of former employees visiting the facility for the express purpose of removing patches from the residents. Patches are commonly diverted for personal use, but some have been sold for up to $50 on the street.

Various methods have been used to extract and abuse the active ingredient. Syringes have been used to extract and withdraw the fentanyl from the underside of the patch. Patches have been boiled, the fentanyl extracted and injected. Some abusers have dried and inhaled the fentanyl. Some chew or suck the patch. Patches have been cut and fentanyl eaten or consumed in a beverage. Some abusers apply patches to their own skin, covering them with a heating pad, or using a hair dryer to increase absorption. These are very dangerous methods, because there is no way of knowing how much fentanyl will reach the abuser's system. Small doses can cause fatal respiratory depression, particularly when combined with heroin and other street drugs. Detecting fentanyl may be difficult because it is administered in such small quantities.[44] Urine drug screens do not routinely detect fentanyl, but assays can be requested to identify it if abuse is suspected.

Methods for reducing the risk of fentanyl diversion

You can reduce the risk of fentanyl diversion by

- Removing packages from the box and inspecting them for signs of tampering during narcotic count.

- Writing the date, time, and your initials on the patch with a marker or pen each time you apply a patch. Compare the information against the medication administration record (MAR) each shift. Initial the MAR to verify you have checked the patch each day.

- Checking new patches for cuts, holes, or a dehydrated appearance suggesting tampering.

- Discarding used patches according to facility policies and procedures. The manufacturer recommends folding the patch with the adhesive side in, then flushing down the toilet.[45] However, in some facilities, the patch is discarded in the sharps container. Your facility may require that you cut the patch into small pieces before discarding it. When using this method, wear gloves to avoid skin contact with the gel.

- Melting the remaining active ingredient in the patch before discarding it by placing the patch (with the medicated side facing up) in the sink, and running hot water over it.

- Having another nurse witness the destruction or disposition of used patches.

- In some facilities, an individual sign-out sheet is issued for each control drug given to each resident. A community sign-out sheet is not used. This is a common practice in long-term care. If an individual record is used, cross through blank lines when the drug is discontinued. Note that the drug has been discontinued on the form, and remove it from the narcotic book. Note its disposition. If the drug will remain in the locked narcotic cabinet overnight or on a weekend, continue to count the drug every shift until it is picked up.

- Being alert to signs of tampering, diversion, and the potential for abuse.

Reported deaths as a result of fentanyl patches

In 2004 and 2005, several lawsuits were filed against the manufacturers of fentanyl patches and the pharmacies that dispensed the drug. These lawsuits allege that manufacturing defects caused overdoses and deaths because the gel leaked from the bottom of the patch and was absorbed into the plaintiff's skin.[46] Generic fentanyl patches are available from several manufacturers. Since up to 60% of the drug remains in a used patch, nurses should make sure old patches are removed when a new patch is reapplied. Be alert to signs of patch leakage. If you suspect a patch is leaking, apply gloves and remove it from the resident. Replace it with a new patch. Document your actions. Place the used patch in a zipper plastic bag and ask the pharmacist to examine the patch and investigate the problem. Remember that the drug is absorbed slowly, and the resident may be affected by drug residual after the patch has been removed. Monitor his or her mental status and vital signs carefully for 24 to 36 hours.

In 2005, the FDA notified healthcare professionals of changes to the prescribing information for Duragesic®. These changes include important safety information in the following areas of the labeling: Use only in opioid-tolerant patients, misuse, abuse and diversion, hypoventilation (respiratory depression), interactions with CYP3A4 inhibitors (ritonavir, ketoconazole, itraconazole, troleandomycin, clarithromycin, nelfinavir, and nefazodone), damaged or cut patches, accidental exposure to fentanyl, chronic pulmonary disease, head injuries and intracranial pressure, interactions with other CNS depressants, and interactions with alcohol and drugs of abuse.

Chapter eighteen

References

1. Tobias DE and Pulliam CC. (1997). General and psychotherapeutic medication use in 878 nursing facilities: A 1997 national survey. American Society of Consultant Pharmacists, Inc. Online. *www.ascp.com/public/pubs/tcp/ 1997/dec/research2.html.* Accessed 01/11/06.

2. Edwards DJ. (2005). Study: two million drug injuries threaten NH residents annually. Nursing Homes. April 2005. Online. *http://www.findarticles.com/p/articles/mi_m3830/is_4_54/ai_n13675115.* Accessed 01/10/05.

3. Austin Community College Diabetes lectures. Online. *www2.austin.cc.tx.us/.* Accessed 8/20/03.)

4. Beers, M. and Berkow, R. (Eds). (2000). Merck Manual of Geriatrics. New Jersey, Whitehouse Station. Merck & Co. Online. *www.merck.com/.* Accessed 8/20/03).

5. Lorber, D. (1995). Nonketotic hypertonicity in diabetes mellitus. Med Clin North Am. 1995 Jan;79(1): 39-52.

6. Delaney, M., Zisman, A., Kettyle, W. (2000). Acute complications of diabetes diabetic ketoacidosis and hyperglycemic hyperosmolar nonketotic syndrome. Endocrinology and Metabolism Clinics. Vol. 29, No. 4, Dec. 2000. W. B. Saunders Company.

7. Kern, M. and Leonard, P. (1999). Warfarin Management Considerations in Long-Term Care Facilities. *Annals of Long-term Care* 1999; 7[3]:98-103.

8. Ansell J, Hirsh J, Dalen J, et al. Managing oral anticoagulant therapy. Chest. 2001;119:22S-38S.

9. Washington University School of Medicine. (2006). Common blood thinner increases risk of bone fracture. Online. *http://mednews.wustl.edu/ news/page/normal/6422.html?emailID=7859.* Accessed 01/24/06.

10. Suvarna, R; Pirmohamed, M; Henderson, L. (2003). Possible interaction between warfarin and cranberry juice. BMJ 2003;327:1454 (20 December), doi:10.1136/bmj.327.7429.1454.

11. American Medical Directors Association and American Society of Consultant Pharmacists. (2000). List of Top Ten Drug Interactions in Long-Term Care. Online. *www.scoup.net/M3Project/topten/.* Accessed 10/15/01.

12. American Heart Association. (Eds). (1994). Guide to Anticoagulant Therapy Part 2: Oral Anticoagulants. (Circulation. 1994;89:1469-1480).

13. Crowther, M. (2003). Inadequate monitoring and management of warfarin places patient at significant risk of harm. July 2003. Morbidity and Mortality Rounds on the Web. Online. *http://webmm.ahrq.gov/case.aspx?caseID=21.* Accessed 8/3/03.

14. Kern, M. and Leonard, P. (1999). Warfarin Management Considerations in Long-Term Care Facilities. *Annals of Long Term Care* 1999; 7[3]:98-103.

15. Crowther MA, Douketis JD, Schnurr T, et al. Oral vitamin k lowers the international normalized ratio more rapidly than subcutaneous vitamin k in the treatment of warfarin-associated coagulopathy. A randomized, controlled trial. Ann Intern Med. 2002;137:251- 254.

16. Shetty HG, Backhouse G, Bentley DP, Routledge PA. Effective reversal of warfarin-induced excessive anticoagulation with low dose vitamin K1. Thromb Haemost. 1992;67:13-15.

17. American Heart Association. (Eds). (1994). Guide to Anticoagulant Therapy Part 2: Oral Anticoagulants. (Circulation. 1994;89:1469-1480).

18. Kern, M. and Leonard, P. (1999). Warfarin Management Considerations in Long-Term Care Facilities. Annals of Long-term Care 1999; 7[3]:98-103.

19. Farrell SE. (2005). Acetaminophen toxicity. Emedicine online. *www.emedicine.com/emerg/topic819.htm.* Accessed 01/14/06.

20. Losch, Philip C. (2000). Acetaminophen toxicity. Kentucky Board of Pharmacy News. December 2000. Online. *www.ncbop.org/jan01-2.asp.* Accessed 12/13/02.

21. Nicolle LE, Strausbaugh LJ, Garibaldi RA. Infections and antibiotic resistance in nursing homes. Clin Microbiol Rev 1996;9:1-17.

22. Strausbaugh LJ, Crossley KB, Nurse BA, Thrupp LD, SHEA Long-term Care Committee. Antimicrobial

resistance in long-term care facilities. Infect Control Hosp Epidemiol 1995; 17:120-9.

23. Crossley K. Long-term Care Committee of the Society for Health Care Epidemiology of America. Vancomycin-resistant enterococci in long-term care facilities. *Infect Control Hosp Epidemiol* 1998;19:521-5.

24. Nicolle LE, Bentley D, Garibaldi R, Neuhaus E, Smith P, SHEA Long-term Care Committee. Antimicrobial use in long-term care facilities. *Infect Control Hosp Epidemiol* 1996;17:119-28.

25. Smith P, Rusnak P. Infection prevention and control in the long-term-care facility. *Am J Infect Control* 1997; 25:488?512.

26. M3 Project. Top ten drug interactions in long-term care. Online. *www.scoup.net/M3Project/topten/*. Accessed 8/1/04.

27. Centers for Disease Control and Prevention Fact Sheet. Falls and Hip Fractures Among the Elderly. Online. *www.cdc.gov/ncipc/factsheets/falls.htm*. Accessed 7/08/02.

28. American Nurses Association. (Eds). (1997). Position Statement on Polypharmacy in the Older Adult. Online. *www.nursingworld.org*.

29. Inouye SK. The dilemma of delirium: clinical and research controversies regarding diagnosis and evaluationof delirium in hospitalized elderly medical patients. Am J Med. 1994;97:278-288.

30. Rudberg MA, Pompei P, Foreman MD, Ross RE, Cassel CK. The natural history of delirium in older hospitalized patients: a syndrome of heterogeneity. Age Aging. 1997;26:169-174.

31. Moore AR, O'Keeffe TO. Drug-induced cognitive impairment in the elderly. Drugs Aging. 1999;15:15-28.

32. Sullivan, E. & Decker, P. (2001). Effective leadership and management in nursing. Upper Saddle River, NJ: Prentice Hall.

33. Trinkoff Storr, S., & Wall, M. (1999). Prescription-type drug misuse and workplace Access among nurses. Journal of Addictive Diseases, 18(1), 9-17.

34. Smith, L., Taylor, B., & Hughes, T. (1998). Effective peer responses to impaired nursing practice. Nursing Clinics of North America, 33(1), 105-18.

35. Burke, J. (1999). Facing up to drug diversion. American Journal of Health System Pharmacy, 56 (18), 1823-27.

36. Smith, L., Taylor, B., & Hughes, T. (1998). Effective peer responses to impaired nursing practice. Nursing Clinics of North America, 33(1), 105-18.

37. Tranbarger, R. (1997). A nurse executive's nightmare, the rogue nurse. Nursing Management, 28(2), 33-6., R.

38. Addiction: from craving to recovery. Online. *http://library.thinkquest.org/*. Accessed 11/03/02.

39. Janssen Pharmaceutica (eds). Transdermal therapy for chronic pain. Online. *www.powerpak.com/CE/transdermal/pharmacy/lesson.cfm*. Accessed 11/03/02.

40. Minutes Indiana Medicaid DUR Board Meeting of April 19, 2002. Online. *www.indianamedicaid.com/*. Accessed 11/03/02.

41. New York State Information for Providers. (10/29/01). Dear Administrator Letter - Fentanyl Alert. Online. *www.health.state.ny.us/nysdoh/provider/nhadmin/fentanyl_ltr.htm*. Accessed 11/03/02.

42. Hardcastle, M. (8/2/02). Drug abusers turning to medical patches for highs. *Dayton Daily News*. Online. *www.mapinc.org/*. Accessed 11/03/02.

43. Caruso, David B. (3/29/02). Abuse rises with spread of painkiller patches. *Buffalo News*. Online. *www.mapinc.org/*. Accessed 11/03/02.

44. Addiction: from craving to recovery. Online. *http://library.thinkquest.org*. Accessed 11/02/02.

45. Physicians' Desk Reference 56th Edition 2002. (2002). Montvale, NJ. Medical Economics Co., Inc.

46. Duragesic patch allegedly caused yet another death. (2004). Pharmaceutical Law & Litigation Report, Vol. III, No. 8, p. 159.

Employee lawsuits

Sexual harassment

Title VII of the Civil Rights Act of 1964, and its amendments, grants employees the right to work in an environment free from discrimination, insult, and ridicule based on the individual's gender, religion, race, skin color, or national origin. The law forbids sexual harassment in the workplace, and requires the employer to take adequate, decisive, and appropriate action to eliminate sexual harassment and to take steps to prevent current and future occurrences.

Sexual harassment usually has little to do with flirtation or normal sexual desire. Like sexual assault, sexual harassment is most commonly a means of exerting power, control, and domination over another individual. Occasionally, it occurs because of the perpetrator's inability to relate in a more appropriate way, or from a lack of understanding of the negative effects of the behavior and the way in which sexually harassing behavior affects others.

The American Psychological Association estimates that 71% of working women will be subjected to sexual harassment during their careers. However, men can also be sexually harassed, although this is not as commonly reported.[1] Sexual harassment in the workplace is a violation of both federal and state laws.

Sexual harassment is influencing, offering to influence, or threatening the career, pay or job of another person (man or woman) in exchange for sexual favors; or deliberate or repeated offensive comments, gestures, or physical contact of a sexual nature at work or in a work-related environment.[2] In a highly technical sense, *"sex discrimination"* is discrimination based on the biological differences between males and females. *"Gender discrimination"* is discrimination based on social or cultural differences between men and women. *However, most courts use these terms (sex discrimination and gender discrimination) interchangeably.* The Supreme Court has determined that "sex" and "gender" are not distinct concepts for purposes of Title VII.[3]

Sexual harassment can take two forms. The first is a person of either gender being subjected to a hostile working environment because of conduct by another. To file a claim based on a hostile work environment, the plaintiff must prove that

- a reasonable person would find the working environment hostile or abusive

- similar discrimination would detrimentally affect a reasonable person of the same sex (gender) in that position

- the employee suffered intentional discrimination because of his or her gender

- the discrimination was pervasive and regular

- the discrimination detrimentally affected the plaintiff

- the employer had a respondeat superior liability

The plaintiff does not have to show direct evidence of harassment, which often occurs privately. The court will accept circumstantial evidence. The employer's response to complaints about a hostile work environment should be quick and decisive, and "reasonably calculated to prevent further harassment."[4]

The second form of sexual harassment is called *quid pro quo*, which is generally a supervisor threatening a subordinate worker with firing, loss of raise, promotion, or other remuneration. This type of claim may also be brought if the employer condones or ignores sexually harassing behavior and fails to act on complaints. To be successful in bringing a quid quo pro claim, the worker must furnish proof of an economic loss as a direct result of refusing to submit to the sexual advances of another. Other components the plaintiff must prove are that

- he or she is a member of a protected class

- he or she was subjected to unwelcome sexual harassment in the form of sexual advances or requests for sexual favors

- the harassment complained of was based on sex (gender)

- the refusal to submit to the unwelcome advances was an express or implied condition

for receiving pay or benefits, and the refusal resulted in loss of these benefits

- the employer had respondeat superior liability and failed to discipline, terminate, or take other remedial action after being notified of the harassment

Legal opinions—sexual harassment by a supervisor

An employer can be sued for the discriminatory acts of an employee if the employer knew or should have known of the employee's offensive conduct and failed to prevent or stop the behavior and eliminate the hostile environment. The United States Circuit Court of Appeals for the Fifth Circuit (Texas) upheld a nurse's sexual harassment claim against her employer, a long-term care facility, for sexual harassment by the male director of nursing. The nurse who made the allegations was the treatment nurse. She complained that the male director of nursing asked about her sexual habits, made numerous offensive and inappropriate sexual remarks, and joked about her sexual behavior, commenting she knew nothing about condoms because she was the mother of seven children. The DON also exhibited sexist behavior by requiring that the nurse do things that were not in her job description, such as making coffee, filling his coffee cup, washing his dirty dishes, and making photocopies that were unrelated to her position.

The nurse asked the DON not to make sexual comments to her. When he persisted, she went to the human resources department, who failed to act on her complaint. The nurse did not use the specific term "sexual harassment" in her complaint, but the court ruled she did not have to in order to be afforded protection. A second nurse made similar complaints to the human resources director, who failed to investigate the situation and encouraged the nurses to "hang in there." After reviewing the evidence the court ruled that this provided substantial evidence that the nurse's employer, the long-term care facility, had failed to take prompt remedial action upon an employee's justifiable complaint of sexually hostile treatment on the job, as required by law.[5]

Legal opinions—sexual harassment by a resident

Female caregivers in a residential facility for developmentally disabled adolescents and adults complained they were being inappropriately grabbed, touched, and fondled by a 17-year-old resident. The teenager was large in stature, more than six feet tall and weighing more than two hundred pounds. However, the resident had the mental capacity of a two- to five-year-old child. The facility failed to address the problem because poor impulse control is expected in a child of his mental age. The resident's aggression toward female staff escalated, and over the course of several months, female staff members complained to management, who took no action. The supervisor eventually asked a female employee to allow him to observe the resident grabbing her so that company executives could view the problematic conduct. She quit instead. The female personnel sued, and the U.S. Circuit Court of Appeals for the Eighth Circuit (Minnesota) ruled that the facility should have addressed their complaints. The court noted that the facility should have done a sexuality assessment and seriously considered assigning male staff to care for the resident. They also advised the facility to hire sufficient caregivers of either gender capable of restraining the resident, if necessary to prevent him from groping female staff. Citing EEOC regulations, the Eighth Circuit reversed a previous summary judgment for the employer, finding that "a fact finder could characterize the facility's response as implicitly or even explicitly

requiring the appellants to endure repeated sexual assaults as an essential part of the job."[6]

In another case in which a home health care client with Alzheimer's disease made infrequent, sexually inappropriate remarks to a nurse, the Fifth Circuit Court of Appeals held that the behavior complained of by the plaintiff did not rise to the level of actionable hostile environment sexual harassment. In this situation, the employer investigated the nurse's complaints and offered to reassign her to other clients. She responded that she did not want reassignment. The sexual harassment case was filed after the nurse was terminated for a situation unrelated to this event. The nurse also alleged her termination was retaliation in violation of Title VII of the Civil Rights Act of 1964. The home care client had been diagnosed with Alzheimer's and Parkinson's disease. The court noted that conditions such as this may result in abnormal behaviors and, "[i]n this context, [the patient's] improper requests and tasteless remarks cannot form the basis of a justiciable claim for sexual harassment [because the patient's conduct was not so severe or pervasive to interfere with the plaintiff's work performance]." The court limited the scope of this ruling to the "unique circumstances of this case." They noted that the plaintiff never complained or alleged that the patient engaged in any physical conduct that threatened her.[7]

Legal opinions—sexual harassment by a peer or subordinate

A long-term care facility dietary assistant complained that a housekeeper made unwanted advances. The dietary assistant informed the supervisor, who changed the housekeeper's schedule to minimize contact with the dietary assistant. The supervisor discreetly asked other department heads to keep an eye on the situation.

The dietary assistant subsequently complained that the housekeeper asked her for a date and approached her from behind, grabbing her breasts. When the administrator confronted the housekeeper, he denied the allegations. There were no witnesses to this situation, but the housekeeper was given a written reprimand and informed he would be terminated if there were further complaints. Because of the potential magnitude of the problem, the written warning was strongly worded, stating, "We have had two written complaint[s] against you for harassment by females. This is your one and only warning. Harassment of any kind by an employee to another employee absolutely will not be tolerated. Any further occurr[c]nce will result in your immediate termination."

After the housekeeper was given the written warning, the episodes stopped, but the dietary assistant said she could not continue working at the facility as long as the housekeeper was there. The facility administrator informed her of all the actions taken to stop the harassment and stated nothing else would be done until or unless the housekeeper persisted in his harassment. The dietary assistant was given the option of staying or resigning. (The housekeeper's work station continued to be physically removed from the dietary aide's, but she did not want to see him at all.) The dietary assistant resigned and sued the facility for sexual harassment based on a hostile work environment. A trial court ruled in favor of the facility, noting that the dietary assistant had failed to prove the facility was responsible for the housekeeper's conduct (under the respondeat superior doctrine).

The dietary assistant appealed the ruling. The appeals court ruled that the district court erred when it noted that the facility could not be held liable under the respondeat superior doctrine. They stated that in cases of sexual harassment by a coworker, the employer's liability is direct. The dietary assistant was a member of a protected class, she was subject to unwelcome sexual harassment, and the harassment was based on her gender. However, the court of appeals ruled she must show evidence that the harassment interfered with her ability to do her job and created a hostile environment. They also noted that they could not validate the complaint unless the facility knew of the harassment and failed or refused to implement prompt and appropriate corrective action. In this situation, the department head and facility administrator were aware of the dietary assistant's allegations, but the harassment was unwitnessed and the housekeeper denied improper conduct, so it was his word against hers. The court of appeals ruled that facility action was determined by the individual circumstances, and in this case, the administrator's actions were prompt and appropriate. The dietary assistant could not force the facility to fire the housekeeper based on her word alone.[8]

Examples of sexual harassment

Sexual harassment can take many forms. Verbal sexual harassment includes

- making comments about your body, clothing, or sexual activities

- telling offensive or sexual jokes, making sexual remarks, or teasing in a sexually-offensive manner

- making requests or demands for sexual favors that hint or suggest your employment status will be jeopardized or threatened if you do not comply.

- making gender-biased comments such as, "women do not belong in this job."

Nonverbal sexual harassment includes

- making offensive or insulting sounds

- leering or staring at your body

- making obscene gestures

- displaying pornographic or sexually suggestive photos, videos, or other materials

- creating a hostile work environment

Physical sexual harassment includes

- physical interference with normal work or movement

- unwanted, inappropriate touching or pinching

- deliberately brushing up or bumping against the body of another

- sexual assault

Sexual harassment can occur as a single behavior or take a multiplicity of forms, including ongoing and unwanted sexual attention that is verbal, nonverbal, or physical. The individual who is perpetrating the harassment is, in effect, creating a hostile work environment by creating an atmosphere that is stressful and causes mental anguish for the coworker(s). The person who is the target of the sexual harassment may suffer from the effects on a daily, hourly, or almost constant basis resulting in an intolerable working environment for the victim.

Actions the targeted employee should take

- Do not ignore sexual harassment; it will not go away!

- Contact your supervisor, personnel manager, or Employee Assistance Program (EAP) and learn about the facility's policies and procedures on sexual harassment.

- Speak up about sexual harassment you experience or witness.

- Keep detailed records, documenting all incidents of harassment you experience. Document names and contact information for witnesses.

- Keep copies of performance evaluations and other documents attesting to the quality of your work. A common tactic is for the harasser to question or criticize your job performance in order to justify his or her behavior.

- Keep copies of all written materials, including notes, letters, and e-mails.

- Inform the harasser verbally and in writing, that his or her behavior is unwelcome, unacceptable, and offensive to you. Mention specific incidents of unwanted sexual attention.

- Report sexual harassment to the proper administrative person, verbally and in writing.

- If the facility has a policy and procedure for filing grievances, initiate the grievance procedure.

- If you are a member of a union, inform the union representative or steward.

ANA recommendations

The ANA believes that sexual harassment negatively impacts the healthcare environment. ANA recognizes that nurses and nursing personnel are sometimes the victims of this insidious form of sex discrimination. They note that under-reporting of the problem is common. In fact, one study found that the greater the nurse's distress, the less likely he or she was to report the incident. ANA also identifies emotional costs of sexual harassment, including anger, humiliation, and fear, in addition to the monetary costs of counseling and lawyers' fees. The combination of emotional and physical costs is an unreasonably high price to pay.[9]

The ANA has long been opposed to *any civil rights violation* and opposes any form of discrimination against individuals or groups of individuals based on race, gender, age, national origin, religion, disability, or sexual orientation. ANA believes that nurses have a right to and responsibility for a workplace free from sexual harassment. Many excellent resources are found in their website at *http://www.nursingworld.org*. The ANA describes a four-step process to deal with sexual harassment:

- *Confront* the person and make it clear that the behavior is unwanted. Repeat, if necessary.

- *Report the harassment* to a supervisor or manager using the chain of command. If a formal grievance system exists in your facility, file a formal complaint. Discuss your concerns with the personnel or human resources department.

- *Document the details* immediately after the event. Do not wait. Documenting promptly will preserve important details while you remember them most clearly. Include what happened, when, where and your responses. Note witnesses' names. If necessary, consider taping phone calls, saving harassing letters and emails, etc. If the behavior persists, consider mailing the harasser a certified, return-receipt letter; Keep a copy. Keep a log or journal and document every incident.

- *Find support* from others you trust, whether it be a friend, colleague, spouse, clergy, or representative from your state nurses' association.

Sexual harassment legal claims

An employer may be sued for sexual harassment by

- workers of the same gender or the opposite gender; sexual orientation is not a consideration

- claims arising from a nurse/patient relationship

or relationship of another professional with a patient

- applicants for employment or independent contractors

- employees who were not harassed but found the work environment intolerable (hostile) because of harassment to (an)other worker(s) in the same workplace

To prove a sexual harassment claim, the plaintiff must have proof that the sexual harassment was severe and/or pervasive enough to create an abusive work environment or change working conditions. He or she must show that another reasonable person would consider the same conduct severe or pervasive. The more egregious the conduct, the less it has to be pervasive. The court will consider the frequency and severity of the conduct, whether the acts were physically threatening or humiliating, and whether the behavior interfered with work performance.

When a plaintiff prevails in a sexual harassment claim, he or she may be awarded damages for medical and psychiatric care, and lost wages. He or she may be awarded damages for emotional distress and punitive damages. To receive an award for punitive damages, the plaintiff should be able to prove that the

- employer hired or retained an individual who was harassing others; the employer took no effective (appropriate) action when he or she became aware of the harasser's behavior

- employer approved of, encouraged, or condoned the wrongful conduct

- employer was personally guilty of oppression, fraud, malice, or other illegal conduct

The laws governing sexual harassment also provide for

attorneys' fees, which may provide an incentive for lawyers considering whether to accept such suits on a contingency basis.

Prevention

In the 1970s and 1980s, facilities thought that having strong policies and procedures would be sufficient to protect them from potential claims. In 1991, congress amended the law and expanded employee protections and illegal behaviors under the act. In the late 1990s, the Supreme Court changed the rules and expanded the definition of sexual harassment. The EEOC and other courts began to take a more aggressive stance on sexual harassment. Because of these changes, employers learned that strong policies are not the end all, be all in this issue. The United States Supreme Court has ruled that strong policies and procedures are virtually worthless unless the department heads and managers receive education regarding how to apply the rules mandated in the manuals, and how to apply basic employment law. The courts have also ruled that the mere existence of a policy and procedure is not adequate.[10] The premise here is that the existence of a written antiharassment or a zero tolerance policy does not guarantee its effectiveness. *The court expects the employer to use reasonable care in implementing the policy.*

When formulating facility policies and procedures, you should specifically state that complainants will be free from retaliation. The court supported one plaintiff claim because the policy failed to make a freedom from retaliation statement. However, the policy warned that false reports of harassment would subject a complainant to disciplinary action, including termination.[11] (The freedom from retaliation statement protects the facility if an employee subsequently files suit and says he or she was afraid to complain for fear of retaliation.) The procedure for filing a complaint must designate an accessible person

with whom employees can file complaints. If an employer has a sexual harassment policy that requires an employee to complain to a person who is not reasonably accessible (such as at a remote location on the other side of town), then the courts will consider the policy to be ineffective.[12] In a unionized facility, filing a grievance with the union may be sufficient to fulfill the reporting requirement. In Watts v. Kroger Co., 170 F.3d 505, 510-11 (5th Cir. 1999), the court ruled that the plaintiff need not complain using the employer's policy and procedure as long as he or she reasonably takes advantage of some corrective opportunity. In Watts, the plaintiff complained by means of filing a union grievance, which the court found sufficient.

Harassment based on race, ethnicity, religion, gender and other protected characteristics is not defined by who does the harassing. It may be a contractor, visitor, supervisor, other employee, or resident. If the offensive conduct is work-related, all the same rules apply if the situation subjects the employee to a hostile work environment or the harassment interferes with the employee's ability to do the job. If either is the case, the employer must act quickly and decisively, regardless of who is doing the harassing.

To prevent potential sexual harassment claims, each facility should have clear, strong policies and procedures regarding professional conduct in the workplace. Develop a decisive, effective procedure for redress of complaints. Also, establish a complaint procedure for non-employee harassment. Doing this places the responsibility on the employee to report the conduct. He or she will have no redress for remaining silent and subsequently filing a lawsuit. Specifically state that discrimination and sexual harassment will not be tolerated. Other considerations include

- making sure the policy is well known and widely distributed

- giving each employee a copy of the policy and procedure during facility orientation and/or inservices, and having each employee sign an acknowledgment that he or she has read and understands the information

- making sure the policy is reaffirmed during any sexual harassment investigation

- ensuring there are adequate provisions for guarding the complainant against retaliation

- ensuring that no one employee has unchecked power to prevent sexual harassment complaints from being reported

- teaching department heads how to interview prospective employees to avoid the illegal questions, including those regarding sexual orientation and behavior; as agents of the facility, department heads have specific responsibilities, including taking immediate and appropriate action in preventing sexual harassment and responding to complaints

- developing a progressive discipline policy and/or sanctions for sexual harassment

- informing and educating employees on their legal rights and action to take if harassment occurs

- conducting periodic inservices on sexual harassment; to be effective, consider including the following information:

  - the legal definition of sexual harassment

  - the legal basis for prohibiting sexual harassment under federal, state and local laws, regulations and ordinances

  - examples of what constitutes sexual harassment

  - the facility policy prohibiting sexual harassment

  - a description of the facility's internal complaint process available to all employees

  - a description of the legal recourse and complaint processes available at the local state and federal levels, (e.g., local and state human rights divisions and EEOC)

  - the state and federal laws protecting employees against reprisal

  - an opportunity to ask questions and clarify information presented

- depending on the workplace and resident population, department heads and other employees may need additional, focused education regarding:

  - identifying populations who are most vulnerable to sexual harassment and abuse

  - potential power abuses that occur in some work environments

  - how to respond to complaints

  - identifying troublesome or potentially offensive behavior patterns

  - preventing or identifying incidents of sexual harassment

  - investigating and documenting charges of sexual harassment

  - assisting or counseling victims of sexual harassment or those who harass others

  - helping victims to cope with the emotional and physical effects of sexual harassment

– assisting those who sexually harass others to change their behavior

– local sources of referral and resources

The ANA recommends that facilities include a policy statement that specifies how confidentiality will be ensured. The policy statement should be visible, generally available, and demonstrate the employer's commitment to the maintenance of a harassment-free work environment. ANA recommends that facility sexual harassment policies:

- provide a clear explanation of the offensive or prohibited conduct

- ensure freedom from retaliation for employees who file good faith complaints

- promise that confidentiality will be protected to the extent possible

- identify individuals who should receive sexual harassment complaints

- outline an investigative process that is free of chain-of-command entanglements

- guarantee that investigations will commence promptly after a complaint is registered (typically, within five business days)

- promise that the investigation of all complaints will be thorough and that all potentially involved parties and appropriate witnesses will be interviewed

- reassure employees that the employer will take immediate and appropriate action when sexual harassment is identified or validated

- identify possible sanctions for harassing behavior

- offer counseling and support to the person complaining of sexual harassment

An additional word of caution to prevent potential sexual harassment entanglements: Supervisors and department heads must be very careful in socializing, mingling, or partying with their staff members (subordinates) to avoid the appearance of impropriety or favoritism.

Responding to complaints

Teach department heads and others the proper steps to take if they receive a complaint about sexual harassment. The facility must respond quickly and decisively, by investigating and taking whatever additional steps are necessary. At the very least, while an investigation is ongoing, protect the harassed employee from harm, retaliation, and further harassment. As much as possible in a small workplace, separate the employee and harasser, or suspend the harasser during the investigation. Be tactful and have an established procedure for doing this. You must separate the employees without giving the appearance you are demoting or prejudicing either employee's position with the facility. Other steps to consider when formulating a plan are

- Tactfully and diplomatically confronting the accused source of the harassment. Inform him or her that an allegation of harassment has been made, and request a response.

- Interviewing all complainants and witnesses known to have knowledge of the event, documenting as appropriate, and requesting these individuals make (or sign) written statements.

- Obtaining any and all other potential documentation relating to the sexual harassment, such as notes, e-mails, love letters, cards, gifts, etc.

- Determining a plan of action in consideration of what a timely, reasonable investigation would have or did reveal.

- Identifying appropriate remedial/disciplinary measures. The corrective measure should be calculated to end the current harassment and deter future harassment. The remedial action may be considered adequate even if it fails to stop harassment, as long as it was reasonably calculated to deter further harassment. If the court cannot determine whether the action was reasonable, they have the authority to refer the situation to a fact finder for further investigation.

- Determining when the magnitude of the offense warrants termination. Although the specific discipline is determined by the employer, he or she need not use the most serious sanction available (usually termination) to punish the perpetrator. However, the court has ruled that the employer cannot ignore reasonable evidence of harassment and instruct the victim and the perpetrator to "work things out."[13]

  – If you are dealing with a repeat offender, however, you are obligated to ensure the response is appropriate. Make sure a reasonable person would agree on the adequacy of your response when it is known to be the second or third complaint. The employer's response may be stronger if this is a second (or subsequent) complaint against the same individual.[14] Occasionally, inadequate repeat discipline strengthens the plaintiff's case and reveals that the initial discipline was also inadequate or unreasonable.[15]

- Carefully documenting each and every action you take and maintaining these records in a confidential file in a secure location. If the facility is subsequently sued for sexual harassment, you will be asked to provide this documentation. Make sure documentation is correct

and accurate at the time of the event. Never go back and create, deliberately alter, or falsify it. Check with your legal counsel before supplying any records to the plaintiff's attorney.

- Documenting preventive opportunities and protection from harm afforded or offered to the employee making the complaint. Document his or her failure or refusal to take advantage of these opportunities. This specific documentation will become an important part of your defense if the plaintiff behaved unreasonably in avoiding or correcting the sexual harassment.

- Handling complaints promptly without betraying confidentiality. If an employee complains of sexual harassment, consider reminding all staff through inservice or other methods (posters, pamphlets, other resources) that sexual harassment will not be tolerated. Avoid mentioning the current complaint or incident.

Potentially discriminatory interview questions

In the United States, department heads and others who interview job applicants are considered agents of the employer. As such, they must be careful to avoid the appearance of discrimination in hiring based on questions asked of the applicant during the application process and personal interview. Questions that may be perceived as discriminatory are those that question the applicant's

- Age
- Color
- Disability, health, or previous medical history
- Gender
- Marital status

- National origin

- Race

- Religion

Interview questions should be relevant to the job and not used to reveal personal information about the applicant. The Equal Employment Opportunity Commission (EEOC) and Age Discrimination in Employment Act of 1967 (ADEA) consider asking an applicant's age or date of birth to be *legal questions*. However, denying employment based on age discrimination *is illegal* if the applicant is 40 years of age or older. Most illegal questions are asked out of ignorance, with no malice intended.

However, the applicant may have civil recourse, even when there was no criminal motive or intent on the part of the facility. Teach those who are interviewing that *asking the questions is not illegal, but asking with a discriminatory motive is*, particularly if the responses are used to deny employment. Since the applicant does not know the interviewer's motive for asking the questions, he or she may perceive that employment was denied because of discrimination. Because of this, avoiding personal questions based on the list above (that are generally perceived as discriminatory) is the best approach to take. However, *after* an offer of employment has been made, asking questions about age, marital status, legal residency or ability to work in the United States, etc. may be appropriate.

The applicant's criminal record is another highly sensitive area. Generally speaking, employers can ask about convictions but not arrests that did not lead to conviction. In health care, make sure criminal history questions are asked to determine whether the applicant is qualified to work in a health care facility according to your state laws. Some facilities get away with asking questions about the criminal history by

adding a disclaimer to the application that states the information will not be used to deny employment. However, facilities should always consult legal counsel before adding questions or disclaimers that may be perceived as sensitive or discriminatory.

Violence in healthcare facilities

The National Institute for Occupational Safety and Health (NIOSH) defines workplace violence as "violent acts (including physical assaults and threats of assaults) directed toward persons at work or on duty."[16] This includes terrorism, such as the terrorist acts of September 11, 2001 that resulted in the deaths of 2,886 workers in New York, Virginia and Pennsylvania. The guidelines do not specifically address terrorism, but OSHA recognizes that this type of violence remains a threat to U.S. workplaces.

Imposters masquerading as surveyors

In April 2005, reports surfaced of individuals masquerading as JCAHO inspectors at hospitals in Boston, Detroit and Los Angeles.[17] Subsequently, reports of phony inspectors surfaced in other areas of the country, and it was theorized that these individuals were attempting to gain access to hospitals for terrorism purposes. All these individuals either implied they were with JCAHO or identified themselves as JCAHO inspectors. Several presented counterfeit identification cards, but when pressed for more information, they were either expelled or left the premises voluntarily.

The Joint Commission was sufficiently alarmed to add notations about potential imposters to all their newsletters, including those sent to long-term care facilities. They have removed inspector names from their state web sites to prevent potential identity theft, and facilities are encouraged to ask each inspector for a

- Joint Commission ID badge
- Letter printed on Joint Commission letterhead and signed by Russell Massaro, M.D., executive vice president, Accreditation Operations, explaining who they are and why they are at the facility

The imposters have been both male and female. Several were Caucasians. Several appeared to be of middle-eastern descent. They were all well dressed, usually in business suits and carrying briefcases. They arrived at off hours, such as during the night or weekend. One was found unattended in the newborn nursery. Others inquired about the pharmacy, laboratory, or overall emergency preparedness for a large-scale disaster. They requested floor maps of the facility. JCAHO recommends that all healthcare facilities make personnel aware that the potential for imposter surveyors exists. However, as of this writing, the true identity of the intruders and their motives are not known.

After the JCAHO warning was issued, other suspicious behavior and individuals were reported in hospitals in Arizona, California, Indiana, Massachusetts, Michigan, New Jersey, New York, and Texas. In May 2005, the government issued a memo advising facilities to take extra security measures, including

- Educating staff concerning the potential of unauthorized personnel presenting seemingly legitimate identification and credentials to gain access to the facility
- Encouraging employees to confront and identify all suspicious individuals
- Controlling and monitoring all entrances and exits with closed circuit television, and imple-

menting card-access technology for areas beyond the main entrance

- Requiring identification badges for all employees, contractors, official visitors, consultants, and others with legitimate business in the facility
- Prohibiting information sharing with purported inspectors or surveyors *without first contacting an administrative person or manager on call* to validate the inspector and purpose of the visit
- Requiring photographic identification and verifying the identities of surveyors
- Securing and locking all areas of the facility that are not open to the public including pharmaceutical storage areas, laboratories, cleaning supply closets and HVAC and utility equipment areas
- Increasing the inspection and inventorying of sensitive materials and equipment in the facility

Although the reported imposters masqueraded as JCAHO surveyors, they could just as easily misrepresent themselves as representatives of your state health department or another survey agency, such as OSHA. Counter-terrorism analysts are concerned that terrorist organizations may attempt to target U.S. medical facilities to cause immediate casualties and disrupt healthcare and emergency medical services. All facilities should be vigilant to the potential for imposters and report suspected intruders to law enforcement officials and the appropriate survey agency. This is an area in which you cannot be too careful. Emphasize the importance of proper surveyor identification with your staff, who may be intimidated if surveyors visit during off-hour shifts. If necessary, role play actions to take during an inservice. *Attempts to identify legitimate surveyors will be respected by the survey agency, who views this as one way the facility protects the residents.*

Requests for surveyor identification will not result in facility deficiencies.

Violence directed at employees

In 2006, two people charged with robbing a Claypool Hill, VA nursing home were given lengthy prison sentences. They pleaded guilty to charges of robbery and possession of schedule II narcotics, and no contest in a charge of using a firearm in commission of a felony. The staff member who was robbed testified she was traumatized by the incident and truly believed they would shoot her if she didn't give them the drugs. Witnesses to the robbery reported that two people entered the facility and demanded a variety of prescription drugs. The perpetrators denied having a gun, but a grainy video shows what appears to be a gun in the waist of one of the robber's pants. The robbers were subsequently arrested while trying to sell the stolen drugs.[18]

Violence against employees is another potential problem area that facilities must view proactively and not reactively. Like sexual harassment, facilities may wish to consider developing and implementing strong, zero-tolerance antiviolence policies and procedures. Orient and inservice all staff on these policies and make sure they are uniformly and consistently enforced. Violence directed at facility employees (while at work) may take many different forms:

- Intruders who have no relationship with or business in the facility (See Chapter 9)

- Residents with cognitive impairment, known mental illness, affective disorders, paranoid delusions, chemical abuse or dependency, dementia, impulse control disorders and personality disorders

- Family members who are upset about some facet of the resident's care

- Horizontal violence from peers and coworkers

- Violence from supervisors or managers

- Violence from a spouse or significant other who comes to the facility with specific intent to harm the employee

To ensure an effective antiviolence program, OSHA recommends that management and employees work together, such as in a team or committee approach. Facilities may wish to organize a safety or violence-prevention team with representatives from all departments. The committee can assist with

- establishing realistic violence prevention goals

- developing viable antiviolence policies and procedures

- assessing and identifying violence potential

- determining what constitutes a threat to employees; making suggestions for employee response in defusing the situation

- assisting with teaching violence prevention and trauma response

- making recommendations to ensure the facility is secure, such as:

  – recommending visitor restrictions, including employee spouses, relatives, and friends

  – drug testing policies and procedures

  – weapons possession policies and procedures

  – extraordinary hazard plans, such as hostage situations

  – conducting violence drills (e.g., a drug hold-up drill) to practice and walk through policies and procedures, as appropriate

  – reviewing policies and procedures annually and after a major event to ensure they

are appropriate, accurate, and fill the
intended need

Education is a key to violence prevention. Inservices
increase employee awareness and promote safe practices. They make employees aware of the need to
be alert to the safety of self and others. Teach all
employees to prevent, disarm, and defuse violence by
using a consistent approach in dealing with the violent individual. OSHA recommends that managerial
commitment to violence prevention includes[19]

- Demonstrating organizational concern for
  employee emotional and physical safety
  and health

- Exhibiting equal commitment to the safety and
  health of workers and residents

- Assigning responsibility for the various aspects
  of the workplace violence prevention program
  to ensure that all managers, supervisors and
  employees understand their obligations and
  responsibilities

- Allocating appropriate authority and resources
  to designated responsible individuals

- Maintaining a system of accountability for
  involved managers, supervisors and employees

- Establishing a comprehensive program of medical and psychological counseling and debrief-
  ing for employees who have experienced or
  witnessed assaults or other violent incidents

- Supporting and implementing appropriate recommendations from safety and health committees

Employee involvement should include[20]

- Understanding and complying with the workplace violence prevention program and other
  safety and security measures

- Participating in employee complaint or suggestion procedures addressing safety and security
  concerns

- Reporting violent incidents promptly and
  accurately

- Participating in safety and health committees
  or teams that receive reports of violent incidents or security problems, making facility
  inspections and responding with recommendations for corrective strategies

- Attending and successfully completing an inservice or comprehensive continuing education
  program that covers techniques to recognize
  escalating agitation, assaultive behavior, or criminal intent, and describing appropriate responses

Facility hiring practices

Your facility can be sued for negligence if you fail to
implement preemployment screening and someone is
hurt as a result of an employee's violence. Thoroughly
screening applicants and checking references (Chapter
2) is one of the best ways of preventing problems. In
addition to reviewing the application, checking licensure and certification, and validating references, consider the following red flags that may come up during
the interview of a prospective employee. The applicant

- has had numerous jobs in a relatively brief
  period of time

- provides vague explanations for gaps in
  employment

- has a history of positions with declining salary

- is seeking a lower position than he or she
  previously held

- forgets (or fails) to sign the release, reference, and
  consent forms accompanying the application

- tries to sidetrack you and provides anecdotes and long stories about previous jobs

- complains bitterly about former employers

- talks rapidly or in circles without providing the specific details you seek

- avoids giving straightforward answers to questions

- cannot remember (does not have, cannot access) former employer information, such as names, addresses, phone numbers, and names of supervisory references

Domestic violence at work

Nursing is a predominately female profession. Many of our workers are involved in dysfunctional relationships. The numbers are probably not disproportionate to other businesses that have a more even distribution of male and female employees. Sadly, some abusive and dysfunctional worker relationships are ended when a spouse or partner comes to the healthcare facility with the intent to harm others.

In 2003, the LVN ADON of a Texas long-term care facility was shot and killed by her estranged husband in the parking lot after her daughter dropped her off at work. The husband ran to Indiana, where he shot and killed himself in a cornfield as authorities approached to arrest him.[21]

In 2005, a male employee at a state school for the mentally retarded in Virginia shot a female co-worker multiple times and then fled before fatally shooting himself. Authorities were investigating the case as domestic violence.[22]

In November 2005, pepper spray and a Taser gun were used on a man who was seeking to confront his wife, an employee of a Wisconsin long-term care facility. He was apparently trying to make good on a promise to hurt her when she went to work. The man entered the facility at supper time, when staff were busy and roamed the halls in search of his wife. The nursing assistant had warned her employer when she arrived at work that her husband had threatened to come to work and harm her. Alert employees saw the man and called police. However, he refused to leave the facility and kept his hands in his pockets, leading officers to believe he had a gun. Because he continued to resist arrest, the officers used pepper spray on him, which was ineffective. They subsequently used a Taser gun to subdue him, and he was arrested without further incident. The facility administrator stated that facility residents were never at risk. The man was charged with resisting arrest, battery to a police officer and disorderly conduct.[23]

Assaults on residents

A January 2004 show on *Dateline NBC* featured a story entitled "Shattered Lives: Shots in the Dark." The show chronicled the lives of a Georgia family with a history of young-onset Huntington's disease (HD). In 2002, a mother fatally shot her two adult sons (both HD sufferers) in their long-term care facility beds. She had cared for their father and his mother until their respective deaths from HD. Although relatively young (ages 41 and 42), both the sons had advanced cases of HD, and were mentally impaired and totally dependent. (The mother had cared for them at home until doing so was no longer possible.) After shooting the sons in the head, she put the gun down and quietly waited for police to arrive. The woman contended that she was honoring her sons' wishes to end their suffering once they reached the later stages of the disease. Previously, she and her sons had entered a suicide pact and simultaneously ingested an overdose of antidepressants and analgesics, but the suicide attempt failed.

The mother was charged with two counts of first-degree murder with malicious intent, but plea bargained a guilty plea to assisting a suicide, which was illegal in her state. She was sentenced to five years in a maximum-security prison and five years of probation.[24] One surviving son, age 38 at the time of the plea agreement, also suffers from HD. Part of the plea bargain involved forbidding her to care for or live with this son upon her release from prison.

In California in April 2004, an 83-year-old man visiting his 78-year-old wife at a long-term care facility shot and killed her, then turned the gun on himself, in an apparent murder-suicide. Facility employees heard gunfire, then found the woman dead in her room near the body of her husband, who had arrived to visit her a short time earlier. No one else was hurt.[25]

Also in April 2004, an elderly man entered a Grapevine, Texas long-term care facility and fatally shot his wife, a resident of the facility in the head, before killing himself. Apparently no one heard the shots, which occurred about 2:40 p.m. The shootings were identified when oncoming staff made rounds shortly after shift change. Facility workers had previously assisted the husband out of his car and up a ramp into the facility with his oxygen tank. They were not aware he had a small handgun in his pocket. A suicide note was found in his wallet, stating he had been given six months to live and he needed to end their mutual suffering while he was still able to do so.[26]

Little can be done to anticipate and prevent injury to residents at the hands of their loved ones. Sadly, incidences of murder-suicide are increasing in long-term care facilities. Although workers and other residents are seldom threatened, the potential for other injuries always exists, particularly if there is a weapon in-volved. Make employees aware that the potential for violence exists. Describe warning signs to report. Facility administration must take threats and warning signs seriously and act on them promptly. Likewise, facility personnel must be alert to the presence of individuals with weapons in the facility and report them promptly to an administrative person and law enforcement. Personnel should avoid placing themselves in a situation in which they could be injured, such as by attempting to disarm an intruder or visitor.

Preventing violence

Violence in the work place is increasing in our society. Long-term care facilities are not exempt from problems, some of which are quite serious. Consider providing inservice classes on violence prevention. Teach workers to reduce their exposure to conditions that can lead to injury. OSHA has developed guidelines for preventing violence in the healthcare facility and many employers use these guidelines to develop and initiate safety programs for their employees. Potential reasons for violence in the healthcare facility include

- the prevalence of handguns and other weapons

- acute and chronically mentally ill residents

- individuals who abuse alcohol and drugs

- the availability of drugs in the facility, making it a likely robbery target

- the increasing prevalence of gangs and gang members in many communities

- unrestricted movement of the public in healthcare facilities

- drug and alcohol abuse in employees, visitors, and others

- distraught family members and other individuals who become angry and frustrated

- low staffing levels during meals and at other times when staff is busy caring for residents and unable to observe activity in the hallways and common areas

- poorly lighted parking lots, garages, and ramps

- staff feel safe and secure at work and overlook special precautions, such as locking doors in the evening

- lack of staff awareness of risk factors and preventive measures, such as locking doors and reporting suspicious individuals

Guidelines for employee safety and security

Facilities should teach employees safety and security policies and procedures and make sure they are enforced. Other methods of preventing potentially violent incidents include

- Reporting suspicious individuals or other potential safety hazards to the appropriate manager.

- Making sure that controlled and secured areas are kept locked. Avoid giving access or keys to employees indiscriminately.

- Following facility policies and procedures for locking all entrance doors at a designated time each evening. Respond quickly if the doorbell rings so incoming employees are not outside alone in the dark. (You may wish to assign someone to the door at shift change.) Identify all who enter.

- Providing information and inservice classes on cultural diversity. Consider classes and activities to teach sensitivity regarding cultural, racial, and ethnic issues and differences.

- Avoiding scarves, necklaces, earrings, and other jewelry that could cause injury if a resident or other individual attacks you.

- Avoiding remote, dark areas when you are alone.

- Exercising caution in elevators, stairwells, and unfamiliar areas. Follow your instincts. If you think a hazard exists, leave the area immediately!

- Requesting security personnel to escort employees outside, in parking lots, basements, or other potentially risky areas, particularly in the dark. If no security personnel are available, require personnel to have another staff member accompany them to isolated areas in which danger may exist.

- Use the "buddy system" any time personal safety may be threatened.

- If a resident or other person is threatening or potentially violent, avoid letting the person come between you and the exit.

Guidelines for dealing with a violent individual

- Remain calm and avoid raising your voice, which may worsen the agitation.

- Speak slowly, softly, and clearly. Be polite and remain calm.

- Call for help, if possible or send someone for help.

- Move away from heavy or sharp objects that may be used as weapons. If you see a potential weapon in the room, avoid staring at it, which may give a perpetrator the idea to use it.

- Monitor your body language; avoid movements that could be interpreted as demeaning or challenging, such as placing your hands on the hips, moving toward the perpetrator, pointing your finger or staring directly at the person. Avoid distractions. Focus your attention on the person so you know what he or she is doing at all times.

- Position yourself at right angles to the perpetrator. Avoid standing directly in front of him or her.

- Maintain a distance of three to six feet from the perpetrator.

- Position yourself so that an exit is accessible.

- Avoid making sudden movements.

- Listen to what the person is saying. Encourage the person to talk; inform him or her that you sincerely care and will do all in your power to help. Validate his or her feelings by acknowledging that he or she is upset or angry. Help him or her reduce large problems into smaller, manageable ones.

- Avoid arguing and defensive statements. Accept criticism in a positive way. If you sincerely feel criticism is unwarranted, ask clarifying questions.

- Ask the person to leave and return when more calm.

- Ask questions to help regain control of the conversation.

- Avoid challenging, bargaining, or making promises you cannot keep.

- Describe the consequences of the abusive or assaultive behavior.

- Avoid touching an angry person.

- If a weapon is involved, ask the person to place it in a neutral location while you continue talking. Avoid trying to disarm the person, which may put you in danger.

Worksite analysis

OSHA recommends an analysis of each worksite to identify existing or potential hazards for workplace violence. The analysis should include a review of actions, procedures, or operations that potentially contribute to hazards. Analysis helps you identify specific areas where hazards may develop. A threat assessment team, or similar task force or coordinator may assess the vulnerability to workplace violence and determine the appropriate preventive actions to take. Team members should represent all levels and categories of facility workers. The QA committee or this team should also review injury and illness records and workers' compensation claims to identify patterns of assaults that could be prevented by workplace adaptation, procedural changes or employee education. As the team identifies appropriate controls, they should be instituted.[27]

Other employee injuries

Long-term care facilities have long been one of OSHA's five target industries because OSHA considers them among the most dangerous places to work. Long-term care facilities also have a high incidence of worker sprains, strains, and other musculoskeletal injuries. The American Nurses Association has also taken an active interest in injury prevention. According to the ANA, nursing personnel are among the highest at risk for musculoskeletal disorders (MSDs), compared with other occupations.[28] The Bureau of Labor Statistics lists nursing assistants (identified as nurses aides, orderlies, and attendants) as being at the top of a list of high risk occupations for strains and sprains. Other top occupations are

- Second—Truck drivers

- Third—Laborers

- Sixth—Registered nurses (RNs)

- Seventh—Stock handlers and grocery baggers

- Eighth—construction workers

MSDs are injuries affecting nerves, muscles, tendons, ligaments, joints or spinal discs. Examples of common MSDs are

- Carpal tunnel syndrome

- Rotator cuff syndrome

- Trigger finger

- Sciatica

- Epicondylitis

- Tendinitis

- Raynaud's phenomenon

- Carpet layers' knee

- Tennis elbow

- Herniated nucleus pulposis (spinal disc)

- Low back pain

- Hand-arm vibration syndrome

- Tension neck syndrome

Signs and symptoms of MSDs include

- Loss of grip strength

- Reduced or limited range of motion

- Loss of muscle function

- Inability to do everyday tasks

- Painful joints

- Pain in wrists, shoulders, forearms, knees

- Pain, tingling or numbness in hands or feet

- Fingers or toes turning white

- Shooting or stabbing pains in arms or legs

- Back or neck pain

- Swelling or inflammation

- Stiffness

- Burning sensation

Ergonomics

Simply stated, *ergonomics* is "fitting the job to the worker." We tend to do the opposite by trying to fit the worker to the job. When there is a mismatch between the job and the worker, injuries often result. An *ergonomic hazard* is any work or workplace condition that increases biomechanical stress on the worker. Examples of conditions and problems that increase biomechanical stress on workers are improper work methods, improper (or inadequate) equipment, poor posture, force, repetition, and inadequate work-rest regimens.

An *instantaneous injury* is an injury that occurs suddenly or spontaneously, such as in an accident. A fall is an instantaneous injury. Many instantaneous injuries are caused by unsafe lifting techniques. The "safe lifting zone" is the area between the knees and shoulders. To lift an item below knee level, bend from the knees, using the leg muscles. To lift from above shoulder height, stand on a stool or ladder. Rearrange cupboards and shelves, if necessary. Move frequently used, heavy items to the center.

Cumulative trauma disorders are injuries to nerves, tissues, tendons and joints that result from repeated stress and strain over a period of months or years. Repetitious tasks are the leading cause of cumulative trauma disorders. In healthcare workers, the greatest offenders are

- Using muscular force to perform a job

- Doing heavy lifting without assistance

- Poor posture

- Standing in awkward positions

- Not taking a break, or inadequate rest caused by not taking short breaks frequently

Workplace MSDs are commonly caused by exposure to the following risk factors:

- *Repetition*, or doing the same motions repeatedly, which increases stress on the muscles and tendons, particularly if the movements are sustained. The severity of risk (or severity of the resulting injury) is determined by frequency (how often the action is repeated), the speed of the movement, the number of muscles involved, the force used by the worker, and unfamiliarity with the task or activity.

- *Forceful Exertions.* Force is the total physical effort needed to do the task or to maintain control of the resident or heavy object being lifted (or equipment or tools). The risk for injury is increased if the force is sustained for a prolonged period of time. The amount of force will probably vary, depending on the weight of the resident or object, type of grip used, the worker's body posture, the nature of the activity, and duration of the task. A forceful exertion injury commonly occurs when trying to catch or stop a resident who is falling, or in lifting the resident from the floor after a fall.

- *Awkward Postures.* Posture is the position of the body. It affects each muscle and muscle group involved in the physical activity. Awkward postures involve repeated or prolonged reaching, twisting, bending, kneeling, squatting, working overhead with the hands or arms, or maintaining a fixed position for a prolonged period of time. A common awkward-posture injury occurs when the wheelchair is too far away for

a pivot transfer, causing the workers to twist rather than moving the feet in the direction of the transfer. Other common causes are bending at the waist and over raised siderails.

- *Contact Stress.* Pressing against a sharp or hard surface increases pressure and stress on nerves, tendons and blood vessels.

- *Vibration.* Although nursing workers seldom use vibrating tools or mechanical devices, workers in maintenance, housekeeping, and laundry are at greater risk of injury by using vibrating tools such as buffers, sanders, grinders, chippers, routers, drills and other saws. Over time, repeated contact with vibrating mechanical devices can cause nerve damage.

Common causes of musculoskeletal injuries

An analysis of accident and injury data provides clues regarding postures and tasks in which the risk of injuries is increased. Many times, injuries occur as a result of confined spaces, such as working in small bathrooms or bedrooms with limited space. Awkward posture also contributes to employee injuries. If the worker's body is not in an efficient neutral position, the risk for injury is always increased. Awkward posture also results in loss of strength, fatigue, and inability to use muscles to their best advantage during the task. It may be difficult to maintain proper posture in the space available. Tasks that have been identified as increasing risk to workers are often tasks workers have already identified as being most difficult, or among tasks they least like to do:

- Lifting over the shoulders

- Lifting below the knees

- Pulling rather than pushing

- Bending at the waist

- Twisting the spine

- Lifting heavy weights (above those listed in NIOSH guidelines)

- Elbows away from the body.

- Forceful, uneven, or sudden movements

- Friction impediments to the task

- Body in other-than-neutral position

Long-term care facility workers perform these tasks many times each day in the course of providing routine resident care. The maneuvers listed above are likely to cause worker injury alone, or in combination. For example, bending at the waist while twisting the spine increases the risk of staff injury when moving a resident. Doing a risk assessment involves detailed analysis and considering manual handling hazards from various viewpoints and a number of different angles. A study of this type provides a full understanding of why a task is a problem and provides potential methods of changing or correcting it to reduce the risk. Safety professionals recommend a "hierarchy of controls" to follow when evaluating a hazardous task. To reduce the risk of injury in any potentially hazardous task, consider

- eliminating the task or any hazardous part of the task

- substituting a less-hazardous task for a more-hazardous one

- modifying the task (or modifying the load) so it is less hazardous

- using equipment and devices to reduce the ergonomic hazards

- modifying the layout or equipment used

- redesigning the task, work patterns, or controlling the environment

- identifying other available administrative methods to reduce the risk to workers

When evaluating the safety of resident care tasks involving lifting, moving, transfers, or mobility, ask yourself the following questions:

- Is the task safe for the nursing assistant (or other worker)?

- Is the task safe for the resident?

- Is the task consistent with principles of restorative nursing (does it maintain or improve the resident) as much as possible?

If the answer to all three questions is affirmative, chances are good that your facility is providing quality care and ensuring employee safety. If not, study the task and find another way of doing it. Modifying the way a task or procedure is done is the best means of relieving stress on the body. For example, when evaluating transfers of a heavy resident or object, answer the following questions:

- Is the resident larger than you are? If so, consider asking another worker to assist, or using a transfer belt or mechanical lift.

- Can the resident follow directions? If not, get help. Do not attempt this transfer alone.

- Can the resident help with the transfer? If so, how much assistance can he or she provide? What about the resident's mental status and ability to follow directions, and impulsiveness? Consider a transfer belt. Two workers may be needed for this transfer despite the resident's ability to help.

- Can a sliding board, lift sheet, mechanical lift, or other device be used?

- Do you need help? If the resident exceeds your body weight by one third ($1/3$) to one half ($1/2$) or is completely dependent, ask for help.

- Does the resident grab at persons or objects? If so, always get help.

- Can you move the resident within the safe lifting zone? A transfer belt may make this possible. If not (such as when a resident is on the floor), get help.

- Can you move the resident without twisting, bending at the waist, or stretching? If the answer is negative, you must find another way to facilitate the transfer. Avoid moving the resident until a satisfactory solution is identified.

- Is special equipment needed to move the resident safely? Is the equipment available and in working order? Has the worker been taught to use the equipment? Is more than one worker needed?

- Is the resident's footwear appropriate for the floor surface? Is yours?

- Are there obstacles on the floor or in your path? If so, move them.

- Are the resident and workers in a confined space? If so, find another way to perform the procedure. The greatest problem here is in bathrooms. Be creative, such as by placing a shower chair or commode chair over the toilet. Transfer the patient to the chair before entering the bathroom. Consider a ceiling-mounted lift.

Involve direct care workers when evaluating work practices. They know the problem areas and residents, and their suggestions may prove invaluable. Follow-up, evaluation, and review are essential aspects of the risk-management and task-analysis process. Review

modifications and control measures promptly after implementation, then periodically to determine if risk factors have been eliminated or controlled and whether new hazards have been introduced.

Back injuries

During the year 2000, the incidence for back injuries involving lost work days was 181.6 per 10,000 full-time workers in long-term care facilities and 90.1 per 10,000 full-time workers in hospitals. In 2001, injuries to healthcare workers recorded a 52% increase in injuries (resulting in lost days) over the previous year. Other incidence rates were 98.4 for truck drivers, 70.0 for construction workers, 56.3 for miners and 47.1 for agriculture workers. Of all employee injuries, lower-back injuries are the most costly. Many of these injuries are unreported. Studies of back-related workers' compensation claims reveal that nursing personnel have the highest claim rates of any occupation or industry.[29] At the time of this writing, the last year for which statistics are available is 2004. The healthcare industry, which includes hospitals, long-term care facilities, and ambulatory care centers continues to lead the pack in the total number of worker injuries, although the numbers have decreased slightly from 2003.

The licensed nurse workforce in the United States is aging, and there is a severe shortage of nursing personnel. There is an estimated increase in demand of 40% annually. However, the supply of available nurses has only increased by approximately six percent.[30] Patients and residents are getting larger, and obesity is a major health problem in the United States. Bariatric care units are becoming common in both hospitals and long-term care facilities. Combine the increased resident size with the loss of agility nurses experience as part of normal aging, and the presence of a nursing shortage. This makes attention to the incidence of back and other musculoskeletal injuries in the U.S. nursing workforce a grave concern. Research regarding the impact of musculoskeletal injuries on nurses reveals:

- 52% of nurses complain of chronic back pain.[31]

- 12% of nurses report that they have left nursing "for good" because of back injuries and/or back pain.[32]

- 20% of RNs requested a transfer to a different unit, position or employment because of low back pain, with 12% considering leaving the profession.[33]

- 38% of RNs have suffered occupational-related back pain severe enough to require taking leave from work.[34]

- 6%, 8% and 11% of RNs reported changing jobs for neck, shoulder and back problems, respectively.[35]

Legislation

In 2005, the State of Texas passed TX SB 1525, the first state legislation signed into law requiring hospitals and long-term care facilities to implement safe patient handling and movement programs. "The Texas Nurses Association has worked long and hard on passage of this important legislation," commented Anne Hudson, RN, BSN. "With Texas the first state to succeed with passage of legislation, a number of other states continue working toward legislative protection of healthcare workers against preventable injury from manual patient lifting." Ms. Hudson views this legislation as a major improvement, and hopes that "eventually all of the United States will mandate safe patient handling practices like those already in place in countries more advanced in protecting nurses and patients against injury from manual lifting."[36]

California assembly bill 2532 would have made con-

cepts like lift-teams, zero-lift policies and lift-assist equipment mandatory components of healthcare in the state, had it been turned into law. However, Governor Schwarzenegger vetoed the bill (which was drafted and supported by the California Nurse's Association [CNA]) because it was too costly for the industry. The CNA noted that hospitals with zero-lift policies had reduced worker back injuries by 39%, and in addition to relieving nurses of the burden of intense pain, back injuries increase workers' compensation costs and exacerbate the nursing shortage.[37] This is obviously an issue that will be ongoing in today's healthcare climate. Facilities should closely monitor their state legislation and long-term care association newsletters for changes in state laws and requirements to prevent worker back injuries. OSHA has an abundance of materials, resources, and educational aids available on MSD prevention. Several of their publications were written specifically for long-term care workers.

Back support belts

Some facilities require workers to wear back-support belts if the worker lifts or moves residents or heavy objects weighing more than 10 to 15 pounds. Some workers wear a back support belt because they prefer it. They state they are more comfortable when wearing the belt for support. Several old studies suggested that workers using the back support had fewer back injuries. However, other studies have shown no difference in the rate of injuries. The belt forces the user to keep the back straight and to use good body mechanics. Improved body mechanics may be the reason for a lower incidence of injuries. Using improper body mechanics when wearing the belt is difficult. For this reason alone, the belt may prove beneficial. Workers also appear to lift more slowly when wearing the belt. Since the back support belt decreases torso movement, it forces the worker to use a squat-lift technique versus a bending or stooping technique.

Some workers believe that using the back support belt makes them stronger. This is not true, and workers must be instructed to avoid lifting more weight than they would if they were not wearing the belt. NIOSH opines that workers wearing back belts have a false sense of security and may attempt to lift more weight than they would without a belt, potentially increasing risk of injury. Back belts should not be regarded as personal protective equipment. In the largest study of its kind, the Centers for Disease Control and Prevention's (CDC)'s National Institute for Occupational Safety and Health (NIOSH) found no evidence that back belts reduce back injury or pain. (This study was done in the retail industry; 9,377 employees were studied at 160 stores. Healthcare workers were not studied.)

This study was conducted over a two-year period, and found no statistically significant difference between the incidence of back injuries among employees who reported using back belts daily, and the incidence rate claims among employees who reported never using back belts or using them infrequently.

Through interviews, data were gathered and detailed information collected on workers' back-belt wearing habits, work history, lifestyle habits, job activities, demographic characteristics, and job satisfaction. The study also examined workers' compensation claims for back injuries among employees over the two-year period. In this study, NIOSH determined workers' habits in wearing back belts in advance of any injuries, and collected data as workers filed back injury claims.

The study also revealed no statistically significant difference between the rate of back injuries in businesses in which use of back-belts was mandatory versus the rate in businesses where back belt use was voluntary. These results are consistent with NIOSH's 1994 finding, that there is insufficient scientific evidence that

wearing back belts protects workers from the risk of job-related back injury. A previous history of back injury was the strongest risk factor for predicting either a back-injury claim or reported back pain, regardless of back-belt use. The rate of back injury among those with a previous history of back pain was nearly twice as high as the rate among workers without a previous history of back pain.[38]

Recommendations of professional organizations

It is theorized that the back-support belt increases intra-abdominal pressure, which in turn redistributes the forces on the back when lifting. The back belt may decrease muscle fatigue and strain due to increased support and through raising the local area temperature. The belt supports and stiffens the back which may decrease the forces on it. It restricts mobility, especially movement at the waist and forward bending. (Interestingly, the ligaments in the back do not support forward bending well, especially if twisting is involved. When pressure increases on the disk in the back, the nucleus of a disk is forced backwards, increasing the risk for bulge or rupture. A rupture or bulge will also damage nerves.) Some authorities recommend tightening the back support belt only during lifting and moving, and leaving it unfastened the remainder of the time. This is to keep the muscles normally conditioned and toned so they are not dependent on the belt.

The American Academy of Orthopaedic Surgeons recommendations on preventing low back pain can be accessed at *http://orthoinfo.org/brochure/thr_report.cfm? Thread_ID=10&topcategory=Spine&all=all* or *www.aaos. org/*. The National Institute for Occupational Safety and Health (NIOSH) information on preventing low back pain can be accessed at *www.cdc.gov/niosh/ homepage.html* or *http://www.cdc.gov/niosh/epstep1.html.*

References

1. Barling, J. (1996) The prediction, experience, and consequences of workplace violence. In G.R. Vanden-Bos & E.Q. Bulatao (Eds). *Violence on the Job* (p29-49). Washington, DC: American Psychological Association.

2. EEO Terminology. Online. *www.usma.edu/EEO/eeo_terminology.htm.* Accessed 0/15/06.

3. Price Waterhouse v. Hopkins, 490 U.S. 228, 250-51 (1989) (plurality opinion).

4. Mincin v. Shaw Packing Co., 989 F. Supp. 710 (W.D. Pa. 1997) (quoting Knabe v. Boury Corp., 114 F. 3d 407, 411 n.8 (3d Cir. 1997)).

5. Farpella-Crosby vs. Horizon Health Care, 97 F. 3d 803 (5th Cir., 1996).

6. Crist vs. Focus Homes, Inc., 122 F. 3d 1107 (8th Cir., 1997).

7. Cain v. Blackwell d/b/a Advanced Respiratory Care, Inc., 246 F.3d 758 (5th Cir. 2001)

8. Blankenship v. Parke Care Centers, --- F.3d --- (1997 WL 475867, 6th Cir.) or 123 F.3d 868 (6th Cir., 1997)

9. American Nurses Association. (1993). *ANA workplace issues: Workplace rights. Sexual harassment: It's against the law.* Washington, DC. American Nurses Publishing.

10. Conto v. Concord Hospital, 2000 WL 1513798 (D.N.H. 2000).

11. Williams v. Spartan Communications, 210 F.3d 364 (4th Cir. 2000).

12. Wilson v. Tulsa Junior College, 164 F.3d 534 (10th Cir. 1999). (This policy required the complainant to report to the director of personnel services, but the director was inaccessible due to hours of duty and location in a separate facility; it bypassed the supervisor entirely.)

13. Mota v. The University of Texas Houston Health Science Center, 261 F.3d 512, 525 (5th Cir. 2001).

14. Curry v. District of Columbia, 195 F.3d 654, 662 n. 17 (D.C. Cir. 1999).

15. Adler v. Wal-Mart Stores, Inc., 144 F.3d 664, 676 (10th Cir. 1998).

16. CDC/NIOSH. Violence. Occupational Hazards in Hospitals. 2002.

17. Brown D. (2005). Fake hospital inspectors probed. *Washington Post.* Friday, April 22, 2005; Page A10.

18. Talbert J. (2006). Robbery suspects get prison time. *Richland News Press.* January 24, 2006. Online. *www.richlands-news-press.com/servlet/Satellite?pagename=RNP/MGArticle/RNP_BasicArticle&c=MGarticle&cid=1137833623932&path=!frontpage.* Accessed 01/24/06.

19. Occupational Safety and Health Administration. (2004). Guidelines for preventing workplace violence for health care & social service workers.

20. Occupational Safety and Health Administration. (2004). *Guidelines for preventing workplace violence for health care & social service workers.* Online. *www.osha.gov/Publications/osha3148.pdf.* Accessed 01/20/06.

21. Associated Press. (2003). State police find man wanted in Texas nursing home shooting. *Fort Worth Star-Telegram.* 08/05/2003.

22. Associated Press. (2005). State school worker shoots colleague, kills himself. *Houston Chronicle.* 01/01/05.

23. Curtis L. (2005). Taser needed to subdue intruder at Lasata. GM Today. November 30, 2005. Online. *www.gmtoday.com/news/local_stories/2005/November_05/11292005_16.asp.* Accessed 11/30/05.

24. HD Blog. (2004). Dateline Synopsis. Online. *http://www.huntingtons.info/MT/archives/2004/01/dateline_synops.html.* Accessed 01/21/06.

25. Associated Press. (2004). Pair dies in Calif. nursing home shooting. *Tallahassee Democrat.* April 17, 2004. Online. *www.tallahassee.com/mld/tallahassee/news/8452339.htm.* Accessed 4/17/04.

26. Dennis D. (2004). Man kills wife, self at her nursing home. *Dallas Morning News.* April 28, 2004.

27. Occupational Safety and Health Administration. (2004). Guidelines for preventing workplace violence for health care & social service workers. Online. *www.osha.gov/Publications/osha3148.pdf.* Accessed 01/20/06.

28. American Nurses Association. (2004). *Handle with Care.* Washington, DC. American Nurses Publishing. Online. *www.NursingWorld.org/handlewithcare.* Accessed 01/20/06.

29. American Nurses Association. (2004). *Handle with Care.* Washington, DC. American Nurses Publishing. Online. *www.NursingWorld.org/handlewithcare.* Accessed 01/20/06.

30. American Nurses Association. (2004). *Handle with Care.* Washington, DC. American Nurses Publishing. Online. *www.NursingWorld.org/handlewithcare.* Accessed 01/20/06.

31. Nelson, A. State of the science in patient care ergonomics: lessons learned and gaps in knowledge. Presented at the Third Annual Safe Patient Handling and Movement Conference. March 5, 2003, Clearwater Beach, FL.

32. Stubbs D.A., Buckle P.W., Hudson M.P., Rivers P.M., Baty D. (1986). Backing out: nurse wastage associated with back pain. *International Journal of Nursing Studies,* 23, 4:325–336.

33. Owen, B.D. (1989). The magnitude of low-back problem in nursing. *Western Journal of Nursing Research,* 11, 2: 234–242.

34. Owen, B.D. (2000). Preventing injuries using an ergonomic approach. *AORN Journal,* 72, 6: 1031–1036.

35. Trinkoff, A.M., Lipscomb, J.A., Geiger-Brown, J., Storr, C.L., Brady, B.A. (2003). Perceived physical demands and reported musculoskeletal problems in registered nurses. *American Journal of Preventive Medicine,* 24, 3: 270–275

36. Texas passes first safe patient handling legislation in U.S. (2005). ErgoWeb. Online. *www.ergoweb.com/news/detail.cfm?id=1140.* Accessed 06/29/05.

37. Attempt to regulate hospital lifts vetoed in California. (2004). ErgoWeb. Online. *www.ergoweb.com/news/detail.cfm?id=1012.* Accessed 06/29/05.

38. Centers for Disease Control and Prevention. (2000). No evidence that back belts reduce injury seen in landmark study of retail users. Online. *www.cdc.gov/niosh/beltinj.html.* Accessed 01/20/06.

Self determination

Need for advance directives

In 2005, the Terri Schiavo case evoked strong feelings from the general public and health professionals regarding the rights of facility residents to die a peaceful and dignified death. Unfortunately, Ms. Schiavo's case was complicated because of her relatively young age (41 at the time of death), an estranged husband who had lived with another woman for years, parents who loved and were very devoted to their daughter, and media who could not seem to get enough of the sad story. Ms. Schiavo was reportedly in a persistive vegetative state for 15 years, and her husband and parents were on opposite sides of a legal and ethical debate about withdrawing the gastrostomy tube that was supporting her nutrition and hydration. The Roman Catholic Church also became involved in advocating for Schiavo, and administered Holy Communion through her feeding tube before it was withdrawn at the request of her estranged husband. Pope John Paul II made a statement on the issue, by noting that feeding tubes are "morally obligatory" for most patients in vegetative states. In fact, several high-ranking cardinals commented that removing a feeding tube could be considered a means of legalized euthanasia. (Ironically, Pope John Paul II also had a nasogastric tube inserted prior to his own death.) Prior to this time, the Catholic church had not taken a strong position or made a definitive statement on tube feeding.

The Governor of Florida and Florida Supreme Court also became involved in the legal wrangling. The United States Supreme Court refused to hear the case. The feeding tube was initially removed and replaced by court order. Eventually, the gastrostomy tube was withdrawn on request of the husband, and Ms. Schiavo died. As the clock ticked down, pro-life organizations, disability-rights groups, and hundreds of other supporters staged round-the-clock protests, demonstrations, and prayer vigils outside Ms. Schiavo's long-term care facility. Although she never put her wishes in writing, her husband contends the resident had stated she would not want to "live like this." The situation turned into a legal battle and media circus because her advance directive status was not initially known and her parents were unwilling to recognize the husband's authority as surrogate decision maker. Her case underscores the need for open and frank discussions about advance directives with all long-term care facility residents and responsible parties.

Misinterpretation and misuse of advance directives

A long-term care facility resident experienced abdominal pain and was sent to the hospital. The facility stated they sent a copy of the resident's advance directive requesting no CPR to the hospital. The hospital admits to receiving the advance directive documentation, but states the doctors forgot to note it.

While in the emergency room, the resident experienced a cardiac arrest and was resuscitated. The resident survived for ten days, during which time a ventilator and advanced life support measures were used. After the resident died, her son attempted to file a medical negligence suit. However, in this state, the estate of a dead person cannot sue for pain and suffering. As a result, the son filed an elder abuse lawsuit, noting the conduct of the hospital and its personnel were so egregious that they constituted abuse.[1]

In another situation, a resident had provided a copy of his living will to the facility. The document stated he did not want resuscitation, a ventilator, a feeding tube or other invasive form of nutrition or hydration, surgery or a variety of other procedures. The resident experienced a stroke that affected his ability to swallow and lost 24 pounds in 18 days. He died shortly thereafter. The resident's family sued, alleging the facility failed to treat him aggressively. They noted that two physicians had not certified the resident as being terminally ill, which was required by law in this state.[2]

Federal law for self determination

The resident is given the opportunity to sign an advance directive upon admission. Presenting this information to the resident or family is usually the responsibility of the social worker. Many facilities will provide the forms, but are not legally obligated to do so. If the facility does not supply the state approved forms, refer the resident or responsible party to a resource where information and forms may be obtained. Facilities should also avoid giving legal advice concerning advance directives. The resident or responsible party should be referred to their attorney for specific legal information. If the resident does not sign an advance directive upon admission, he or she is free to sign one at any time.

The Patient Self Determination Act (PSDA) became federal law effective in 1991. The purpose of the law is to ensure that individuals entering a healthcare facility are given information about their right to execute an advance directive. An *advance directive* may be either a *living will*, a *durable power of attorney for healthcare*, or both. Some states have additional, state-specific directives available:

- *Durable Power of Attorney for Healthcare*—gives the person designated as the agent or proxy the authority to make any and all health care decisions for the resident in accordance with the resident's wishes, including the resident's religious and moral beliefs, when the resident can no longer make sound decisions. The designated person is obligated to follow the resident's instructions when making healthcare decisions. He or she may consent, refuse to consent, or withdraw consent to medical treatment and may make decisions about withdrawing or withholding life-sustaining treatment. In some states, the person with durable power of attorney for healthcare *may not* consent to voluntary inpatient mental health services, convulsive treatment, psycho-surgery, or abortion. A physician must comply with the resident's agent's instructions or allow the resident to be transferred to another physician. The agent's authority begins when the doctor certifies that the resident lacks the competence to make healthcare decisions. In some situations, loss of decision-making ability will be temporary. After a recovery period, the resident may be able to resume responsibility for making his or her own healthcare decisions.

- *Living Will*—is a form that communicates the resident's wishes about medical treatment in the event that he or she becomes unable to make these wishes known because of illness or injury. The wishes are usually based on the resident's beliefs, ethics, religion, and personal values. In particular, the person signing the document should consider what burdens or hardships of treatment he or she would be willing to accept for a particular amount of benefit obtained if he or she were seriously ill. *A living will does not take effect until a physician certifies that the resident is terminally ill.* In some states, two physicians must verify the terminal illness. When signing this document, the resident may specify the type of care he or she desires, whether it be aggressive, limited, or comfort care only.

- Some states have additional, state-specific forms, such as those used for out-of-hospital cardiac arrests, or a healthcare surrogate directive form for use when a critically ill person has not previously signed a directive and is incompetent or incapable of communication.

The PSDA requires hospitals, long-term care facilities, and other healthcare providers who receive federal Medicare or Medicaid funds to offer written informa-tion explaining the patients' legal options for accepting or refusing treatment in the event they are incapacitated. Most facilities provide a brochure that meets state requirements.

The PSDA laws vary from state to state. The significant provisions of the federal act are

- Each state is required to develop written descriptions of the law concerning advance directives in their jurisdiction, and provide this material to healthcare providers.

- Hospitals, long-term care facilities, home health care agencies, hospice, and HMOs are required to maintain written policies and procedures guaranteeing clients written information explaining their involvement in treatment decisions. The information must supply state-specific data, and written policies of the facility regarding implementation of these rights. The medical record must contain documentation regarding whether the individual has implemented an advanced directive.

- The healthcare facility must provide for education of staff and the community regarding advance directives.

Nurses' responsibility

Advance directives have been an issue in lawsuits filed by family members of long-term care facility residents. In 2005, a Florida woman sued a long-term care facility over her husband's death, alleging that a DNR order in his medical record was meant for his roommate. The resident collapsed, but nurses took no aggressive action because of the DNR order, and the resident died.[3]

The American Nurses Association (ANA) published a statement describing the nurses' responsibilities in implementation of the PSDA. The ANA recommendations state that nurses should be familiar with the laws of the state in which they practice, and should understand the strengths and limitations of each form of advance directive. They note that the nurse has the responsibility to facilitate informed decision making, including, but not limited to advance directives.

Nursing personnel must adhere to a resident's advance directive. Resuscitating a resident who has a DNR order could lead to a lawsuit alleging battery. The opposite is also true. Failure to initiate CPR on a resident who is a full code, or not starting CPR in a timely manner can lead to negligence charges. Various other charges have been filed, such as mental and physical abuse.

The legal documents—designating a nurse as durable power of attorney

All states have laws providing for designation of a durable power of attorney, developing a living will, or both. The individual state laws will specify who may witness the execution (signing) of these documents. Again, the rules vary from one state to the next. The nurse must be aware of specific laws for the state in which he or she practices. In many states, a caregiver who is *related to the resident by blood or marriage may be designated* as the durable power of attorney for health care. Caregivers who have no blood or marital relationship may not accept this designation. (However, friends and acquaintances of the resident who are licensed healthcare professionals *may be designated* as the agent because they do not have a caregiving or nurse-patient relationship with the individual.)

Over time, states have modified and changed their rules and advance directive forms. Because of this, you should carefully read the form the resident gives you. The language on the form may be different than

it is today. Follow the instructions on the form signed by the resident unless he or she wishes to sign a newer version of the form. Unless specified by state law, older versions of the form do not expire and must be honored unless revoked by the resident.

Also, resident needs sometimes change, causing the need to revisit a living will or durable power of attorney (DPOA) with the resident or responsible party. A resident who is admitted as a full code may subsequently be diagnosed with terminal cancer, or a chronic condition may worsen. A designated healthcare proxy may die or move away. Review the advance directive status at care conferences or other designated intervals to make sure the advance directives remain current and reflective of the resident's wishes.

Witnessing an advance directive

State laws vary regarding who can witness the signing of these documents. Individuals, such as the administrator, may be prevented from witnessing them because of a financial interest in the operation of the facility. Nursing personnel also cannot witness the signing of advance directives in many states. The best option may be to ask another alert resident, another resident's family, or a facility visitor to witness the signing of the document, unless this is prohibited by state law. If these individuals are not available, asking a housekeeping or dietary worker may be permissible. Check your state requirements.

A DNR order is not an advance directive

An advance directive is a verbal or written statement made by an alert resident or other qualified individual that lists information and instructions about the extent to which the resident wants life-sustaining treatment in certain situations. The directive is implemented through a physician order, such as a "do not resuscitate" (DNR) order. Thus, the DNR order is a treatment decision. Having a DNR order on a resident's medical record does not confirm or create an advance directive.

Physician's orders and facility policies

The long-term care facility should keep a photocopy of the signed directive on the medical record. Return the original to the resident or responsible party. If the resident is transferred to the hospital or other healthcare facility, send a copy of the directive with the transfer form. Notify the ambulance service transporting the resident of the directive.

An advance directive requesting the facility to withhold CPR requires a physician order in most states. If the directive states the resident does not want CPR or other life-sustaining measures, contact the physician for a DNR (do not resuscitate) order, if appropriate. Most facilities require this order to be written in the physician's handwriting. Some require two nurses to witness a DNR order. Follow your facility policy. However, keep in mind that this is a potential legal risk if the resident is not terminally ill at the time the document is signed. Old age is not considered a terminal condition! Other common problems such as dementia are not considered terminal. The DNR applies only to terminal conditions, according to the terms written in the document. If you are unsure, read the language on the directive and take the appropriate action.

Do not assume that the presence of an advance directive means you must automatically get a DNR order. Also, remember that a DNR order is not an order to withhold all treatment. These are common lapses in nursing judgment made as a result of misunderstanding the state laws for advance directives. It is also an area of potentially significant legal exposure. Facilities should consider and address the nursing routine for requesting

DNR orders when presented with a "no heroics" directive in their policies, procedures, staff orientation and education. Ideally, the person receiving the DNR request should discuss the ramifications of the order with the resident and find out what his or her wishes are with respect to other types of care, such as tube feeding, IV, antibiotics, and others. When presented with an advance directive, do the following:

- *Read the directive.* Consider whether the resident has been diagnosed with terminal illness. Make sure that withholding CPR is in keeping with the resident's wishes today, and as stated on the form. If the resident experienced a cardiac arrest today, would the DNR be appropriate?

- *See if the directive contains a statement* that says something to this effect: "If, in the judgement of my physician, I am suffering with a terminal condition from which I am expected to die within six months, even with available life-sustaining treatment provided in accordance with prevailing standards of medical care."

  – A statement such as this suggests that the physician must document the presence of a terminal condition with a six month prognosis on the medical record. If the directive requires the physician to certify the resident as being in terminal condition, you will need further clarification. For example, a resident with an advance directive specifies no CPR. He has a DNR order. However, at this time the resident has *no known terminal illness*. If he chokes on food in the dining room, you should perform CPR. This is an accident/emergency that is unrelated to terminal illness. By getting a DNR order, are you depriving the resident of emergency care to which he or she is entitled? Not necessarily.

However, the answer to this question would be determined by how well your nursing personnel understand the rules for advance directives. If the DNR order was obtained specifically because of the provisions of the advance directive, you may be on shaky legal ground because the resident has *specified he does not want CPR if he is terminally ill*. Thus, the DNR order applies only to complications of terminal illness. It would not apply to accidental choking in a resident who is not known to be terminally ill. As you can see, blanket DNR orders can be very confusing with a high potential for error in the absence of known, diagnosed, and documented terminal illness.

– This situation becomes even more complicated if you have residents in the facility who have DNR orders, but no advance directive. Nursing personnel may not know when to implement the DNR and when to start emergency care. Clarify your policies and procedures before you are faced with such an emergency. You will find that nurses have widely divergent opinions regarding what constitutes heroic care. Rather than allowing for opinions to dictate nursing action, facility policies should identify appropriate nursing responses, and define what constitutes life-sustaining care.

• Consider a resident who has no known terminal illness who becomes dehydrated and requires an IV and antibiotics for a serious urinary infection. If the resident has a DNR order, will you provide IV therapy, or is this considered life-sustaining treatment? In some facilities, IV therapy is withheld in the presence of a DNR order, whereas in others, an IV is considered routine care. Are antibiotics a routine treatment measure or do they constitute life-sustaining care? This may be another gray area that makes the facility legally vulnerable. You will find nursing opinions that weigh in on both sides of the scale. Do not allow for chance. Define your facility's position on such treatments. Also consider feeding tubes and similar measures that may be considered routine measures and also life-sustaining treatments.

• *Facility policies should clearly define "life-sustaining care" or "heroic care."* Remember, if the resident is not in terminal, irreversible condition, as certified by one or more physicians, you should probably not withhold routine care or emergency care because of the presence of an advance directive. Clarify whether each resident would want a DNR order in this type of emergency before routinely obtaining blanket orders that may or may not be in keeping with the residents' wishes. Make sure your nursing personnel know the appropriate action to take in various types of treatment situations. If you are not sure, or if the policies do not specify, do not withhold routine care or emergency care because of the presence of a DNR order unless the resident is in terminal, irreversible condition, as certified by a physician.

• Review and become familiar with the language on the various advance directives used by your state, at various times from 1991 to date. Getting blanket DNR orders whenever the resident has a "no heroics" directive is not the answer, and may greatly increase your legal vulnerability. Many lawsuits have been filed as a result of erroneous advance directive actions.

- Depending on your state laws, this may be an issue that you will need to have the medical director and/or QA & A committee review and put policies and procedures in place. Your facility may need to consult a lawyer or your corporate legal/risk-management department.

Revoking the advance directive

A resident can revoke the advance directive at any time. Often, a resident will verbally revoke the advance directive by telling the nurse of his or her wishes. Follow your state laws for revocation of the directive. In some states, the nurse may not be able to witness the revocation. This could become a nasty legal issue if the resident verbally revokes the directive during the night, and dies before morning. At the very least, the revocation should be in writing, if possible, and supported by the signatures of two witnesses. In some states, an oral revocation may be made to any healthcare practitioner. In other states, requests for revocation must be made to a physician. In some states, a second witness must also be present at the oral revocation. The healthcare practitioner and witness should both document the substance of the oral revocation in the resident's medical record. The best approach is to be proactive. Learn your state laws regarding advance directives before you are in this position.

Another consideration is to check the resident's transfer form and hospital discharge orders. They may have a DNR order or contradict information in the long-term care facility's record. A DNR order may have been appropriate in the hospital, but inappropriate in the long-term care facility. Likewise, the order may contradict the resident's wishes, as stated in the advance directive. Always clarify discrepancies such as

this immediately.

Advance directives have been an issue in lawsuits filed by family members of long-term care facility residents. Know and follow your state laws and facility policies to protect yourself and your facility. State laws are always changing. Keep up with changes mandated by the legislature in your state.

Special situations

A geriatric resident with mild mental retardation and developmental disability was admitted to a long-term care facility. He required sliding scale insulin and could not be managed properly in a group home. Upon admission, the physician wrote a DNR order. Family members did not want the DNR order, but it was not rescinded, and they sought legal assistance. The court ruled that persons who are mentally retarded and developmentally disabled are not second-class citizens. By permitting the DNR order to stand, the facility negatively affected the resident's quality of life. The court noted that although a mentally retarded person's life may seem like an insignificant possession, *it is the resident's possession*, and no physician or court has the right to substitute its judgment regarding what is an acceptable quality of life for any person. Without calling the good faith of the physician or the loving devotion of the resident's sister into question, the resident's right to life is unquestionably implicated in any decision to deny him essential medical care. They ruled that a DNR order may not be written for the resident.[4]

A resident with senile dementia who has been declared mentally incompetent by a court and been given a court-appointed guardian cannot sign a valid advance directive expressing his or her wishes regarding artificial feeding, hydration, CPR, or endotracheal intubation. However, if the resident wants to sign an advance directive, the court should take his or her wishes into consideration. The Superior Court of New Jersey ruled that the court can issue an advance directive to the facility on behalf of the incompetent resident. In making this decision, the court noted that although a resident has been adjudicated incompetent, the very act of attempting to execute an advance directive has shown that the resident is capable of expressing a meaningful personal preference.[5]

Expectations of the resident and family members

Some chronically ill residents are admitted to the facility after illness or injury at home. Family members anticipate the resident will recover and return home. They do not always know or consider the total effect of the illness or injury on the resident's mortality. If the resident suddenly or progressively worsens and dies, the family may blame the facility. For example, hip fractures are associated with increased mortality in the elderly. Consider the resident with a hip fracture who has been admitted for therapy, with plans to return home eventually:

- Falls are the leading cause of injury-related deaths in the elderly. Of all fall deaths, at least 60% involve individuals who are over age 73. Of all fractures from falls, hip fractures cause the greatest number of deaths and lead to the most severe health problems. Only one in four patients recovers completely, 40% will require nursing facility care, 50% will need a cane or walker, and 24% of those over age 50 will die within twelve months of complications.[6] Women sustain 75% to 80% of all hip fractures. However, fall-related deaths are higher in men than women and differ by race. Caucasian males have the highest death rate, followed by

Caucasian females. African American males have the third highest death rate, followed by African American females.[7]

Rehabilitation potential

Most facilities ask the admitting physician to specify the resident's rehabilitation (rehab) potential upon facility admission. If the physician rates the rehab potential as being poor or fair, additional information will be needed. Thoroughly assess the resident and review the documentation sent from the transferring institution, if any. Question the physician about anticipated outcomes and determine what he or she has told the resident and his or her family members regarding prognosis and expectations for recovery. Next, request a meeting with the resident and family members (as appropriate) to clarify their understanding of the situation and identify their goals. Having both a nurse and social worker present for this meeting is a good idea. Some facilities do this at the first care conference, but this may leave you vulnerable and expose the facility to potentially serious problems during the first three weeks if the care conference is not held until day 21 of admission. A 2005 Sixth Circuit Court of Appeals decision upheld civil monetary penalties against a facility who was hospitalized as a full-code patient. Upon her return to the facility, the transfer form specified that she was a "no-code" resident. The physician did not write a DNR order, and the facility failed to seek clarification at the time of admission. There was no advance directive to guide them. The resident subsequently became unresponsive, pulseless, and respirations ceased. Rather than calling EMS or starting CPR, the nurse contacted the physician. The total length of the phone call was fifteen minutes. When questioned by surveyors about the resident's code status, the nurses told the inspectors the resident should have been a full code in absence of a DNR order, in keeping with their facility policies. The court viewed the failure to clarify code status as substandard care planning and upheld the citation and monetary fine.[8]

When meeting with the resident and/or family, discuss the disease process, prognosis, expectations for complete recovery, knowledge of potential complications, facility actions, services, notifications, and so forth. Determine whether a hospice evaluation is wanted or needed. Ask the resident and family to outline their goals and expectations and find a common ground on which to establish your initial plan of care. Be sensitive, compassionate, and honest. If the resident or responsible party are in denial, unreceptive to teaching information, unwilling to have such a frank discussion, or family members cannot agree, involving other professionals may be necessary, such as the physician, facility administrator, clergy, mental health and others. Pamphlets, videos, and other teaching aids are available on a wide variety of subjects and may be useful for resident and family teaching.

If a resident has multiple children and/or other interested family members, ask them to select one to be the designee for facility communications. This person will be notified of changes in condition and is expected to notify other interested family members. Ideally, this individual is the designated healthcare proxy, if the resident has named a durable power of attorney for healthcare.

Maintain a master listing of advance directives and DNR orders, and ensure the list is kept current. Some facilities use visual identifiers as well, such as blue wrist identification bands indicating the resident is a "Code Blue" in the event of cardiac arrest. Consider the speed with which nurses can access these data. In an emergency, they must quickly ascertain the resi-

dent's code status and take the appropriate action. Consider the need for an identifier on the resident's person. A resident may not be in his or her room at the time of an emergency. This is why wristbands are usually an effective method.

Some facilities use two colors such as blue, noted above, and red (or any other color) for those residents with no code (DNR) order.

Facility policies and procedures

There will be times when a resident's condition is emergent and he or she requires prompt treatment in the acute care hospital. Contacting the physician to request a transfer order may not be a realistic option and serves to delay the transfer further. Some facilities have standing orders, guidelines, policies, and procedures that permit nurses to immediately transfer residents to the hospital in an emergent situation. Reasons to implement this type of order may vary from situations such as uncontrolled bleeding to lack of immediate physician availability. Each facility should consider the need for standing orders authorizing nurses to send a resident to the emergency department based on nursing judgment, in certain circumstances. Solicit information from nursing personnel about how and when nurses should send a resident to the ER, and develop criteria, policies, and procedures. Present the information to the medical director and quality assurance committee for approval. Develop a method for notifying the physician and designated family member after the transfer. These notifications should always be made if the resident leaves the facility, even if they are made after the fact.

Special situations

You may have residents with special requests that must be fulfilled at or immediately after the time of death. For example, some residents may donate their bodies to science. Some donate organs, such as the brain to groups like the Huntington's Foundation for research into the cause and treatment of specific diseases. Although not common in long-term care facilities, some residents may wish to donate specific tissues or organs for various purposes. To be viable for the intended purpose, specific preparations, storage, and shipping are usually required. For example, the brain must be removed by a qualified individual before the body is embalmed. It must be preserved properly and shipped under refrigeration. The facility must probe the receiving organization in advance and obtain specific instructions regarding how to manage the body immediately after death to preserve organs and tissues for their intended purpose. List these instructions on a form or other document inside the chart and note the presence of special information on the care plan. Specify the steps for staff to take and notifications to make when death is imminent, or at the time of death. Do not leave anything to chance. If the body is not properly prepared, it may not be useful for the resident's intended purposes after death, and the cause is usually extremely important to the resident and family.

More than 400,000 Americans have joint-replacement surgery each year. Rush University in Chicago gratefully accepts post-mortem donations of artificial joints for medical research. This program has been in existence since 1990. The research is part of a study on joint replacement funded by the National Institutes of Health and other private philanthropic sources. There is no cost to the family for this valuable service, which has increased in popularity in recent years. Most families have expressed great satisfaction in the ability to honor their loved one's wishes in this manner. The researchers note that post-mortem retrieval is the only effective way to study joints that have

worked well enough to outlast the patient. Additionally, post-mortem studies enable the physicians to retrieve tissues surrounding the joint to determine whether they have been affected by the implant. For example, researchers found that screw holes and uncoated surfaces are susceptible to migration of debris generated by wear and tear on the joints. The presence of debris triggers a local immune response, causing pain, loosening of the implant, and further loss of natural bone. This research has revealed new information, showing that human bone continues to grow into the porous-coated surfaces, strengthening the joint, for years after surgery.

Rush University always has retrieval teams on call, and they respond quickly when a donor dies. The team travels to the community with its own surgical instruments, collection containers and protective apparel. If the deceased is a long distance from Chicago, they work with the funeral director and a physician or pathologist from the local community on the logistics of removing the joint and surrounding tissue, and packing and shipping the items via a refrigerated carrier to the Chicago facility. This does not delay funeral or burial plans. Since joint-replacement surgery has improved the quality of life for so many individuals, studying joints post mortem will help to improve the prostheses to benefit future generations. Most donors volunteer the joints in gratitude for their improved ability to move, reduction in pain, and an overall improved quality of life. Although much is known about using prosthetics inside human tissue, scientists continue to seek information about how the devices interact with joint tissues and how to improve them.[9]

Provide relevant information to the funeral director, as well. For example, if a resident has been diagnosed with a disease such as HIV or infectious hepatitis, the funeral home may need to take additional special precautions because the body remains infectious after death. Residents with implanted medication pumps, pacemakers, radioactive implants, electro-mechanical devices, and special external implants may need to have these items removed if cremation is planned. These devices may explode in the crematorium, causing damage to the equipment and increasing the risk of injury to crematory personnel. Artificial joints, such as knees and hips, are usually not removed prior to cremation. In case of an implanted pump, the manufacturers provide prepaid mailers upon request, so the explanted pumps can be returned to them for further research and study upon removal. They will provide directions and assistance if removal is necessary. As you can see, providing complete information to the funeral director shows respect for the resident and family and helps ensure the safety and well-being of your colleagues working in the mortuary and crematory.

RN pronouncement of death

In some states, an RN can make a legal pronouncement of death in certain situations. Although state laws vary, RN pronouncement is usually limited to natural death in which criminal conduct and suspicious circumstances are not suspected. There may also be prohibitions to pronouncing death in situations if the resident was being supported by artificial means, such as a ventilator that precludes determination that spontaneous respiratory and circulatory functions have ceased.

Before permitting nurses to pronounce death, each facility should develop policies and procedures for pronouncement of death. These should be approved by the quality assurance committee and medical director. The policy and procedure should be all inclusive, such as listing assessments to make and findings to document. Documenting a vague state-

ment, such as "pronounced by RN" are too imprecise for the reader to determine the actions taken, and may be considered inadequate in a court of law. Consider adding information about notifications to the policy and procedure, such as reporting to the attending physician and guardian or legal representative. Other notifications, such as the county coroner or justice of the peace may also be necessary, to maintain compliance with state and local laws. Some states require a physician's order to release the body if the pronouncement of death was made by an RN. In some municipalities, a coroner or justice of the peace must be notified of all long-term care facility deaths.

Death certificates and cause-of-death statements

In 1999, an Arkansas coroner did an extensive study of 100 questionable long-term care facility deaths that occurred from 1993 to 1999. The researchers interviewed families and nurses and reviewed all available documentation and clinical information for the deceased, including medical records and long-term care facility records. As part of the study, seven bodies were exhumed and autopsied. The researchers determined that more than 30% of the death certificates listed an incorrect cause of death. "The families were being told that their loved ones died of heart attacks, strokes and other natural causes, but what we actually found was that about a third were wrongful and preventable deaths, either caused by or exacerbated by dehydration, malnutrition, including choking, or from sepsis from bedsores," said the coroner, who had just been appointed to the U.S. Department of Justice's newly formed forensic working group at the time the findings were published. As a result of this study, the State of Arkansas passed a law requiring facilities to notify the coroner of every death. In a follow-up, the *St. Louis Post-Dispatch* reviewed the death certificates and the physicians' evaluations of 55 long-term care facility residents in Missouri and Illinois whose survivors were suing for neglect. In 42 of these cases, the newspaper found that the cause of death listed on the death certificate differed from what physicians said the medical records actually showed.[10]

Although the long-term care facility has little to do with identifying the cause of death, you may find an inaccurate or imprecise cause of death is problematic if the facility is sued. It is critical that the full sequence of events leading to the resident's death is documented and provided to the physician, including information about the initiating condition, or underlying cause of death. Subsequent morbid events ending with death are also identified on the death certificate as secondary or tertiary causes of death. You may be surprised to learn that the death certificate is often a key piece of evidence in the medical malpractice trial. The studies above offer cause for alarm. If the cause of death is not accurately identified, the opposing attorney may suggest the facility was negligent in some manner. For example, the cause of death is listed as "sepsis," suggesting a massive, overwhelming infection. This may be secondary to long-term catheterization for a condition such as multiple sclerosis. However, by not identifying this treatment on the death certificate, there is room for an attorney to create reasonable doubt in the minds of a jury that the sepsis resulted from negligence. Some physicians commonly list "cardiac arrest" as the cause of death. In fact, everyone ultimately dies of cardiac arrest, so this diagnosis is uninformative and of little

value. The cause of death information for each resident is coded and entered into state and federal mortality databases, such as those maintained by the National Center for Health Statistics. The information is used for research, statistics, public-health decision-making, policy setting, and lawmaking. It also provides information for the family and others who use the death certificate for legal purposes.

Since most long-term care facility residents are not autopsied, an accurate physician's determination of the cause of death is critical. The facility must be familiar with state laws, as well as information the physician will need in order to identify the cause of death accurately. A major goal when identifying the cause of death is to report an underlying cause that is as etiologically specific as possible. Each state has standards and guidelines for completing the death certificate. Some have a specified time frame, such as five to 10 days. Excellent tutorials are available on identifying the cause of death and writing it correctly at

- The National Association of Medical Examiners
  www.thename.org/

- Texas Department of Health
  www.tdh.state.tx.us/ (see continuing medical education programs)

Few physicians receive formal education in medical school or elsewhere about proper completion of the death certificate, so this is very useful information. You may wish to become familiar with the tutorial information and pass it on to your medical director and other attending physicians.

References

1. Saillant C. (2004). Hospital fights elder abuse lawsuit. *Los Angeles Times.* September 9, 2004

2. Living will confusion prompts lawsuit. (2004). *Nursing Home Law and Litigation Report.* 4,8, 252.

3. Associated Press. (2005). Widow: Florida nursing home's error caused husband's death. *South Florida Sun Sentinel.* 1/11/05.

4. New York Supreme Court, 1995.

5. Matter of Roche, 687 A. 2d 349 (N.J. Super. Ch., 1996).

6. AAOS Fact Sheet. Hip Fracture. Online. *http://orthoinfo.aaos.org/fact/thr_report.cfm?Thread_ID =229&topcategory=Hip.* Accessed 7/08/02.

7. Centers for Disease Control and Prevention Fact Sheet. Falls and Hip Fracture Among the Elderly. Online. *www.cdc.gov/ncipc/factsheets/falls.htm.* Accessed 7/08/02.

8. Omni Manor Nursing Home v. Thompson, 2005 WL 2508547 (6th Cir., October 11, 2005).

9. Associated Press. (2006). Volunteers bequeath their artificial joints to science. *Quad City Times.* January 29, 2006. Online. *www.qctimes.net/articles/2006/01/ 29/news/state/doc43dc52b43f851502615491.txt.* Accessed 01/29/06.

10. Schneider A and O'Connor P. (2002). Nation's nursing homes are quietly killing thousands. *St. Louis Post-Dispatch.* 10/12/02. Online. *www.stltoday.com/ stltoday/news/special/neglected.nsf/0/D99DA8A06D2CB A8C86256C500057AAC5?OpenDocument.* Accessed 10/24/06.

Quality assurance/benchmarking

> The Director of Nursing (DON) in long term care advocates for the assessment and evaluation of outcomes in the long term care facility and develops implementation strategies for negative outcomes. The DON realizes the critical importance of Quality Assurance or any other type program which serves to seek out problems and strategize their solutions.[1]

The quality assessment and assurance committee

The OBRA regulations introduced long-term care facilities to a new requirement in the form of a mandate to establish a comprehensive quality assessment and assurance (QA & A) program. Our colleagues in hospitals and other branches of health care had been working under a similar mandate from the JCAHO for at least ten years. The current federal rules state:

F520 §483.75(o) Quality Assessment and Assurance

(1) A facility must maintain a quality assessment and assurance committee consisting of—

  (i) The director of nursing services;

  (ii) A physician designated by the facility; and

  (ii) At least three other members of the facility's staff.

The intent of this regulation is to ensure the facility has an established quality assurance committee that identifies and addresses quality issues and implements corrective action plans as necessary. Facility QA & A committees may be referred to by other names such as Performance Improvement or Continuous Quality Improvement committees but the functions and goals are the same. The quality assessment and assurance committee is responsible for identifying issues that necessitate action of the committee, such as issues that negatively affect quality of care and services provided to residents. In addition, the committee must develop and implement plans of action to correct identified deficiencies. The medical director may be the designated physician who serves on this committee.

Some facilities have been spared deficiencies because they were able to show that they had already identified and corrected problems through their QA program which were later identified by surveyors. The importance placed on quality assurance committees is seen in the Guidelines to Surveyors which states "If the facility has been out of compliance with a regulatory requirement between two surveys in which they were in compliance, that past noncompliance will not be cited by the survey team if a quality assurance program is in place and has corrected the noncompliance. An exception to this policy may be made in cases of egregious past noncompliance."

Almost every process reviewed by the QA & A committee can be explained in terms of four basic parameters: cost, time, customer (or employee) satisfaction, and errors or defects. Individual state rules have modified the original federal requirement for committee composition. In some states, facilities are required to expand their membership to include the facility administrator, a representative of the facility's governing body, and an individual who represents the residents. The frequency of the committee meetings may also be stipulated by individual state laws, but in most facilities the committee meets quarterly.

A commitment to quality

The keys to achieving quality are an organizational commitment, benchmarking data, and risk management. Promoting a culture of quality is helpful, but you must believe in it and commit to high quality care to be successful. Once you have committed to providing quality care, make quality improvement a priority.

Use the quality assurance committee to review incidents, pressure ulcers, restraints, catheters, infections, and other problem areas. However, do not limit the committee to these topics. Any potential problem may be reviewed. When evaluating incidents, pressure ulcers, and infections, remember to look at the big picture. Determine whether a dysfunction in the system caused the problem or set the stage for individual failure.

When evaluating quality, you must have a system for evaluating your activities and determining whether they have been successful. Facilities who emphasize teamwork, communication, and encourage direct care staff involvement into resident plans of care are often successful with quality improvement efforts. These assets set the stage for quality care. Change is a constant in health care. Although there are many quality improvement models, the goals are essentially the same—to identify areas in which change is needed and implement changes to improve processes of care delivery. You may want to develop checklists for doing quality review audits. List the current standards of care for the area you are evaluating. Review the state and federal rules and make sure to include all the requirements. In some situations, record review may provide all the information you need to determine whether services are delivered effectively. In others, you must do direct observation on the units, and interview staff and residents or responsible parties. Much will depend on the subject you are studying. When auditing for quality, try to think of all related factors and do not leave any stones unturned. **You will find an example audit and a blank template form on the CD-ROM that accompanies your book.**

In 2002, the CMS took quality improvement one step beyond the QA & A Committee when they introduced the quality measures. In 2004, a set of advanced quality measures was released. *Quality indicators* (QI) (also called *quality measures* (QM)) are identified by using data on the MDS assessments. MDS data are transmitted to the state long-term care survey office, then sent to the federal government. The government collects information concerning the residents' physical and clinical conditions and abilities, preferences, and life care wishes. After the assessment data are converted into quality measures, they are posted on the Medicare web page so they can be used as a source of information with which to evaluate facility services. When facilities consider "reportable events" they often think of abuse, neglect and misappropriation of property. In reality, because of the MDS system, every fall, weight loss, pressure ulcer and numerous other data are reported to the state through the MDS submission process. Most of the quality measures reflect a resident's condition for the seven days before the MDS was completed, so they may not represent the resident's condition accurately. For example, residents were assessed for pain over the past seven days. Pain that was subsequently relieved will not be reflected until the assessment is updated. Because of this, facilities should have mechanisms to monitor current data on an ongoing basis.

Monitoring quality indicators has become popular in health care. Quality indicators are a benchmark of sorts. There are many free tools for research and decision-making available online. These can be used for identifying and recognizing potential problem areas, tracking changes in performance and outcomes, and identifying areas that need further study and research. Indicators that reflect facility services can be measured. Since facilities are required to have systems in place for recording and reviewing events such as falls, skin tears, med errors etc., they should put these data to work as a part of their QA program. This develops the facility's own benchmarks and a basis upon which to initiate improvement. How many falls did you have last month, last year? Are you utilizing the data to develop a culture of safety awareness in your facility? Stepping from reactive to proactive involves incorporating the information from risk assessments into the QA process. Instead of waiting for a resident to fall and developing an intervention, you act upon the risk assessment to prevent the fall in the first place.

The quality measures used by CMS were selected because the issues are important to resident care. All of the QI's reflect conditions that can be modified or corrected, so facilities have a means of changing and/or improving their scores. Comparing the indicators also provides a means of comparing your facility and its residents with other facilities. They provide a snapshot of how facilities and their residents are different from one another, and how they are alike. The online quality measures have been validated and are research-based. Statistical methods have been applied to adjust measures that are out of a facility's control, so as not to lower the score unfairly. The quality measures are posted on the Nursing Home Compare Web site at *www.medicare.gov* so that any interested person can access the data. Facilities are encouraged to check the information posted on the web site. If you find errors in your facility's data, inform CMS of the problem and ask them to correct it.

Benchmarking

Benchmarking is part of the quality improvement process. A benchmark is a standard reference point against which performance is measured. Benchmarking is an activity in which a facility establishes "best practices" by comparing what they are doing with similar facilities. The supply of data that can be benchmarked is limitless. Any aspect of the organization can be benchmarked. To make a comparison, you must be familiar with the standard of care for the clinical area being compared. If you are unsure of the current standards, benchmarking is helpful in identifying the applicable standard of care. By benchmarking with other organizations, the facility can improve its processes and achieve excellence.

Critical thinking is an essential skill for quality assurance. It is used for problem solving, brainstorming potential solutions, drawing conclusions, combining information, separating fact from opinion, or identifying potential outcomes. Benchmarking involves applying critical thinking to learn what other facilities are doing, and using the information to solve problems in your own facility. This does not involve copying what others are doing. Once a problem has been identified, you apply practices that are likely to work. This may mean employing many approaches from several different facilities, and modifying them to fit your situation.

Root cause analysis

Root Cause Analysis (RCA) is used for identifying the cause or contributing factors associated with untoward events. It employs critical thinking to identify solutions to problems. Your facility will have guidelines for conducting a root cause analysis investigation. Root cause analyses:

- Should involve an interdisciplinary team, making sure that personnel are knowledgeable about the processes involved

- Emphasizes systems and processes rather than individual performance

- Focuses on determining what happened and why it happened; it asks questions repeatedly until all aspects of the process are reviewed and contributing factors identified

- Makes recommendations for procedural changes to reduce the risk of untoward events and incidents

After the root cause analysis is done, the team will write a root cause statement. The root cause statement:

- Identifies the cause and effect of the incident or event being studied.

- Answers all obvious questions.

- Operates on the premise that most incidents have multiple potential underlying causes; there is seldom only one cause of an untoward event.

- Avoids negative terminology; uses only

positive terms.

- Recognizes that each human error has a cause. Procedure violations are usually not considered root causes. Each violation must have a preceding cause. Failure to act is only a root cause if the staff member has a duty to act.

- Determines whether workplace or system redesign will reduce the risk of incident recurrence.

- Is consistent and not contradictory.

- Considers relevant literature and standards.

- Includes recommendations for corrective actions and outcome measures.

Root cause analysis focuses on learning how an incident occurred. It is not a punitive process and does not place blame. The team uses what they have learned to make recommendations for preventive measures and solutions. *Transparency* is essential to root cause analysis. This means the information is available to others. The results of an investigation are not useful unless they are accessible and understandable. Facility staff and interested others should know how and where to access the information.

Lack of root cause analysis opened the door to a dozen lawsuits for one hospital. Newborn infants and one mother spontaneously developed respiratory distress as a result of surreptitious Lidocaine injections by a technician. The United States District Court for the Middle District of Alabama scrutinized the incident reports and other documentation in great detail. The jurists determined there was an obvious pattern to the incidents. The presence of a pattern should have caused the hospital to investigate to determine whether the incidents were random or isolated, or if a pattern of personnel or other circumstances existed.

The court ruled the hospital had a legal responsibility to identify and eliminate the cause of the problem long before a dozen patients were injured.

The court stated that one purpose of quality assurance is to be aware of the possibility of suspicious patterns in adverse episodes. If a potential pattern of ongoing intentional criminal misconduct exists, the QA committee must take steps to identify it. A good place to start is matching up the personnel on duty with the incidents, then reviewing and/or investigating their backgrounds. The court noted that a hospital can be liable for negligence if patients continue to be harmed after events have provided an opportunity for the QA committee to notice the problem and act on it.[2]

Customer and employee satisfaction

In addition to improving quality of care, some facilities are reviewing consumer satisfaction and have borrowed ideas from the retail industry to ensure the residents and families are happy. Staff turnover reduction is also an area of intense study. Facilities realize that turnover is expensive, so the quality assurance program studies and implements new methods for employee satisfaction and staff retention.

Best practices

Best practices are procedures, programs, or activities that are successful and can be readily adopted by other individuals or organizations. These practices may be considered leading edge, or exceptional models for others to follow. Many facilities share best practices that have been effective and have been successful in improving some aspect of facility life or services. Several states and quality improvement organizations post this information on their web pages for others to download. Many tools are available to help you evaluate care. You may wish to check

your state nursing facility regulatory web page, state health department, and any of the many best practice and quality information web sites.

The governing body

The governing body or board of directors has been named as a party to many lawsuits. The generally low reimbursement rate, intensive regulatory scrutiny, and overall demands of facility operations have made it difficult for the individual or family-owned facilities to survive. Most facilities have corporate ownership. Plaintiffs often allege that the corporate approach has reduced the quality of care. However, without the corporately-owned facility some communities would not have long-term care services available. Plaintiffs commonly allege corporate greed. Sympathetic juries have awarded millions in punitive damages to send the corporate owners a message. Without taking a position in this argument, facilities must be aware that the governing body has a responsibility for quality, and thus they have a stake in the activities of the QA & A Committee. The QA & A Committee should have some means of communicating with and reporting their activities to the governing body.

The requirements for the governing body are interspersed with information about survey compliance, as well as billing fraud and abuse. However, the governing body clearly also bears a responsibility for regulatory compliance and quality of care. In a document providing guidance to members of the governing body, the General Accounting Office (GAO) summarizes the responsibilities of the facility directors.[3] The governing body's responsibilities include determining the mission, goals and objectives of the facility. These important functions set the tone for quality care. The facility must have policies, procedures, and written standards of conduct and professional services that have been endorsed by the governing body. The standards should be binding on all employees and other professionals, independent contractors, and volunteers performing services for the nursing facility, as well as other providers operating under the nursing facility's control, such as therapy companies, durable medical equipment suppliers and laboratories. The code of conduct describes the facility's commitment to ethical behavior, and identifies expectations of employees. The code should also make a commitment to legal compliance. It helps define the facility's culture by detailing the fundamental principles, values, and framework for action within the facility. You would expect the general operating policies to derive from its principles. The code represents the facility's ethical philosophy, and the policies and procedures represent the organization's response and methods of managing the daily operations and problems the facility confronts.

The code of conduct should be implemented by written policies and procedures that facility staff should follow. The compliance officer is usually assisted by the QA & A Committee, who analyze problems and advises on strategies for improvement and promoting regulatory compliance. The board of directors should satisfy itself that management has developed a system that establishes accountability for proper implementation of the compliance program. The GAO notes that the experience of many organizations is that program implementation lags where there is poor distribution of responsibility, authority and accountability beyond the Compliance Officer. They note that facilities must act on deficiencies or suspected noncompliance promptly. Failure to respond to a known deficiency may be considered an aggravating circumstance in evaluating the organization's potential liability for the underlying problem. In addition, the Board should receive sufficient information to evaluate the appropri-

ateness of the organization's response.[4] Since the governing body is often the legal entity licensed by the state to operate the facility, final responsibility for facility operations rests with this body. This body must be kept informed of quality assurance activities and approve changes in operating policies and procedures. Additional information about the responsibilities of the governing body is found in Chapters 3 and 22.

Confidentiality of QA & A committee data

Surveyors are expected to question facility staff and review documents only for the purpose of determining whether the facility has a quality assurance committee, and whether the committee is used for the intended purpose of identifying and addressing problematic (or potentially problematic) issues. Surveyors are not to use QA committee minutes or findings as a basis for writing deficiencies. The rules imply that the QA data are protected and need not be disclosed:

§483.75(o) (3) A State or the Secretary may not require disclosure of the records of such committee except insofar as such disclosure is related to the compliance of such committee with the requirements of this section. (4) Good faith attempts by the committee to identify and correct quality deficiencies will not be used as a basis for sanctions.

Because of this rule, facilities tend to place a great deal of potentially damaging information under the auspices of the QA & A committee. For example, they consider all investigations of alleged abuse and neglect, incident reports, information about in-house pressure ulcer development, and nosocomial infections to be protected quality assurance information that is not disclosed to surveyors, or anyone else. The protected information privilege has been the subject of a number of court rulings in many states. In many rulings, the various courts have required facilities to release the information they considered protected. Court opinions from one state are not necessarily limited to the state of origin. If a similar issue comes before the court in any state, documents and opinions on related subjects from other states are likely to be reviewed and considered. Court opinions are often lengthy and copying them is beyond the scope of this book. However, relevant parts are snipped from several court rulings. The source document can be readily accessed for additional, more comprehensive information.

"The Legislature recognized the chilling effect that would be engendered by enfeebling confidentiality. . . . We agree that, "[o]nce a state has made the policy decision to afford privileged status for certain records, the Legislature and the courts should not undermine the policy objective by circumventing or weakening the privileged status with exceptions not mandated by constitutional considerations or the long-term interests of justice. Nothing is worse than a halfhearted privilege; it becomes a game of semantics that leaves parties twisting in the wind while lawyers determine its scope." (Quoting Charles David Creech, The Medical Review Committee Privilege: A Jurisdictional Survey, 67 N.C.L. Rev. 179, 179-80 (1988))."

"Texas courts have not carved out new exceptions to the peer-review committee privilege but have simply applied the peer-review privilege to prevent what the appellant now attempts to do—namely, *cloak public information in confidentiality by first filtering it through the peer-review process*. In Irving, the court limited the privilege to those documents created by the committee itself. Texas courts have consistently limited the peer-review committee privileges to those documents generated by the committee as a result of the committee's deliberative processes and to those submitted to the committee at their direction and in

furtherance of committee business. See Memorial Hosp.—The Woodlands v. McCown, 927 S.W.2d 1, 9 (Tex. 1996); Barnes v. Whittington, 751 S.W.2d 493, 496 (Tex. 1988); Jordan v. Court of Appeals, 701 S.W.2d 644, 647-48 (Tex. 1985); Texarkana Mem'l Hosp., Inc. v. Jones, 551 S.W.2d 33, 34-36 (Tex. 1977); Ebony Lake, 62 S.W.3d at 869; see also Creech, supra at 184 (noting that the privilege is limited to what the committee produces). *Just because a report may deal with a nursing home's quality of care and has been reviewed by a peer-review committee does not necessarily mean that the report is cloaked with a committee privilege."* (*Capital Senior Management 1, Inc. v. Texas Department of Human Services 03-02-00615-CV [Tex.App. Dist.3 03/11/2004]*)

In a lawsuit against a long-term care facility, the plaintiffs filed a writ to compel the facility to release their surveys. The appeals court addressed the issue of whether a long-term care facility investigation report prepared by the state survey agency, the facility's plans of correction, and the testimony of surveyors regarding their investigations are excluded from lawsuit discovery under the peer review privilege. The plaintiff asked the appellate court to order the trial court to permit use of the survey reports during discovery and at trial. The facility resisted, claiming peer review privilege. They argued that the surveyors' reports were prepared from confidential information that the facility's peer review committee provided. (This is not necessarily true, because the surveyors reviewed resident records and data that may also have been reviewed by the QA & A Committee.) As a result, they contended the information was privileged and should not be released. The facility stated that surveys were part of the peer review process. (In this facility, the QA & A Committee also reviewed survey findings.) The court noted that there was no evidence that the survey reports disclosed any confidential information. The opinion stated that *the mere fact that the facility's peer review committee may have reviewed the documents did not make them privileged*. The Court of Appeals noted that the civil statutes that protect the peer review privilege do not apply when records are required or authorized by law to be disclosed. In this case, surveys and plans of correction must be posted in the facility and are considered a public record. The court determined that the peer review privilege extends to documents prepared by or at the direction of a peer review committee for committee purposes. Other documents, such as surveys that are submitted to a committee or that are created without committee impetus and purpose are not protected. *(In re Donna Pack, 996 S.W.2d 4 [Tex. App.—Fort Worth 1999 n.w.h.])*

State Supreme Court opinions

Supreme court opinions are also quite lengthy. The Texas court system has also addressed the confidentiality of records and peer-reviewed documents at many levels, and their decisions provide helpful information and guidance on this issue. The Supreme Court of Texas heard a case in 2004 in which the facility had filed a *Writ of Mandamus*. This is an extraordinary action that is used to command an official to perform an act as an absolute duty that is not left to the individual's discretion. A writ of mandamus action is typically used only when all other judicial remedies have failed. In Texas, a person may obtain mandamus relief only if (1) the trial court clearly abused its discretion and (2) the party requesting mandamus has no adequate remedy by appeal. In this case, the trial court had previously ordered the facility to produce documents that lacked a "QA & A privilege" stamp, and privilege log documents that did not have the word "committee" in the name to the plaintiff.

The issue reviewed on appeal was brought by a long-term care facility that was being sued for wrongful death and providing negligent care. After being served with discovery, the facility withheld many internal documents, asserting the medical peer review privilege and the quality assessment and assurance (QA & A) privilege. The plaintiff filed a *motion to compel* (demand) production of the documents. The facility was required to submit various documents for judicial review, including an affidavit from the director of nursing. An *affidavit* is a formal sworn statement or written declaration made under oath. It is witnessed, usually by a notary public or other person who is legally authorized to administer an oath. The affidavit described the QA & A committee activities and explained that the privileged documents were logged. The documents submitted for review were of two types:

(1) information and reports prepared for the committees to review

(2) reports generated by the committee

The facility's QA & A Plan stated that documents prepared or reviewed by the QA & A committee will be stamped with a confidentiality statement that reads, "This report has been generated as part of the facility's quality assessment and assurance process and constitutes confidential Quality Assessment and Assurance Committee records." However, not all the documents submitted for judicial review were stamped. The QA & A Plan noted that four privileges were protected by the peer review process under the auspices of the quality assurance committee. These were the:

- medical committee privilege

- medical peer review committee privilege

- nursing peer review committee privilege

- quality assessment and assurance privilege

In deciding this case,[5] the Supreme Court of Texas referred to several previous opinions, which stated that both "the medical committee privilege and the medical peer review privilege extended to initial credentialing by medical committees." It also applied to other confidential documents that are "generated" by a committee or "prepared by or at the direction of the committee for committee purposes." Privileged documents included the "minutes and recommendations" of medical committees, inquiries about a physician to other sources and the sources' responses, and communications between the physician and the facility. They added that *simply passing a document through a peer review committee does not make it privileged."* In the previous opinions, the justices noted that the statutes did not protect documents that were "made or maintained in the regular course of business by a hospital or extended care facility." They interpreted this to mean that medical records should be evaluated to determine whether they were made "in the regular course of business." Business records excepted from the peer review privilege include a "patient's medical records" and "business and administrative files and papers apart from committee deliberations." The justices noted that the QA & A Committee was authorized to evaluate the quality of health care services, so it was comparable or similar to a medical peer review committee. As a medical committee, QA & A committee documents are privileged, *except as limited by the business records exception.*

The Texas Occupations Code[6] is a legal statute that defines regulated occupations, such as physicians and nurses, in which state licensure or registration is required. The justices previously ruled that a medical peer review committee has the authority "to evaluate the quality of medical and health care services, such as the administration of drugs by a nurse at the instruc-tion of a physician." They noted, *"The purpose of medical peer review is protection of an evaluative process, not mere recordkeeping."*

A nursing peer review committee is also defined by the Occupations Code.[7] The justices noted that, "Separate from the medical committee and the medical peer review committee, a "nursing peer review committee" is the entity authorized to engage in nurse peer review." *To qualify as a nursing peer review committee, nurses must comprise at least three-fourths of the membership of the committee. Thus, the long-term care facility may only assert the nursing peer review privilege if the committee meets the narrow and rigorous membership requirements defined in the occupations code.* Since the facility's QA & A Plan defined its nursing peer review committee as consisting of the Administrator, Director of Nursing, Medical Director or other designated physician, social service representative, dietary representative, and a Certified Nursing Assistant, it did not meet this definition. The facility did not submit proof that three-fourths of the membership consisted of nurses. Because of this, the justices ruled that the nursing peer review privilege *did not apply* in this case.

Although the facility clearly won some concessions, the justices ruled that many of the documents at issue in this case fell outside the range of documents protected by the medical committee and medical peer review privileges. The documents withheld by the facility included surveys and documents that concern licensing and investigation by state agencies. Records included information about employees, as well as incident logs and other reports referencing the plaintiff. Additional documents withheld by the facility included governing body meeting minutes, personnel records including documentation of training, and policy and procedure documents. The judicial opinion noted that, *"The peer review privilege is intended to extend far enough to foster candid internal discussions for the purpose of making improvements in the quality of care, but not so far as to permit the concealment of "routinely accumulated information."* [T]he privilege [does] not prevent discovery of material that ha[s] been presented to a committee if it [is] otherwise available and 'offered or proved by means apart from the record of the committee.' The privilege extends only to the products of the peer review process: reports, records (including those produced for the committee's review as part of the investigative review process), and deliberations.

The plaintiff in this case alleged that the facility waived its claim of privilege by failing to follow its own policies because it had not stamped the documents with a QA & A privilege statement. The court disagreed, noting that under the current rules of discovery, inadvertent disclosure does not automatically waive a claim of privilege. Similarly, they held that a party's inadvertent failure to utilize its own internal procedure for identifying privileged documents does not automatically waive the privilege. They noted, however, that the absence of the confidentiality stamp may also be relevant, so the trial court would not abuse its discretion by weighing the lack of stamp, in addition to considering the reason for its absence, along with the DON's affidavit, the QA and A privilege log, and the sample documents, in determining whether the facility met its burden to demonstrate that the documents at issue were part of the peer review process. They noted further *in camera review* should be done by the trial court. An *in camera review* is done by submitting the documents in question to the judge, who will review them privately. The information is not made public or submitted to the jury until the judge has rendered a decision on its admissibility.

Of all the sample documents submitted in this case, the Supreme Court of Texas noted that the only ones that *may possibly* be privileged were the "Incident Report QA & A logs" and the "Weekly Pressure Ulcer QA & A logs." The trial court had previously limited its in camera review to only those documents that were stamped with the QA & A committee stamp, and these had not been stamped. The justices noted that further review of the documents was needed, and left the final determination of privilege for the sample Incident Report logs and Weekly Pressure Ulcer logs to the trial court. All other documents submitted were determined to be clearly outside the privilege because:

(1) they do not pertain exclusively to physicians

(2) they pertain to nurses, but the facility did not establish a nurse peer review committee consistent with the statutory requirement; or

(3) they were contemporaneous resident records made in the ordinary course of business and were not specifically created for committee review, evaluation, or investigation.

The court opinion noted that "the trial court considered only the name of the documents or whether the documents were stamped with the QA & A indicia, and failed to consider other determining factors, including the purpose for which the documents were created. The trial court must determine:

(1) whether the existing evidence establishes the privileged status of any documents without the need for an in camera inspection

(2) whether to conduct an in camera inspection of additional documents or categories of documents in light of this opinion

(3) whether the additional documents, if furnished, are privileged; and

(4) whether the long-term care facility, by failing to produce all documents for in camera inspection, failed to satisfy its burden to prove privilege

They concluded that the facility was entitled to mandamus relief because the trial court abused its discretion by using only superficial indicators to deny the facility's privilege claim as to nearly all the documents at issue. They directed the trial court to vacate its original discovery order and determine whether, upon further examination, any documents withheld by the facility may be considered privileged.[8]

This is a complex opinion that draws on many other judicial opinions, but the implications for facilities in every state are clear:

- Simply passing a document through a peer review (QA & A) committee does not make it privileged.

- Recordkeeping of meetings and committee business should be precise enough to determine what type of information is being reviewed, deficiencies identified, and action or recommendations taken as a result of this review.

- If numerous documents, such as incident reports are reviewed, some type of log should be maintained with committee records.

- Facilities should follow their policies and procedures regarding maintaining QA & A Committee logs and stamping items as confidential.

- Facilities should learn if their state has legal definitions of peer review, nursing peer review, and other committees and determine whether their in-house committees function according to the legal definitions. If not, the privilege protections may not apply.

- Facilities should learn whether peer review protections in their state apply only to organizations such as hospitals, physician practices, and others. The law should specify whether long-term care facilities are also afforded peer review protection.

- Facilities should learn if the state law exempts any documents from peer review privilege, and if so, how these exceptions apply.

> "Identifying opportunities for change generally represents a departure from traditional patterns and methods of doing business. Examining the purpose of health care and re-directing commitments toward new goals, demands strong partnerships, not only internally, but externally with the community. A well conceived and developed planning process can build and strengthen these alliances. The outcome: health care success."[9]

Effective quality assurance

Do not allow the legalities of disclosure or immunity of information to alter your plan for quality assurance. Effective quality assurance programs may be your best investment into avoiding lawsuits in the first place. A team approach and root cause analysis can reduce pressure ulcers, falls, psychoactive medications, weight loss and a myriad of other issues often cited as the basis for lawsuits. In the end an effective quality assurance program may well be your best defense and your resident's best friend.

References

1. National Association of Directors of Nursing Administration/Long Term Care (NADONA) (eds). (2000). Standards of Practice (4th edition). Cincinnati, OH. National Association of Directors of Nursing Administration/Long Term Care.

2. Gess vs. U.S., 952 F. Supp. 1529 (M.D. Ala., 1996).

3. Office of Inspector General and American Health Lawyers Association (Eds.). (2003). Corporate responsibility and corporate compliance: a resource for health care boards of directors. Rockville, MD. U.S. Department of Health and Human Services. Online. *http://oig.hhs.gov/fraud/docs/complianceguidance/040203CorpRespRsceGuide.pdf.* Accessed 01/20/06.

4. Office of Inspector General and American Health Lawyers Association (Eds.). (2003). Corporate responsibility and corporate compliance: a resource for health care boards of directors. Rockville, MD. U.S. Department of Health and Human Services. Online. *http://oig.hhs.gov/fraud/docs/complianceguidance/040203CorpRespRsceGuide.pdf.* Accessed 01/20/06.

5. In Re Living Centers of Texas, Inc., D/B/A Wharton Manor, Relator. No. 04-0176. In the Supreme Court of Texas. October 14, 2005.

6. Texas Statutes. Occupations Code. Online. *www.capitol.state.tx.us/statutes/octoc.html.*

7. "Nursing peer review committee" means a committee established under the authority of the governing body of a national, state, or local nursing association, a school of nursing, the nursing staff of a hospital, health science center, nursing home, home health agency, temporary nursing service, or other health care facility, or state agency or political subdivision for the purpose of conducting peer review. The committee includes an employee or agent of the committee, including an assistant, an investigator, an intervenor, an attorney, and any other person who serves the committee in any capacity. (5) "Peer review" means the evaluation of nursing services, the qualifications of a nurse, the quality of patient care rendered by a nurse, the merits of a complaint concerning a nurse or nursing care, and a determination or recommendation regarding a complaint. The term includes: (A) the evaluation of the accuracy of a nursing assessment and observation and the appropriateness and quality of the care rendered by a nurse; (B) a report made to a nursing peer review committee concerning an activity under the committee's review authority; (C) a report made by a nursing peer review committee to another committee or to the board as permitted or required by law; and (D) implementation of a duty of a nursing peer review committee by a member, an agent, or an employee of the committee. (Acts 1999, 76th Leg., ch. 388, § 1, eff. Sept. 1, 1999. Amended by Acts 2003, 78th Leg., ch. 553, § 2.018, eff. Feb. 1, 2004.)

8. In Re Living Centers of Texas, Inc., D/B/A Wharton Manor, Relator. No. 04-0176. In the Supreme Court of Texas. October 14, 2005.

9. Zagury CS. Making a difference: Strategic planning for the director of nursing in long term care. The Director. Online. *www.nadona.org/media_archive/media/media-238.pdf.* Accessed 08/25/04.

Financial Fraud and Abuse

Fraud and abuse

Medicare has become very profitable for some individuals. Both Parts A and B have been subject to abusive practices. Although most healthcare facilities, suppliers, and businesses comply with the letter of the law, some have taken advantage of every available loophole. To ensure that the program remains solvent in the future, the government is aggressively attempting to reduce costs. Simultaneously, oversight and enforcement measures and programs have been implemented to prevent fraud and abuse. Claims submitted for payment are being scrutinized more closely than in the past.

Do not be fooled into believing that financial fraud and abuse are responsibilities of the administrator and bookkeeper. Protecting against fraud and abuse are important nursing responsibilities. This protection is provided by ensuring facility personnel are familiar with and adhere to acceptable standards of long-term care nursing practice. The state or federal government pays the facility for care that meets a certain standard of care. In making payment, they expect the residents to receive care that meets their standards. If care is found to be substandard or not delivered at all, nurs-

ing personnel are also considered parties to financial fraud and abuse.

The BCD Nursing Center failed to improve Nancy Smith's condition and they certainly did not maintain her condition. They failed to inform the resident, the resident's interested family member and/or the resident's legal representative and arrange for the resident's transfer to a facility that was willing and able to provide nursing home care that meets the standard of care. They failed to provide an organizational structure and methodology to detect, intervene and correct widespread patterns of neglect in the care being provided. They failed to ensure that Nancy Smith received care in a manner and in an environment that maintained or enhanced her quality of life without abridging her health, safety, and welfare. They failed to ensure that policies were in place to see that Nancy Smith received necessary medical and nursing care and services. They failed to ensure that Nancy Smith was promptly assessed and her treating physi-

> cian notified of acute illness, complications, and ongoing problems in a timely manner. They failed to ensure physician orders were followed. They failed to ensure that Nancy Smith received services for which the facility was being paid, including assistance with activities of daily living, turning and repositioning, pressure relief, hygienic care, using infection control practices that meet accepted standards, and providing proper diabetes management, yet they billed the Medicare program and state Medicaid agency and accepted payment for providing these services. They failed to promptly secure a higher level of care when it was apparent that resident's needs were beyond the scope of the facility to care for them. They failed to recognize the magnitude and severity of the resident's condition in November and December. They failed to stabilize the resident's condition.
>
> *(From an actual lawsuit report alleging progressive failures and omissions of care.)*

CMS has stated they are committed to fighting fraud and abuse of the Medicare and Medicaid programs. Fraud and abuse divert dollars that could otherwise be spent to safeguard the health and welfare of beneficiaries. Medicaid is the largest source of funding for medical and health-related services for people with limited income. The individual states are primarily responsible for policing fraud in the Medicaid program, but CMS provides technical assistance, guidance and oversight. Medicare, Medicaid and other government healthcare programs can impose a wide range of sanctions against healthcare businesses that engage in fraudulent practices. At the very least, the facility will be required to repay overpayments and will be monitored to ensure its billing practices are compliant in the future. At most, there are civil monetary penalties and criminal prosecution, including prison time for offenses the government considers egregious.

In 2005, a federal grand jury indicted several long-term care facility owners, alleging they conspired to defraud Medicare and Medicaid by collecting payments for services they did not provide to the residents. The U.S. Attorney alleged that they provided a "level of care so deficient as to be non-care." The indictment says inadequate staffing resulted in residents suffering from malnutrition, dehydration and pressure ulcers, as well as going without bathing. It further notes that some residents were physically abused or were so poorly supervised they eloped. One resident was said to have been left in excretions for hours at a time, and in the weeks before death was found covered with ants. The indictment covers a period from 1998 to 2001, during which the facility is accused of restricting nursing staff to dangerously low levels. However, they allegedly continued to bill Medicare and Medicaid for services that were inadequate or not performed at all. The indictment contends the defendants allegedly enriched themselves with Medicaid and Medicare reimbursements while concealing the poor conditions in the facilities. Although state inspectors cited the facilities repeatedly, they were unsuccessful in their attempt to revoke facility licenses.[1]

Examples of fraud and abuse

The term abuse is used to describe practices that, either directly or indirectly, result in unnecessary costs to the Medicare (or Medicaid) program. Abuse appears similar to fraud except that it is not possible to establish that abusive acts were committed knowingly, willfully, and intentionally. Providers have an obligation to conform to the requirements of the Medicare and Medicaid programs. Medicare fraud may be prosecuted under various provisions of the United States Code and could result in the imposition of restitution, fines, and, in some instances, imprisonment. In addition, there is a range of administrative sanctions (such as exclusion from participation in the program) and civil monetary penalties that may be imposed when facts and circumstances warrant. Medicaid fraud may be prosecuted by your state Attorney General's office. When a facility is charged with fraud and/or abuse, it is usually the result of billing for services that were not delivered.

CMS applies three standards when determining abusive acts in billing were committed against the Medicare program. They attempt to determine if the billed services

- were reasonable and necessary

- conform to professionally recognized standards

- were provided at a fair price

Other examples of abuse include, but are not limited to

- Charging excessive amounts for services or supplies

- Providing medically unnecessary services or services that do not meet professionally recognized standards of practice

- Billing Medicare based on a higher fee schedule than used for non-Medicare residents

- Submitting bills to Medicare that are the responsibility of other insurers under the Medicare secondary payer (MSP) regulation

- Violating the participating physician/supplier agreement

- The facility is cited for quality of care issues, and the government alleges they paid the facility to provide a level of quality that was not delivered

Although these types of practices may initially be categorized as abusive in nature, under certain circumstances they may develop into fraud if there is evidence that an individual or facility was knowingly and willfully conducting an abusive practice. The OIG, CMS, the Department of Justice, and state enforcement agencies have developed various flags and indicators for identifying quality-of-care risk areas. Issues and areas of special concern include

- Absence of a comprehensive, accurate assessment of each resident's functional capacity

- Absence of a current, comprehensive care plan that includes measurable objectives and timetables to meet the resident's medical, nursing, and mental and psychosocial needs

- Inappropriate or insufficient treatment and services to address residents' clinical conditions, including pressure ulcers, dehydration, malnutrition, incontinence of the bladder, and mental or psychosocial problems

- Failure to accommodate individual resident needs and preferences

- Failure to properly prescribe, administer and monitor prescription drug usage

- Inadequate staffing levels or insufficiently trained or supervised staff to provide medical, nursing, and related services

- Failure to provide appropriate therapy services

- Failure to provide appropriate services to assist residents with activities of daily living (e.g., feeding, dressing, bathing, incontinence care, etc.)

- Failure to provide an ongoing activities program to meet the individual needs of all residents

- Failure to report incidents of mistreatment, neglect, or abuse to the administrator of the facility and other officials as required by law

The OIG believes that facilities should have a strong commitment to compliance, and notes each facility should have a compliance plan that meets its individual needs. (Also see information on compliance in Chapter 21). They note that attention to billing practices is part of maintaining compliance, and require each facility to "continually reassess its billing procedures and policies to ensure that unanticipated problems are promptly identified and corrected."[2] Reimbursement risk areas that facilities should consider addressing as part of its written compliance policies and procedures include

- Billing for items or services not rendered or provided as claimed

- Submitting claims for equipment, medical supplies and services that are medically unnecessary

- Submitting claims to Medicare Part A for residents who are not eligible for Part A coverage

- Duplicate billing

- Failing to identify and refund credit balances

- Submitting claims for items or services not ordered by the physician

- Knowingly billing for inadequate or substandard care

- Providing misleading information about a resident's medical condition on the MDS or otherwise providing inaccurate information used to determine the Resource Utilization Grouping (RUG) assigned to each resident

- Upcoding the level of service provided

- Billing for individual items or services when they either are included in the facility's per diem rate or are of the type of item or service that must be billed as a unit and may not be unbundled

- Billing residents for items or services that are included in the per diem rate or otherwise covered by the third-party payor

- Altering documentation or forging a physician signature on documents used to verify that services were ordered and/or provided

- Failing to maintain sufficient documentation to support the diagnosis, justify treatment, document the course of treatment and results, and promote continuity of care

- Filing false cost reports

(Please note that most of the areas listed directly or indirectly affect nursing services.)

Kickbacks and other inducements

The OIG believes that facility policies and procedures should prohibit kickbacks and other inducements to services, and comply with numerous state and federal laws. Potential areas of risk that facilities should address in the policies and procedures include

- Routinely waiving coinsurance or deductible amounts without a good-faith determination that the resident is in financial need, or absent reasonable efforts to collect the cost-sharing amount

- Agreements between the facility and a hospital, home health agency, hospice, or other individual or agency that involve the referral or transfer of any resident to or by the nursing home

- Soliciting, accepting or offering any gift or gratuity of more than nominal value to or from residents, potential referral sources, and other individuals and entities with which the nursing facility has a business relationship

- Conditioning admission or continued stay at a facility on a third-party guarantee of payment, or soliciting payment for services covered by Medicaid, in addition to any amount required to be paid under the State Medicaid plan

- Arrangements between a nursing facility and a hospital under which the facility will only accept a Medicare beneficiary on the condition that the hospital pays the facility an amount over and above what the facility would receive through PPS

- Financial arrangements with physicians, including the facility's medical director

- Arrangements with vendors that result in the nursing facility receiving non-covered items (such as disposable adult diapers) at below market prices or no charge, provided the facility orders Medicare-reimbursed products

- Soliciting or receiving items of value in exchange for providing the supplier unlimited access to residents' medical records and other information needed to bill Medicare

- Joint ventures with entities supplying goods or services

- Swapping; this situation occurs when a supplier gives a facility discounts on Medicare Part A items and services in return for referrals for Medicare Part B business; with swapping, there is a risk that suppliers may offer a SNF an excessively low price for items or services reimbursed under PPS in return for the ability to

service and bill nursing facility residents with Part B coverage[3]

Sometimes it is difficult to differentiate a business service from a kickback. For example, if the pharmacy or laboratory provides a dedicated personal computer or fax machine that is used only for the purpose of sending, receiving, and printing information from the facility to the pharmacy or lab, this is a business service. If the pharmacy or laboratory provides a regular personal computer that may be used for many purposes in addition to sending and receiving data to and from the external provider, or a fax machine that may be used to transmit data anywhere, these items may be viewed as inducements or kickbacks. In this situation, the computer or fax machine has a definite added value to the facility.

Creation and retention of medical records

The OIG guidelines recommend developing and implementing medical records policies and procedures that ensure complete and accurate medical record documentation as part of the compliance program. The policies and procedures should address the creation, distribution, retention, and destruction of documents. Policies should provide for the complete, accurate, and timely documentation of all nursing and therapy services, including subcontracted services, as well as MDS information. Privacy concerns and regulatory requirements also should be taken into consideration. They recommend including

- All records and documentation, including billing and claims documentation required for participation in federal, state, and private healthcare programs, including the resident assessment instrument, comprehensive plan of care and all corrective actions taken in response to surveys

- All records, documentation, and audit data that support and explain cost reports and other financial activity, including any internal or external compliance monitoring activities

- All records necessary to demonstrate the integrity of the nursing facility compliance process and to confirm the effectiveness of the program

Policies and procedures should

- Support the medical necessity of the services provided as well as the level of service billed

- Prohibit falsification and backdating of records

- Have clear guidelines, consistent with applicable professional and legal standards, that set out those individuals with authority to make entries in the medical record and the circumstances when late entries may be made

While conducting compliance activities and daily operations, the nursing facility should document its efforts to comply with applicable statutes, regulations, and federal healthcare program requirements. If you ask for advice from a government agency or Medicare intermediary, document and keep a record of the conversation. They further recommend

- Securing the information and documentation in a safe place

- Retaining hard copies of all electronic or database documentation

- Limiting access to this documentation to avoid accidental or intentional fabrication or destruction of records

- Conforming document retention and destruction policies to applicable laws

Employee performance

Part of the compliance program involves evaluating adherence to the compliance policies and procedures as part of the routine employee performance appraisal. Provide education for key employees to ensure their knowledge is current and keeps up with new changes. Maintain copies of

- employee certifications relating to training and other compliance initiatives

- compliance training materials

- hotline logs and any corresponding reports of investigation, outcomes, and employee disciplinary actions

- relevant correspondence with carriers, fiscal intermediaries, private health insurers, CMS, and state survey and certification agencies

Policies should require that managers, especially those involved in direct resident care and in claims development and submission

- discuss with all supervised employees and relevant contractors the compliance policies and legal requirements applicable to their function

- inform all supervised personnel that strict compliance with these policies and procedures is a condition of employment

- inform all supervised employees of the penalties for noncompliance, including disciplinary action, up to and including termination (however, OIG also notes that positive reinforcement is usually more effective than punitive measures in conditioning behavior; managers should be given mechanisms to reward employees who promote compliance)

Compliance officer and compliance committee

OIG notes that each facility must have a compliance officer who is responsible for all compliance activities. This individual may be assisted by others who are specialists in their areas of expertise, such as a billing or payroll clerk. In most facilities, the administrator serves as the facility compliance officer. The department heads assist him or her in fulfilling compliance responsibilities.

The compliance committee also assists with the overall facility compliance program. The QA & A Committee usually fulfills compliance committee functions. This includes teaching personnel applicable rules and laws, and conducting audits and other activities to ensure the facility adheres to the regulations.

The facility must also have a method or chain of command for communicating issues and problems to the compliance officer. Again, this is usually established by facility policies, and department heads or other designated individuals may serve as intermediaries to relay information to the compliance officer. Employees should be familiar with the reporting structure. Likewise, employees should be permitted to complain anonymously through proper channels. The compliance officer or designee should maintain a log of complaints, investigations, and resolution of incidents. Individually identifying information should be redacted from the log, whenever possible. However, they should inform employees that in certain situations, it will be necessary to reveal the identity of the employee making the report. Under most circumstances, facilities should strive to protect employee privacy and confidentiality.

Employee discipline

The OIG makes clear that sometimes it is necessary to discipline employees to maintain regulatory com-pliance. However, discipline as a result of an action should not be a surprise. Disciplinary policies and procedures should be clearly defined and available to all employees. Disciplinary action should be fair and consistent with these policies and procedures. Likewise, to avoid the appearance of impropriety or favoritism, discipline should be consistent from one employee to the next. All employees in all positions should be subject to the same punitive action for similar offenses. If an employee complains, avoid being tempted to retaliate. Some individuals have filed *qui tam* lawsuits after being disciplined, isolated, harassed, or tormented after reporting problems to upper management. Take complaints seriously and attempt to investigate and resolve all employee concerns.

The Federal False Claims Act makes it illegal to terminate an employee who blows the whistle on the employer for fraudulent Medicare billing practices. If the employee is terminated, he or she can subsequently file a retaliatory discharge lawsuit. Conducting (and documenting) exit interviews with departing employees helps identify problems that are troubling the employee. This is evidence that the facility is making a good-faith attempt at identifying and resolving problems.

Self-reporting

When the compliance officer, compliance committee, or a management official identifies credible evidence of misconduct that he or she believes violates criminal, civil or administrative law, the facility should promptly investigate the matter. If the investigation reveals violation of the law, the facility must self-report the problem to the appropriate federal and state authorities within a reasonable period, but not more than 60 days after determining that there is credible evidence of a violation. The OIG notes that timely voluntary reporting demonstrates the facility's good faith and willingness to work with governmental authorities to correct and remedy the problem. Self-reporting is considered to be a mitigating factor by the OIG in determining administrative sanctions (e.g., penalties, assessments, and exclusion), if the facility is the target of an OIG investigation. Although self-reporting is required, facilities may wish to consult legal counsel if reporting becomes necessary. Repayment will be expected if billing fraud is identified.

Qui tam actions

A *qui tam* lawsuit occurs when a private party sues the facility on behalf of the government for fraud committed against the government. If successful, the lawsuit can net the individual filing suit (called the *relator*) from 10 to 25% of the recovery. In the past, this type of lawsuit has been used exclusively by the federal government to recover monies paid due to fraud and abuse. However, recently, the Attorney Generals in some states have also made use of this action when whistleblowers report violations of the various state Medicaid Fraud Prevention Acts.

An effective corporate compliance plan with employee policies and procedures will help reduce the risk of *qui tam* actions. Making sure that employees are taught their job responsibilities, and know facility rules and regulations further reduces the risk. Promptly investigating reports of wrong-doing and following self-reporting policies and procedures further reduces the risk and removes the inducement for a *qui tam* lawsuit.

Hospice services

When a hospice provides care and services to residents in long-term care facilities, the hospice will be paid the normal Medicare home care rate. This is a flat daily fee, regardless of the services needed by the resident. A private pay facility resident remains responsi-

ble for payment of the room and board charges. If the resident is a Medicaid recipient, the state Medicaid program pays the hospice at least 95% of the regular facility rate. The hospice is responsible for paying the resident's room and board. The state Medicaid program will determine specific services that must be included in the daily rate. The hospice should pay the facility a rate that does not exceed what the facility would otherwise have received if the resident had not been a hospice recipient. Additional payments should not exceed the fair market value of services actually provided *that are not normally included in the Medicaid rate.*[4] When hospice assumes care of a facility resident, there is usually an overlap in the types of services that both the facility and hospice provide. This provides an incentive for one or the other to reduce costs. OIG has done studies which show that hospice recipients in long-term care facilities receive fewer services than they do in a home care environment. Because the hospice receives a fixed daily rate, the potential for higher profits exists.

In some situations, providing hospice services in the long-term care facility can be very profitable. This poses somewhat of a dilemma to the facility, which is responsible for ensuring quality services are delivered to the residents. On one hand, hospice services may be reasonable, necessary, appropriate, and beneficial to terminally ill residents who desire palliative care. On the other hand, having an exclusive agreement between one or two hospices and the nursing home provider makes it appear as if the facility is requiring the residents to use a specific hospice. This type of arrangement is valuable to the hospice, which usually makes more money caring for residents in the facility compared with home care clients. Residents in facilities tend to use hospice services for longer periods of time than home care clients. The nursing facility represents a large source of potential client referrals for the hospice. This type of exclusive agreement ensures the facility can coordinate care, screen hospices, and maintain control. It also represents a real value to the hospice. In this situation, some facilities have requested illegal inducements to influence the selection of a hospice. Likewise, hospices have provided kickbacks to the facility to ensure the arrangement remains exclusive. As you know, kickbacks and inducements for referrals and services are illegal. When contracting with a hospice, keep this in mind. You may wish to consult legal counsel before entering into a hospice contract.

Additional information

For additional information regarding the OIG compliance program requirements, consult the *Federal Register*, Vol. 65, No. 52, March 16, 2000, pages 14289 to 14305.

Internet fraud against long-term care facilities

For several years, a variety of money order scams have made their way around the internet. There are several themes, but typically a buyer mails a money order to a seller of an online auction as payment for goods. The buyer usually sends more than the asking price (auction ending price), then asks the seller to use part of the overage for expedited shipping of the item. The seller is instructed to keep a percentage of the proceeds for his or her trouble, then return the remaining money to the buyer, who often has a foreign address and plausible, legitimate-sounding reason for sending extra money.

Many online auction sellers lost money in this scam before it was widely publicized. When it stopped working, the perpetrators changed their method of operation. They began sending cashiers' checks to private individuals, many of whom are elderly. They com-

monly send a large check, which is often alleged to be from a local business, such as a hospital.[5] The recipient is informed the hospital entered a European lottery in his or her name and won. Buying or selling tickets for a foreign lottery across state lines or international boundaries is illegal. Some of the recipients do not question why the hospital would enter a foreign lottery using someone elses' name. In some instances, the recipients had never been a patient in the hospital and had no business relationship with the facility.

The victim is told he or she has won a large amount, such as $100,000. All he or she must do is cash or deposit a $3000 to $5000 check, then remit the cash or money order to the "claims office" at a distant or foreign address to pay the "terrorism taxes," transfer fees, or some similar tax on the winnings. A letter promises that upon receipt of the taxes, a check for the remainder of the prize will be mailed to the victim. Some recipients brought the checks to their banks, who verified the checks were valid. Because the bank verified the check, the recipient cashed it and followed the instructions he or she received, sending the money to an address outside the United States. Subsequently, the bank notified the individual the check was no good and he or she was expected to repay the money immediately. Several unfortunate elderly victims were arrested and spent the night in jail for cashing (or attempting to cash) the fraudulent checks.

In another variation of the scam, people send spam emails at random stating they are self employed and live outside the US. Most claim to be writers or illustrators, which is a plausible reason for being self employed. They claim they are having trouble collecting money from US businesses whom they do freelance work for because they live out of the country. They appeal to the email recipient for help by having the US checks direct-deposited into the recipient's bank account. The account holder is promised a percentage (typically 10%) of the money for their trouble.

Long-term care facilities

In 2006, a variation of this scam made its way to the long-term care market. Unfortunately, it has received no media attention, so facilities are largely unaware of the problem. At the time of this writing, a scammer is targeting facilities with web sites. He sends prepayment for a short stay in the facility, noting he will be out of the area for a period of time and plans to admit his mother for respite care.

Alternately, he will be visiting the area and needs the services of the facility to care for his elderly mother (who is traveling with him) during the stay. Of course, the payment submitted is well above the normal facility fees. The perpetrator then contacts the facility before the check clears the bank, requesting repayment of the overage. Since the original check is fraudulent, the facility loses money if it issues a refund.

High quality checks and money orders

The individuals using this scheme have one thing in common. All of their checks and money orders are very good, authentic-looking forgeries. Some are regular checks, some are cashiers' checks, and others are US Postal Service Money orders. The money orders are an older style that was used in the recent past, but are so realistic-looking they are difficult or impossible to differentiate from valid money orders. Many of these individuals use foreign addresses, but some are in the US. In this case, the forger uses a proprietary mail service (which has a regular street address) or (less commonly) a post office box. Interestingly, many of the fraudulent checks and money orders are sent to the recipient via Federal Express or another courier service, instead of through postal mail. The post office claims this is to prevent them from detecting the fraud and confiscating the checks from the mail.

In any event, facilities should be alert to this scam. Census is the lifeblood of the facility, and most administrators are delighted to accept respite admissions. The scammers appear to have no conscience, and are sadly unconcerned that they are stealing from individuals and facilities who can ill afford the loss. It is sad to see the deterioration in morals, ethics, and principles of some individuals. Phony lotteries and sweepstakes are one of the most devastating frauds facing consumers today. Senior citizens and business serving them are increasingly being targeted by unscrupulous crooks willing to say just about anything to get their money.

References

1. Wittenauer C. (2005). Nursing home fraud alleged in indictments. *Jefferson City News Tribune.* Online. *www.newstribune.com/articles/2005/11/18/news_state/ 0111805031.prt.* Accessed 11/18/05.

2. Department of Health and Human Services Office of Inspector General. (2000). OIG Compliance Program Guidance for Nursing Facilities. *Federal Register* Vol. 65, No. 52. Thursday, March 16, 2000. Pages 14289-14306.

3. OIG Advisory Opinion 99–2 (February 1999).

4. Office of the Inspector General. (1998). Special Fraud Alert. Fraud and abuse in nursing home arrangements with hospices.

5. University of Texas Medical Branch. (2006). Fraud alert. Online. *www.utmb.edu/alert/euro_lotto_scam.htm*

Documentation

Documentation standards

Most lawsuits involving long-term care facilities and their nurses are civil cases that attempt to prove that negligent nursing care resulted in injury to a resident. Negligence is failure to provide a resident with the standard of care that a reasonably prudent nurse would exercise under the same or similar circumstances. To prove that a nurse (or facility) was negligent, the resident's attorney must prove these four elements:

- The nurse (or facility) had a duty to provide care to the resident and to follow an acceptable standard of care.

- The nurse (or facility) failed to adhere to the standard of care.

- The nurse's (or facility's) failure to adhere to the standard of care caused the resident's injuries.

- The resident suffered damages as a result of the nurse's (or facility's) negligent actions.

> The long-term care nursing facility must maintain clinical records on each resident, in accordance with accepted professional health information management standards and practices, that are complete; accurately documented; readily accessible; and systematically organized. It is my opinion that the EFG Care Center records were negligently kept or the records were deliberately scrambled and disorganized prior to my receiving them. The record was in a mess as far as its organization; it was not provided in the same manner as usually kept in the ordinary course of business. It did not meet the standard for closed records. As stated previously, some photocopies were illegible, and many parts appear to have been redacted.
>
> *(From an actual lawsuit report alleging progressive failures and omissions of care.)*

The professional practice standard for long-term care requires nursing facilities to maintain clinical records for each resident, in accordance with accepted professional health information management standards and practices, that are complete; accurately documented; readily accessible; and systematically organized. Jurors often expect healthcare professionals to be above reproach. Think about it. Healthcare workers are entrusted with peoples' lives. They make life-and-death decisions. When a case goes before a jury, jurors generally expect documentation to be factual and honest. As you can see, documentation can be very important when an individual or facility are facing allegations of negligence. Naturally, all parties involved will contend that they provided care that met the applicable standard, and that it is always their practice to do so. This position may be markedly weakened if documentation does not reflect that the applicable standards were met. During a trial, expect the plaintiff's attorney to use the medical record to prove that the standard of care was not met.

In healthcare, there is a maxim, "If it's not charted, it wasn't done." Although what is written in the medical records could harm you in court, omissions can make the damage seem insurmountable. Without proper documentation, a reader may assume that no care was provided. Although some facilities use a system called "charting by exception," most adhere to the age-old maxim and chart all care given. Charting by exception (CBE) is a formal documentation system. It has formal, written policies and procedures and well-designed flow sheets and forms. It is not an excuse for haphazard charting. Even in a charting-by-exception system, the state nurse practice act always prevails. Most states have a clause similar to this one: *"The nurse shall accurately and completely report and document the client's status including signs, symptoms and responses; nursing care rendered; physician, dentist or podiatrist orders; administration of medications, and treatments; and client response(s); contacts with other healthcare team members concerning significant events regarding client's status."*[1] Thus, even in a charting-by-exception system, the nurse must have a means of documenting care given and the resident's response, as well as the other elements listed above.

Documentation is a critical part of nursing practice, not an afterthought. Some nurses say, "The residents come first; paperwork is secondary." This is probably a good practice to ascribe to, assuming that the paperwork is completed after residents are cared for. Omitting paperwork entirely is never a good practice. American Nurses Association (ANA) standards of nursing practice require that documentation be based on the nursing process and that it should be ongoing and accessible to all members of the healthcare team.[2] View documentation as an important part of the care you give. A medical-legal chart reviewer will be able to identify the various aspects of the nursing process during a documentation review. The purpose of documentation is to communicate care. Documentation is a true, complete, objective record of the care given and the residents' response. It is the first line of defense in proving accountability.

If a facility and/or its personnel are sued, all verbal testimony will be considered, contrasted, and compared with documentation on the medical record. The nurses can testify that their normal practice is to turn residents every two hours and provide other preventive skin care. However, the jury is not obligated to believe this testimony, especially if the medical record does not show evidence of regular turning and repositioning. In this case, documentation skips most probably support the injuries that the resident and/or family are alleging. This situation occurred in a 2004 lawsuit against a Kentucky hospital. The family filed suit for nursing negligence based on a patient who fell and sustained a fracture, then subsequently developed a Stage III pressure ulcer. Her condition deteriorated to the point where the healthcare proxy decided to withhold her regular dialysis treatments and the patient died. Despite verbal nursing testimony, documentation on the medical record was erratic, inconsistent, and did not show evidence of routine turning or preventive skin care. When skin breakdown became evident, a wound care nurse consultation was ordered, but the nurse did not respond in a timely manner. The physician ordered a special pressure-relieving bed. Nurses' notes confirmed the bed was not provided for more than 48 hours after the order was written. The jury did not believe the nurses' testimony about routine preventive skin care in light of the erratic documentation and delays in consultation and special pressure-relieving equipment. They found in favor of the plaintiff, and the Court of Appeals upheld the jury verdict.[3]

Nursing personnel failed to collect pertinent information using the nursing process. They failed to observe or assess Donnie Jones. They failed to plan his care based on that assessment, and failed to intervene on his behalf. The staff failed to properly evaluate his condition and risk factors. His medical status and nursing information should have been accessible, communicated, and recorded. The facts could have been obtained by simply reading records, reports, etc. and looking at, listening to, and touching the resident. By not doing this, the nurses failed to use the nursing process. They consistently failed to use the nursing process to observe and assess the resident, they failed to analyze the data, and they failed to make accurate nursing diagnoses so that an appropriate care plan could be formulated. They did not update the plan promptly when his condition changed. Their care was not individualized for Donnie Jones, and no consistent plan of care was followed by the staff. Furthermore, the staff did not evaluate the effectiveness of their care by observing the resident's response to their interventions. The process

was not systematic and ongoing. Diagnoses were not derived from the assessment data and were not validated by other healthcare providers. Documentation has been removed from the medical record. There are no nursing documents on the medical record for January 12, 2001, and the record is silent regarding the resident's mental and physical condition prior to the hip fracture event. The dates of the consultations are left blank. The record is not accurate or complete. Omissions and questionable entries call the veracity and credibility of the entire record into question.

(From an actual lawsuit report alleging progressive failures and omissions of care.)

Requirements for nursing documentation

American Nurses Association (ANA) standards of nursing practice require that documentation be based on the nursing process and that it should be ongoing and accessible to all members of the health care team.[4] Nursing documentation should be

- Based upon the requirements of your state's Nurse Practice Act

- Objective—not critical or subjective

- Clear, concise and comprehensive

- Accurate, truthful, and honest—does not appear self-serving, especially if an incident or injury occurs

- Relevant and appropriate

- Reflective of observations, not of unfounded conclusions

- Reflective of resident education

- Reflective of resident response to care and actions taken to rectify unsatisfactory response

- Timely and completed only during or after giving care

- Chronological

- Internally consistent

- A complete record of nursing care provided, including assessments, identification of health issues, a plan of care, implementation and evaluation

- Legible and non-erasable

- Unaltered

- Permanent

- Retrievable

- Confidential

- Resident-focused

- Outcome-based

- Completed using forms, methods, systems provided or methods and systems consistent with these standards, facility policies, and state laws

Confidentiality of medical records and identifiable resident information

As you know, each resident has a right to privacy with regard to his or her medical information. The residents' medical records are always privileged and confidential documents. All staff are responsible for protecting resident information and data from access by unauthorized persons. Medical records and other resident data should be accessed only by those with a need to know the information. Staff should not be permitted to read resident charts out of curiosity.

In 1996, congress passed the *Health Insurance Portability and Accountability Act (HIPAA)*. This law has many provisions. *Protected health information*

(PHI) is the nucleus of the HIPAA privacy regulations. The purpose of the HIPAA rules is to

- increase resident control over their medical records

- restrict the use and disclosure of resident information (however, residents cannot refuse to permit state and federal access to electronically-transmitted RAI information)

- make facilities accountable for protecting resident data

- require the facility to implement and monitor the effectiveness of their information-release policies and procedures

The HIPAA rules ask providers to analyze how and where resident information is used, and develop procedures for protecting confidential data. This includes the areas where resident charts are stored, the places where private or identifying resident information is discussed, and how residents' personal health information is distributed. The HIPAA policies and procedures are written by and individualized to the facility.

The HIPAA regulations describe

- what information is considered PHI

- the circumstances in which PHI may be disclosed

- the rights of an individual who is the subject of the PHI

Under the HIPAA rules, residents have the right to:

- know about uses and disclosure of their own PHI

- inspect their medical records

- decide whether their PHI can be disclosed and to whom

- correct inaccurate information in their medical records

 The Long-Term Care Legal Desk Reference

Anything that potentially reveals the resident's identity is PHI. This includes:

- names on a roster posted on the wall or by the doorway to the room (unless the resident consents)

- lists (such as supplement lists, restraint lists, BM lists, etc.) posted at the nurses' station in public view

- photographs of residents (unless the resident consents)

- admission and discharge data

Since the HIPAA regulations protect all individually identifiable health information in any form, the rules apply to paper, verbal, and electronic documentation, billing records, and medical or clinical records. They cover virtually all communications made by the long-term care facility. Resident information is provided to staff on a "need to know" basis. The premise of this requirement is that information is disclosed only if staff need it to carry out their duties. For example, the dietary department would need to know if a resident was on a diabetic diet. They would not need to know that the resident has an infectious disease. The nursing staff would need to know about both the diabetes and the infection. The MDS nurse may need to read the entire chart to complete the RAI. However, other employees such as the pharmacist, dietitian, nursing assistant, social worker, activities, and others should be given access to limited areas of the medical record. Vendors should not be given free access to resident charts because of the potential for Medicare and Medicaid fraud. The facility should not allow access to a resident's clinical record unless a physician's order exists for supplies, equipment, or services provided by the entity seeking access to the record. Facilities must monitor how and where they use resident information. Policies

must protect resident charts, conversations and reports about resident information, faxing resident documents, emailing or using a wireless transmitter to send electronic information, and disclosing other personal information. Examples of violation of the HIPAA rules are

- disclosing personal resident details on computer monitors facing public areas

- discussing residents in areas in which conversations can be overheard

- misdirecting mail

- discarding PHI in the regular trash without shredding

- discarding feeding tube, catheter, or IV bags with resident names in the regular trash

- leaving computerized diet sheets on resident trays and dumping them into the general trash after meals

- posting the documentation form for meal intake on a clipboard on the wall for all to see

- leaving the meal-intake documentation form unattended in the dining room after meals even though the resident names are covered by a piece of construction paper

- disclosing identifiable information such as name, address, contact information, medications, medical condition, room number, vitals, etc. (disclosure may be deliberate or inadvertent, such as leaving the computer monitor facing a public area)

- placing complete names on resident chart covers and leaving the charts in an area in which the public can read resident names

- taking photos in which residents inadvertently appear in the background

Penalties for violations of the HIPAA rules can be very substantial. The amount and type of penalty are determined by the situation, the safeguards and controls the covered facility has implemented, and the demonstrated and documented compliance efforts made by the facility. Civil monetary penalties (CMP) are enforced by the Department of Health and Human Services. The U.S. Department of Justice enforces criminal penalties. The fines range from no more than $100 per person for failure to comply with a single regulation up to $25,000 per calendar year per person for recurrent or multiple violations. The penalties increase if violations of multiple regulations or by multiple individuals are identified. Criminal penalties may apply for wrongful disclosure of protected health information.

How to chart

- Always follow the documentation policies and procedures established by your employing facility. Most facilities develop policies and procedures based on state law, professional standards of practice, and other requirements, such as those of accrediting organizations. The documentation policies should identify how often documentation should be done, who is responsible for charting in each part of the medical record and what abbreviations, techniques, and procedures are acceptable. If the facility's requirements are less stringent than those of your state nurse practice act, always adhere to the higher standard of the nurse practice act.

- Follow your facility policy for ink color. Most facilities use blue or black ink.

- Follow facility policy for documenting time. Many facilities use military time.

- Chart the exact time treatments, medications, and other procedures were administered, and nursing notes were written. Never document these by using shift times, such as "6-2." Document as soon as possible after care is given.

- Always document the exact time of nursing observations and actions, and physician and family notifications.

- Spell terms correctly, and use proper grammar.

- Illegible entries may adversely affect care and hinder attempts to demonstrate that a reasonable course of treatment was identified and followed. The reader of an illegible entry may infer the care was haphazard or did not meet standards.

- Chart legibly: Sloppy or illegible handwriting can be catastrophic in a lawsuit. If your handwriting is not legible, print.

- Close all entries with your first name or initial, last name, and title. Make sure your signature and title are legible.

- If you initial some entries, such as the medication record, make sure you sign the key with your full signature to match the initials.

- Write the resident's name and other identifying information on each page.

- Avoid skipping lines.

- Chart events in chronological order.

- Be truthful.

- Do not chart in advance or prior to giving care. The only component of the nursing process that may be documented in advance is the plan of care. Document all other observations and activities only after you assess the resident or implement a nursing intervention.

- Document information as close to the time of the event or nursing intervention as possible. If you wait until the end of the shift to document, you may forget important details or eliminate potentially important information because you are pressed for time. If necessary, make notes of important events, and destroy them after documenting in the medical record.

- Use only those abbreviations accepted by your facility. These should be listed in the policy and procedure manual, or other facility manual.

- The JCAHO and Institute for Safe Medication Practices (ISMP) maintain lists of potentially unsafe abbreviations **(see your CD-ROM for a list of these abbreviations)**. Consider these abbreviations and the rationale for not using them when approving abbreviations for facility documentation.

- Make sure your documentation is in keeping with acceptable nursing practice. Use nursing diagnosis, but avoid making medical diagnoses. Make sure documentation reflects use of the nursing process.

- Document only what you are qualified to do, based on your education, experience, and licensure.

- If a documentation form is more than one page, make sure that all pages are numbered and/or dated so they can be matched up if the chart is dropped, or pages are out of sequence.

What to chart

In the long-term care facility, a complete assessment is not usually done every shift unless the resident is ill or is being monitored. Policies and state laws vary on the frequency of charting, but in stable residents, this is generally weekly or monthly. Daily care, treatments, and medications are usually documented on flow sheets. This is acceptable unless a problem occurs or abnormality develops.

Clinical documentation is the element of resident care that contributes to identification and communication of residents' problems, needs and strengths, that monitors their condition on an ongoing basis, and that records treatment and response to treatment, is a matter of good clinical practice and is an expectation of licensed healthcare professionals.[5] Note that documentation cannot be separated from resident care. It is an element (or part) of comprehensive resident care.

Assessment

- Residents who are in the long-term care facility under the Medicare payment program must have a notation on the medical record at least once every 24 hours. However, many facilities require documentation and assessment of the resident's skilled condition and needs each shift. The reason for the policy is usually related to skips in documentation, which is a problem that plagues many long-term care facilities. If a note is required once in 24 hours, and the nurse gets busy, forgets, or otherwise fails to write this note, there is no documentation for the 24-hour period. Thus, most facilities require a note each shift, even if the resident is stable. *Remember that the note should reflect the nursing assessment, nursing action, resident response, and evaluation related to the resident's Medicare-covered condition.*

- If your assessment reveals an abnormality, documentation should describe what nursing action was taken. Simply describing an abnormality is inadequate. In most cases, a notation that simply says, "will continue to monitor" is also inadequate. The nursing process and the plan of care should guide care and documentation. Vague notes referring to ongoing monitoring are not sufficient to describe care or necessary monitoring. Review the steps in the nursing process. Avoid documenting an abnormal observation without documenting the other steps in the nursing process related to this observation. For example, do not document "crackles in lungs" without documenting nursing actions, physician notification, resident response, and follow up evaluation and care. This is a significant issue in many lawsuits.

- Record information about allergies and past health history.

- If the resident has a condition such as arthritis or a pressure ulcer that is potentially painful, document regular pain assessments and nursing interventions to relieve pain. Use an appropriate pain-assessment tool. Avoid random statements, such as, "Smiling. Does not appear to be in pain." For residents with painful or potentially painful conditions, regular assessment is necessary. *Failure to assess for, document, or report pain does not mean that residents do not have pain.* A quarterly MDS assessment of untreated pain is not adequate.

Care given

- Remember, you are talking about a person. Review a medical record of a resident with a gastrostomy tube, pressure ulcer, or other chronic condition. Does most of the documentation address the gastrostomy tube or chronic condition to the exclusion of other information about the resident? If so, staff are not documenting holistically. Address the entire person.

The condition is always secondary to the person. Use the nursing process.

- Nursing facilities are required to document the resident's care and response to care during the course of the stay, and it is expected that this documentation would chronicle, support and be consistent with the findings of each MDS assessment. Always keep in mind that government requirements are not the only or even the major reason for clinical documentation.[6] Charting care that you did not give or assessments you have not done is fraud.

- Make sure your care and documentation are consistent with acceptable professional standards of practice, state laws, facility policies and procedures, and the resident's plan of care.

- Record all nursing care given, including the resident's response to treatment.

- Describe teaching, as well as the resident's response and understanding. List specific instructions you have given.

- Document all safety precautions taken to protect the resident. This may be done on a flow sheet. Be specific. Stating "fall precautions" does not tell the reader what you did. However, listing specific fall precautions on the care plan, then writing "fall precautions per plan of care" may be considered acceptable. However, make sure the plan does not list generic precautions such as "call signal within reach." The plan must be individualized to the resident's needs and updated when necessary.

- Always document the reason for giving a PRN medication and the resident's response.

- When following a physician's order, always leave a "paper trail," e.g., assessment of resident, implementation of valid orders, notification of the physician (and responsible party) and outcome.

Refusals, noncompliance, behavior problems, documenting about the resident and family

- If you document a resident's or family member's comments, place their words in quotation marks and attribute the comment to them. Avoid paraphrasing.

- Document all resident refusals or noncompliance. Cite specific behaviors or statements. The resident has a right to refuse care, but the nurse has a responsibility to explain the consequences of the refusal to the resident in terms he or she can understand. Documentation should reveal adequate teaching.

- Avoid labeling or stereotyping the resident in the medical record.

- Avoid criticizing or expressing animosity toward a resident or family. Describing a resident or family as uncooperative, difficult or manipulative or being sarcastic suggests you do not value or respect the individual. Negative labels, descriptions, and stereotypes may reflect your frustration, but you should make every effort to describe residents and family members factually, in an impartial manner.

- Document the presence of any unauthorized items in the resident's room and action taken.

- Document any actions of the resident or family that contribute to the resident's illness or injury, including refusals of care.

- Refusals of care are often thinly disguised behavior problems. Do adequate teaching to ensure the resident understands the situation completely. Consider trying behavioral approaches. Modify the plan of care to identify and address the behavior. Contact the social worker to see if the resident would benefit from behavior management or mental health services. Don't give up! Document your efforts and results.

- Document tampering with medical equipment, such as oxygen concentrator, IV pump, etc.

- Document the existence and disposition of important personal belongings, large sums of money, and valuables. Add items to the inventory list and ask the resident to sign the list if he or she sends items home. If the family takes items home, remove them from the inventory list and ask the resident or family member to sign the inventory.

- Avoid labeling events and behaviors. Be specific. For example, avoid charting the resident was "uncooperative," or "acting in an unruly manner." Specifically describe the behavior without making judgments. Document conclusions that can be supported with data. You may document observed behavior, such as "refuses bath, shouts and shakes fists."

- Avoid referring to other residents by name. Use words such as "roommate," or refer to the other resident by initial, medical record number, or room number, according to your facility policy.

- If you use an interpreter when instructing a resident, state who the interpreter was and exactly what was discussed. State that you had the resident's consent to communicate the information through the interpreter. Keep explanations simple. Most lay interpreters do not have a medical background and may become confused by technical terminology.

- Document all comments or threats by residents and families, such as, "calling the state," complaining to a professional licensure board, or filing a lawsuit.

Test results, consultations

- Document your review of laboratory, radiology, and other reports and note the date, time, and method of physician notification. If you fax an abnormal report to the physician, documentation should reveal that you followed up by telephone in a timely manner. Update the care plan to reflect any monitoring needed for the abnormality. Ask the physician whether follow-up lab is needed.

- The facility must provide or obtain laboratory services to meet the needs of its residents. *The facility is responsible for the quality and timeliness of the laboratory services.*[7] If laboratory or other test results and reports are not received in a timely manner, document that you notified the appropriate agency, department, or person, and followed up on the situation.

- If the consultant dietitian, pharmacist, or other consultant visits, make sure to read his or her notes. Follow up on recommendations. Add changes to the care plan. Contact the physician if orders are necessary. Document his or her response.

> The EFG Care Center failed to read the notes and test results authored or written by other health care providers and consultant personnel. They failed to recognize the significance of these providers' observations. They apparently overlooked diagnostic reports on the record. They failed to include appropriate management techniques, preventive care, and consultant recommendations on the care plan. They failed to solicit interventions from the consultants for problems experienced by the resident. These failures deprived the resident of collaborative, interdisciplinary care.
>
> *(From an actual lawsuit report alleging progressive failures and omissions of care.)*

Intake and output

- Intake and output (I & O) monitoring does not require a physician's order. However, if the physician orders it, documentation is essential, not optional. Intake and output monitoring, as well as any special approaches or resident preferences are listed on the written care plan. If you list "encourage fluids" as a care plan approach, or if the physician orders increased fluids, you must have a means of evaluating the effectiveness of your approaches. Without a means of evaluation, this approach is meaningless. When documenting I & O, ensure that:

  - Fluid intake is planned so that approximately 65%–75% of the total daily intake is delivered at meals, and 25%–35% delivered during non-meal times, such as medication passes and planned nourishment or snack times. Fluid with medication administration may be standardized to a prescribed amount; e.g., 180 mL (6oz.) per administration pass.

  - All fluid the resident consumes during each shift is recorded in metric measurements (cc or mL) on an intake and output flow sheet or worksheet. This includes fluids consumed on the nursing unit, fluids consumed with medications, fluids consumed during meals, and fluids consumed during activities.

– All fluid excreted is also recorded in metric measurements. For the most part, this is urinary elimination. However, emesis, wound drainage, and liquid stools may also be included in output recording.

– The nurse reviews each resident's fluid intake at the end of each shift. If he or she determines that the fluid intake and output are inaccurate or inadequate, he or she will question the accuracy of the recorded information and attempt to reconcile the record. He or she may also instruct the nursing assistant to administer fluids immediately. Low liquid intake may also be reported to the next shift, who will increase fluid intake. Both nurses document the assessment and nursing interventions. Update the plan of care.

• Take intake and output (I&O) monitoring seriously. Make sure the flow sheet is complete. The midnight shift nurse or other designated person should cumulate and assess the 24-hour fluid intake each day. Compare these values with the dietitian's calculations of the resident's minimum fluid requirements. If the resident consumes less than his or her minimum requirements, act on the information! Modify the plan of care to ensure sufficient intake.

EFG Care Center neglected to provide an organizational structure and methodology for the Nursing Services Department to ensure that clinical records were complete, accurate, and contained all necessary information for the care of Donnie Jones. They neglected to develop, maintain, and evaluate a format for documentation that facilitated desired outcomes for Donnie Jones. Documentation is a means of communication with other healthcare providers. EFG Care Center failed to ensure that nurses' notes were informative and descriptive of the resident's condition, care provided, and response to care. They failed to ensure that records were completely and accurately documented. They failed to ensure that nurses assessed intake and output values and compared them with the resident's daily fluid requirements. They failed to ensure that documentation reflected that care was provided within the confines of acceptable professional standards of practice.

(From an actual lawsuit report alleging progressive failures and omissions of care.)

Skin condition

Pressure ulcers and skin breakdown are a leading cause of lawsuits against long-term care facilities and their personnel.

• Document the skin risk assessment on admission, quarterly, and according to facility policy. If the resident is at risk, begin a preventive care plan. If the resident experiences new breakdown, repeat the skin assessment promptly.

• If the resident's skin is fragile and at risk for bruises and/or skin tears, implement a protective care plan to prevent injury.

- The standards for monitoring and documenting skin condition include

    – To prevent pressure ulcers, individuals at risk should be identified so that risk factors can be reduced through intervention. The condition of an individual admitted to a healthcare facility is not static; consequently, pressure ulcer risk requires routine reexamination. Accurate and complete documentation of all risk assessments ensures continuity of care and may be used as a foundation for the skin care plan.[8]

    – All individuals at risk should have a systematic skin inspection at least once a day, paying particular attention to the bony prominences. Results of skin inspection should be documented.[9]

    – Assess the pressure ulcer initially for location, stage, size (length, width, depth), sinus tracts, undermining, tunneling, exudate, necrotic tissue, and the presence or absence of granulation tissue and epithelialization.

    – Reassess pressure ulcers frequently. If the condition of the resident or wound deteriorates, reevaluate the treatment plan as soon as any evidence of deterioration is noted.[10]

    – To achieve successful wound healing, the nurse must carefully follow every step in wound management, including critical assessment, planning, implementation, evaluation, and documentation.[11]

- Facilities should assess and document high-risk residents' skin conditions at least weekly, or more often if breakdown occurs.

- For residents with pressure ulcers or other open skin areas, weekly documentation should reflect at least

    – diameter and depth of area, in metric measurements

    – stage

    – color

    – odor (presence or absence of)

    – drainage (presence or absence of, characteristics, appearance)

    – necrosis (presence or absence of)

    – appearance of the surrounding skin (periphery)

Consistency and objectivity

- Documentation must be consistent with the care plan. Avoid documenting information that contradicts the approaches listed on the plan.

- Charting should be descriptive. Provide accurate descriptions of information you can see, hear, touch, and smell. Avoid generalizations and vague expressions. Avoid documenting feelings, opinions, or judgments about the resident or his or her family.

- Always document objectively. Avoid terms such as "normal," or "good," "resident had a good night," or "appears" or "seems" which are subjective and can be interpreted many different ways. If you document information such as, "wound healing," or "condition improved," be sure to state facts to support your observation. Give exact measurements and state the observations supporting the opinion.

- Ensure that information about the resident's level of function on the nurses notes' and weekly/monthly summary does not conflict with information in the Minimum Data Set, or other areas of the record. If documentation reflects a change in level of function, clearly state this in the notes. Consider updating the MDS and care plan.

- If a resident is receiving physical, occupational, or speech therapy, make sure that your documentation is consistent. Read what the therapist has written before writing your notes. Conflicting documentation between nursing and therapy is a significant legal and financial issue. It commonly occurs because nurses do not read therapy notes and are not aware of mobility goals. For example, if the therapist notes the resident can safely ambulate in her room with a walker, nursing documentation should not state the resident is routinely restrained in a chair "for safety and to prevent falls." In this case, restraining the resident is effectively reversing the skilled care therapy is providing. If you have concerns about resident safety, meet with the therapist and find a middle ground.

- If a resident is on fall precautions, hip precautions, anticoagulant precautions, or some other type of monitoring, all personnel should be doing the same thing. The facility should have policies and procedures addressing the actions to take. The care plan should state individualized approaches to use for the resident. For example, each nurse notes the resident is on "hip precautions." Without a specific policy or care plan, the reader does not know what precautions were used to protect the resident. This may become an issue if the resident's prosthesis dislocates and he or she is hospitalized and promptly dies of a pulmonary embolus.

- Documentation in one part of the medical record should be consistent and not contradict information in other parts. For example, a resident's weight is recorded as 123 pounds on the October 1 MDS. The October 3 dietitian note documents the resident's weight as 92 pounds. The nursing summary of October 5 states the resident weighs 114 pounds. The flow sheet of October 7 states the resident weighs 98 pounds. The magnitude of the inconsistencies makes it clear that no one knows the resident's true weight. In extreme cases, facilities may be charged with Medicare or Medicaid fraud because they were paid for care that was not provided. At the very least, the personnel in this facility do not appear credible, based on the erratic, inconsistent, contradictory documentation, and there is no clear benefit to the resident.

- When charting, emphasize quality of content, not quantity of words.

EFG Care Center failed to maintain accurate and complete medical records on Donnie Jones. Numerous documents are missing from the record. Minimum Data Sets and care plans are missing from the record. There is no paper trail to verify that some physician orders were followed. Laboratory reports are missing. Facility personnel failed to chronicle physical findings and circumstances leading to Donnie Jones's declines, denying the resident medically necessary care and services. These examples are not all inclusive; nursing assessment is erratic and largely absent on this record. The medical record is silent relative to a narration of events leading up to the resident's hospitalizations. It is evident from the documentation that nurses were not practicing preventive care or following any type of care plan. Care was inconsistent. Acute conditions were not monitored or acted upon. Care was so fragmented and communication so poor, it appears no one knew what anyone else was doing. The records were not accessible, information was not communicated and valuable information was not recorded. The record did not give the treating physician sufficient information to make accurate clinical decisions for the resident's care. Examples include, but are not limited to absence of an accurate height measurement, numerous gaps and lack of assessment of intake and output data, numerous care omissions in nursing notes and flow sheets, failure of nursing personnel to address observations made by other providers and documented in the record, and lack of assessment and ongoing monitoring of acute conditions. Weight monitoring is inconsistently documented, erratic, and not done often enough to track the resident's rapid weight loss so it could be promptly addressed and reversed. Weights are contradictory for various documents in the record, such as the MDS, weight record, dietitian's notes, and nursing notes. There is no evidence that nursing personnel were evaluating and assessing the meaning and significance of the intake numbers they were recording, which is the purpose for monitoring intake and output.

(From an actual lawsuit report alleging progressive failures and omissions of care.)

Co-signing and documenting for others

- As a rule, do not document for someone else.

- Avoid adding information to someone else's notes.

- Do not change or correct someone else's charting. If you discover that a co-worker has made an error, do not correct it. Inform that person about the error. Correcting someone else's documentation is a legal issue that can cause serious problems if the medical record goes to court.

- Avoid co-signing documentation if you cannot attest to the accuracy of the information.

- Documentation must reflect who performed the action. If it is absolutely necessary to document care given by another person, document factual information. For example, the nurse from the previous shift calls and states she gave a resident acetaminophen for arthritic pain several minutes before her shift ended and forgot to document it. In this case, making a narrative note explaining the details of the nurse's notification is appropriate. Assess and document the resident's current level of pain. Initial the medication record with "your initials for (the other nurse's initials)." When the nurse arrives for her next shift, she should co-sign this documentation.

- Countersigning someone else's documentation generally means the nurse has verified that all required resident care has been provided. In some facilities, nursing assistants are not permitted to write in the narrative notes. Their care and observations are documented on flow sheets, with additional narrative information entered on nurses' notes by the licensed nurse. Activities of daily living flow sheets are commonly completed by nursing assistants each shift. The forms may be reviewed and counter-signed by a nurse. Facility policies should address the meaning of countersigned documentation; i.e., whether by documenting on a flow sheet the licensed nurse is verifying the care was provided, or simply that the nursing assistant had the authority and competence to perform the procedure.[12]

- Some facilities require nurses to complete the ADL flow sheets because of problems with documentation errors and skips by nursing assistants. *Consult the facility legal counsel about this practice.* It is virtually impossible for the nurse to know that each item he or she signs off represents care that was given as documented. This is an example of *documenting care that is supposed to be given without knowing it was actually given.* It may cause the reader to question the veracity, integrity, and credibility of the nurses' documentation. Document care only if you gave it personally, or *directly and personally observed* an unlicensed worker providing the care.

The Nursing Assistant Plan of Care on your CD-ROM may help you solve the problem related to gaps in flow sheet documentation.

Master signature legends for flow sheets

Unless prohibited by state law, facilities are permitted to maintain master signature legends as a key to the initials on flow sheets. This eliminates the need for personnel to sign a signature key for each flow sheet every month. However, in facilities with heavy turnover, tracking the signatures of employees daily to ensure the master signature legend is accurate may be impossible. The federal requirements state that use of a master signature legend in lieu of the legend on each form for nursing staff signatures of medication,

treatment, or flow sheet entries is acceptable under the following circumstances:[13]

- Each nursing employee documenting on medication, treatment, or flow sheets signs his full name, title, and initials on the legend.

- The original master legend is kept in the clinical records office or director of nurses' office.

- A current copy of the legend is filed at each nurses' station.

- When a nursing employee leaves employment with the facility, his name is deleted from the list by lining through it and writing the current date by the name.

- The facility updates the master legend as needed for newly hired and terminated employees.

- The master signature legend must be retained permanently as a reference to entries made in clinical records.

If your facility maintains a master signature legend, consult your legal counsel to determine whether you must furnish a copy of the legends for the relevant time frame when a resident requests a copy of his or her medical record. If lawsuit is filed, the plaintiff attorney will most probably subpoena these records if you have not previously furnished them. He or she may also subsequently subpoena time cards, assignment sheets, schedules, personnel files, and other employee data. The medical-legal reviewer will compare initials on the signature legends with the flow sheets. If he or she questions the veracity of the record or suspects falsification of the flow sheets or other information, the reviewer may compare the initials, names, handwriting, signatures, or other data with schedules, assignment sheets, time cards, and payroll data to confirm whether certain individuals were employed and on duty during the days in question.

Staffing problems, problems with other workers

- Keep comments about other staff members or allegations of inadequate care out of the record.

- Avoid documenting information about staffing shortages, criticisms of the employer, problems, or conflicts in the resident's medical record, such as "Treatment not done due to lack of staff."

- Avoid criticizing other healthcare workers in the record.

- Avoid stating you have "informed" a supervisor, physician, or other healthcare provider of an event if you have barely mentioned it, or mentioned it briefly in passing.

Transfers and discharges

- When a resident leaves your care, document the time, the condition of the resident upon leaving, and any other information necessary to reflect the situation accurately. For example, if the resident is at risk for skin breakdown, document the complete condition of the skin.

- When transferring a resident, state the date and time, resident condition, who accompanied the resident, who provided the transfer, where and to whom the resident is transferred, and manner of transfer (wheelchair, stretcher, ambulance, and so forth). Document the disposition of the resident's personal possessions and medications. List instructions given to the resident, and teaching in anticipation of discharge.

Readmissions

If a resident is discharged for 30 days or fewer and readmitted to the same facility, the medical record must be updated upon readmission. To update the clinical record, staff must

- obtain current, signed physicians' orders

- completely assess the resident's condition using the facility admission assessment form and/or write a descriptive nursing note, giving a complete assessment of the resident's condition

- note changes in diagnoses, if any

- obtain signed copies of the hospital or transferring facility history and physical and discharge summary, if applicable. A signed transfer form containing this information is acceptable, but may not be as complete as the other documents

- complete a new RAI and update the comprehensive care plan if evaluation of the resident reveals a significant change that appears to be permanent. If no significant change has occurred, then update only the comprehensive care plan

If the resident has been discharged from the facility for more than 30 days, a new clinical record must be initiated.

Late entries, addendums, clarifications

- Late entries are acceptable if the delay is justified by the circumstances. The documentation should never appear to be self-serving.

- If you forget to document, follow your facility policy for making a late entry. Specify the exact date and time the entry was recorded, as well as the exact date and time the event occurred. Clearly mark your documentation as a "Late entry for (date, time)."

- Avoid making late entries or rewriting new pages of the record to make the details sound more favorable. This is usually a transparent attempt to cover up negative outcomes. You may add late entry information if it pertains to information and missing details. However, making details sound favorable in a late entry gives the reader the impression that you are hiding something. An attorney or jury may assume that the information was added for damage control purposes.

- A clarification note is a late entry that is written to prevent incorrect interpretation of information that has been previously documented. For example, after reading an entry, you can see how it could be easily misinterpreted. Write the clarification note as soon after the original entry as possible. To make a clarification entry, note the current date and time. Write "clarification." State the reason for the clarification and refer to the entry being clarified. Identify any additional documents or sources of information that support the clarification.

- If you must add something to a previously written entry, go to the next available line and write, "Addendum to note of (date and time of prior note)." An addendum is a late entry that provides new or additional information related to a previous entry. The addendum refers to the previous note and provides additional information to address a specific situation or incident. Refer to information supporting the addendum, if any. Do not use this type of note if you forget to chart something. (Use a late entry for forgotten information.) To make an addendum, note the current date and time. Write "addendum" and state the reason, referring to the previous documentation. Complete the addendum entry as soon as possible.

Errors, omissions, and corrections

- If you make an error, do not erase it, use correction fluid, or otherwise obliterate it. Avoid writing over the entry to correct it. The original

entry must be visible. Draw a single, thin line through the entry, and write "error." Sign your name, and initial and date the change. State the reason for the error, such as "wrong chart" in the margin or above the note. Then write the correct information. If someone else has made a subsequent entry, skip down to the next available line and write the correction as a late entry, referring to the previous incorrect entry.

- Check the medication record, treatment record, and flow sheets at the end of your shift to make sure you have documented all information for which you were responsible.

- Be aware that there are many pitfalls with checklist and flowsheet charting. Initial care only if you personally completed it. Don't follow the previous nurse's check marks and don't chart care unless you know it was actually done. Be aware that blank spaces in flow sheets raise doubts about whether or not something was done. If a resident is in the hospital or out of the facility, remove the sheet from the notebook or turn it over or upside down until the resident returns.

- Do not chart care because it is supposed to be done. Chart only if care was actually given. For example, avoid blanket statements, such as "turned q two hours," "peri care after each incontinence," "toileted q2h," "call light within reach," etc. unless you personally know that this was done as documented throughout the shift. Many nurses document this information because it is "supposed to be done." The medical record is a true, complete, and accurate record of care given. Thus, care that is "supposed to be done" does not belong in the record, and may undermine the nurses' credibility. In some facilities, nurses complete ADL flowsheets. This, too, is a questionable practice because in most cases, the nurse does not give this care and does conclusively know what care has been provided. In a courtroom, you can expect this type of documentation to be scrutinized and questioned by the plaintiff attorney.

- If you make an omission or mistake, it must be documented. Document only the facts, which will speak for themselves. Avoid making statements such as, "I made a mistake," or "the nursing assistant made an error." Other words to avoid are "accidentally," "somehow," or "inadvertently."

- Practice defensive documentation, but avoid lying or selectively omitting potentially damaging information.

- Document omitted medications and treatments. Circle them on the flow sheet to indicate they were not given. State the reason in a narrative note or on the back of the flow sheet.

- Occasionally, documentation is lost. If you must recreate an entry because of missing or lost information, clearly mark the entry as a replacement for lost information. If you cannot recall the event or care, state that information for the specific time frame has been lost.

- When documentation spans two pages (continues from one page to the next), always sign your name and title at the bottom of the first page. Note that the entry will "continue on the next page." Begin the new page by noting the date and time from the previous page. Note that the entry is "continued from previous page." Write the resident's identifying information in the appropriate space on the new form.

You have asked that I review the medical records of Donnie Jones, which your office provided. These records were made and maintained by the EFG Care Center. No other medical records were received or reviewed in connection with the care of this resident. The EFG Care Center records are incomplete. They begin on December 29, 2004. The nursing notes end on March 3, 2005. Notes for March 4, 2005 are missing. The progress notes and physician orders end on March 4, 2005, which appears to be the actual date of discharge from the facility. The dates of service are missing from the various consultation reports on the record. The resident sustained a fall and serious hip fracture in the facility on January 12, 2005. All nursing notes for this day have been removed from the record. When a medical record is altered, sanitized or tampered with, it calls the credibility/integrity and veracity of the entire document into question.

(From an actual lawsuit report alleging progressive failures and omissions of care.)

Falsification

- Be truthful in your documentation. Although you may practice defensive documentation do not omit or alter relevant details of any event.

- Tampering with, altering, or falsifying the medical record in any manner is fraud. Any individual tampering with a medical record is subject to criminal, civil, and licensure action. Fraud has a longer statute of limitations than medical malpractice in some states. The nursing licensure board is not bound to the statute of limitations when investigating and punishing nurses for fraudulent documentation.

- Never record care you have not given. Avoid making up or overstating information. Avoid documentation that is obviously self-serving.

- Do not alter or destroy the medical record.

- Do not remove and rewrite pages of the medical record. On rare occasions, liquid or another substance may be spilled on a medical record, or a page may be damaged so it is illegible. If this is the case, retain the original page. Make the reason for recopying clear. Mark it as damaged and on what date. Recopy the page exactly like the original. Place both pages in the chart, or note where the damaged original is located. This prevents concern that a page was recopied to conceal or add information.

- You may feel pressured to fill in gaps in flow sheet charting. This is a dangerous practice because you may not remember what occurred several weeks after the fact. Completing flow sheets during your shift is always best. If gaps in flow sheets are a problem in your facility, assign someone to audit them each shift. Going back and completing or "filling holes" in the medication, treatment, or ADL flow sheets is considered willful falsification and is illegal. Facility policies should address how to correct omissions on flow sheets, but only if the person making the correction has complete and total recall of the care given. Some states have time frames in which omissions may be completed. Usually, you cannot go back and correct a flow sheet. Writing a late entry narrative note describing the care given is probably the best approach.

- Charting medication administration, treatments, or other care in advance is falsification of records.

- Writing your initials on a medication record indicates the medication has been given, not just removed from the drawer. (The same principle applies for all other flow sheet charting.)

- If you place your initials on the record before giving the medication, you are increasing your risk of legal exposure. (The same principle applies for all other flow sheet charting.)

- Evidence of tampering with a chart not only is illegal, it can cause the entire medical record to be inadmissible as evidence in court.[14]

Medical record accuracy

- Medical records and documentation are not only part of the resident's care, they are the validation of that care. Without accurate and complete documentation, no one can really determine what has been done or what should be a future clinical approach to resident care.[15] If you are involved in a lawsuit or questioned by an attorney, avoid using the excuse that documentation is a bureaucratic requirement that adds nothing to the resident's care or well-being. The opposing attorney is bound to have an expert witness who will persuasively explain why properly maintained medical records are important and essential to the residents' welfare.

- Make sure that your documentation is accurate. Errors, omissions, and questionable or inaccurate entries diminish your credibility. This is an issue if the nursing care is questioned or negligence is alleged, affecting both the reliability of your chart and the strength of your case if you end up in court. Covering up minor errors that were not negligent damages your credibility. An accurate and concise record shows you are conscientious. It implies that you have given quality care. Errors suggest you are careless. If you are careless with your documentation, the reader may assume you are careless with the care you give.

Medical record retention

The facility is required by law to safeguard clinical records against loss, destruction, or unauthorized use. The facility must keep confidential all information in the resident's records, regardless of the form or storage method of the records, unless release is required by

- law

- transfer to another healthcare institution

- third-party payment contract

- the resident

Formal facility medical record retention policies are determined by state law. If your state law does not specify a period of time for which to retain records, the facility must keep them for five years after the date of the resident's discharge. If the resident is a minor, retain records for at least three years after the resident's 21st birthday, or the legal age according to state law.

Thinning charts

Nursing personnel are often required to "thin" the active medical records to fit in the charts. Forms that have been removed are sent to the medical records department, where they are maintained in each resident's permanent file. If a record is requested by a resident or law firm, check the thinning pile to make sure the resident's thinned records have all been filed in the resident's permanent file. Certain forms must remain on the open chart permanently, whereas others may be removed and filed after a period of time. Most facilities retain three to six months of departmental notes on the open record. Facilities are strongly encouraged to provide written guidelines for staff

for thinning their open charts. The following items must remain in the active clinical record (open chart):

- current history and physical

- current physicians' orders

- current physician progress notes

- all RAIs and Quarterly Reviews for the previous 15-month period

- current care plan

- most recent hospital discharge summary and/or transfer form

- current nursing and therapy notes

- current medication and treatment records

- current lab and x-ray reports

- the admission record

- the current permanency plan

Example guidelines for thinning medical records are on the CD that accompanies this book.

Index of admissions and discharges.

The facility must maintain a permanent, master index of all residents admitted to and discharged from the facility. This index must contain at least the following information:

- name of resident (first, middle, and last)

- date of birth

- date of admission

- date of discharge

- social security, Medicare, or Medicaid number

Destruction of records

When resident records are destroyed after the retention period is complete, the facility should shred or incinerate the records in a manner that protects resident confidentiality. At the time of record destruction, maintain a log to document the following for each record destroyed:

- resident name

- date of birth

- medical record number

- social security number, Medicare/Medicaid number. **A master index can be found on your CD-ROM.**

- date and signature of person disposing of the record

- method of record disposal

Facility closure

In the event the facility closes, changes ownership, or changes administrative authority, the new management must maintain documented proof of the medical information required for all residents. This documentation may be in the form of copies of the resident's clinical record or the original clinical record. In a change of ownership, the two parties will agree and designate in writing who will be responsible for the retention and protection of the inactive and closed clinical records.

Communication books, shift reports, anecdotal records

- Communication books and shift reports are used to alert the health care team to critical information. These tools should note where the relevant information is documented. Relevant health information documented in these tools must also be documented in the health record.

- Nurses may use personal or anecdotal notes to record personal reflections and resident information. This information must also be documented in the residents' charts. Personal

and anecdotal notes can be requested during legal proceedings.

- Use communication books and shift reports only for information that must be passed on to other members of the healthcare team.

- Pertinent information from communication books and shift reports must also be included in the residents' records.

- Maintain resident confidentiality when storing or disposing of communication books, shift reports, anecdotal records, such as by destroying or shredding the documents.

- Follow facility policies for retaining and storing communication books, shift reports, schedules, assignment sheets, and other internal documents in a secure area for a specified period of time.

Evaluating your documentation

Since nurses are responsible for assigning and delegating to nursing assistants, the nurse is responsible for monitoring nursing assistant documentation to ensure it is accurate and complete. All facilities should set a goal for random chart audits quarterly. This shows staff that management is concerned with documentation substance, accuracy, and completion. When trying to determine whether your charting meets acceptable professional standards, ask yourself

- Are your medical records as complete as they should be to fully document what you did and why, including the resident's response?

- Does your documentation reveal each element of the nursing process?

- Does your documentation reveal that the residents' risks and needs were identified, and care was given to meet these needs?

- Does your documentation reveal you followed the care plan?

- Does your documentation contradict information elsewhere on the record, including the MDS?

- Does your documentation reflect care that was actually given (versus care that is supposed to be given)?

- Does your documentation clearly show evidence of evaluations and outcomes (even if outcomes differ from stated goals or include deviations from normal)?

- Would a plaintiff attorney or expert be able to criticize you?

- Would a defense attorney or expert be able to defend you?

- Would Medicare or Medicaid agree that your note justifies the care they paid for?

- Does documentation validate a higher level of care and a higher payment rate?

Contents of the medical record

Information in the medical record falls into six general categories:

- medical findings, and/or information about the resident's condition

- assessments and identification of risk factors and problems requiring care

- the care plan and documentation of care treatment given to meet the residents' basic needs and address the problems

- evidence that care follows applicable standards and the care/treatment plan

- goals of care and evaluation of outcomes achieved/resident response to care

- effectiveness of the care/treatment plan and modification of the plan when needed

The information is located in many different places in the medical record. Most long-term care facilities use a system called *source oriented medical records (SOMR)*. The SOMR is divided into categories, such as physician orders and progress notes, nurses' notes, vital signs and weights, medications, treatments, laboratory and other diagnostic data, dietary, therapy, social services, and activities. Each category or discipline has a separate divider in the chart in which their records are stored. The sequence of the record is determined by facility or corporate policy and varies from one facility to the next. Most file forms are backwards chronological order, with most recent records on top.

Some facilities use the *problem-oriented medical record (POMR)*. This type of record is divided into general categories, such as history, encounters, orders, progress notes, and test results. In some facilities, the record is subdivided into anatomic categories. All disciplines chart in each category, as appropriate. Facilities that use this system believe it improves communication and makes finding information easier. The structure of the POMR readily translates to electronic documentation, and has been used efficiently in many electronic medical record environments, including those that are highly specialized.

See your CD-ROM for a description of documentation formats and systems.

Discharge planning

Nursing facilities are required to develop a post-discharge plan of care when the resident will be transferred to another facility, or to his or her own home. This requirement is the source of a great deal of confusion, and many deficiencies on surveys. The requirement does not apply if the resident is transferred to the acute care hospital in an emergency and does not return to the facility.

Discharge planning begins on facility admission and continues throughout the resident's stay in the facility. If the resident subsequently transfers to another facility or to his or her own home, the facility should

- Prepare a post-discharge plan of care.

- Teach the resident and/or responsible party about the care plan, as applicable. Give them a copy of the plan of care. Also provide written instructions, if needed, and essential phone numbers to call for problems or questions.

- Send a copy of the most recent MDS and other relevant documents if the resident is being transferred to another long-term care facility.

The standard

F283 (e) Discharge Summary: When the facility anticipates discharge a resident must have a discharge summary that includes—

F283 (1) A recapitulation of the resident's stay;

(2) A final summary of the resident's status to include items in paragraph (b)(2)* of this section, at the time of discharge that is available for release to authorized persons and agencies, with the consent of the resident or legal representatives; and

F284 (3) A post-discharge plan of care that is developed with the participation of the resident and his or her family, which will assist the resident to adjust to his or her new living environment.

The interpretive guidelines, which are guidance for surveyors in determining whether a deficiency exists, state at §483.20(e)

- A post-discharge plan of care for an anticipated discharge applies to a resident whom the facility discharges to a private residence, to another nursing facility or skilled nursing facility, or to another type of residential facility such as a board-and-care home or an intermediate care facility for mentally retarded individuals. Resident protection concerning transfer and discharge are found at 42 CFR 483.12. A "post-discharge plan of care" means the discharge planning process that includes assessing continuing care needs and developing a plan designed to ensure the individual's needs will be met after discharge from the facility into the community.

- "Anticipates" means the discharge was not an emergency discharge (e.g. hospitalization for an acute condition) or due to the resident's death.

- "Adjust to his or her new living environment" means the post-discharge plan, as appropriate, should describe the resident's and family's preferences for care, how the resident and family will contact these services, and how care should be coordinated if continuing treatment involves multiple caregivers. It should identify specific resident needs after discharge such as personal care, sterile dressings, and physical therapy, as well as describe resident/caregiver education needs to prepare the resident for discharge.

In plain language, surveyors often interpret this to mean that a discharge care plan will be developed and reviewed with the resident and/or responsible party. A copy of the plan is sent to the receiving facility or agency, or home with the family caregiver. For legal purposes, the facility should retain a copy of the discharge care plan, transfer form, and all related documents on the resident's closed medical record.

- The items referred to include information about the resident's medical condition and previous medical history, physical and mental status, sensory and physical impairments, nutritional status and requirements, special treatments or procedures, mental or psychosocial status, dental condition, activities, cognitive status, rehabilitation potential, discharge potential, and drug therapy.

- Another caveat that may be overlooked is "Any time a resident is admitted to a new facility (regardless of whether or not it is a transfer within the same chain), a new comprehensive assessment must be done within 14 days. When transferring a resident, the transferring facility must give the new facility necessary medical records, including appropriate MDS assessments, to support the continuity of resident care."[16]

Records from other facilities

If the resident transferred from your facility to a hospital or another long-term care facility, you can expect the plaintiff attorney to request their records as well. The resident's condition upon arrival is very important to the initial medical-legal record review.

The electronic medical record

Facilities that use electronic documentation are required to have a backup system from which records can be reconstructed in the event the computer goes down. They are also required to have a secure system so unauthorized individuals cannot access the resident information. Each person using the computer must have an individual electronic identifier. This is usually done by maintaining a user name and password.

When documenting electronically, a few additional precautions are in order:

- Don't be afraid of computerized charting.

- Keep in mind that audit trails track the computer, user, date, time, and exactly which medical records are accessed based on the user identification. In many programs, the computer's internal clock automatically documents the date and time of the entry.

- When documenting on a specific resident, double check to make sure you have entered the correct identification code.

- Some computers display a greeting when you log on. The greeting will note the last date and time you logged onto the computer. Always read this message. If the greeting shows you logged on for a day when you were not on duty, report this security breach immediately.

- Use only your own identification and password. Never use someone else's.

- Select a password that is not easily deciphered. Avoid dates such as your birth date or anniversary. A combination of letters and numbers is very effective, such as "83PF211UTK."

- Do not give your identification code or password to others. Do not write it down and leave it under the mouse pad, keyboard, or in an electronic file. Change your password periodically. Change the password immediately if you suspect it has been compromised. Remember it!

- Do not let someone look over your shoulder when you are logging on or accessing resident data.

- Protect confidential information displayed on monitors (e.g., location of monitor, use of screen saver, privacy screens).

- Access only information you are authorized to obtain, and is necessary for you to know.

- Document only in areas you are authorized to use.

- Protect resident confidentiality if information is also reproduced in hard copy. Do not print information unnecessarily. Destroy printed copies that are not part of the permanent record.

- Never delete information from the computerized record.

- Many computer programs place expert reminders or error codes on the screen. Read and follow the directions given.

- The procedure for late entry and addendum documentation will be different than it is in a narrative system. Know and follow your facility policies for this type of charting.

- To correct an error in an electronic medical record, you will follow the same basic principles as a manual system. The computer will be able to track corrections or changes after documentation has been authenticated. Enter the current date and time, identify yourself, and state the reason for the change. If a hard copy has been generated, it must also be corrected.

- The facility must maintain a hard copy of each resident's MDS, even if the clinical record system is entirely electronic. The MDS must be signed by the RN and each individual who has completed a portion of the assessment.

- Always log off when you have finished using the computer.

- Always wash your hands immediately after using the computer. Many people use it, so the keyboard is a potential source of cross contamination.

- Some facilities cover the keyboard with a plastic cover. Users type through the plastic. If this is the case, the cover should be routinely disinfected. (However, prompt handwashing is still necessary after you have used the computer.)

- When cleaning the computer and accessories, avoid products containing alcohol. Use only products that are recommended for the surface being cleaned.

- The electronic record must note whether manual records are also being used. Likewise, if a manual record is used during an electronic system failure, the records must cross reference each other.

- When data from a manual record is entered into a computerized record, the entry should identify who documented and who provided the care.

- Electronic documentation must be signed by the person providing care. Electronic signatures are valid provided that they are accessible only to the person identified by that signature.

- Protect resident data transmitted electronically, such as by using an e-mail encryption service.

- Stay current. Attend continuing education programs to learn how to maximize the use of computerized charting and information systems.

Electronic data transmission

Electronic data transmission via fax (facsimile) or e-mail (electronic mail) is acceptable for sending and receiving healthcare information, documents, laboratory reports, physician notifications, and physicians' orders. Most facilities routinely transmit RAI information to a state regulatory office over the internet.

If the nature of an electronic communication is urgent, you may want to notify the receiving party by phone to expect the arrival of an urgent fax transmission. With a non-urgent fax, it is also a good idea to call the intended recipient to notify him or her to expect a facsimile. You may also want to consider asking the recipient to send a return fax to verify the information was received. When sending information by electronic means, long-term care facilities should

- Implement safeguards to assure that faxed documents are directed to the correct location to protect confidential health information.

- Sign all faxed documents before transmission.

- Set your fax machine to print a verification report for each fax transmission; maintain a file or log of these reports.

- Check to make sure you have the correct fax number before dialing. Read the number on the fax machine display after you have entered it. Recheck the number again before pressing the send button.

- If you believe the fax went to the wrong number, contact the recipient and apologize for the inconvenience, or send another fax asking the recipient to destroy the material.

- Never transmit insecure, identifiable resident information.

- Use the subject line of the email or cover sheet for the fax to warn the receiver that the transmission contains confidential data. On the fax cover sheet, clearly note in large, bold letters that the accompanying material is confidential.

- Place a disclaimer in the body of the e-mail or in large letters at the bottom of the fax cover sheet. **Examples of disclaimers to use can be found on your CD-ROM.**

Handheld computers and HIPAA compliance

Personal digital assistants (PDAs) and *Tablet PCs (TPCs)* are handheld computers that have become quite popular in recent years. Some staff members have purchased the units for personal use, but also use them to record data while at work. In addition to using the computer as an information resource at work, most individuals use them as a source of personal information, such as their appointments, important addresses, and list of phone numbers. Most also have a calculator function. Computers are very beneficial, and the portability of handheld models has made them a popular alternative.

In some facilities, handheld computers are used to transmit data using wireless internet technology. Thus, the facility may transmit sensitive information such as ADL flow sheet data, neuro checks, intake and output values, pain-scale ratings, nursing notes and vital signs to the mainframe computer. Before handheld computer technology was available, nursing personnel commonly scribbled notes on the backs of their hands, on paper towels, and scraps of paper. If the data were not subsequently lost, they were transferred to resident charts later in the shift. By using the handheld computer, personnel can record important data by typing on the keypad with a stylus, then transmitting it to the main computer. Light pens and touch-screen data entry are also useful tools with some models. The handheld device is not practical for long entries, but as you can see, the unit can hold a wealth of PHI for each resident. It can be plugged into a regular keyboard for typing longer narrative entries.

The handheld computer is portable, and operates by using a rechargeable battery. Hot-syncing is a term that refers to linking the handheld computer to a full-size computer to update the information on both. The PDA is placed in a cradle and a button is pushed to upload data to the mainframe. Placing the unit into the cradle also recharges the battery.

HIPAA affects all healthcare communication, and

information technology (IT) contains a wealth of information. Because of this, facilities usually have layers of access to resident medical records. The IT department will have a system for tracking who is accessing any resident's record, and will be able to identify misuse of the system.

When PDAs and TPCs are used in the facility, the following potential problems must be anticipated and addressed:

- Important resident data will be lost if the unit is not regularly charged and maintained. Anticipate battery use in advance and make sure data is transferred to the mainframe before the battery goes dead.

- Since PDAs and TPCs usually have the ability to access the Internet wirelessly, the facility must construct and maintain a firewall that is strong enough to ensure that sensitive resident data are not being broadcast into cyberspace.

- Although PDAs and TPCs have enormous benefit and many potential applications in healthcare facilities, protection of resident confidentiality and maintaining HIPAA compliance may be a drawback. Make sure wireless internet transmissions are protected by a firewall. Policies

and procedures must address personal use of the devices outside of the facility. Taking PHI home in the computer and inadvertently allowing family members and others to access it is a serious HIPAA violation. Personal computers used at work must have encryption, passwords, and other safeguards to prevent others (including your own family members) from accessing the resident data.

Example Electronic Media Policy

When electronic communication devices are used by facility personnel, an overall policy and procedure should address their use. All employees with access to electronic media should be asked to read and sign the policy. Figure 23-1 is an example policy.

Some facilities have had problems with inappropriate photos being taken of residents in various stages of undress, using cell phone cameras. Because of this, facility policies should limit availability of personal cell phones on the nursing units, and prohibit their use for the purpose of taking still photographs or making videotapes.

Figure 23-2 is an example of a policy and procedure for use of personal communication devices.

Figure 23-1   *Example Electronic Media Policy*

1. Employees have access to various forms of electronic media and services (computers, e-mail, telephones, voicemail, fax machines, external electronic bulletin boards, wire services, online services, and the Internet (hereinafter called "media").

2. The facility encourages the use of electronic media. However, media provided by the facility are facility property and the purpose of the devices is to transact facility business.

3. The following procedures apply to all media that are:

   • accessed on or from facility premises

   • accessed using facility computer equipment or via facility-paid access methods

   • individually identifiable, including communications that make reference to the facility in any manner; and/or

   • used in a manner that identifies the employee with the facility

4. Media may not be used for transmitting, retrieving, or storing any communications that are of a discriminatory or harassing nature; derogatory to any individual or group; obscene; of a defamatory or threatening nature; for "chain letters"; for personal use; illegal or against facility policy; or contrary to the facility's interest.

5. Electronic information created and/or communicated by an employee using media will not generally be monitored by the facility. However, the facility routinely monitors usage patterns for both voice and data communications (e.g., number called or site accessed; call length; times of day called) for cost analysis/allocation and the management of the Internet server. The facility also reserves the right, in its discretion, to review any employee's electronic files and messages and usage to the extent necessary to ensure that media are being used in compliance with the law and with facility policy. Therefore, employees should not assume electronic communications are private and confidential.

6. Employees must respect other people's electronic communications. Employees may not attempt to read or "hack" into other systems or logins; "crack" passwords; breach computer or network security measures; or monitor electronic filings or communications of other employees or third parties except by explicit direction of facility management.

7. Every employee who uses any security measures on a facility-supplied computer must provide the facility with a sealed envelope containing a hard copy record of all passwords and encryption keys (if any) for facility use if required.

Figure 23-1   *Example Electronic Media Policy*

8. No e-mail or other electronic communications may be sent that attempt to conceal the identity of the sender or represent the sender as someone else or someone from another facility.

9. Media may not be used in a manner that is likely to cause network congestion or significantly hamper the ability of other people to access and use the system.

10. Employees may not copy, retrieve, modify, or forward copyrighted materials except as permitted by the copyright owner or except for a single copy for reference use only.

11. Any information or messages sent by an employee via an electronic network are statements identifiable and attributable to the facility. All communications sent by employees via a network must comply with facility policy, and may not disclose any confidential or proprietary facility information.

12. Network services and World Wide Web sites monitor access and usage and can identify at least which facility and often which specific individual is accessing their services. Accessing a particular bulletin board or Web site leaves facility-identifiable electronic "tracks" even if the employee merely reviews or downloads the material and does not post any message.

13. Any employee violating this policy will be subject to corrective action and/or risk losing the privilege of using media for him/herself and possibly other employees.

14. Employees are responsible for keeping virus protection up to date by downloading weekly computer updates. Employees must virus-scan all file attachments before opening them.

15. Employees must use discretion in opening files. Avoid indiscriminate opening of files attached to email. In general, do not open files with the suffix ".exe." Notify the information technology manager if a file with this suffix is received. You must avoid all files if you are not familiar with the sender or are not expecting the file. Employees may be held responsible for the cost of repairs for damage to computers caused by opening files infected with viruses. Employees will be subject to disciplinary action if data is lost as a result of viral infection of the computer.

16. Follow all HIPAA rules, facility policies and procedures for protecting individually identifiable resident health information.

Figure 23-2 | *Example Policy for Personal Communication Devices*

It is the policy of this facility to prohibit the use by staff and students of non-work related personal communication devices, including but not limited to cell phones, pagers,
text messaging units, PDAs, and TPCs. Safety and care of the residents is paramount.
The cessation of work, even briefly, to make or answer telephone calls or to check an
electronic pager or other wireless communication device is not consistent with this
goal. In non-clinical departments, use of personal communication devices may represent a safety hazard and interferes with your work. Honesty demands that time paid by
the employer will be used profitably. If the work assigned is insufficient to occupy the
time, report to the nurse in charge or other supervisor for additional duties. Please plan
to make and return all personal communications and phone calls during breaks only.

In addition to being a distraction, the use of camera phones present opportunities for
serious violations of residents' rights to confidentiality, dignity, and privacy. Taking still
photographs or making videotapes of residents with camera phones or other personal
electronic equipment is strictly prohibited.

Generally speaking, do not bring personal communication devices to the work area.
These may be accidentally lost, damaged, or broken when on duty. Some radio frequency devices will interfere with medical equipment and may jeopardize resident
health and safety, as well as facility operations. Employees must accept responsibility
for informing family and friends and asking them to comply with this policy. Disruptions of
work or resident care by personal communication devices is grounds for discipline or
termination. The facility is not responsible for damage to or loss of personal communication devices.

We understand that emergencies may occur, and these will be accommodated, if possible. If a situation arises in which communication is critical, speak with your supervisor.
He or she has the discretion to approve a one-time, acceptable compromise to this
policy. (Situations such as "the babysitter may need to get ahold of me" are generally
not considered emergencies, and may be handled by calling the facility in the usual
manner.) In extraordinary circumstances, the supervisor may agree to the temporary
use of an electronic pager or cellular phone set for silent alert that is imperceptible to
others. In these situations, the staff member will not interrupt resident care to respond
to calls, but rather will respond after resident comfort and safety are assured.

Requests for medical records

Each facility should have specific policies, procedures, consents, and authorization forms for medical record release upon request of the resident or responsible party. You may wish to write a sentence into your policies, such as notifying the facility administrator or facility legal counsel any time a record has been requested. Do not send the records out until he or she gives approval. However, you have a tight time frame to respond, so do not delay making contact. The resident or his or her legal representative has the right

- Upon an oral or written request, to access all records pertaining to himself or herself including current clinical records within 24 hours (excluding weekends and holidays)

- After receipt of his or her records for inspection, to purchase at a cost not to exceed the community standard photocopies of the records or any portions of them upon request and two working days advance notice to the facility.

In addition to clinical records, the term "records" includes all records pertaining to the resident, such as trust fund ledgers, admission agreements, and contracts between the resident and the facility. "Purchase" is a charge to the resident for photocopying. If state statute has defined the "community standard" rate, facilities should follow that rate. In the absence of state statute, the "cost not to exceed the community standard" is that rate charged per copy by organizations such as the public library, the Post Office or a commercial copy center, which would be selected by a prudent buyer in addition to the cost of the clerical time needed to photocopy the records. Additional fees for locating the records or typing forms/envelopes may not be assessed.[17] When determining what to charge, make sure to recover your costs for the mate-

rials. A large, high-volume commercial copy center buys products in bulk and often gets a discounted rate. You may find you cannot recover the cost of toner when charging the rate a commercial copy center charges.

Some facilities charge for each page, such as 10 to 50 cents a page. Others charge 75 cents to a dollar a page. Some have package prices, such as

- A basic retrieval or processing fee not to exceed $30.00 for first 10 pages of records; then,
    a. $1.00 per page for pages 11-60
    b. $.50 per page for pages 61-400
    c. $.25 per page for any remaining pages
    d. Plus actual cost of mailing or shipping
    e. In addition, a reasonable fee not to exceed $10.00 is charged for execution of an affidavit or certification of records.
    f. Microform or electronic medium copy processing fee can be up to $45.00.
    g. You may also charge for the costs of mailing if it is being mailed to another location.

Although most facilities prefer a signed release to produce medical records, the federal rules state that an oral request may be sufficient to produce the current record for review. You may still request a written release, but do not withhold records if the individual requesting the records does not sign it. Most facilities use a records release form such as, "Authorization for Release of Medical Information." The release must be dated and signed before records are provided. Make sure the form is time-limited, with an expiration date for medical record release, such as 30 days, 60 days, or 90 days. If another copy is requested after the specified time period, a new authorization should be signed and dated by the appropriate party. The written consent must specify the

- information or specific medical records covered by the release

- reasons or purposes for the release

- person to whom the information is to be released

When a resident, responsible party, or family member requests a medical record, make sure the person requesting the information is legally entitled to it. For example, the confused resident's adult daughter is designated as the durable power of attorney for health-care. However, the son requests a copy of the medical record. He is not entitled to a copy of the record unless the daughter named the resident's health care proxy signs a record release.

Example record releases and other documents are on the CD-ROM that accompanies this book. However, before using them, consult the facility's legal counsel to make sure the authorization and release form complies with HIPAA, certification of medical records provisions, and any other idiosyncrasies in your state law. In some states specific laws apply to provision of mental health, HIV testing, and substance abuse treatment records. Some release forms have a checklist for the records being requested, such as nurses' notes, physicians' orders, laboratory reports, progress notes, medication records, etc. The requesting party may check which sections they want. One of the items listed may be "entire chart" or "chart in entirety" or "all of the above."

When "all records" are requested, you must copy records from the open chart, permanent medical records file, unfiled thinnings, and all business office and billing records. If some records are from the hospital, physi-cian, or other provider, you should copy them as part of the request. However, you are under no obligation to request or obtain records from other facilities for the purpose of furnishing them to the resident.

Make sure that both sides of two-sided forms are copied and collated together. You can staple them, but this may be very time consuming. This writer recommends stapling the MDSs and other long documents together individually. If these become separated, it is difficult or impossible to put them back together. Make sure the name and dates at the top and bottom are not cut off in copying. Make sure you do not cut off the sides of the MDS information. This is easily done because data is written close to the page margins.

In some facilities, chart forms are designed for binders that hold the records at the top. The forms are right side up on the front of the page and upside down on the back side. (This is called *"top to tail."*) Copy these records on single pages or make sure two-sided copies both face the same direction (*"top to top"*). Copy each telephone order and small-size laboratory report individually, or three to a page so they are legible. Avoid copying a page of documents filed with one order on top of the other. If this is the case, only the top document will be legible. There is no obligation to sort the record in a particular order, but avoid deliberately scrambling it.

When records have been requested, be honest and forthright. Avoid body language and demeanor that make it appear as if you are hiding something. Offer to interpret the information. An untrained observer comes up with many purported deficiencies because they do not understand the recordkeeping requirements. For example, the untrained reviewer may complain that there is "no nurse's note every shift," or "Doctor ordered MOM at bedtime PRN" and nurses seldom gave it, or a nurse gave it one day at 3:00 p.m. instead of HS. (The individual reviewing the record probably does not know the meaning of the PRN abbreviation.) Explaining these things to the reviewer may save you time, trouble, and grief over the long term.

A formal records request from a current or former resident, responsible party, or attorney usually means that someone is dissatisfied with care outcomes and they are considering a lawsuit. You may wish to notify your legal counsel if you have not already done so. You may also wish to review the record to determine whether care-related problems exist. However, you should avoid tampering with the record, removing pages, scrambling or rearranging the pages of the record. Some facilities try to tamper with flow sheets by filling in documentation gaps at this stage. Falsification causes the reader to question the credibility of the entire record. It is unlikely that filling in the boxes to show the resident had a shower three times a week will affect the plaintiff's allegations. In order to prove negligence, the plaintiff must have damages. Facilities do not always understand this, and focus on filling in documentation errors that are unrelated to the plaintiff's allegations.

Occasionally, the resident or responsible party will request and obtain a copy of the medical records involved before a lawsuit has been filed. This is usually done immediately after discharge. These records are provided to the attorney and are used as the basis for the initial review for merit screening. If a lawsuit is subsequently filed, the attorney will typically request a complete set of records from the facility. These records will be compared with the family's copy of the records to determine if the record was subsequently altered or if certain documents are missing. Discrepancies found during this review are used to damage the credibility and veracity of the medical record, the facility, and its personnel.

Clinical records service supervisor

Some states require facilities to designate a clinical records supervisor in writing. For example:

- The facility must designate in writing a clinical records supervisor who has the authority, responsibility, and accountability for the functions of the clinical records service. The clinical records supervisor must be (1) A registered health information administrator (RHIA) or registered health information technician (RHIT); or (2) An individual with experience appropriate to the scope and complexity of services performed as determined by the Texas Department of Human Services, and who receives consultation at a minimum of every 180 days from an (RHIA) or (RHIT).[18]

If a medical record is subpoenaed or requested by an attorney, the person responsible for medical records in your facility may be asked to sign an affidavit or declaration of authenticity attesting that the records provided are a true and complete copy of the medical records used and maintained by the facility during the usual course of business. If another individual, service, or business has photocopied the records, the responsible person may also have to sign a declaration related to the photocopying. **Example declarations are included on the CD-ROM that accompany this book.** You will most likely need to sign the form in front of a notary public. The declaration or affidavit is governed by the laws of your state, but generally speaking, the person certifying the records does so under penalty of law, such as making a false statement in an official proceeding. The affidavit or declaration must be signed in a manner that, if falsely made, would subject the maker to criminal penalties under the laws where the declaration is signed. A party who subpoenas the records or enters the record into evidence must provide written notice of intention to all adverse parties, and must make the record and certification available for inspection sufficiently before their offer into evidence to give an adverse party a fair opportunity to challenge them.

If the subpoena names a specific person or position, such as the clinical records supervisor, he or she may be required to produce the records in person. If a subpoena states the custodian of records must appear and produce the records in person, then the facility may designate a person to make the appearance. Consult with your legal counsel if you are unsure. A subpoena is a legal document that should never be ignored, under penalty of law.

Requests for records related to litigation

Do not release records to an attorney, law firm, or other party until you have a properly signed release for production of the records, or a court ordered subpoena. A facility (Facility A) released a resident's medical records upon the request of an attorney who was defending another facility (Facility B) in a lawsuit filed by the resident. The resident subsequently filed suit against Facility A for releasing the records without proper consent. He sought damages for embarrassment and humiliation because the records were released to the opposing attorney. Facility B and its attorney sought to have the case dismissed, since the records were needed in a court proceeding. The Court of Appeal of Louisiana upheld the suit, noting that it is a breach of medical confidentiality for a healthcare facility to release a resident's records before being served with a court subpoena or with a proper medical-records release executed by the resident. The court noted in its opinion that the attorney could

have sought a court order compelling the resident to sign a release, or could have accessed the records by other means, such as issuing a subpoena. The fact that this was not done was a clear-cut violation of the resident's right to medical record confidentiality.[19]

Legal record reviews

Before a lawsuit is filed, the plaintiff attorney usually asks a legal nurse consultant or nursing expert to do a preliminary review of the medical records to determine whether the prospective lawsuit is meritorious. *"The primary role of a legal nurse consultant (LNC) is to evaluate, analyze, and render informed opinions on the delivery of health care and its outcomes. For nearly 20 years, legal nurse consultants have acted as collaborators, strategists, and educators by offering support in medically related litigation and other medical-legal matters. An LNC is a registered nurse, unlike a paralegal or a legal assistant, and is a unique and valuable member of the litigation team. LNCs bring their health science education and clinical expertise to healthcare-related issues in the litigation process. The practice of legal nurse consulting is performed in collaboration with attorneys and others involved in the legal process. The LNC's scope of practice does not include the independent practice of law. Legal nurse consulting is a specialty of nursing. Nursing education and experience set the LNC apart from other members of the legal team."*[20]

The attorney will obtain information from the nurse about each of the four elements listed on the first page of this chapter to determine whether a potential lawsuit has merit. Although the attorney decides whether the case has merit, he or she does so after consultation with the nurse and other health professionals, as appropriate. The nurse reviewer will analyze the record for both strengths and weaknesses. He or she will provide a preliminary report to the attorney, who will decide whether to file a lawsuit. If so, additional medical records may be requested, more comprehensive chart reviews will be done, and written chronologies and reports may be generated. The mechanics of this process are determined by attorney preference and strategy. The process is also limited by record availability. An incomplete record may produce inaccurate results, so having complete facility records is necessary. Although having a complete set of records (medical, billing, pharmacy, physician, hospital, long-term care, etc.) is ideal, reviewers may have to evaluate records in batches as they become available. Some attorneys prefer verbal reporting only, whereas others require exhaustive chronologies and written reports. State laws apply to discovery of this nursing information. In general, all written information developed by a testifying expert must be disclosed to the other party. Written information developed by behind-the-scenes experts (called consulting experts) and legal nurse consultants are not disclosed unless an expert witness has reviewed the information and used it in formulating his or her opinion. Because of the disclosure rules, many attorneys do not share this information with testifying expert witnesses.

A record request is also a tip-off that the survey team may visit soon for a complaint investigation. Plaintiff attorneys often encourage disgruntled families to call the abuse and neglect reporting hotline. The results of the complaint survey may harm or help you if the case proceeds to trial, depending on the surveyors' findings. In any event, be prepared for visitors. If the resident was discharged a long time previously, the attorney may prepare a written report and attach parts of the medical record for the family to send to the state survey agency.

Record analysis

Each resident's medical record is a legal source of evidence of services provided by the facility, its physicians, and consultant personnel. The medical record is an objective source of care given and the resident's response. A thorough and concise medical record suggests that adequate care was given.[21] An inadequate, incomplete chart suggests inadequate care was given. Since the medical record represents the nucleus of the residents' care, a thorough record review is the core of any legal action. In a lawsuit, attorneys and others will review all facility records pertaining to the resident, including billing information. They will also review hospital records, physician office records, and records from other facilities in which the resident lived.

When the determination has been made to progress to a lawsuit, the attorney will retain licensed professionals who are experienced in the care given and documentation standards to review and analyze the medical records. These reviewers are usually physicians and/or nurses who are familiar with long-term care facility standards and documentation requirements. Like yourself, they have the education and experience to determine whether the applicable standards of care were met. The reviewer analyzes the record for information that is included as well as omissions in documentation. In fact, omissions are often very important to the legal review. This may be as simple as a skip on a flow sheet, or as complex as checking each MDS for a five-year residency period to ensure all are present and were completed when indicated. The reviewer will read and compare information on the medical record with other data available, such as Medicaid and Medicare documentation, bills, ambulance, and hospital records. He or she is looking for consistencies and contradictions.

The record reviewer may sort the record so that like documents are together. Ideally, the record will be received in this order, but often it is not. Working from a sorted record saves expert time and money, and greatly improves accuracy because of the detailed nature of the review and large amount of cross checking necessary. Each medical record reviewer has their own preference for chart order. Many sort the record in a manner similar to the open medical record, except that the various sections are arranged chronologically, by date, from oldest to most recent. Charts reviewed in this manner read like a book, and finding information is relatively simple. In a long-term care facility lawsuit, the reviewer usually reads every word of the nursing home record.

Always avoid the temptation to repair or alter a medical record. Provide it to the requesting party replete with skips and documentation problems. Checking for signs of alteration or falsification is a routine part of the record review. However, most reviewers will tell you they have never reviewed a mistake-free medical record. The reviewer is not looking for a perfect record, isolated flow sheet skips or harmless documentation errors. He or she evaluates patterns of skips and errors and compares them with the injuries sustained by the resident. For example, in a given month, one would expect to find documentation of the resident's food consumption for at least 90 meals. In our example record, documentation omissions were made and only 60 meals were documented. If there was no weight loss or related nutritional problem, this is most likely a non-issue. However, if the resident experienced a significant weight loss during the month, you can expect the skips to be problematic as the lawsuit progresses. The implication may be that the resident was not given 30 meals during the month. There appears to be a direct relationship between the documentation skips and the weight loss.

However, the reviewer will also consider the skips in the context of the resident's diagnoses, physician orders, care plan, labs, dietitian notes, and other related information. The flow sheet will not stand on its own when drawing conclusions about resident injuries. Thus, the documentation skips are a small part of a much larger puzzle.

Minimum data sets

The minimum data sets (MDS) and care plans are especially important in long-term care lawsuits, related to evaluating resident improvement, declines, and overall nursing care. These documents are the foundation of the nursing process, as well as all resident care. The medical record reviewer will be addressing the resident holistically, and looking for patterns of excellent care, as well as poor care. The remainder of the record will be compared with the MDS for consistencies and inconsistencies. Accurate completion of the MDS is particularly important. If the facility misses an item that is a potential trigger, a care plan problem may be missed. If the facility states the resident is terminally ill and the decline was unavoidable, the reviewer will review the terminal illness section of the MDS. He or she will depend on the MDS to determine whether problems such as contractures were present on admission and compare these data with the time of discharge. Again, the MDS is reviewed in the context of the information elsewhere in the record. The data are not isolated. Putting it bluntly, the government has handed you a wealth of information to use in providing quality care for the residents. If the facility does not use it as intended, a legal reviewer may find a way to use the information to show the facility did not meet the applicable standards of care.

Care plans

The care plan is a source of great consternation for many facilities (Chapters 4 and 10). Each resident is unique and facility staff must maintain a commitment to individualized care that meets the resident's needs. The legal reviewer uses critical thinking and the nursing process when evaluating the care plan and comparing it with information on other parts of the record. He or she will try to determine whether the care plan provides a representative snapshot of the resident during his or her stay in the facility. The reviewer is not looking for a perfect care plan. He or she may consider some care plan omissions significant and others insignificant. The concern here is whether the plan provides an overview of the resident's strengths and needs and whether the plan is used to drive the care provided by the facility. If the reviewer finds evidence of adequate care elsewhere on the record, a care plan omission is often considered a harmless documentation error. However, if the reviewer finds evidence of substandard care resulting in harm to the resident, care plan omissions suggest serious breaches of duty.

Facilities often have difficulty keeping care plans current. Having a temporary care plan form initiated at the time of admission is a helpful tool. Include obvious problems and potential problems. When the MDS and care plan are completed, incorporate the relevant information, then file the temporary plan. A temporary plan may also be useful between care plan reviews. If a resident experiences a change in condition, injury, infection, or other problem, the nurse discovering the problem should add the information to the temporary plan of care. In this case, the temporary plan is used as a supplement to the full care plan. The temporary plan is updated when necessary, and filed when the condition is no longer problematic. Updating temporary care plans usually requires the knowledge of a nurse who works on the unit. A facility MDS nurse or care plan coordinator may not be immediately aware of incidental changes

in each resident's condition that should be care planned.

The care plan is reviewed and updated quarterly and whenever a change in condition occurs. However, if a resident experiences a change in a high risk condition, such as a fall or pressure ulcer, it is a good idea to evaluate and update the plan of care immediately. Likewise, if a resident experiences recurrent problems, such as skin tears, falls, urinary infections, etc., the reviewer will evaluate how these are managed on the plan of care. The plan should be adjusted when problems occur. If the resident has a fall prevention plan and experiences recurrent falls, the plan is ineffective. Change it immediately. Do not wait for the quarterly care conference! Even minor problems, such as recurrent skin tears warrant care plan adjustments. The reviewer will look to see if the plan was changed in a timely manner. He or she will look elsewhere in the record to determine whether the care listed on the plan was being delivered. Having a perfect written plan is purposeless. The reviewer will use critical thinking and healthcare knowledge to determine whether the nursing process was used and the resident benefitted from the plan adjustments and updates. He or she will also determine whether the resident's problems were unavoidable based on this review.

Physician orders

A legal record reviewer will read each physician order and telephone order on the medical record. A great deal of cross checking is done with physician orders to determine whether they were implemented, evaluated, and the physician notified of the resident's progress (or lack of progress), as necessary. Part of the chart audit involves cross-checking information from the nurses' notes, care plan, medication and treatment records to ensure facility response to resident problems was appropriate and timely, and that physician orders were implemented reasonably soon after a problem occurred. He or she will look for notification of the closest family member or other responsible party. The reviewer will check to ensure follow-up monitoring was appropriate if the resident had a medical (or other) problem. Depending on the nature of the problem, the reviewer may audit additional records, such as laboratory reports and social service notes. The reviewer will also look for evidence of the physician's involvement in the plan of care. If the attending physician was not available to respond to a nurse's call, the reviewer will determine whether subsequent nursing action and notifications were appropriate.

If the nurse reviews a telephone order suggesting an incident, injury, or other problem, he or she will refer to the nurses' notes to find documentation of the problem, as well as follow-up care. A common problem is finding telephone orders for obvious problems with no corresponding nurses' note.

Falsifying telephone orders

Some nurses feel secure in knowing what various physicians commonly order in usual situations. They fill out telephone orders listing the physician's "usual" practices and preferences without actually contacting the physician. *This is never a safe practice unless you are writing a telephone order to implement approved facility protocols, standing orders, or policies and procedures.* If a medical record is involved in a lawsuit, the physician will most likely testify that he or she did not approve the nursing order. This exposes the nurse to potentially serious criminal penalties and adverse licensure action.

Reading back orders

One JCAHO requirement for accredited facilities is that telephone and verbal orders must be "read back" to the person who originated the order for confirma-

tion. Although most long-term care facilities are not JCAHO accredited, this is still an important safety policy to consider and adopt. The readback requirement applies to all orders and "critical test results." A "critical test result" is any lab or other diagnostic test, such as imaging studies and electrocardiograms ordered stat or returns with a panic value.

Readbacks of telephone and verbal orders

The readback rule applies whenever a nurse takes a telephone or verbal order. Simply repeating the order is not sufficient. According to the JCAHO, the intent of the rule is for the nurse to receive and document the *complete order*, then read it back to the physician who gave the order.

Readbacks for critical test results

When reporting critical test results, the JCAHO expects the facility to establish a procedure in which the physician (or other healthcare professional) "reads back" the critical test results to the person who reported them. Facility staff should request the "readback" whenever communicating critical test results verbally, including over the telephone.

Voice mail and electronic messages

The JCAHO will not accept a voice mail or verbal electronic message for satisfying the readback requirement. They note that "most state laws require nurses and pharmacists to obtain the order directly from the prescriber or his or her agent." When the order is not received directly, the nurse (or pharmacist) must call the prescriber back to obtain the order directly, including a "readback."

Verification of readbacks

The JCAHO requires verification of readbacks, but leaves the method to the facility. Some facilities have added "RB" to their accepted abbreviation list, denoting the order was "read back." The person receiving the order notes "RB" when he or she signs the verbal or telephone order. For example, the nurse writes the following on the order sheet:

"TO/Dr. Kritzberg/S. Lovewell, RN/RB/SL"

This means: Nurse Lovewell received a telephone order ("TO") from Dr. Kritzberg, read it back ("RB") to him or her, and initialed the documentation ("SL").

Surveyors may ask how the facility tracks readback performance to ensure it is being done consistently. Many facilities are doing audits of phone and verbal orders each month. If compliance is less than a designated percentage (such as 95% of the orders comply, 5% do not), the facility should consider remedial action.

A medical-legal reviewer will also consider presence or absence of readback documentation when making determinations about the credibility and veracity of the medical record.

Progress notes

The physician must write a progress note each time he or she visits the resident. The physician must see the resident once every 30 days for the first 90 days, then every 60 days after that. After the initial visit, the physician may alternate face-to-face visits with a nurse practitioner, clinical nurse specialist, or physician assistant. The reviewer will determine whether physician visits were made in the specified time frame and whether the resident was also seen by a nurse practitioner or other professional. If so, he or she will look for evidence that the physician was managing the care. The medical-legal review involves reading every detail of the physicians' progress notes. He or she will cross check information against nursing notes and other records, as appropriate.

If the physician has ordered routine monitoring, such as vital signs and intake and output every shift or weights daily, the reviewer will look for evidence that this was done. If the physician writes an order such as, "Encourage fluids," the reviewer will look for evidence that this was added to the care plan and done consistently every shift. Nurses do not have the authority to omit basic procedures ordered by the physician, or to pick and choose which physician orders they will follow. All physician orders must be followed and many warrant a care plan note or addition.

The reviewer will weigh and consider physician progress notes stating that certain declines were unavoidable. However, other factors must also be considered when determining whether a problem was unavoidable. The physician note is an important consideration, but is not taken at face value without additional supportive information about the problem. The presence of a high-risk condition does not make certain problems inevitable. If a high-risk condition is noted, the chart reviewer will determine whether the facility has provided effective prevention and treatment of the condition, based upon consistently providing routine and individualized interventions.

A condition such as a pressure ulcer is determined to be "unavoidable" if the problem occurred despite the facility's best prevention efforts. This means the facility has identified and acted on the risk by taking steps to reduce or ameliorate risk factors, and providing preventive care. They have implemented interventions that are consistent with resident needs, goals, and recognized standards of practice. The facility must effectively and consistently monitor and evaluate the effectiveness of their interventions; and revise the approaches to care, when appropriate. If these things have not been done, the reviewer will most likely consider the skin breakdown or other problem to be avoidable with proper care.

Nursing notes

The nurse reviewer will read every nursing note in the record. Depending on the resident's outcome, he or she will evaluate various aspects of the care given. The nurse reviewer wants to know about the resident. He or she does not want to read several years worth of notes describing the care of a gastrostomy tube (such as, "G-tube patent.") You are caring for a person, not a tube! Make sure narrative documentation describes the resident and his or her condition. Normal observations, such as "G-tube patent" can be easily documented on a flow sheet.

Use the nursing notes to describe:

- medical or behavior problems

- discovery of or change in skin condition, such as skin tears and pressure ulcers

- incidents and accidents such as falls

- abnormal vital signs leading to focused system assessments

- documentation of notifications made on the resident's behalf

Ongoing monitoring of abnormalities is important, as is the evaluation of the effectiveness of treatment. For example, if the resident has a URI, the reviewer may expect to find a note about lung sounds, nasal congestion, or cough. If the only entry states, "No side effects to antibiotic," there is no way to evaluate the resident's condition and corresponding nursing actions. If a reviewer finds a pattern of recurrent documentation of like problems (such as recurrent UTIs, falls, or skin tears) in the nurses' notes, he or she will look for recognition of high risk for this condition,

and will review the care plan to determine whether the problem is being addressed. He or she will also determine whether illnesses were identified and monitored appropriately, in a timely manner.

Residents with high-risk conditions, changes in condition, or signs of acute illness require complete assessment and frequent monitoring. The assessment and implementation information must be thoroughly documented. If the chart ends up in court, the jury may not believe monitoring was appropriate unless it is documented. Verbal testimony indicating nurses checked the resident is viewed with suspicion in absence of proper documentation. Often, family members will contradict nursing testimony by stating that no one assessed the resident despite their pleas. If their testimony is consistent with the resident's outcome, jurors will likely accept it as the truth.

If a nurse documents numeric observations such as a resident's weight, appetite or bowel movement on the nurses' notes, you can expect the reviewer to cross check these data on the flow sheets. Finding contradictions, such as "Appetite 15%" in nursing notes and "100%" on the flow sheet is not uncommon. If the nurses' notes indicate the physician was called, the reviewer will check the telephone orders. If a medication or treatment was ordered, he or she will also check the appropriate flow sheet and care plan to determine if and when the order was implemented.

If the resident transferred from your facility to a hospital or another long-term care facility, you can expect the plaintiff attorney to request their records as well. They may also subpoena transportation providers, such as the ambulance service. When a resident is transferred to the acute care hospital, the nurse reviewer will expect to find an assessment of the problem in the nursing notes, as well as the action taken, notifications, monitoring, and transfer. The reviewer will also compare, contrast, and evaluate the data on the transfer form, ambulance run sheet, and hospital admitting record to determine whether the information is consistent or contradictory. He or she will also compare the resident's condition on admission with documentation of the resident's condition upon discharge from the long-term care facility. For example, a facility nurse documents the resident's foley is "draining clear amber urine." The ambulance run sheet notes the drainage bag is empty. The ER nurse notes "gross hematuria with mucous shreds and sediment in catheter drainage bag." Another typical example is the long-term care facility documenting a 1-centimeter Stage I ulcer on the coccyx, with the hospital documenting a malodorous 4-centimeter Stage IV ulcer in the same location. The records of the ambulance service and emergency department sometimes reflect poorly upon the long-term care facility.

When a resident is transferred to the hospital, labs are usually drawn on admission. The legal reviewer will study the laboratory reports to determine whether preventable abnormalities are present. He or she will review the time of the facility discharge note, ambulance arrival and departure, and ambulance arrival at the hospital, and time of emergency department or hospital admission to determine whether they are all within the same approximate time frame. Prolonged delays may be questioned.

Laboratory, x-ray, and related reports

The nurse reviewer will evaluate the laboratory reports. If the physician orders routine labs, such as a CBC monthly, the nurse will determine whether the labs were done as ordered. He or she will determine when the sample was drawn, and when the result was phoned or faxed to the facility. If the laboratory values are abnormal, he or she will try to determine

whether facility personnel recognized and acted on the abnormality by making phone contact with the physician, notifying other professionals such as the dietitian, as appropriate, and updating the plan of care. If the laboratory reports were not returned in a reasonable period of time, the reviewer will try to determine why. He or she will also look for evidence that the facility was aware that lab reports were missing, and action taken to rectify the problem. If the lab reports suggest correctable medical problems, he or she will also review the care plan. For example, the BUN value is elevated by two points suggesting early (mild) dehydration. Other values are normal. The legal nurse consultant will look for facility recognition of the problem and prompt physician notification. Nursing observations, actions, and special monitoring should be listed on the care plan and implemented when appropriate, such as by adding I&O monitoring and placing an I&O flowsheet in the record.

Dietitian notes

The dietitian's assessment and notations are an important part of the medical-legal review. Many long-term care facility residents have problems related to nutrition and hydration. The dietitian also plays an important role in the management of various medical problems, such as diabetes and pressure ulcers. The dietitian will document the resident's height and weight on admission. He or she will use these data to perform certain mathematical calculations, such as the resident's minimum daily caloric and fluid needs. The dietitian will review the available laboratory reports and may make recommendations for care (such as increasing fluids) or additional monitoring, such as repeating the hemoglobin and hematocrit in thirty days. He or she may also make nutritional recommendations, such as adding a vitamin or high-calorie nutritional supplement. The dietitian will review the diet order and resident food consumption for appropriateness and adequacy, and may also make recommendations for changes in this area. Nursing personnel are expected to read the dietitian's documentation and consult the physician for a change in orders, when necessary. Omissions of this nature are often significant.

The medical legal reviewer will compare the dietitian's calculations of the resident's minimum fluid and caloric needs with the intake and output record, meal consumption record, weight records (including weights documented on the MDSs.) He or she will review documentation of supplements and nourishments, and calculate caloric values of the products being given. The reviewer will determine whether the facility has been attentive to providing sufficient fluids and nutrients. If not, he or she will consider information on care plans, nursing notes, and other records to determine whether problems such as weight loss, malnutrition, and dehydration were avoidable.

A surprising number of tube-fed residents develop malnutrition and dehydration as a result of nursing failure to provide fluid and supplement solutions as ordered by the physician and dietitian. Documentation of care for residents with feeding tubes is often in good order, with no skips or apparent documentation problems. If the tube-fed resident experiences dehydration, malnutrition, or significant weight loss, the reviewer will probably question the credibility, integrity, and veracity of the documentation unless the resident has terminal cancer or another medical condition to account for the problem.

Other documentation

The medical-legal reviewer will read, review, compare, and contrast all other documents on the facility record, including flow sheets, therapy evaluations and notes, pharmacist notes (if any), social services, and activities

records. These may or may not be important to the review, depending on the resident's medical problems and injuries alleged. They may also become important if they reflect problems or observations with no nursing follow-up. Contradictions between these records and the MDS and nursing records may also be significant. The reviewer will check to see that these departments have provided consultation and participation to relevant resident problems. He or she will consider the care plan and flow sheets to determine whether care given is in keeping with the recommendations of therapists, the social worker, and other professionals, when indicated.

As you can see, the determination to go forward with a lawsuit is based on this initial review of the medical records. The facility has a very limited time frame in which to produce the records. Making sure that documentation is accurate and concise when the record is open and ongoing is the best protection you can provide. After the record has been closed, sorting it and putting it in facility-designated order will make it much easier to review. Once again, the facility is being evaluated based on external appearances. A complete, concise, accurate and organized medical record will help project a positive image of the facility, and reduce the risk that a lawsuit will proceed. Keep this in mind as you review the common injuries and changes-in-condition information in this book.

Theories of recovery

If a lawsuit is filed as a result of this record review, it will probably contain one or more of these theories of recovery:

- General negligence. (Allegations of negligent hiring, negligent supervision, negligent retention of staff and understaffing.)

- Aggregate (pattern) of poor care, including

recurrent incidents and injuries, such as skin tears, pressure ulcers, falls, or fractures.

- Medical malpractice.

- Negligence Per Se (statutory violation of OBRA, state laws, and/or federal regulations).

- Breach of contract (breach of the admission agreement and care plan)

    - In assisted living facilities, this is breach of the service plan. Assisted living facilities have fewer regulations to provide substance to complaints alleging breach of the standard of care. For this reason, many lawsuits emphasize the importance of breach of contract and failure to have or follow the service plan.

- Failure to fulfill promises on marketing brochures and advertising materials, such as "24-hour nursing care provided." The facility does not provide 24-hour nursing care to each resident. A more appropriate statement may be, "Nursing personnel on duty 24 hours a day."

- The plaintiff may also approach "breach of contract" from the opposite direction. The

facility also contracts with the state agency who administers the Medicaid program. As part of the contract with this agency, the facility pledges that it will comply with the agency's rules and regulations on a continual basis. The facility promises to correct all deficiencies in a timely manner. These provisions establish a cause of action for breach of contract in facilities with an ongoing history of relevant deficiencies.

The lawsuit may also request an award for punitive damages. A claim for punitive damages is appropriate if the facts of the case are considered egregious. In most states, the plaintiff must demonstrate gross, wanton, or willful misconduct to recover punitive damages.

Most lawsuits are filed in state court. Occasionally, long-term care cases are filed in federal court. The plaintiff is not required to file in federal court, even if he or she alleges a breach of federal laws. However, occasionally cases are filed in federal court for other reasons, such as circumventing state medical malpractice caps. Sometimes the charges result in criminal prosecution of individuals, if allegations of abuse and neglect are proven.

Chapter twenty three

References

1. Texas Board of Nurse Examiners. (2006). *Nurse Practice Act*. Online. http://www.bne.state.tx.us. Accessed 02/11/06.

2. *Better Documentation*. (1992). Springhouse, Pa.: Springhouse Corp., 39.

3. Thomas v. Greenview Hosp., Inc., __ S.W. 3d __, 2004 WL 221198 (Ky. App., February 6, 2004).

4. *Better Documentation*. (1992). Springhouse, Pa.: Springhouse Corp., 39.

5. Morris, JN, Murphy, K., Nonemaker, S. (2002). *Long-term care facility resident assessment instrument (RAI) user's manual*. Des Moines. Briggs Corp.

6. Morris, JN, Murphy, K., Nonemaker, S. (2002). *Long-term care facility resident assessment instrument (RAI) user's manual*. Des Moines. Briggs Corp.

7. State Operations Manual. §483.75(j)(1) Laboratory Services.

8. U.S. Department of Health and Human Services (Eds). (1992). *Pressure Ulcers in Adults: Prediction and Prevention*. Rockville, MD. Agency for Health Care Policy and Research.

9. U.S. Department of Health and Human Services (Eds). (1992). *Pressure Ulcers in Adults: Prediction and Prevention*. Rockville, MD. Agency for Health Care Policy and Research.

10. U.S. Department of Health and Human Services (Eds). (1994). *Pressure Ulcer Treatment*. Rockville, MD. Agency for Health Care Policy and Research.

11. Hess, Cathy Thomas. (1998). *Nurse's Clinical Guide Wound Care*. Springhouse, PA. Springhouse Corporation.

12. Tscheschlog, B. et al (Eds). (1995). *Mastering documentation*. Pennsylvania, Springhouse. Springhouse Corporation.

13. *State Operations Manual*. §483.10(b)(2)

14. *Chart Smart: The A-to-Z guide to better nursing documentation*. (2001). Springhouse, Pa.: Springhouse Corp., ix, 203, 301.

15. Richards, M. (2001). Documentation - a vital and essential element of the nursing process. Survey Savvy. Des Moines, Briggs Corporation.

16. Morris, J.N., Murphy, K., Nonemaker, S. (2002). *Long-term care facility resident assessment instrument (RAI) user's manual*. DesMoines. Briggs Corp.

17. *State Operations Manual*. §483.10(b)(2)

18. *Texas Administrative Code*. §19.1913.

19. Sanders vs. Spector, 673 So. 2d 1176 (La. App., 1996).

20. American Association of Legal Nurse Consultants. (1999). Getting started in legal nurse consulting: An introduction to the specialty, second edition. Chicago. American Association of Legal Nurse Consultants.

21. This statement is made assuming that the reviewer is analyzing the original open or closed medical record; not a record that was subsequently altered or corrected.